Oxford Textbook of

Neuromuscular Disorders

Oxford Textbooks in Clinical Neurology

Oxford Textbook of
Neuromuscular Disorders

Edited by

David Hilton-Jones
Nuffield Department of Clinical
Neurosciences, West Wing, John Radcliffe Hospital, Oxford, UK

Martin R. Turner
Oxford University Department of Clinical
Neurosciences & Oxford University Hospitals NHS Trust,
John Radcliffe Hospital, Oxford, UK

Series Editor

Christopher Kennard

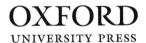

OXFORD
UNIVERSITY PRESS

OXFORD
UNIVERSITY PRESS

Great Clarendon Street, Oxford, OX2 6DP,
United Kingdom

Oxford University Press is a department of the University of Oxford.
It furthers the University's objective of excellence in research, scholarship,
and education by publishing worldwide. Oxford is a registered trade mark of
Oxford University Press in the UK and in certain other countries

Published in the United States of America by Oxford University Press
198 Madison Avenue, New York, NY 10016, United States of America

British Library Cataloguing in Publication Data
Data available

Library of Congress Control Number: 2014930244

ISBN 978-0-19-969807-3

Printed in the UK by
Bell & Bain Ltd, Glasgow

Preface

There is a view that the traditional medical textbook is dead—replaced by immediate accessibility to the latest literature and the availability of cheap electronic mobile devices to enable the reading or presentation of data in, literally, any environment. It is undoubtedly wonderful to be able to view the latest paper or systematic review on the management of, say, Churg–Strauss vasculitic neuropathy in a matter of milliseconds, but only if that is the correct diagnosis. The ready accessibility of the primary literature is a boon to the specialist, but it is a potential minefield for the tyro.

We firmly believe that there is still a role for the textbook, but its aspirations need to be clearly defined and understood. This volume on neuromuscular disorders is not primarily intended for neuromuscular specialists. However, given the ultra-specialization that sometimes exists, we hope they may still find it helpful to have a comprehensive summary from an expert in a parallel field. Although individual chapters cover specific disorders in detail, there is an overarching aim, reflected particularly in the first three chapters, to help the novice navigate the pathway from first seeing the patient, to establishing the correct diagnosis, and optimal management.

We have been honoured to be able to assemble many of the opinion leaders from the various specialist fields of neuromuscular disorders. Throughout the volume the reader will benefit from their pearls of wisdom (as we did), many of which are never aired in formal scientific papers.

We hope that you will enjoy reading this book as much as we have enjoyed working with our friends and colleagues internationally to bring it to you. We warmly extend our thanks to the contributors, and to Oxford University Press for making the venture possible.

Contents

Abbreviations

AAV	ANCA-associated vasculitis/ adeno-associated virus		BM	Bethlem myopathy
ABC	ATP-binding cassette		BMD	Becker muscular dystrophy
ABD	actin-binding domain		bpm	beats per minute
ABG	arterial blood gases		BVVL	Brown–Vialetto–Van Laere [syndrome]
ACE	angiotensin-converting enzyme		CADM	clinically amyopathic dermatomyositis
ACh	acetylcholine		CAN	cardiac autonomic neuropathy
AChE	acetylcholinesterase		c-ANCA	cytoplasmic ANCA
AChR	acetylcholine receptors		CANOMAD	chronic ataxic neuropathy, ophthalmoplegia,
A-CIDP	CIDP with acute onset			monoclonal protein, cold agglutinins, and
ACTH	adrenocorticotropic hormone			disialosyl antibodies
AD	autosomal dominant		CASQ	calsequestrin
ADA	American Diabetes Association		CB	conduction block
ADG	α-dystroglycan		CBC	complete blood cell count
ADM	abductor digiti minimi		CCD	central core disease
ADQB	abductor digiti quinti brevis		CFTD	congenital fibre-type disproportion
AFO	ankle–foot orthosis		CGH	comparative genomic hybridization
AGEs	advanced glycation endproducts		ChAT	choline acetyltransferase
AIDP	acute inflammatory demyelinating		CHN	congenital hypomyelinating neuropathies
	polyneuropathy		CI	confidence interval
AIMG	autoimmune myasthenia gravis		CIAP	chronic idiopathic axonal polyneuropathy
AIN	anterior interosseous nerve		CIDP	chronic inflammatory demyelinating
AKI	acute kidney injury			polyneuropathy
ALD	adrenoleucodystrophy		CIM	critical Illness myopathy
ALS	amyotrophic lateral sclerosis		CIP	critical illness polyneuropathy
ALT	alanine aminotransferase		CIPA	congenital insensitivity to pain and anhidrosis
ALSFRS	ALS Functional Rating Scale		CK	creatine kinase
AMAN	acute motor axonal neuropathy		ClC-1	muscle-specific chloride channel 1
AMC	arthrogryposis multiplex congenita		CMAP	compound muscle action potential
AMCBN	acute motor conduction block neuropathy		CMD	congenital muscular dystrophy
AMN	adrenomyeloneuropathy		CMS	congenital myasthenic syndromes
AMSAN	acute motor and sensory axonal neuropathy		CMT	Charcot–Marie–Tooth [disease]
ANA	antinuclear antibody		CNM	centronuclear myopathy
ANCA	antineutrophil cytoplasmic antibody		CNS	central nervous system
AON	antisense oligonucleotide		ColQ	collagen-Q
APB	abductor pollicis brevis		CoQ$_{10}$	coenzyme Q10
APL	abductor pollicis longus		COX	cytochrome c oxidase
AR	autosomal recessive/androgen receptor/aldose		COX-2	cyclooxygenase-2
	reductase		CPAP	continuous positive airway pressure
ARB	angiotensin receptor blocker		CPEO	chronic progressive external ophthalmoplegia
ARDS	acute respiratory distress syndrome		CPK	creatine phosphokinase
ARS	aminoacyl-tRNA synthetase		CPN	common peroneal neuropathy/common
AST	aspartate aminotransferase			peroneal nerve
ATGL	adipose triglyceride lipase		CPT	carnitine palmitoyltransferase
BiPAP	bilevel positive airway pressure		CSF	cerebrospinal fluid
			CSS	Churg–Strauss syndrome

CTD	connective tissue disorder
CTS	carpal tunnel syndrome
CV	conduction velocity
CYC	cyclophosphamide
DADS	distal acquired demyelinating symmetric polyneuropathy
DAG	diacylglycerol
3,4-DAP	3,4-diaminopyridine
DELTA-P	Dutch–English LEMS Tumor Association Prediction [score]
DEXA	dual-energy x ray absorptiometry
DG	dystroglycan
DGC	dystrophin–glycoprotein complex
DHA	docosahexaenoic acid
DHEA	dehydroepiandrosterone
dHMN	distal hereditary motor neuropathy
DLRPN	diabetic lumbosacral radiculoplexus neuropathy
DM	diabetes mellitus/dermatomyositis
DM1/DM2	myotonic dystrophy Type 1/Type 2
DMD	Duchenne muscular dystrophy
DML	distal motor latency
DPA	D-penicillamine
DRPN	diabetic radiculoplexus neuropathy
DSD	Dejerine–Sottas disease
dSL	desoxysphingolipid
dSMA	distal spinal muscular atrophy
DSPN	diabetic sensorimotor polyneuropathy
EAST	Elevated Arm Stress Test
ECG	electrocardiography/electrocardiogram
ECM	extracellular matrix
ECRB	extensor carpi radialis brevis
ECRL	extensor carpi radialis longus
ECU	extensor carpi ulnaris
EDB	extensor digitorum brevis
EDL	extensor digitorum longus
EDM	extensor digiti minimi
EDMD	Emery–Dreifuss muscular dystrophy
EDS	excessive daytime sleepiness
EEG	electroencephalogram
EFNS/PNS	European Federation of Neurological Societies/ Peripheral Nerve Society
EGRIS	Erasmus GBS Respiratory Insufficiency Scale
EHL	extensor hallucis longus
EIM	electrical impedance myography
ELISA	enzyme-linked immunosorbent assay
EMG	electromyogram/electromyography
ENMC	European Neuromuscular Centre
EOM	extraocular muscles
EPB	extensor pollicis brevis
EPL	Extensor pollicis longus
EPP	endplate potential
EPS	electrophysiological studies
ER	endoplasmic reticulum
ERT	enzyme replacement therapy
ESR	erythrocyte sedimentation rate
ETF	electron transfer flavoprotein
ETFDH	electron transfer flavoprotein dehydrogenase
FAD	flavin adenine dinucleotide
FADS	fetal akinesia deformation sequence
FAO	fatty acid oxidation
FAP	familial amyloid polyneuropathy
FCMD	Fukuyama congenital muscular dystrophy
FCR	flexor carpi radialis
FCU	flexor carpi ulnaris
FD	Fabry disease
FDB	flexor digitorum brevis
FDG	fluorodeoxyglucose
FDI	first dorsal interosseous
FDL	flexor digitorum longus
FDM	flexor digiti minimi
FDP	flexor digitorum profundus
FDS	flexor digitorum superficialis
FEV	forced expiratory volume
FFA	free fatty acid
FGF	fibroblast growth factor
FHB	flexor hallucis brevis
FHL	flexor hallucis longus
FOSMN	facial-onset sensory and motor neuropathy
FPB	flexor pollicis brevis
FPL	flexor pollicis longus
FRAFO	floor reaction ankle–foot orthosis
FSH	facioscapulohumeral
FSHD	facioscapulohumeral (muscular) dystrophy
FTD	frontotemporal dementia
FUS	fused-in-sarcoma
FVC	forced vital capacity
GAA	α-1,4-glucosidase
Gb3	globotriaosylceramide
GBS	Guillain–Barré syndrome
GDE	glycogen debranching enzyme
GGT	gamma-glutamyl transferase
GH	growth hormone
GHRH	growth hormone releasing hormone
GNE	UDP-N-acetylglucosamine 2-epimerase/N-acetylmannosamine kinase
GSD	glycogen storage disease
GT	Gomori trichrome [stain]
HAART	highly active antiretroviral therapy
HDAC	histone deacetylase
H&E	haematoxylin and eosin
HGA	hereditary gelsolin amyloidosis
HIBM	hereditary inclusion body myopathy
HIV	human immunodeficiency virus
HKPP	hypokalaemic periodic paralysis
HMGCR	3-hydroxy-3-methylglutaryl-coenzyme A reductase
HMSN	hereditary motor and sensory neuropathies
HNA	hereditary neuralgic amyotrophy
HNPP	hereditary neuropathy with liability to pressure palsies
HRV	heart rate variability
HSAN	hereditary sensory and autonomic neuropathy
HSN	hereditary sensory neuropathy
HSP	hereditary spastic paraplegia/Henoch–Schönlein purpura
HTLV-1	human T-lymphotropic virus type 1
IB	immunoblot
IBM	inclusion body myositis

IC	immune complex	MEPP	miniature endplate potential
ICD	implantable cardioverter defibrillator	MERRF	myoclonic epilepsy with ragged-red fibres
ICU	intensive care unit	MFM	myofibrillar myopathy
ICU-AW	ICU-acquired weakness	MFS	Miller Fisher syndrome
IDMC	International Myotonic Dystrophy Consortium	MG	myasthenia gravis
IENF	intra-epidermal nerve fibre	MGFA	Myasthenia Gravis Foundation of America
IF	immunofluorescent	MGUS	monoclonal gammopathy of undetermined significance
Ig	immunoglobulin		
IGF-1	insulin-like growth-factor-1	MGUSP	MGUS polyneuropathy
IGT	impaired glucose tolerance	MH	malignant hyperthermia
IHC	immunohistochemical	MHC	major histocompatibility complex
IIM	idiopathic inflammatory myopathy	MIRAS	mitochondrial recessive ataxia syndrome
ILD	Interstitial lung disease	MLPA	multiplex ligation-dependent probe amplification
INA	idiopathic neuralgic amyotrophy	MM	multiple mononeuropathy/Miyoshi myopathy
INEM	isolated neck extensor myopathy	MmD	multiminicore disease
INFα	interferon-α	MMN	multifocal motor neuropathy
INM	inner nuclear membrane	mNCV	motor nerve conduction velocity
iNOS	inducible nitric oxide synthase	MND	motor neuron disease
IPV	inactivated polio vaccine	MNGIE	mitochondrial neurogastrointestinal encephalopathy
IRIS	immune restoration inflammatory response		
IVF	*in vitro* fertilization	MNSI	Michigan Neuropathy Screening Instrument
IVIg	intravenous immunoglobulin	MPA	microscopic polyangiitis
KAFO	knee–ankle–foot orthosis	MPO	myeloperoxidase
L	litre	MPZ	myelin protein zero
LCHAD	long chain 3-hydroxy/acyl-CoA dehydrogenase	MRC	Medical Research Council
LDH	lactate dehydrogenase	MRI	magnetic resonance imaging
LDM	Laing distal myopathy	MRS	magnetic resonance spectroscopy
LEMS	Lambert–Eaton myasthenic syndrome	MSA	myositis-specific autoantibody
LFCN	lateral femoral cutaneous nerve	MSM	myosin storage myopathy
LGMD	limb-girdle muscular dystrophy	mtDNA	mitochondrial DNA
LH	luteinizing hormone	MTP	mitochondrial trifunctional protein
LHON	Leber hereditary optic neuropathy	MUGA	multigated cardiac radionuclide ventriculography
LMN	lower motor neuron	MUNE	motor unit number estimation
LOS	lipo-oligosaccharide	MuSK	muscle-specific kinase
LRP4	low-density lipoprotein receptor-related protein 4	NA	neuralgic amyotrophy
LRPN	lumbosacral radiculoplexus neuropathy	NADH-TR	nicotinamide adenine dinucleotide tetrazolium reductase
LSDs	lysosomal storage disorders		
MAC	membrane attack complex	NAM	necrotizing autoimmune myopathy
MADD	multiple acyl-CoA dehydrogenase deficiency	NARP	neurogenic muscle weakness, ataxia, and retinitis pigmentosa
MADSAM	multifocal acquired demyelinating sensory and motor neuropathy		
		NCS	nerve conduction studies
MAG	myelin-associated glycoprotein	NCV	nerve conduction velocity
MB-DRM	desmin-related myopathy with Mallory body-like inclusions	NDS	Neuropathy Disability Score
		NEM	nemaline myopathy
MCAD	medium chain acyl-CoA dehydrogenase	NF-1	neurofibromatosis type 1
MCT	medium-chain triglyceride	NFTs	neurofibrillary tangles
MCTD	mixed connective tissue disorder	NGF	nerve growth factor
MCV	mean corpuscular volume	NGS	next-generation sequencing
MDC	Muscular Dystrophy Campaign	NIS	Neuropathy Impairment Score
MDC1A	merosin-deficient congenital muscular dystrophy Type 1A	NIV	non-invasive ventilation
		NLDSI	neutral lipid storage disease with ichthyosis
MDDG	muscular dystrophy–dystroglycanopathy	NMDA	*N*-methyl-D-aspartate
MDNS	Michigan Diabetic Neuropathy Scale	NMJ	neuromuscular junction
MDSG	Myotonic Dystrophy Support Group	^n NOS	neuronal nitric oxide synthase
MEB	muscle-eye-brain disease	NSP	Neuropathy Symptom Profile
mEGOS	modified Erasmus Guillain–Barré Outcome Score	NSVN	non-systemic vasculitic neuropathy
MELAS	mitochondrial encephalomyopathy with lactic acidosis and stroke-like episodes	NT3	neurotrophin 3
		OCTN2	sodium-dependent carnitine transporter
MEMSA	myoclonic epilepsy, myopathy, sensory ataxia	ODM	opponens digiti minimi

2OME	2'O-methyl phosphothiorate
OMG	ocular myasthenia gravis
OMIM	Online Mendelian Inheritance in Man
ONM	outer nuclear membrane
OPV	oral [live attenuated] polio vaccine
ORF	open reading frame
OT	occupational therapy
PAN	polyarteritis nodosa
p-ANCA	perinuclear ANCA
PARP	poly(ADP-ribose) polymerase
PBG	porphobilinogen
PbP	progressive bulbar palsy
PCD	primary carnitine deficiency
PCR	polymerase chain reaction
PE	plasma exchange
PEEP	positive end-expiratory pressure
PEG	percutaneous endoscopic gastrostomy
PEO	progressive external ophthalmoplegia
PET	positron emission tomography
PFKD	phosphofructokinase deficiency
PFS	pulmonary function score
PGD	preimplantation genetic diagnosis
PGK	phosphoglycerate kinase
PGAM	phosphoglycerate mutase
PGM	phosphoglucomutase
PHK	phosphorylase b kinase
PHYH	phytanoyl CoA hydroxylase
PIN	posterior interosseous nerve
PIRCS	percussion-induced rapid contractures
PKC	protein kinase C
PLP	pyridoxal-5'-phosphate
PLS	primary lateral sclerosis
PM	polymyositis
PMA	progressive muscular atrophy
PME	progressive myoclonic epilepsy
PMO	phosphorodiamidate morpholino oligomer
PNH	peripheral nerve hyperexcitability
PNHD	peripheral nerve hyperexcitability disorder
PNPLA2	pastatin-like phospholipase domain-containing protein 2
PNS	peripheral nervous system
POEMS	polyneuropathy, organomegaly, endocrinopathy, monoclonal protein, and skin changes
polyA	polyadenylation
PROMM	proximal myotonic myopathy
PQ	pronator quadratus
PR3	proteinase 3
PT	pronator teres
PTH	parathyroid hormone
QMG	Quantitative Myasthenia Gravis [test]
QSART	quantitative sudomotor axon reflex testing
RA	rheumatoid arthritis
RCE	respiratory chain enzyme
RCS	Rosenberg–Chutorian syndrome
RCT	randomized controlled trial
RF	respiratory failure
RIG	radiologically inserted gastrostomy
RNS	repetitive nerve stimulation
ROS	reactive oxygen species
RRFs	ragged red fibres
RSMD	rigid spine muscular dystrophy
RyR	ryanodine receptor
SANDO	sensory ataxia, neuropathy, dysarthria, ophthalmoplegia
SAP	sensory action potential
SBMA	spinal and bulbar muscular atrophy
SCAE	spinocerebellar ataxia with epilepsy
SCAIP	single-condition amplification/internal primer
SCIg	subcutaneous immunoglobulin
SCLC	small cell lung cancer
SDH	succinate dehydrogenase
SFEMG	single-fibre electromyography
SFN	small fibre neuropathy
SGC	sarcoglycan complex
SHA	strategic health authority
sIBM	sporadic inclusion body myositis
SIMV	synchronized intermittent mandatory ventilation
SIRS	systemic inflammation response syndrome
SLE	systemic lupus erythematosus
SMA	spinal muscular atrophy/smooth muscle antibody
SMARD	spinal muscular atrophy with respiratory distress
SNAP	sensory nerve action potential
SNARE	soluble NSF attachment protein receptor
SNP	single nucleotide polymorphism
snRNP	small nuclear ribonucleoprotein
SPMA	scapuloperoneal muscular atrophy
SPT	serine palmitoyltransferase
SRP	signal recognition particle
SSRI	selective serotonin reuptake inhibitor
STIR	short TI inversion recovery
T3	triiodothyronine
T4	thyroxine
TAG	triacylglycerol
TD	temporal dispersion
TDP-43	TAR (transactive response) DNA-binding protein
TGFβ	transforming growth factor β
TL	terminal latency
TMD	tibial muscular dystrophy
TMS	transcranial magnetic stimulation
TNF	tumour necrosis factor
TNM	transient neonatal myasthenia
TOS	thoracic outlet syndrome
TPMT	thiopurine methyltransferase
TPP	thyrotoxic periodic paralysis
TSH	thyroid-stimulating hormone
TTR	transthyretin
TTS	tarsal tunnel syndrome
UCMD	Ullrich congenital muscular dystrophy
UENS	Utah Early Neuropathy Scale
UMN	upper motor neuron
UTR	untranslated region
VAPP	vaccine-associated paralytic poliomyelitis
VCP	valosin-containing protein
VCPDM	vocal cord and pharyngeal distal myopathy
VGCC	voltage-gated calcium channel
VGKC	voltage-gated potassium channel
VGSC	voltage-gated sodium channel

VDP	vaccine-derived poliomyelitis		WDM	Welander distal myopathy
VEGF	vascular endothelial growth factor		WG	Wegener granulomatosis
VF	ventricular fibrillation		WHO	World Health Organization
VLCAD	very long chain acyl-CoA dehydrogenase		WWS	Walker–Warburg syndrome
VLCFA	very long chain fatty acid		XLDC	X-linked dilated cardiomyopathy
VT	ventricular tachycardia		XMPMA	X-linked myopathy with postural muscle atrophy

Contributors

Zohar Argov Department of Neurology, Hadassah-Hebrew University Medical Center, Jerusalem, Israel

Michaela Auer-Grumbach Department of Orthopaedics, Medical University Vienna, Vienna, Austria

Dirk Bäumer Nuffield Department of Clinical Neurosciences, West Wing, John Radcliffe Hospital, Oxford, UK

David L. H. Bennett Nuffield Department of Clinical Neurosciences, John Radcliffe Hospital, Oxford, UK

Kate Bushby Institute of Human Genetics International Centre for Life, Newcastle upon Tyne, UK

Patrick F. Chinnery Institute of Genetic Medicine, Newcastle University, and Directorate of Neurosciences, Newcastle upon Tyne Hospitals NHS Foundation Trust, UK

Nigel F. Clarke Institute for Neuroscience and Muscle Research The Children's Hospital at Westmead & Sydney Medical School, University of Sydney, Sydney, NSW, Australia

Emma Clement Department of Clinical Genetics, Great Ormond Street Hospital, London, UK

Peter Connick Department of Clinical Neurosciences, Cambridge Centre for Brain Repair, Cambridge University, UK

Maxwell S. Damian Department of Clinical Neurosciences and Neurocritical Care Unit, Cambridge University Hospitals, UK

Pieter A. van Doorn Erasmus MC, University Medical Center, Department of Neurology, Rotterdam, The Netherlands

Judith Drenthen Erasmus MC, University Medical Center, Department of Neurology, Rotterdam, The Netherlands

Baziel G.M. van Engelen Professor of Neuromuscular disorders, Department of Neurology, Radboud University Medical Centre, Nijmegen, The Netherlands

Eva L. Feldman University of Michigan, Department of Neurology, Ann Arbor, MI, USA

Sarah Finlayson Nuffield Department of Clinical Neurosciences, West Wing, John Radcliffe Hospital, Oxford, UK

Kenneth Fischbeck Neurogenetics Branch, NINDS, NIH, Bethesda, MD, USA

Kevin M. Flanigan Departments of Pediatrics and Neurology, The Ohio State University and Principal Investigator, Center for Gene Therapy, Nationwide Children's Hospital, Columbus, OH, USA

Lionel Ginsberg Department of Neurology, Royal Free Hospital, London, UK

Stephen A. Goutman Department of Neurology, University of Michigan, Ann Arbor, MI, USA

Christopher Grunseich Neurogenetics Branch, NINDS, NIH, Bethesda, MD, USA

Michael G. Hanna MRC Centre for Neuromuscular Diseases and Department of Molecular Neurosciences, National Hospital for Neurology and Neurosurgery and Institute of Neurology, London, UK

David Hilton-Jones Nuffield Department of Clinical Neurosciences, West Wing, John Radcliffe Hospital, Oxford, UK

Robin S. Howard Lane-Fox Unit and Department of Neurology, St Thomas' Hospital, London, UK

Saiju Jacob Department of Neurology, Queen Elizabeth Neurosciences Centre, University Hospitals of Birmingham, Birmingham, UK

Heinz Jungbluth Department of Paediatric Neurology, Evelina Children's Hospital, St Thomas' Hospital, London, UK

Matthew C. Kiernan Brain and Mind Research Institute, University of Sydney, NSW, Australia

Anneke J. van der Kooi Department of Neurology, Academic Medical Center, University of Amsterdam, Amsterdam, The Netherlands

Elly L. van der Kooi Department of Neurology, Medical Center Leeuwarden, Leeuwarden, The Netherlands

Nigel G. Laing Harry Perkins Institute of Medical Research, The Centre for Medical Research, University of Western Australia, Nedlands, WA, Australia

J. Gareth Llewelyn Department of Neurology, Royal Gwent Hospital, Newport, Wales, UK

Silvere van der Maarel Department of Human Genetics, Leiden University Medical Center, Leiden, The Netherlands

Mohamed Mahdi-Rogers National Hospital for Neurology and Neurosurgery, London, UK

Eleanor A. Marsh Neurology Department, Royal Gwent Hospital, Newport, Wales, UK

Frank Mastaglia Western Australian Neuroscience Research Institute, Centre for Neuromuscular and Neurological Disorders, University of Western Australia, Nedlands, WA, Australia; Institute of Immunology and Infectious Diseases, Murdoch University, Murdoch, WA, Australia

Emma Matthews MRC Centre for Neuromuscular Diseases and Department of Molecular Neurosciences, National Hospital for Neurology and Neurosurgery and Institute of Neurology, London, UK

Merrilee Needham Australian Neuromuscular Research Institute, University of Western Australia and Murdoch University, Department of Neurology, Fremantle Hospital, Perth, WA, Australia

Fiona L.M. Norwood King's College Hospital, London, UK

Mette C. Ørngreen Neuromuscular Research Unit, Department of Neurology, University of Copenhagen, Copenhagen, Denmark

Jacqueline Palace Nuffield Department of Clinical Neurosciences, West Wing, John Radcliffe Hospital, Oxford, UK

Gerald Pfeffer Institute of Genetic Medicine and Department of Neurology, Newcastle, UK

Violaine Planté-Bordeneuve Department of Neurology, University Hospital Henri Mondor, Hôpitaux de Paris, Créteil, France

Gianina Ravenscroft Harry Perkins Institute of Medical Research, The Centre for Medical Research, University of Western Australia, Nedlands, WA, Australia

Mary M. Reilly MRC Centre for Neuromuscular Diseases and Department of Molecular Neurosciences, National Hospital for Neurology and Neurosurgery and UCL Institute of Neurology, London, UK

Alexander M. Rossor MRC Centre for Neuromuscular Diseases and Department of Molecular Neurosciences, National Hospital for Neurology and Neurosurgery and UCL Institute of Neurology, London, UK

Stacey A. Sakowski Alfred Taubman Medical Research Institute, University of Michigan, Ann Arbor, MI, USA

Ivo N. van Schaik Department of Neurology, Academic Medical Center, University of Amsterdam, Amsterdam, The Netherlands

Neil G. Simon Prince of Wales Clinical School, University of New South Wales; and, Neuroscience Research Australia

Andrea L. Smith Department of Neurology, University of Michigan, Ann Arbor, MI, USA

Kevin Talbot Nuffield Department of Clinical Neurosciences, University of Oxford, John Radcliffe Hospital, Oxford, UK

Maarten J. Titulaer Department of Neurology, Erasmus Medical Center, Rotterdam, The Netherlands

Chris Turner MRC Neuromuscular Unit, National Hospital for Neurology and Neurosurgery, London, UK

Martin R. Turner Oxford University Department of Clinical Neurosciences & Oxford University Hospitals NHS Trust, John Radcliffe Hospital, Oxford, UK

Bjarne Udd Neuromuscular Research Center, Tampere University Hospital, Tampere, Finland

Camiel Verhamme Department of Neurology, Academic Medical Center, University of Amsterdam, Amsterdam, The Netherlands

Jan J. G. M. Verschuuren Neuromuscular Diseases, Department of Neurology, Leiden University Medical Centre, Leiden, The Netherlands

Stuart Viegas Department of Neurology, St Mary's Hospital, London, UK

Marianne de Visser Department of Neurology, Academic Medical Center, University of Amsterdam, Amsterdam, The Netherlands

John Vissing Neuromuscular Research Unit, Department of Neurology, University of Copenhagen, Copenhagen, Denmark

SECTION 1

Approach to the Patient

CHAPTER 1

Eliciting the history

David Hilton-Jones and Martin R. Turner

Introduction

With the introduction of non-invasive neuroimaging, many non-specialists assumed there would be a move away from detailed history-taking and the methodical (some might say obsessive) clinical examination considered characteristic of the neurologist. All that would be needed was the ability to complete an imaging request form and the solution would soon be forthcoming. It rapidly became apparent that the new technology created almost as many problems as it solved, revealing incidental 'abnormalities' of uncertain significance begetting potentially hazardous further assessment, sometimes incorrect diagnoses, and filling neurology clinics with the 'worried well'.

Many neuromuscular disorders, and the majority that require long-term follow-up, have a genetic basis. Diagnosis, previously based solely on a detailed clinical assessment of phenotype, has more recently led to the ability to identify causative genes through linkage studies and whole-genome or exome sequencing in cohorts of patients with specific features. Clinical appraisal thus leads to a 'gene shortlist', and targeted DNA testing can be undertaken. Molecular biologists promise a holy grail of a DNA 'chip' which will detect all of the known 'neuromuscular genes' and allow a genetic diagnosis within hours of phlebotomy, with the expectation (once again) of obviating the need for rigorous clinical assessment. However, the issue of interpretation of sequence variants of unknown significance, the fact that only a small number of genes are being assessed, and the possibility of mutations in two or more genes related to neuromuscular disease having additive effects ('double trouble') suggest that accurate clinical appraisal remains paramount. The practise of medicine relies on Bayesian logic, in which the clinical assessment leads to an appropriate differential diagnosis that may (or may not) be refined by appropriate investigation.

The first three chapters of this book are intended to hone the skills of clinicians who do not have regular exposure to neuromuscular disorders. This chapter deals with taking the history, with an emphasis on eliciting and interpreting the relevant symptoms. Chapter 2 is devoted entirely to genetic considerations, the importance of the family history, and potential pitfalls for the unwary. Chapter 3 deals with the physical examination. Despite the important distinction between symptoms and signs in medicine there is of course an overlap—the history may suggest a particular pattern of weakness, and examination may confirm, refute, or extend that observation.

The presenting complaint and related features

There are relatively few ways in which the peripheral nervous system can react to disease, and the presenting symptom is likely to relate to one of the following: weakness, fatigue, sensory disturbance, autonomic dysfunction, pain, stiffness and muscle hyperactivity, muscle wasting or enlargement, or myoglobinuria.

Detailed questioning of the patient is intended to elicit the often subtle variations on a theme that will aid precise diagnosis. Sometimes, the history alone will strongly suggest a specific diagnosis. More often, the history will lead to a relatively short differential diagnosis which examination will help to shorten further. Then, specifically directed investigation will confirm the diagnosis.

Weakness

Weakness is the most common presenting symptom for neuromuscular disorders. In peripheral neuropathies it is frequently accompanied by some form of sensory disturbance, whereas in motor neuronopathies, neuromuscular junction disorders, and myopathies, 'true' sensory disturbance (see section Sensory disturbance) is notably absent. With respect to weakness the history should determine: age of onset/duration, rate of progression, constancy or variability, and distribution.

Patients do not always use the word 'weakness' to describe what a neurologist understands the word to mean. Common synonyms include 'heaviness' (e.g. 'heavy head' for neck weakness), 'deadness', 'aching', and even 'numbness' in the absence of any sensory change. Conversely, they may use the word 'weakness' to describe restriction of movement due to pain or mechanical dysfunction, and occasionally for sensory dysfunction that is otherwise difficult to describe.

Age of onset is highly important in that it may immediately limit the differential diagnosis. The symptoms of Duchenne muscular dystrophy never appear for the first time after the age of 5 years, whereas oculopharyngeal dystrophy and inclusion body myositis (IBM) do not present before middle age. On the other hand, many neuromuscular diseases can present at any age.

The rate of progression must be determined, and whether the weakness is constant or variable. Marked variability, with evidence of fatigability, is characteristic of myasthenic neuromuscular transmission disorders, and episodic weakness of periodic paralysis. However, many patients with amyotrophic lateral sclerosis (ALS) report diurnal variation to their weakness, so this should not be interpreted in isolation.

The specific distribution of the weakness is of the utmost importance with respect to diagnosing both neurogenic and myopathic disorders. Although physical examination may be more discriminating than the history, the latter still provides important clues. Asymmetry is a feature of focal peripheral neuropathies, ALS, multifocal motor neuropathy with conduction block, and mononeuropathy multiplex (although the latter may mimic a symmetrical polyneuropathy). Acquired polyneuropathy and inherited neuropathies are usually associated with symmetrical weakness, an exception being hereditary neuropathy with a liability to pressure palsies. Symmetry is the norm in most myopathies, but frequent exceptions include facioscapulohumeral dystrophy and IBM.

A major simplification is that myopathic disorders tend to present with proximal weakness whereas neurogenic disorders present with distal weakness. Indeed, most acquired myopathies (e.g. dermatomyositis, polymyositis, endocrine myopathies) are characterized by weakness of the muscles of the pelvis and shoulder girdle, and most neuropathies (e.g. diabetic and nutritional neuropathies, hereditary motor and sensory neuropathies) by distal (lower limb) weakness. Notable exceptions, however, include:

- ♦ distal weakness (of the hands) in two of the more common myopathies (myotonic dystrophy and IBM) and the much rarer distal myopathies (e.g. desminopathy and myotilinopathy);
- ♦ proximal weakness in acquired demyelinating neuropathies (e.g. chronic inflammatory demyelinating polyradiculoneuropathy) and the common (*SMN*-related) forms of spinal muscular atrophy.

Muscular dystrophies are often characterized by highly selective muscle involvement, which in itself may be diagnostic. In facioscapulohumeral dystrophy there is weakness of the scapular fixator muscles, and possibly biceps and triceps, whereas the deltoid is normal. In acquired myopathies, such as polymyositis, there is weakness of all of the shoulder girdle muscles. Focal peripheral neuropathies are associated with highly selective muscle involvement and, often, well-defined patterns of sensory loss.

Extraocular muscle weakness typically presents with diplopia, but in some chronic disorders it is absent, even in the presence of marked restriction of eye movements. Symptomatically the latter may be evidenced by patients having to turn their head to change their direction of gaze. Ptosis is usually commented upon because of the cosmetic appearance, and less commonly because it obscures vision. *Variable* diplopia and ptosis are highly suggestive of myasthenia. Across the range of neuromuscular disorders, involvement of the extraocular muscles is relatively uncommon and therefore highly discriminatory when present (Table 1.1).

Weakness of neck flexion presents as difficulty in lifting the head off a pillow. It is common in the inflammatory myopathies and myotonic dystrophy. Weakness of the neck extensors causes the head to fall forwards ('dropped head syndrome') and is seen in myasthenia (typically in older men rather than younger patients of either sex), ALS, and sometimes idiopathically in isolation (isolated neck extensor myopathy, INEM). It should never be attributed to cervical spine spondylosis, although this is frequently coincident. Patients with neck weakness complain of problems when they travel as passengers in a vehicle because their head lolls in response to movement. Those with myasthenia may say that they have to support their head by placing a hand on their chin.

Weakness of the shoulder girdle causes difficulty with activities performed above shoulder height, such as grooming and hair washing, reaching up to a shelf, and putting on a shirt or pullover. Peri-scapular weakness causes scapular winging, which is often first noticed by others. It is characteristic of facioscapulohumeral muscular dystrophy but is also seen in other dystrophies. Unilateral scapular winging may be seen in facioscapulohumeral dystrophy,

Table 1.1 Neuromuscular disorders associated with extraocular muscle (EOM) involvement

Neuromuscular junction disorders
Myasthenia gravis (EOM involvement common)
Congenital myasthenic syndromes:
• Acetylcholine receptor subunit mutations (EOM involvement common)
• DOK7 mutations (typically limb-girdle weakness without EOM involvement)
• Rapsyn mutations (non-paralytic strabismus)
Lambert–Eaton syndrome (EOM rare)
Botulism (EOM involvement common + pupillary involvement)
Mitochondrial cytopathy
Chronic progressive external ophthalmoplegia (CPEO)
Oculopharyngeal muscular dystrophy
Mainly ptosis
Congenital myopathies
For example ryanodine [*RYR1*] and dynamin2 [*DNM2*] mutations
Thyroid ophthalmopathy
CANOMAD syndrome

CANOMAD, chronic ataxic neuropathy, ophthalmoplegia, M-protein, agglutination disialosyl antibodies.

neuralgic amyotrophy, and with isolated long thoracic nerve palsy (where there may be a history of trauma, e.g. seat-belt injury, or secondary to prolonged compression under anaesthetic during surgery).

Weakness around the pelvic girdle is probably the most common presentation of myopathy. The typical initial complaint is difficulty in either running or climbing stairs. As the weakness progresses there is difficulty in getting up from a squatting position, then from a low chair, and finally problems with walking, initially going up a slope and then on the flat. Preferential weakness of quadriceps (as opposed to weakness of the pelvic muscles), as is seen in IBM or with femoral neuropathy, characteristically presents with falls due to an inability to lock the knee in extension. In IBM and ALS, both of which typically develop in late middle age, the problem is often initially attributed to degenerative disease of the hip or knee, with a consequent delay in diagnosis.

Distal weakness in the upper limbs takes three main forms. Weakness of grip, in the absence of significant weakness of the small hand muscles, is highly characteristic of myotonic dystrophy and IBM. Weakness of the small hand muscles, with little or no weakness of the long finger flexors and extensors, impairs dexterity and is seen in focal and generalized peripheral neuropathies. Weakness of finger extension ('finger drop') can be seen in myasthenia gravis, slow-channel myasthenic syndrome, Laing distal myopathy (*MYH7* mutation), *GNE* mutations (hereditary inclusion body myopathy, quadriceps-sparing myopathy), multifocal motor neuropathy with conduction block, and radial nerve palsy (with wrist drop).

The most common presenting symptom of distal lower limb weakness is foot drop, due to weakness of tibialis anterior, with patients complaining of tripping and catching their toes on the ground (this may be visible to the keen-eyed clinician as a scuff mark on one shoe). Severe acquired or inherited peripheral neuropathies may eventually lead to the loss of all movements around the ankle. Much less common is presentation with weakness of gastrocnemius, causing difficulty in pushing off when walking; this is characteristic of Miyoshi myopathy.

The presenting symptoms of ventilatory muscle weakness will depend in part on the patient's general mobility. Rare presentations in otherwise active individuals can include the inability to descend into water above the level of the diaphragm without feeling acutely breathless. In many myopathies ventilatory muscle weakness is a late feature of the disease and does not present until long after the patient has become completely wheelchair dependent. As a result of their relatively minimal exertions, breathlessness is therefore not a common complaint. Rather, the presentation relates to nocturnal hypoventilation with sleep fragmentation. Patients frequently erroneously attribute sleep fragmentation as due to 'waking to urinate', while in reality this is just a natural consequence of waking for whatever primary reason. Other symptoms of nocturnal hypoventilation include waking feeling groggy, which may be accompanied by headache, and excessive daytime sleepiness. In Duchenne muscular dystrophy common additional complaints include fear of going to sleep and anorexia (eating further inhibits ventilation). In a few conditions (e.g. acid maltase deficiency, limb-girdle muscular dystrophy Type 2I, rigid spine syndromes) ventilatory muscle weakness is an early feature of a generalized neuromuscular disorder. Patients are more likely to note breathlessness and orthopnoea. In any patient with moderately impaired ventilatory function there may be a history of delayed recovery from anaesthesia or ventilatory failure precipitated by chest infection. Ventilatory failure, usually in association with marked generalized weakness, is a feature of myasthenia gravis and acute inflammatory demyelinating polyradiculoneuropathy (Guillain–Barré syndrome).

Progressive dysphagia due to neuromuscular disease is frequently erroneously referred by primary-care physicians to stroke or otolaryngology clinics. It is not an uncommon presentation of myasthenia, but in the absence of ptosis and with dysarthria preceding the dysphagia it is much more likely to be ALS. This is important as the electromyogram (EMG) may appear normal, even in the tongue, and a small number of people with ALS may have incidental acetylcholine receptor antibodies. The presence of pseudobulbar affect (which the patient recognizes as an exaggerated, often explosive, emotional response to minor stimuli) in this context is probably pathognomonic. Other neuromuscular diagnostic considerations for dysphagia include IBM and oculopharyngeal dystrophy.

Fatigue

Few words in the neuromuscular field cause more confusion and miscommunication between patients and doctors than 'fatigue'. Arguably, doctors would like to restrict the word to true physiological fatigue but patients used it in a far broader, less specific, sense. True fatigue, with reduced strength on attempted sustained effort, both as a symptom and a sign, is almost pathognomonic of myasthenic disorders. In its more general sense, the perception of tiring during attempted activity, or increased effort to achieve a particular end, it is highly non-specific and seen in virtually any disorder causing weakness, whether peripheral neuromuscular or more central (e.g. multiple sclerosis). A sense of fatigue, often profound, without demonstrable weakness or neurophysiological

abnormality, is a major feature of chronic fatigue syndrome and related conditions.

Sensory disturbance

As noted in the section Weakness, patients may complain of sensory disturbance when in fact they have predominantly motor dysfunction. A common example is the patient with idiopathic facial (Bell's) palsy who complains of facial numbness—it is best understood as a cortical misperception. True sensory disturbance due to peripheral nerve disease may present as loss of sensation (numbness), abnormally heightened sensation (hyperalgesia and allodynia), or abnormal sensations (dysaesthesia). Focal peripheral nerve lesions, including mononeuropathy multiplex, cause localized areas of sensory disturbance, commensurate with the area of supply of the relevant nerve. Most inherited neuropathies and acquired length-dependent neuropathies cause distal sensory symptoms ('glove and stocking'). As with weakness, age of onset and the time course of progression provide vital diagnostic clues.

Autonomic dysfunction

Symptoms of autonomic dysfunction include postural hypotension, altered sweating, erectile dysfunction, sphincter dysfunction, constipation, and diarrhoea. They may be the presenting symptom of a primary autonomic neuropathy, or be additional features, elucidated from the history, in acquired and inherited sensorimotor polyneuropathies (diabetes most commonly) and in Lambert–Eaton syndrome.

Pain

With respect to neuropathies, the perception of pain may overlap with complaints about sensory disturbance. A number of generalized neuropathies may be painful, notably diabetic neuropathy and idiopathic small-fibre neuropathies. Focal neuropathies such as carpal tunnel syndrome are often associated with pain (which may be reported by the patient as extending proximally in the forearm), and post-herpetic neuralgia is common. The common inherited neuropathies are generally considered to be painless, but many patients with Charcot–Marie–Tooth disease complain of pain, although it is often difficult to determine its precise nature.

Although muscle pain is a very common symptom, it can only infrequently be attributed directly to primary muscle disease. Two critical discriminants are whether the pain is localized or generalized, and whether it is constant or episodic. If episodic, then it is important to establish if it is triggered by any specific circumstance, such as exercise. Generalized continuous muscle pain, with an essentially normal clinical examination, normal serum creatine kinase, negative inflammatory markers, and normal EMG, is a common clinical problem. Causes include chronic fatigue syndrome and arbitrarily defined chronic pain syndromes such as fibromyalgia. Referred pain from orthopaedic and rheumatological disorders is usually localized, and is common. Knee, hip, and back pain, in varying combinations, are almost universal in any neuromuscular disorder that causes lower body weakness and abnormality of gait. The simple assumption is that the abnormal posture and gait place abnormal stresses and strains on joints, ligaments, and associated structures. Patients with facioscapulohumeral dystrophy seem particularly prone to fairly widespread pain, and certainly their lumbar lordosis is frequently a major source of back pain.

Table 1.2 Disorders associated with generalized muscle pain*

Acute myositis (e.g. dermatomyositis)
Infections • Viral (e.g. coxsackie) • Toxoplasmosis
Drug induced (see Table 1.5) • Steroid withdrawal • Metabolic disorders • Hypothyroidism
Metabolic bone disease (osteomalacia)
CPT deficiency
Polymyalgia rheumatica
Parkinson's disease
Kennedy syndrome
Porphyria

CPT, carnitine palmitoyltransferase.
*May be generalized, but mostly proximal limbs.

Tables 1.2–1.4 list specific disorders that can be associated with generalized pain (Table 1.2), localized pain (Table 1.3), and exercise-induced pain (Table 1.4). Drugs that may cause muscle pain are shown in Table 1.5. Exercise-induced pain is a classical feature of metabolic myopathies, with glycogenoses (e.g. McArdle's disease) typically presenting with pain early in exercise and disorders of fatty acid metabolism (e.g. carnitine palmitoyltransferase deficiency) with pain on sustained exertion. An important catch is dystrophin-related disorders. Both Duchenne and Becker muscular dystrophies may present with exercise-induced calf pain, mimicking a glycogenosis, but later develop weakness. Some dystrophin mutations, and other dystrophy-related genes (e.g. *ANO5*) may cause exercise-induced pain without weakness, and this is sometimes referred to as a pseudo-metabolic presentation.

Table 1.3 Disorders associated with localized muscle pain

Neuralgic amyotrophy
Focal neuropathies
Infections • Bacterial (pyomyositis) • Parasitic
Inflammation • Sarcoidosis
Acute alcoholic myopathy
Metabolic myopathies
Tumours (primary muscle tumours, infiltration from other tumours)
Secondary to local joint/rheumatological problems
Compartment syndromes

Table 1.4 Causes of exercise-induced pain

Intermittent claudication
Muscular dystrophies • Duchenne • Becker • Anoctamin 5 (limb-girdle dystrophy Type 2L)
Metabolic myopathies • Glycogenoses (e.g. McArdle's disease) • Disorders of lipid metabolism (e.g. CPT deficiency) • Mitochondrial cytopathies • Brody's syndrome
Dermatomyositis

CPT, carnitine palmitoyltransferase.

Stiffness and muscle hyper-excitability

The terms contracture, cramp, and spasm are misunderstood by patients and doctors alike. Contracture may mean one of two things. Permanent muscle shortening due to fibrosis is an inevitable late sequela of numerous neuromuscular disorders associated with marked weakness and muscle atrophy. Typical examples are fixed flexion contractures at the hips, knees, and elbows. These contractures are in themselves painless, but may contribute to discomfort because of difficulty with positioning. They are rarely a presenting symptom. In some muscle disorders contractures develop as an early feature, when there is little muscle weakness and generally good mobility. The commonest include Emery–Dreifuss syndrome, which is genetically heterogeneous, with early contractures affecting the neck (limiting flexion), elbows and ankles (Achilles tendon tightening), Bethlem myopathy, and the various forms of rigid spine syndrome. The second meaning of contracture is a transient, painful shortening of a muscle due to failure of relaxation,

Table 1.5 Drugs causing muscle pain (not a complete list—see also Chapter 33)

Statins
Amiodarone
Cimetidine
Clofibrate
Emetine
Gemfibrozil
Heroin
Beta blockers
Nifedipine
D-Penicillamine
Procainamide
Vincristine
Zidovudine

and overlaps with the term cramp used by patients. EMG would be silent, and it is due to failure of relaxation secondary to metabolic factors that impair calcium reuptake and thus the end of the contraction process. The commonest example is that seen in McArdle's disease, where it is precipitated by exercise.

Cramps (which may be referred to as spasms by patients) are due to peripheral nerve hyper-excitability and consist of brief painful contracture most commonly affecting gastrocnemius. EMG would show high-frequency motor unit discharges. In the more widespread cramping syndromes (see Chapter 21) cramps may affect the feet, hands, proximal limb and trunk muscles, and axial muscles, and can also be associated with muscle twitching and rippling. The latter is due to peripheral nerve hyper-excitability and must be distinguished from rippling muscle due to caveolin mutations and autoimmune rippling muscle disease, in which the rippling is electrically silent.

Myotonia is due to repetitive depolarization of the muscle fibre membrane and is perceived by the patient as muscle stiffness. Grip myotonia means that after squeezing something tightly there is difficulty in opening the hand (e.g. wringing out a cloth, releasing anything held tightly, releasing after a hand-shake). The most common association is with myotonic dystrophy. In the very much less common myotonia congenita, proximal muscle myotonia causes stiffness when first trying to move after sitting or standing still, and an attempt to move quickly may cause a fall.

Fasciculation, often with frequent cramps, may be the presenting symptom of ALS, and of the much rarer Kennedy disease. It is also a feature of multifocal motor neuropathy and chronic inflammatory demyelinating polyradiculoneuropathy. In ALS, fasciculations are surprisingly rare as the first reported symptom, frequently going unnoticed by the patient until they are pointed out. Benign fasciculation is, by definition, the principal symptom reported and is without weakness. It is a diagnosis of exclusion in those with no abnormality on examination, and does not require EMG to be certain. Benign fasciculations have generally been present in an individual for many years (rather than the more sinister explosive fasciculations of recent onset), but do not have to be confined to the calf muscles. For practical purposes it includes the commonly seen twitching of the peri-orbital muscles, sometimes also referred to as myokymia.

Muscle wasting or muscle enlargement

Muscle wasting or muscle enlargement are rare presenting symptoms. Wasting tends to be a late feature of myopathies, and so presentation is more likely to be with weakness. By contrast, in neurogenic disorders, wasting may be the presenting symptom. Examples include the patient noticing wasting of the dorsal interossei in ulnar neuropathy, and wasting of the first dorsal interosseous and thenar eminence with relative preservation of the medial hand muscles in ALS (the so-called split hand). Progressive and bilateral wasting of the tongue, typically the lateral borders, and especially with visible fasciculations, is essentially pathognomonic for ALS. Focal muscle wasting due to radiculopathy in either the cervical or lumbar regions is rare, e.g. calf atrophy with a S1 lesion where the patient notices that a boot on that side is loose-fitting.

Muscle hypertrophy, other than in response to physical training, is uncommon and is rarely a presenting symptom. Generalized muscle hypertrophy may be a feature of myotonia congenita,

caveolin mutations (often associated with rippling muscles), and primary amyloidosis (typically also with tongue enlargement). More restricted hypertrophy may be seen in dystrophinopathies (calves, quadriceps, and less commonly deltoid, but rarely more generalized) and limb-girdle dystrophies (often the quadriceps appears wasted in some parts and hypertrophic in others). Tongue hypertrophy may be seen in Duchenne muscular dystrophy and limb-girdle muscular dystrophy Type 2I. Focal muscle hypertrophy may be seen with local infection (abscess, cysticercosis) or tumour, but is also seen rarely in response to peripheral nerve or nerve root irritation (e.g. calf hypertrophy with S1 radiculopathy).

Myoglobinuria

Extensive breakdown of muscle fibres (rhabdomyolysis), with disruption of the plasma membrane, leads to the release of cytoplasmic contents into the circulation, evidenced by a marked increase in the serum creatine kinase level and myoglobinaemia (not routinely estimated). Excretion of myoglobin into the urine gives rise to myoglobinuria, which the patient reports as the passage of very dark or apparently blood-stained urine (importantly, cross-reactive with the blood detection region of many routine urinalysis sticks). It carries with it the risk of acute tubular necrosis/renal failure. There are numerous causes of myoglobinuria (Table 1.6).

Table 1.6 Causes of myoglobinuria

Metabolic myopathies:
• Glycogenoses (e.g. McArdle's disease)
• Disorders of lipid metabolism (e.g. CPT deficiency)
• Malignant hyperthermia
• Neuroleptic malignant syndrome
Muscular dystrophies:
• Duchenne
• Becker
• Limb-girdle (rare)
Acquired myopathies:
• Myositis
• Infections (viral or bacterial)
Ischaemia and trauma:
• Crush injury
• Status epilepticus
• Electric shock
Drugs and toxins:
• Opiates
• Alcohol
• Statins
• Snake venom
• Bacterial toxins
Others:
• Heat stroke
• Idiopathic
• Extreme exercise in normal individuals

CPT, carnitine palmitoyltransferase.

Systems review

A detailed systems review is required and fulfils several purposes:

1. If the diagnosis is not evident from the foregoing assessment then such a review may point to an underlying cause for the neuromuscular disorder. Examples include features of hormonal dysfunction establishing a diagnosis of endocrine myopathy, haemoptysis from small cell lung cancer presenting with Lambert–Eaton syndrome, cutaneous features suggesting dermatomyositis, or psychiatric or bowel symptoms associated with porphyritic neuropathy.

2. Evidence of multisystem involvement in conditions such as mitochondrial cytopathy (e.g. heart, liver, bowel, skin, central nervous system) or myotonic dystrophy (e.g. cataracts, excessive daytime sleepiness, heart, bowel) may be found.

3. Problems that may complicate management of the neuromuscular disorder can be identified. For example, in a patient with an inflammatory myopathy steroids may be problematic against a background history of diabetes, obesity, hypertension, cataracts, osteoporosis, or affective disorder.

The systematic enquiry thus needs to be thorough and must also be considered alongside the patient's past medical, social, and medication history. The potential links between systemic disease and the presenting neuromuscular complaint are limitless. Associations will be considered further in the chapters dealing with specific disease areas.

Past medical history

The potential relevance of the past medical history to the presenting neuromuscular complaint is largely as discussed in the section The presenting complaint and related features. Identifying a pre-existing condition that is known to be associated with neuromuscular disease may provide answers, but is also subject to false associations. A past history of alcoholism does not prove that that is the cause of the presenting neuropathy, nor does a history of malignancy necessarily mean one is dealing with a paraneoplastic disorder.

Drug and social history

As discussed in detail in Chapter 35, and in other chapters relating to specific forms of neuropathy and myopathy, drugs (therapeutic and recreational) and toxins are a common cause of neuromuscular disorders. The history will readily elicit details of therapeutic drug usage, but more specific enquiry is needed to identify drug and substance abuse, and the possibility of exposure to toxins within the workplace or home environment. Traditional, herbal, or complementary therapies and dietary products, which neither the patient nor the physician may consider important, are in fact a significant potential source of toxicity (e.g. L-tryptophan and eosinophilia-myalgia syndrome) and potential interactions with therapeutic drugs (e.g. grapefruit juice causing drug toxicity by blocking intestinal cytochrome P-450 3A4 and the increased risk of rhabdomyolysis from statins).

Alcohol is an important and ubiquitous neuro- and myotoxin and patient-reported levels of consumption is notoriously unreliable.

Family history

This is so important that the whole of Chapter 2 is devoted to genetic considerations.

CHAPTER 2

Genetic considerations

David Hilton-Jones and Martin R. Turner

Introduction

Many neuromuscular disorders have a specific genetic basis; that is, they are linked to mutation within a single gene. Even those considered to be acquired may be the consequence of as yet poorly understood polygenic factors that predispose the individual to the disorder, possibly triggered by environmental factors [e.g. myasthenia gravis, in inclusion body myositis (IBM), idiopathic inflammatory myopathies, motor neuron disorders, polyneuropathies]. The genetic basis of virtually all of the more common neuromuscular disorders, and indeed of many vanishingly rare disorders, is now known and information is available from many readily accessible on-line databases (e.g. <http://www.musclegenetable.fr>, supported by the World Muscle Society). In some instances, especially for rarer disorders, there is a frustrating lag between a specific gene being identified by researchers and the availability of routine testing in the clinical arena. For some diseases associated with multi-exonic genes and no common mutations, analysis may be extremely time-consuming and costly, limiting routine availability. However, it is likely that in the very near future DNA chips and new-generation sequencing technology will advance to allow relatively cheap and simultaneous analysis of many neuromuscular disease-related genes. Advantageous though this will undoubtedly be, it will also generate in a few patients difficulties with the interpretation of variants of uncertain significance.

Specific aspects of the genetic and molecular features of individual disorders will be discussed throughout this book, but the present chapter will address some general issues that need to be considered when dealing with neuromuscular disorders that might have a genetic basis. It assumes that readers are familiar with the principles of autosomal, sex-linked, and mitochondrial inheritance. Specific issues that commonly arise in clinical practice relating to each of these are noted in Table 2.1 and discussed in more detail in the section Issues relating to specific inheritance patterns.

Relationships between genes and diseases—heterogeneity

It would simplify matters greatly if mutations in one gene always caused a specific disorder, and if a characteristic inherited clinical disorder was only associated with mutations in one specific gene. It has long been recognized that that is not the case, and neuromuscular disorders provide numerous examples of both genetic and phenotypic heterogeneity.

Genetic heterogeneity

This describes the situation of a common phenotype which can be caused either by different mutations within the same gene locus (allelic heterogeneity) or by mutations in completely different gene loci (locus heterogeneity).

Allelic heterogeneity is common in all forms of autosomal inheritance. Some mutations are relatively common, and even traceable to a single founder. Screening tests can be devised to look for these specific common mutations. However, in many diseases, for example ryanodine receptor-associated disorders, collagen VI-related disorders, and motor neuron disease (MND) linked to superoxide dismutase-1, many different mutations at the same allele are recognized. Diagnosis may then require sequencing of the whole gene, which is currently time-consuming and expensive. Different mutations within the same gene, e.g. the chloride channel gene in myotonia congenita, may behave in either a recessive or a dominant fashion.

Locus heterogeneity is perhaps best reflected in two major groups of neuromuscular disorders, namely Charcot–Marie–Tooth (CMT) disease and limb-girdle muscular dystrophy (LGMD). Numerous different genes, relating to nerve and muscle proteins respectively, give rise to essentially the same, highly characteristic, phenotype. In both disorders one may see examples of autosomal dominant and autosomal recessive inheritance, and, in the case of CMT disease, X-linked inheritance. Identifying the specific mechanism for an affected individual is essential for genetic counselling for the patient and wider family

Phenotypic heterogeneity

This term is, arguably, less precise than genetic heterogeneity, and encompasses a range of factors. In essence it refers to the fact that mutations in one gene may produce more than one phenotype. Related issues, discussed in the section Issues relating to specific inheritance patterns when considering autosomal dominant inheritance, include penetrance, expressivity, pleiotropy, and anticipation.

It is not surprising that mutations in different parts of the same gene may have different phenotypic consequences relating to different functional domains within the protein being coded for. Depending on the site and type of mutation, mutations in the lamin A/C gene (*LMNA*) can produce a diverse range of often overlapping phenotypes, including Emery–Dreifuss syndrome, LGMD, cardiomyopathy, CMT disease, lipodystrophy, and progeria. Mutations in one region of the *MYH7* gene cause early onset distal myopathy, and in another cardiomyopathy.

What is more surprising is that the same mutation may produce different phenotypes in different individuals, even within the same family. Thus, certain mutations of the caveolin gene (*CAV3*) can produce either LGMD, distal myopathy, isolated hyperCKaemia, or rippling muscle disease.

Mutations in the dystrophin gene (*DMD*), depending upon their site and whether or not the reading frame is disrupted, may cause Duchenne or Becker muscular dystrophy, isolated cardiomyopathy, or a cramp/myalgia syndrome.

Issues relating to specific inheritance patterns

As indicated in Table 2.1, despite the relative simplicity of the general rules there are a number of potential catches relating to each pattern of inheritance.

Autosomal dominant inheritance

In general, those with an autosomal dominant disorder will have inherited the condition from one or other parent and will themselves have a 50% chance of passing the condition on to each of their offspring, all independent of the sex of the individual. The family history is thus likely to be highly informative. Catches to be aware of include the following:

* Non-paternity: rates vary widely according to the population studied (1–10%, and even higher in some). Estimates are much higher for studies where disputed parentage was the reason for testing.

* New mutations: neither parent has the mutation but it arises in meiosis giving rise to the affected offspring, who may then transmit it to the next generation. In some disorders this is quite common [e.g. facioscapulohumeral (FSH) muscular dystrophy]. This will not necessarily cause difficulty if the phenotype is as characteristic as FSH muscular dystrophy, and DNA analysis is readily available. However, if the phenotype is one associated with genetic heterogeneity, such as LGMD, then it may not be immediately apparent whether the individual has a dominant disorder due to a new mutation or has an autosomal recessive disorder, and DNA-based diagnosis may not be readily available. This presents major difficulty with genetic counselling.

* Germline (gonadal) mosaicism: this is sufficiently common to be problematic in everyday clinical practice and, as with non-paternity and new mutations, is also relevant to X-linked disorders (and, extremely rarely, recessive conditions as well). In this situation an individual has two populations of cells in their gonads, one normal (as in the rest of their body) and the other carrying the mutation. The individual is clinically unaffected and standard (blood and any tissue other than gonad) DNA testing would be normal. However, a fetus arising from the mutated cell line would be affected, and of course then be at risk of passing on the abnormality to future generations in standard Mendelian fashion. It is not easily possible to distinguish between a new mutation and germline mosaicism as the cause of a 'normal' individual having a child with an autosomal dominant disorder, but the distinction is hugely important in terms of advising about recurrence risk. In the case of a new mutation the recurrence risk is essentially zero. With germline mosaicism the risk depends largely on the proportion of germline cells with the mutation, and that is impossible to measure. For a few more common diseases risk estimates are available.

* Penetrance: not everybody carrying a dominant mutation develops clinical symptoms. In those who do not the mutation is said to be non-penetrant. When considering penetrance, age must be taken into account. The expression of many diseases is age dependent. For those who do not present before middle age, penetrance may appear to be near zero at age 20 years but may be 100% by 80 years.

* Expressivity: this is often confused with penetrance, but rather than indicating whether or not there is clinical expression of the mutation it describes quantitative and qualitative manifestations of that expression in an individual in whom the disorder is penetrant. It covers the relative severity of expression, and is also often related to that to the age of onset of symptoms. It also covers variation in the different phenotypic features that might be associated with the condition. Both penetrance and expressivity need to be considered alongside pleiotropy and anticipation discussed next.

* Pleiotropy: this term describes multiple phenotypic traits arising from a mutation in one gene, because that gene product is used by different cell types, or is involved in signalling pathways affecting various targets. An example already alluded to is *LMNA* mutations.

* Anticipation: this describes the earlier age of onset of symptoms in subsequent generations. It is best understood in relation to unstable trinucleotide-repeat expansion disorders, most strikingly exemplified by myotonic dystrophy Type 1 (DM1). In addition to earlier age of onset in subsequent generations it is often blandly stated that the severity of symptoms also increases, but in DM1 that hides a more complex picture. Not only is the age of onset earlier, but the pattern of symptomatology changes strikingly, discussed in detail in Chapter 25. In brief summary, in a three-generation family one might see a grandparent who is of normal intellect and develops cataracts at a slightly earlier age than average, but is otherwise asymptomatic. The daughter develops distal weakness and myotonia in adolescence/early adulthood, and may have an IQ in the normal range or slightly reduced. She then has a child with congenital disease, who is hypotonic at birth, has transient feeding and breathing difficulties, dysmorphic facial features, and subsequent learning difficulties that prevent independent existence.

Table 2.1 Some issues relating to different inheritance modes

Autosomal dominant	New mutations
	Germ-line mosaicism
	Penetrance
	Expressivity
	Pleiotropy
	Anticipation
Autosomal recessive	Many cases appear 'sporadic'
	Pleiotropy
	Pseudodominant inheritance
X-linked	Manifesting carriers/dominant expression
	New mutations
Mitochondrial	Non-transmission of the 'common deletion'
	Many 'mitochondrial' disorders are autosomally inherited

Autosomal recessive inheritance

Most individuals with an autosomal recessive disorder have no family history of the condition and thus appear to be sporadic. This manifestation is sometimes referred to as 'horizontal inheritance' as a family tree shows affected members in a horizontal line, with vertical family members (parents and subsequent generations) being unaffected. This is in contrast to the 'vertical inheritance' pattern of dominant disease with parent-to-child transmission.

Penetrance and expressivity are generally considered only to be features of autosomal dominant disease. Although as a general rule recessive disorders tend to have an earlier onset than dominant disorders, there are many exceptions. Another generalization, again with exceptions, is that recessive phenotypes tend to show less variability than dominant ones.

Pseudodominant inheritance describes the apparent 'vertical transmission' of a disorder that is autosomal recessive in nature. McArdle's disease is an autosomal recessive disorder, and thus affected individuals have two mutated alleles and carriers of one mutated allele are asymptomatic. If an affected individual has offspring with an asymptomatic partner who happens to have one mutated allele, then each child has a 50% risk of developing McArdle's disease and the family tree suggests dominant inheritance (Fig. 2.1). Consanguinity of course greatly increases the likelihood of seeing pseudodominant inheritance, so the ethnic background and traditions of the parents need to be considered.

X-linked inheritance

Mutations on the X chromosome, as on an autosome, may behave in recessive or dominant fashion, but the distinction between the two becomes a little blurred due to a variety of factors.

Dominant X-linked disorders are relatively rare but in the neuromuscular field include *FHL1* mutations which can cause a range of phenotypes including scapuloperoneal syndrome, X-linked myopathy with postural muscle atrophy, and reducing body myopathy. As with any dominant disorder, penetrance and expressivity can vary. Despite being dominant, severity tends to be greater in males. Similarly, CMT disease type 1X is inherited as an X-linked dominant trait but almost invariably females are less affected, both clinically and electrophysiologically, than males. Indeed, some females show no clinical features, indicating low penetrance.

The X-chromosome mutations causing Duchenne and Becker muscular dystrophy are considered to be recessive, which classical teaching suggests should mean that females are asymptomatic

carriers and only hemizygous males are affected (cf. haemophilia). However, up to 10% of female carriers may show mild skeletal muscle involvement (most commonly calf hypertrophy, less commonly proximal weakness which very rarely is severe) and are referred to as manifesting carriers. A small number of female carriers may develop cardiomyopathy with or without evidence of skeletal muscle involvement. These 'exceptions' have been attributed to skewed inactivation (or lyonization) of the X chromosome. If there is preferential inactivation of the chromosome carrying the normal gene, then the effects of the mutated gene on the other allele become apparent, but the evidence for this remains inconclusive and other factors may be relevant. Other rare causes of females manifesting disease include the female inheriting two affected X-chromosomes (with a new mutation on one being possible), Turner's syndrome (XO), and X–autosome translocation.

As with autosomal recessive disorders, many affected individuals are seen with no family history, or an affected male sibling (apparent 'horizontal transmission'). One explanation for the apparent absent family history is that in preceding generations the mutation may only have been carried by 'asymptomatic' females. Sometimes the family history has simply not been taken back far enough, and more detailed enquiry will reveal, for example in the case of Duchenne muscular dystrophy, death of an adolescent male several generations ago without the family being aware of the precise diagnosis. For Duchenne and Becker muscular dystrophies, the greatest catches are new mutations and germline mosaicism (both discussed in the section Autosomal dominant inheritance). New mutations are responsible for about one-third of cases. Germline mosaicism is less common, but presents particular difficulties for counselling about recurrence risk.

Mitochondrial inheritance

'Mitochondrial myopathy' was first defined by the demonstration of accumulations of structurally abnormal mitochondria in muscle biopsy specimens. It was then shown that respiratory chain function was impaired in some (e.g. complex 1 or complex 4 deficiencies). Subsequently abnormalities of mitochondrial DNA (mtDNA) were identified, initially deletion of a large section of the circular mtDNA molecule (the so-called common deletion), and later point mutations within mtDNA. The clinical diversity of mitochondrial disorders rapidly became evident, leading to the preferred term 'mitochondrial *cyto*pathy' as in many mitochondrial disorders there is no evidence of muscle involvement. mtDNA is maternally inherited and encodes for only a small number of mitochondrial (respiratory chain) proteins, the rest being autosomal in origin. Thus, mitochondrial cytopathy does not necessarily imply maternal inheritance, and indeed the majority of mitochondrial disorders are either sporadic, and not inherited (e.g. the 'common' deletion of mtDNA, causing late-onset chronic progressive external ophthalmoplegia), or are the result of a dominant or recessive autosomal mutations and behave as already described. A precise molecular diagnosis is clearly essential for correct genetic counselling, which is particularly difficult for maternally inherited mtDNA point mutations, as discussed in detail in Chapter 32.

Family history

Little encouragement is needed to take a detailed family history if the patient spontaneously volunteers information about other

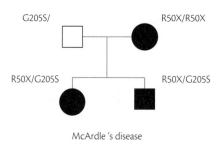

Fig. 2.1 Pseudodominant inheritance. The affected mother (black circle) is homozygous for the most common mutation associated with McArdle's disease. Her asymptomatic partner (open square) carries another recognized mutation on one allele, whereas the other allele is normal. Each child is a compound heterozygote for the two mutations.

affected family members, or the patient's clinical history and examination clearly indicate a genetic neuromuscular disorder. In the absence of such clues, a cursory family history may miss potentially relevant information. Most acquired neuromuscular disorders are sporadic, and thus there will indeed be no relevant family history, but inheritable disorders frequently occur in an isolated individual. Family histories may be misleading or incomplete. Not infrequently, the clue to a genetic disorder may only come after further clinical and laboratory assessment (e.g. finding neurophysiological evidence of a demyelinating neuropathy in a patient initially thought to have an acquired peripheral neuropathy—the correct diagnosis being autosomal dominant CMT disease with incomplete penetrance). One then has to return to the family history. The patient may have inadequate knowledge about their family, and other family members may need to be interviewed. The history-taking may need to be extended to physical assessment of other, apparently unaffected, family members, thus overlapping with issues discussed in the section Genetic counselling later.

It is worth noting that many highly educated individuals will not understand the concept of a condition that 'runs in the family'. Neither should questioning be limited to 'has anybody else in the family had the same problems'; more directed enquiry should be made, such as the use of walking aids, mobility problems, 'undiagnosed' problems leading to disability, and details of potentially erroneous diagnoses such as 'arthritis' as a cause of walking impairment, etc. Recently, an autosomal dominant intronic hexanucleotide repeat expansion in *C9orf72* has been associated with cases of MND (also known as amyotrophic lateral sclerosis, ALS) and frontotemporal dementia (FTD) occurring in members of the same family. MND was often historically termed 'creeping paralysis', and may be labelled erroneously as MS or stroke (in the case of the elderly with bulbar onset). FTD may be considered generically as 'Alzheimer's' or even as simply eccentric behaviour. Such factors have undoubtedly led to cases of MND being labelled erroneously as sporadic.

As emphasized in Chapter 1, many inherited neuromuscular disorders have multisystemic manifestations, and many acquired disorders are secondary to an underlying disorder, so the family history needs to extend beyond neurological problems. Examples of relevant 'general medical' associations are too legion to list, but one example, shown in the section Illustrative family histories, might be a mitochondrial disorder presenting as a myopathy in one individual but as deafness, cardiomyopathy, or diabetes in other family members.

Consanguinity substantially increases the risk of autosomal recessive disorders. This is recognized as being common in certain ethnic and religious groups but may be overlooked in populations in whom consanguineous relationships are rare. The question needs to be asked despite any discomfort that may arise. A related issue is having knowledge of the frequency of particular disorders in the local population as some show considerable regional variability. A classic example relating to ancestral issues is the high prevalence of myotonic dystrophy type 1 in Quebec, Canada.

Taking an adequate family history requires time and patience and may need to be undertaken in more detail at a later date than the initial clinic assessment. Depending upon the experience of the clinician, help may need to be sought from a geneticist or genetics nurse specialist, both of whom may have a subsequent role in genetic counselling.

The next subsection (Illustrative family histories) gives some examples of 'diagnostic', 'missing', 'inadequate', and 'misleading' family histories, all based on real-life examples.

Illustrative family histories

With dominant disorders in particular the family history is often straightforward and highly informative. FSH muscular dystrophy is inherited in an autosomal dominant fashion and is associated with a deletion in the D4Z4 repeat sequence in the telomeric region of chromosome 4. Figure 2.2 illustrates a family in which the patient presented with typical features of FSH muscular dystrophy. His mother and maternal grandfather were known to have had the condition, and his mother had been shown to have the relevant mutation. Arguably, the patient does not require DNA confirmation of the diagnosis.

In the family shown in Fig. 2.3(a) the patient presented with unilateral scapular winging, a well-recognized presentation of FSH muscular dystrophy, and the diagnosis was confirmed at a molecular level. However, neither parent was known to be affected by the condition. There are five possible explanations for what is a common scenario:

1. One parent may be found on examination to have features of the condition but was either not aware of any symptoms or chose to ignore/deny them.

2. One parent carries the mutation but it is non-penetrant and they have no signs of the condition.

3. One parent is a germline mosaic.

4. There has been a new mutation.

5. Non-paternity (Fig. 2.3b).

A patient presented with features consistent with Duchenne muscular dystrophy (Fig. 2.4a) but enquiry back to his grandparents revealed no family history of the condition. Taking the history back (Fig. 2.4b) further identified a male predecessor who died during the Second World War at the age of 16 years from a muscle-wasting condition, without any more detail being available (a common scenario). The patient was shown to have a dystrophin mutation and his mother to carry the mutation. The presumption

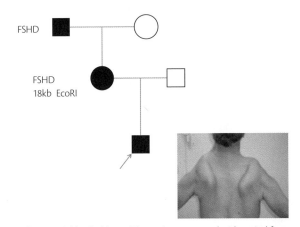

Fig. 2.2 'Diagnostic' family history. The patient presented with typical features of facioscapulohumeral muscular dystrophy. His mother (black circle) and maternal grandfather (top black square) were known to have had the condition, and his mother had had confirmatory DNA analysis.

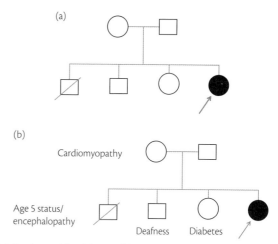

Fig. 2.5 'Inadequate' family history. (a) Enquiry into the family history must go beyond questions about neuromuscular problems, as shown by this family with a maternally inherited mitochondrial cytopathy (b).

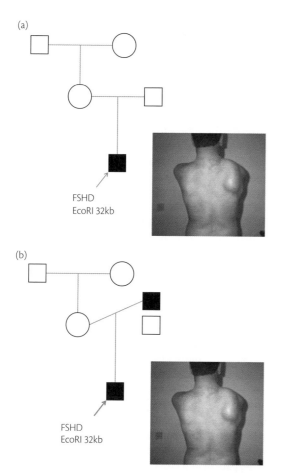

Fig. 2.3 'Missing' family history. The patient presented with unilateral scapular winging (a common presenting feature in milder cases of facioscapulohumeral muscular dystrophy, FSHD) and DNA analysis confirmed the diagnosis. See text for discussion of paternity.

is that his ancestor also had Duchenne muscular dystrophy with intervening female carriers.

Particularly in conditions associated with multisystemic involvement, specific enquiry must be made about non-muscular manifestations. This is exemplified by a family with a maternally inherited mtDNA mutation in whom initial enquiry about muscle problems revealed no relevant family history (Fig. 2.5a), but more detailed enquiry revealed an extensive history of related clinical expression (Fig. 2.5b).

Finally, one must be wary of being misled by the family history. In the family shown in Fig. 2.6, three generations were known to be affected by FSH muscular dystrophy, with DNA confirmation of the diagnosis. In addition, patient III.1 presented with features of myotonia congenita and was shown to be a compound heterozygote for *CLCN1* chloride channel mutations, confirming a diagnosis of autosomal recessive myotonia congenita. At the age of 21 years, patient III.2 presented complaining of weakness and muscle stiffness. She realized that she had a 50% risk of inheriting the FSH mutation, and a 25% risk of developing myotonia congenita, and

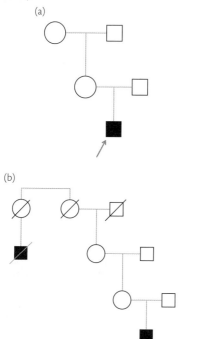

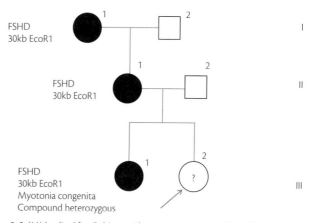

Fig. 2.6 'Misleading' family history. Three generations had clinical features of facioscapulohumeral muscular dystrophy (FSHD) with molecular confirmation of the diagnosis. One member, III.1, in addition had features of myotonia congenita and was shown to have compound heterozygous mutations affecting the chloride channel gene, *CLCN1*, indicating recessive inheritance. Her sibling, III.2, presented at the age of 20 years complaining of muscle stiffness and weakness.

Fig. 2.4 'Inadequate' family history. (a) A male presented with early childhood onset weakness and became wheelchair dependent early in the second decade. (b) Initial family history was 'negative' for neuromuscular disease, but became positive on more detailed enquiry.

believed that she had been twice unlucky. However, examination showed no abnormality, and DNA testing showed that she had not inherited the FSH mutation and was a carrier for only one of the two myotonia congenita mutations.

The last example relates to another common clinical problem, whereby parents knowing that their children have a risk of inheriting a neuromuscular disorder may perceive problems that do not exist. For example, knowledge of a family history of CMT disease may lead to parental anxiety that every trip and fall in the school playground heralds the onset. Another common example is concern that normal scapular prominence in a relatively thin child is the first evidence of FSH muscular dystrophy. These issues are highly relevant when considering genetic counselling issues.

Genetic counselling

In brief, genetic counselling refers to the process of informing individuals about genetic risks and, by extrapolation, advising them about reproductive options. Although potentially complex in the minutiae, the major issues relevant to neuromuscular disorders are summarized in Table 2.2. Genetic counselling should ideally be provided by a clinician who not only has the requisite genetic knowledge but also has widespread experience in the diagnosis and management of neuromuscular disorders, both genetic and acquired. This might be a geneticist who has subspecialized in the field of neuromuscular disorders, or a paediatric or adult neuromuscular specialist who has undertaken appropriate genetic training. In many centres the goal is achieved through collaboration between the relevant clinical service responsible for diagnosis and management, and the department of genetics.

A common clinical problem is an individual who comes from a family known to have a specific neuromuscular disorder and who wishes to know their risk of developing the 'familial condition'. If the mode of inheritance of that condition is known (e.g. dominant, recessive, X-linked, mitochondrial) then it is a simple paper exercise to determine the specific risk of that individual having inherited the relevant mutation(s). And even simpler in principle, if the specific mutation is known, DNA analysis can determine, essentially with 100% accuracy, whether or not that individual has inherited the mutation. In practice however, the question of whether they will develop the familial condition is far more complex.

Table 2.2 Issues relating to genetic counselling

Informing individuals of genetic risks:
- The risk to an individual who has a family history of genetic disease
- The risk of a parent with a genetic disorder having an affected child
- The recurrence risk in subsequent pregnancies if a child has been born with a genetic disorder

Reproductive options:
- Sperm or egg donation
- Pre-implantation genetic diagnosis
- Prenatal diagnosis (e.g. by chorionic villus sampling)

As discussed in the section Illustrative family histories, carrying a mutation does not necessarily mean that an individual will express it, or if they do how severe it will be (including the age of onset) or which organ system(s) it will involve. Counselling of the individual must take into account all of these considerations. Adequate counselling can only be given if the counsellor has intimate knowledge of the condition and all of its potential manifestations.

One special issue relates to the testing of the children of a parent with an inheritable neuromuscular disorder. If the condition was known about prior to conception, then appropriate counselling should have been given beforehand and reproductive options discussed. However, a common scenario is that a parent is diagnosed with such a condition after they have already conceived. Considering the simplest example of an autosomal dominant disorder they will realize that each child has a 50% risk of having inherited the mutation and may enquire about testing. As a general principle, testing asymptomatic children (who, by definition, cannot provide informed consent) is *not* indicated unless a specific therapeutic intervention is available, or knowledge of the mutation might directly affect overall management. If the child develops symptoms or signs that might be attributable to the mutation, then testing may be indicated, but otherwise the general principle is to counsel the child to enable to make their own decision about pre-symptomatic testing once they have reached the age of consent. The parental anxiety is readily understandable. Counselling should help them deal with those anxieties and should include advice to be open in discussions with their children as they mature and might ask questions about their parent's health issues. No rule is absolutely rigid, and the relationship between the patient and clinician over the years should allow constant review of relevant genetic issues.

For all patterns of inheritance, after the birth of an affected child a major issue is the risk of recurrence in subsequent pregnancies. Where the mutation is known, this gives rise to the possibility of prenatal diagnosis in future pregnancies, or pre-implantation genetic diagnosis. Other options, even when the mutation is not known, include egg or sperm donation.

Individual disorders are associated with specific genetic counselling issues, which will be addressed in more detail in the relevant chapters. Myotonic dystrophy presents a number of issues relating to anticipation, and the disease tends to manifest itself in different ways in different generations. It is one of the few neuromuscular disorders where there are good grounds to actively seek out asymptomatic family members to offer genetic testing. An important potentially preventable situation is an asymptomatic mother giving birth to a child with the severe congenital form of the condition.

The principles of genetic counselling seem inherently simple, but the practice is complex and a rashly sent test has the potential to cause irreparable and far-reaching emotional harm. All counselling, by definition, is non-directional. There are enormous sensitivities relating to specific religious and cultural issues. Clinical assessment and DNA testing take place against the background of informed consent, and that is inherently dependent upon provision of the right information, presented in an appropriate fashion.

CHAPTER 3

Examination

David Hilton-Jones and Martin R. Turner

Introduction

Despite the traditional concept of distinguishing rigidly between symptoms and signs, in reality there is substantial overlap, which will have been readily evident from the discussion in Chapter 1. For example, careful elucidation of the history will give a strong indication of the distribution of weakness, which is so critical in establishing the differential diagnosis, and then examination will further refine that distribution. Not infrequently, an observation on examination may lead to further questioning of the patient to elucidate additional features of the symptomatology. Contrary to the established dogma of 'history first, and then examination', the reality is that examination comes first—as one watches the patient walking from the waiting room into the clinic, and observes the patient whilst he or she is relating their history.

Those reading this book will be familiar with the general approach to physical examination, and the purpose of this chapter is to offer some focused observations in relation to neuromuscular disorders.

General examination

The purpose of the general physical examination is to determine whether:

1. There is evidence of a primary general medical disorder that might cause secondary neuromuscular problems. For example:

    (a) endocrinopathy such as hypothyroidism [causing proximal myopathy, or focal neuropathy (carpal tunnel syndrome)] or Cushing's syndrome (proximal myopathy),

    (b) malignancy causing paraneoplastic neuromuscular disorder.

2. There are systemic features associated with a primary neuromuscular disorder. For example:

    (a) myotonic dystrophy—cataracts, hair loss, irregular pulse, pilomatrixomata,

    (b) mitochondrial cytopathy—skin (lipomatosis), pigmentary retinopathy, cardiomyopathy, irregular pulse, movement disorder,

    (c) an association with cardiac arrhythmia and/or cardiomyopathy.

3. There are 'general' medical problems that may complicate a primary neuromuscular disorder or its management. For example:

    (a) rheumatological/orthopaedic problems that will further exacerbate mobility and posture issues relating to a primary neuromuscular disorder (e.g. hip and knee arthritis exacerbating problems relating to quadriceps weakness in inclusion body myositis, or further impairing mobility in hereditary neuropathies),

    (b) cardiorespiratory problems (e.g. asthma, chronic obstructive pulmonary disease, ischaemic heart disease/cardiomyopathy) that may exacerbate ventilatory muscle insufficiency and cardiac problems directly related to the primary neuromuscular disorder.

The findings on general physical examination, or the identification of a primary neurological disorder that is known to be associated with multisystemic features, may require more detailed specialist investigations. Amongst the most common are cardiorespiratory studies. Electrocardiography (ECG) should be an integral part of the initial assessment if a disorder known to affect the heart is suspected (e.g. myotonic dystrophy, laminopathy, dystrophinopathy) and in any patient with an as yet unidentified generalized neuromuscular disorder. A resting tachycardia may be a clue to dysautonomia, and bradycardia to hypothyroidism. More detailed cardiac assessment (echocardiography) is needed at initial assessment and on long-term review in those patients with conditions known to be associated with cardiomyopathy (e.g. dystrophinopathies). More detailed respiratory studies (pulmonary function, sleep studies) may be indicated, but initial assessment should include measurement of erect and supine forced vital capacity in those conditions known to be associated with ventilatory muscle weakness [e.g. Guillain–Barré syndrome, motor neuron disease (MND), myasthenia gravis, and acid maltase deficiency].

Motor examination

Inspection and palpation of muscle and nerves

Adequate physical observation in the setting of neuromuscular symptoms requires the patient to be undressed to their underwear. The distribution of any atrophy or hypertrophy should be noted, together with any spontaneous involuntary movements (e.g. fasciculation, rippling, twitching, myokymia). Fasciculations in MND may be sparse, and are most often missed over the shoulder region and back. Facial fasciculation (especially of the chin) is particularly prominent in Kennedy disease. Tongue fasciculations are best observed with the tongue relaxed. Forced protrusion leads to false positive assignation. In the setting of bilateral tongue wasting and dysarthria, tongue fasciculations are highly suspicious for MND.

Peripheral nerve hypertrophy is seen, or rather felt, in some demyelinating polyneuropathies (including the most common form of hereditary motor and sensory neuropathy, Type 1A), leprosy, and neurofibromatosis. However, it is inconsistent, and there is often not a clear distinction from normality.

Muscle palpation may help detect subtle atrophy. Various textures described in different clinical settings include hardness, 'woody feeling', 'doughy feeling', and 'fibrotic', but we have not found such assessment contributory.

An assessment of limb tone is vital in establishing a central component to a neuromuscular disorder, e.g. amyotrophic lateral sclerosis (ALS). This may range from a subtle 'catch' in forced supination of the forearm, to sustained clonus of the ankle and even patella. Passive movement of joints and the spine are required to identify contractures (see Chapter 1). Common sites include the neck and spine (as in rigid spine syndromes), elbows, finger flexors (e.g. Bethlem myopathy), hips, knees, and ankles.

Strength assessment

Whilst the term *strength assessment* is obviously readily applicable to axial and limb muscles, it is not so appropriate for evaluation of the extraocular or ventilatory muscles. Even when considering limb muscles, in the clinical setting it is often most helpful to think in terms of functional ability than ascribing a numerical value.

Cranio-cervical muscles

With the notable exceptions of myasthenia gravis and myotonic dystrophy, extraocular muscle involvement is uncommon in neuromuscular disorders, but when present is very useful in shortening the differential diagnosis (see Table 3.1). Assessment for ptosis and of the eye movements should be made even in the absence of suggestive symptoms.

Ptosis may be subtle, and is equally a frequent false positive sign. When ptosis is marked the patient may tilt their head back to enable them to see ahead. There may be persistent over-activity of the frontalis muscle to try to compensate (Fig. 3.1). Ptosis is often asymmetric. This is the norm in myasthenia gravis, but even in conditions such as oculopharyngeal muscular dystrophy there may be striking asymmetry. Fatigability, seen as the eyelid progressively drooping either spontaneously or on attempted sustained up-gaze, is virtually pathognomonic of myasthenia gravis.

Weakness of any of the six muscles moving each globe typically presents with diplopia. There may be obvious underactivity of one or more muscles when testing eye movements, but minor weakness causing diplopia may not be readily visible and requires cover testing to determine the muscle(s) involved. A striking feature

Table 3.1 'Minimum' assessments of limb and trunk strength

Neck flexion and extension
Scapular fixation
Shoulder abduction
Elbow flexion and extension
Wrist flexion and extension
Finger flexion, extension, and abduction
Hip flexion and extension
Knee flexion and extension
Ankle dorsiflexion and plantar flexion
Trunk—sitting up from lying supine
Gait

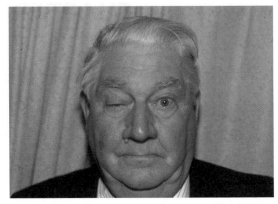

Fig. 3.1 Myasthenia gravis. Ptosis/frontalis over-activity. Asymmetry.

of mitochondrial chronic progressive external ophthalmoplegia (CPEO) is that diplopia is uncommon, despite often gross restriction of eye movements and sometimes with very evident divergence of the ocular axes (Fig. 3.2).

Temporalis muscle atrophy is often striking in myotonic dystrophy and contributes to the characteristic facies (Fig. 3.3). Weakness of the masseter and temporalis is often seen as part of the bulbar weakness in myasthenia gravis.

Mild unilateral weakness of the facial muscles is usually very obvious because of the asymmetry on movement. Conversely, even marked bilaterally symmetric facial weakness may not be obvious and is frequently missed. The first impression of facial weakness may be suspected from the failure of the patient's face to respond to the normal pleasantries exchanged at the start of a consultation, or as they give their history. Arguably, the best sign is the failure to completely bury the eyelashes on attempted forceful closure (Fig. 3.4), and there is no additional information to be gained from attempting forced eye opening. Not all incomplete burying of the eyelashes indicates weakness—those with contact lenses and those with lashings of mascara may be reluctant to attempt the manoeuvre! Weakness of lip closure may be suggested during speech, and can be demonstrated by failure to keep the lips closed when 'blowing up the cheeks' or when the examiner tries to forcibly separate the lips with their thumbs. Patients with facioscapulohumeral muscular dystrophy often have a rather characteristic bulbous appearance to their lips (Fig. 3.5).

The strength of the tongue and soft palate are best assessed by listening to speech (asking the patient to recite a nursery rhyme may be useful), perhaps aided by getting the patient to attempt to produce specific sounds, e.g. saying k and producing a hard g are problematic with palatal weakness, whereas tongue weakness is revealed by difficulty producing d, l, n, and t.

Swallowing can be assessed qualitatively by observation and quantitatively by timing the swallow of a specified amount of water.

Several neuromuscular disorders cause weakness of the neck flexors and extensors (Fig. 3.6), and this often neglected sign can be highly discriminatory in conjunction with other findings. It is often asymptomatic, but marked weakness of flexion causes difficulty lifting and throwing the head forwards in the normal action of sitting up from the supine position (Fig. 3.7). Marked weakness of extension causes the 'dropped head' appearance mentioned in Chapter 1. Weakness of flexion, which may be marked, with normal or only minimal weakness of extension is seen commonly in myasthenia gravis in both sexes and at all ages, myotonic dystrophy, and

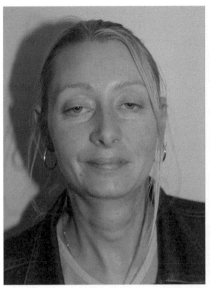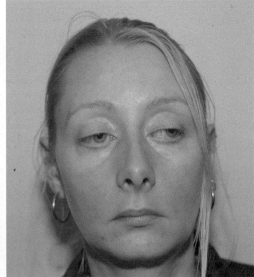

Fig. 3.2 Mitochondrial chronic progressive external ophthalmoplegia.

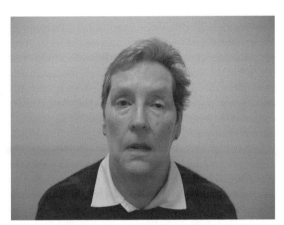

Fig. 3.3 Myotonic dystrophy facies—wasted temporalis.

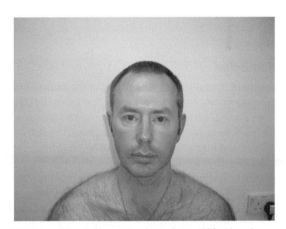

Fig. 3.5 Facioscapulohumeral muscular dystrophy—mild facial weakness and bulbous lips.

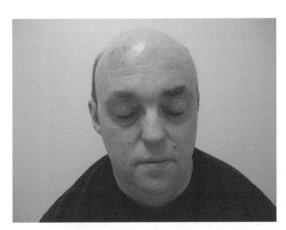

Fig. 3.4 Myotonic dystrophy. Bilateral facial weakness—incomplete burying of the eyelashes.

the idiopathic inflammatory myopathies. Causes of dropped head syndrome include myasthenia gravis in older men, MND, and, rarely, inflammatory myopathies and myotonic dystrophy. Overall, neck weakness is rather uncommon in most dystrophies except in advanced stages.

Axial and limb muscles

Involvement of the axial muscles in the neck has been described (see the section Cranio-cervical muscles). Weakness of the para-vertebral muscles is seen in *FHL1* myopathies (XMPMA; X-linked myopathy with postural muscle atrophy), acid maltase deficiency, and ALS. Marked involvement of the lumbar paravertebral muscles in FSH muscular dystrophy leads to an exaggerated lordosis (Fig. 3.8) and is frequently associated with lumbar pain.

All readers will be familiar with assessment of limb muscle strength, but it is appropriate to make some comments concerning which muscles should be assessed, how strength can be

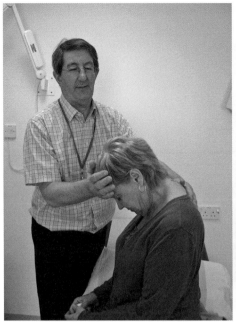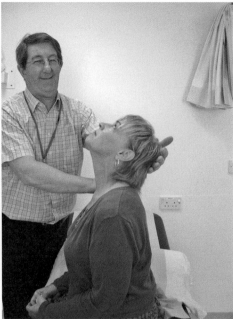

Fig. 3.6 Demonstration of positions for testing neck flexion and extension.

measured and recorded, and the importance of simple functional assessments.

Which muscles?

From the more than 600 skeletal muscles in the human body, the history provides vital clues to the approach that should be taken during examination. A history suggestive of a focal mononeuropathy indicates the need to assess the muscles innervated by that nerve, to confirm one's suspicions but also to look at nearby muscles to show that those innervated by other nerves are unaffected. Symptoms of peripheral neuropathy make distal rather than proximal weakness most likely. A history of generalized weakness may be associated with proximal, distal, or combined weakness, and the examination must look in detail to complement the history to try and identify the exact pattern of weakness which, as stressed in Chapter 1, may greatly shorten the differential diagnosis. As a minimum, the movements listed in Table 3.1 should be assessed in all patients, but the history and preliminary observations on examination will direct

further assessments. The finding of a so-called 'pyramidal' pattern of weakness, whereby there is preferential weakness of upper limb extensors and lower limb flexors, offers little discriminatory value for central versus peripheral neuromuscular disorders in reality.

The position of the limb is critical when assessing strength. Most clinicians use the approaches outlined in the classic *Aids to the Examination of the Peripheral Nervous System*, with personal variations learnt from experience.

Recording strength is easy in principle, but proves to be harder in practice. In routine clinical practice most clinicians use the Medical Research Council (MRC) scale, despite its limitations. The problem with the original scale is that grade 4 covers a wide range, encompassing minimal to substantial weakness. To try to deal with this various expansions have been tried (Table 3.2), but then inter- and intra-observer variations become more apparent. On the basis of Rasch analysis it has recently been proposed that the scale should be reduced to only four items. Whilst this may reduce observer variability, it is less useful for noting small changes in strength over

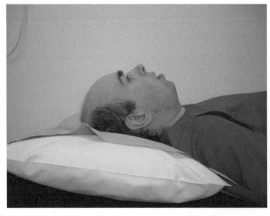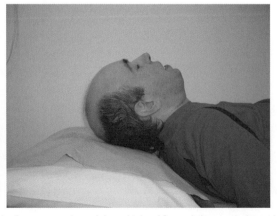

Fig. 3.7 Neck flexion weakness. The patient is trying to get up from the supine position but cannot raise and throw his head forwards (myotonic dystrophy).

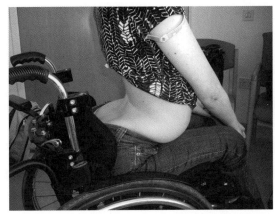

Fig. 3.8 Facioscapulohumeral muscular dystrophy—exaggerated lumbar lordosis due to weakness of the lumbar paravertebral muscles.

time, which may be vital for assessing improvement or deterioration. As noted, in clinical practice it is often more helpful to use quasi-objective functional assessments rather than numbers.

In the research setting MRC scores may be used as well as summed scores from assessing particular groups of muscles, often trying to reflect the particular pattern of muscle weakness associated with a particular disease. In addition to such manual muscle testing, various forms of dynamometry, hand-held or static, are used for quantification. A few diseases have well-validated assessment scales, e.g. the Quantitative Myasthenia Gravis (QMG) test.

A number of simple bedside functional tests provide a powerful tool to record the patient's current status, and readily allow the same clinician or others to note change over time, either deterioration reflecting the natural progression of the disorder or improvement in response to treatment (Table 3.2). For example, a patient with myositis and hip flexion weakness may, when lying supine, be able to raise their leg to get their heel 5 cm off the sheet. A month later they can raise it to 40 cm—a clear demonstration of improvement and yet on both occasions the MRC grade would be recorded as 4. Similarly, being able to rise from a standard height chair without using the arms

Table 3.2 Functional assessments

Standing up from a standard height chair—whether or not the arms need to be used
Rising from a squat
Timed walk: distance within a specific time (6-min walk), or time to walk a specific distance (10-m test), or timed up and go (TUG)

Lying supine
    ability to lift the head
    straight leg lift (heel–sheet distance, time able to maintain)
    sitting up from lying

Ability to run and hop
Ability to walk on heels and tip-toe
Ability to climb stairs in an 'adult' or 'child' (one step at a time) fashion
Height to which arms can be raised (and time able to maintain)

on one occasion but needing to use the arms a month later suggests deterioration.

Manual dexterity relates to both strength and sensory function. A variety of tests have been devised to quantify such function, of which the most commonly used is the nine-hole peg test. They have some value in routine practice, e.g. monitoring progress in multifocal motor neuropathy with conduction block.

Ventilatory muscles

Severe weakness is evidenced by orthopnoea, dyspnoea at rest, use of the accessory muscles of ventilation, ability to speak in only short sentences, and, in extremis, cyanosis. Mild weakness may be asymptomatic and easily overlooked, yet important to establish and monitor regularly in rapidly evolving conditions, e.g. Guillain–Barré syndrome and myasthenic crisis. Chronic nocturnal hypoventilation gives rise to excessive daytime sleepiness and waking with a headache and drowsiness. At the bedside the best assessment of ventilatory muscle strength is measurement of the forced vital capacity (FVC). This needs only a simple, relatively cheap, hand-held spirometer. Devices for measuring peak expiratory flow are totally inadequate for assessment of the neuromuscular patient. As a rule of thumb in an adult, a decline in FVC to 1 L necessitates urgent anaesthetic review for possible admission to an intensive care unit, although earlier transfer for rapidly progressing conditions may also be appropriate.

Many neuromuscular disorders specifically affect the diaphragm, leading to two important additional physical signs. Normally inspiration leads to the diaphragm descending and the abdominal wall moving outwards, but with weakness of the diaphragm it is drawn upwards during inspiration and the abdominal wall moves inwards ('abdominal paradox'). More sensitive is a fall in forced FVC on lying supine compared with when erect. Upon lying, the abdominal contents push the weak diaphragm cranially and reduce the FVC. In normal individuals there is some fall, more marked if they are obese. A fall of more than 10% is likely to be significant, and more than 20% certainly is.

Abnormal relaxation and movements

The most common form of delayed muscle relaxation is myotonia. Myotonic dystrophy is the most often encountered cause, and Type 1 is generally much more prevalent than Type 2. Electromyography may demonstrate myotonia when it is not obvious clinically. Cold tends to exacerbate myotonia. The classical textbook finding is of grip myotonia, whereby after shaking the examiner's hand, or forcefully gripping the examiner's fingers, there is delayed relaxation (Fig. 3.9). This may be severe, taking 10 s or more to achieve full relaxation, but it is frequently very mild and easily missed, especially as the 'warm-up' phenomenon means that it tends to lessen on repeated effort. More sensitive is the demonstration of percussion myotonia, whereby a sharp tap with a tendon hammer of the thenar eminence muscles leads to exaggerated contraction and delayed relaxation (Fig. 3.10).

Muscle stiffness and delayed relaxation are features of severe, long-standing hypothyroidism, and in adults are associated with Hoffman syndrome and in children with Kocher–Debré–Semelainge syndrome. Both are now extremely rare.

Brody's syndrome, due to sarcoplasmic reticulum ATPase deficiency, is also extremely rare and is characterized by impaired relaxation after repeated contractions, evidenced by difficulty opening the hand after repetitive finger flexion.

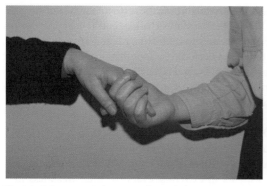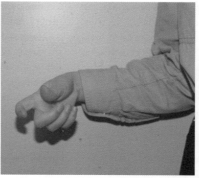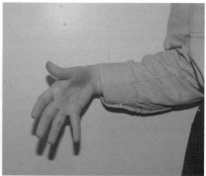

Fig. 3.9 Grip myotonia (myotonic dystrophy).

Rippling muscle describes an extraordinary phenomenon of wave-like contractures traversing a particular muscle. It may occur spontaneously but is often triggered by either stretching or percussion. The movements are electrically silent and their mechanism is not fully understood, but is presumed to relate to disordered membrane function. It was first noted in patients with caveolin mutations, also associated with limb-girdle muscular dystrophy, but is also seen, even more rarely, in association with myasthenia gravis and has an immune basis. Dysfunction of caveolae, membranous lipid rafts associated with various signalling functions, appears to underlie both forms.

Reflexes

As a general rule reflexes are lost late in the course of myopathies, when muscle wasting has become evident, and early in the course of neuropathies, when muscle bulk is still normal, although with some important exceptions. Reflexes are lost, even in clinically apparently unaffected muscles, in Lambert–Eaton syndrome, but may reappear transiently after sustained contraction of the muscle. In acquired demyelinating neuropathies reflexes may be lost over the course of several hours, and preceding weakness. In the common inherited neuropathies (e.g. Charcot–Marie–Tooth disease) generalized areflexia is the norm, but in mild cases may be restricted to the ankle jerks. Curiously, in some patients the ankle jerks are preserved even in the presence of significant distal weakness.

Delayed relaxation of a reflex is characteristically associated with hypothyroidism; although usually considered with respect to the ankle jerk, it is often more impressive with the supinator jerk.

As well as identifying pathologically brisk reflexes in the limbs, demonstration of a brisk jaw or facial jerks in the presence of tongue wasting has important diagnostic value in ALS.

Sensory examination

A distinguished former Oxford Professor of Neurology, Bryan Matthews, advised against 'trying to demonstrate sensory signs in public' (e.g. at a grand round), which appropriately emphasizes the inherent difficulties of sensory testing. With respect to the common sensory modalities of touch, pain, and temperature it is arguable that as much will be gleaned from the patient's description of the distribution and nature of the sensory disturbance as from examination. It is common for a patient with an acquired peripheral neuropathy to describe sensory dysfunction up to the mid-shins, but then be able to distinguish light touch and pin-prick sensation in these regions. Arguably more refined testing techniques may demonstrate a sensory level, but little more is likely to be revealed. Conversely, those with inherited neuropathies may present no sensory symptoms but have readily demonstrable 'stocking' sensory loss.

The history is likely to suggest either a focal peripheral or a generalized peripheral neuropathy, and thus whether examination is directed to look for sensory loss in the distribution of a specific nerve or glove-and-stocking distribution. The history may indirectly suggest disturbance of proprioception or vibration sense, but these are modalities that must be assessed specifically in all suspected neuropathies. In many cases of Charcot–Marie–Tooth disease vibration sense is absent below the knees or ankles, but joint position sense is usually preserved.

Bedside tests of autonomic function are limited in scope and few centres have access to autonomic function laboratories.

Specific tests of autonomic function must be considered where there is suspicion, e.g. diabetic, amyloid, and paraneoplastic autonomic neuropathies, and acutely in Guillain–Barré syndrome where it is a significant cause of mortality. Assessment includes

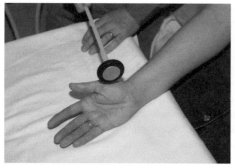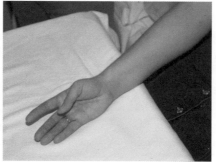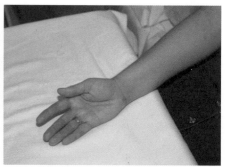

Fig. 3.10 Percussion myotonia (myotonic dystrophy).

measurement of supine and erect blood pressure and pulse rate, and beat-to-beat variation on ECG. Sudomotor testing, both electrical and physiological, is essentially a specialist laboratory activity, but dysfunction may be readily apparent at a simple observational level.

Conclusion

Whilst history-taking should establish a limited differential diagnosis, examination should then be used to exclude some of those possibilities and add support to others. Each informs the other, and as further information is gleaned it may be appropriate to go back to the history, both personal and family, to tease out further points. Seeing other family members, rather than relying on the observation of others, may be extremely helpful.

Appropriately directed further specialist investigations will be discussed in the context of specific disorders.

SECTION 2

Anterior Horn

CHAPTER 4

Amyotrophic lateral sclerosis

Kevin Talbot and Martin R. Turner

Introduction

Amyotrophic lateral sclerosis (ALS), the commonest form of motor neuron disease (MND), remains one the most devastating of the acquired neurological disorders. A progressive degenerative disorder, principally but not exclusively affecting the motor system, ALS is currently beyond the reach of clinically significant disease-modifying therapy [1].

The existence of a large number of neurological diseases in which motor neurons are the focus of pathology suggests that these cells and their associated neuronal networks may have a specific set of vulnerabilities. Whether the biological basis for this selectivity is best explained by defects in specific aspects of cellular biochemistry, abnormalities in synaptic function, or perturbations in higher-level network organization in the motor system is uncertain. Current evidence suggests that the disease is a consequence of the interaction of highly complex genetic risk variants, environmental factors, and age-related stochastic changes in cellular homeostasis. Intensive study of *in vitro* and *in vivo* models based on genetic forms of MND, indicates that these cells, characterized by extreme length and high energy requirements, may be vulnerable through a variety of mechanisms [2], including disturbances in excitotoxicity, axonal protein transport, mitochondrial dysfunction, protein misfolding, oxidative stress, and most recently RNA transport and splicing [3].

Convergent evidence from clinical, neuropsychological, neuroimaging, neuropathological, and genetic studies indicates that ALS is part of a disease continuum with specific forms of frontotemporal dementia (FTD), characterized neuropathologically by the presence of ubiquitinated intracellular inclusions [4]. The disease can therefore be regarded as a multisystem degeneration with motor predominance.

The core features of ALS

In essence, ALS is a progressive motor syndrome of insidious onset with clinical evidence of upper motor neuron (UMN) dysfunction (spasticity, brisk reflexes, extensor plantar responses) and lower motor neuron (LMN) denervation (muscle wasting, weakness, and fasciculations). The common end point is death from respiratory insufficiency, but there is wide variation in overall length of survival. Typically asymmetrical in onset, ALS follows a non-random pattern of development from the site of initial symptoms, suggesting a focal pathological process with anatomically contiguous spread. This is supported by autopsy studies, which indicate a radial reduction in pathological burden away from the anatomical areas most severely affected clinically [5]. Although predominantly a motor disorder, extramotor involvement, especially impairment of executive cognitive function, is detectable in a significant proportion of patients [6]. Sensory or autonomic dysfunction occurs in a minority of ALS patients, but is never the dominant feature.

The incidence of ALS is approximately 2 per 100 000 population each year, without convincing evidence of geographical variation. The apparent exception is the 'ALS–Parkinsonism–dementia complex' prevalent in isolated Pacific populations (Guam, the Kii Peninsula of Japan, and areas of Papua New Guinea), though this entity is characterized by tau pathology distinct from typical ALS, and its aetiology remains obscure [7]. There is no indication that ALS is increasing in absolute frequency, but with progressive increases in life expectancy and improved ascertainment the prevalence (5–7/100 000) and overall lifetime risk (1/300) are rising [8]. Primary-care physicians can expect to encounter a patient with ALS less than once every 10 years.

The most consistently observed risk factor for ALS is aging. The average age of onset is 67 years, though approximately 15% of patients present before the age of 50. It is still a matter of debate whether the incidence of ALS declines after the age of 85. The observed excess of males over females (1.5:1) with ALS is almost completely accounted for by spinal (limb)-onset cases [9].

Approximately 5% of patients report a history of ALS in a first-degree relative, so that it has been largely regarded as a predominantly sporadic disorder. However, in genetic screening studies apparently sporadic cases have been found to carry mutations in genes associated with familial ALS, so that the distinction between familial and sporadic ALS is not absolute [10].

Diagnosis and investigation

Although the identification of novel sensitive and specific biomarkers from cerebrospinal fluid (CSF), serum, neuroimaging, or neurophysiology is a major priority for research [11], the diagnosis of ALS is currently made on clinical grounds, and supported by the judicious use of imaging and neurophysiology (Table 4.1) [12]. Population-based studies have suggested that as many as 8% of patients who are initially thought to have ALS eventually turn out to have another condition, but misdiagnosis in specialist neurological clinics is very uncommon [13]. Despite this, neurologists often feel insecure about making the diagnosis, perhaps because of its grave implications. Case reports of rare conditions that can mimic ALS are frequent in the neurological literature, and probably contribute to inappropriate investigation and delay in diagnosis, which is on average approximately 1 year from first symptoms. However, the insidious nature of symptom onset and the difficulty, in a primary-care setting, of recognizing the significance of subtle early physical signs remain the greatest barriers to identifying patients at an earlier phase of disease [14].

Table 4.1 Clinical patterns of amyotrophic lateral sclerosis (ALS), differential diagnosis, and selected investigations

Clinical pattern	Differential diagnosis	Selected relevant investigations	M:F*	Mean survival from onset (years)*
Typical 'Charcot' ALS	Compressive myeloradiculopathy	MRI spine, NCS/EMG	1.65:1	2.6
Isolated corticobulbar ALS (PBP)	Cerebrovascular disease	MRI brain	1:1	2.0
UMN-predominant ALS	B_{12} deficiency, PPMS, adrenomyeloneuropathy, hereditary spastic paraplegia	B_{12}, VLCFAs, focused genetic testing	1:1	13.1
LMN-predominant ALS	Inflammatory demyelinating neuropathies, inclusion body myositis, distal motor neuropathies	NCS/EMG, muscle biopsy, focused genetic testing	2:1	7.3
'Flail arm' ALS	Compressive myeloradiculopathy, conduction block neuropathy, brachial neuritis	MRI, NCS/EMG	4:1	4
Lower limb-predominant ALS	CIDP, conduction block neuropathy, radiation lumbar plexopathy	NCS/EMG, LP	1:1	3
Respiratory onset ALS	Phrenic nerve palsy	NCS/EMG	6:1	1.4

MRI, magnetic resonance imaging; NCS, nerve conduction studies; EMG, electromyography; PBP, progressive bulbar palsy; UMN, upper motor neuron; LMN, lower motor neuron; PPMS, primary progressive multiple sclerosis; VLCFA, very long chain fatty acid; CIDP, chronic inflammatory demyelinating polyneuropathy; LP, lumbar puncture.

*Data adapted from Chio A et al. *J Neurol Neurosurg Psychiatry* 2011; **82**: 740–6.

Fundamental to the diagnosis in life is progressive weakness in the presence of mixed UMN and LMN signs. Approximately 30% of patients present with asymmetrical or unilateral upper limb dysfunction, 35% with lower limb symptoms, and 30% with disordered speech and swallowing ('bulbar onset'). Only 1–2% of patients present, usually to chest physicians, with isolated respiratory failure. Rarely, the first symptoms are axial weakness leading to non-specific gait disturbance or head drop. Occasionally, symmetrical spastic paraparesis of the lower limbs develops into ALS. As the disease develops into a progressive pure motor syndrome affecting more than one anatomical region (lumbar, thoracic, cervical, cranial), with clear UMN and LMN signs, the diagnosis becomes inescapable. Generalized wasting and fasciculation of the tongue, at any stage, is almost pathognomonic.

In limb-onset ALS, patients may report weakness, clumsiness, wasting, and more rarely stiffness. Typical initial complaints are tripping due to foot drop or loss of grip strength in a hand, which often shows disproportionate wasting of the thenar aspect [15] (Fig. 4.1). In contrast to benign fasciculations, which can be intrusive, ALS-related fasciculations frequently go unnoticed by the patient, and though often florid at diagnosis are only rarely the initial complaint. They tend to fade as the illness progresses. A common site is over the anterior shoulders, but any muscle group can be involved. A brisk reflex, or increased muscle tone, in an otherwise wasted limb is a strong clue, though this may require a subjective clinical judgement. It is useful to extend the conventional neurological examination to include pectoral and trapezius jerks, as well as crossed adductor reflexes of the thigh muscles. Unequivocally pathological reflexes, including ankle clonus and the Hoffman reflex, are important clinical signs. Extensor plantar responses may provide evidence of UMN involvement in a wasted leg, but are curiously an inconsistent finding in ALS [16].

In corticobulbar-onset ALS speech is affected before swallowing in nearly all cases (indeed the onset of dysphagia before dysarthria should prompt a search for an alternative diagnosis). Patients

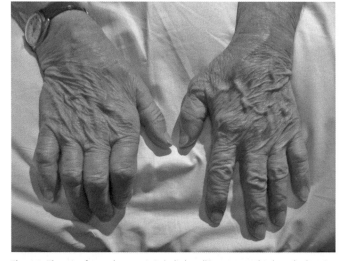

Fig. 4.1 There is often a characteristic 'split-hand' in amyotrophic lateral sclerosis, with disproportionate wasting of the first dorsal interossei.

typically describe slurred speech or a difficulty in articulating certain sounds. This is often variable in the early stages and confusion about the onset may result in referral to stroke services [17]. Difficulty chewing and swallowing in those with bulbar involvement is often worse towards the end of the day, but true fatigability as seen in myasthenia gravis does not occur. The majority of 'bulbar' patients have a mixed UMN and LMN syndrome, and bilateral wasting of the lateral tongue is the rule (Fig. 4.2). Corticobulbar reflexes such as a brisk jaw jerk, jaw clonus, and facial jerks are extremely useful physical signs. Although at least 80% of ALS patients overall go on to develop clinically significant bulbar involvement during the course of the disease, this is not inevitable and even when present may not necessarily require gastrostomy.

Emotional lability (emotionality) is due to loss of the normal suppression of reflex crying (and to a lesser extent also laughing),

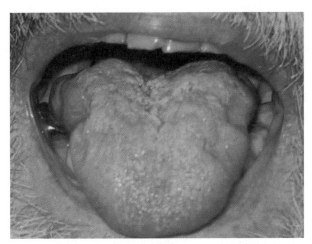

Fig. 4.2 Wasting of the tongue in amyotrophic lateral sclerosis. Typically dysarthria precedes dysphagia, and the lateral borders of the tongue tend to waste first and symmetrically. Reduced movement may exacerbate coating of the tongue surface as seen, which requires focused oral hygiene measures. (See also figure in colour plate section)

arising from involvement of corticobulbar pathways. It is very common in those with frank bulbar involvement and can be a useful supportive diagnostic symptom in the history (though it is often misinterpreted as a sign of depression or cognitive impairment, which are independent phenomena). The emotional response is characteristically mood incongruent, explosive in onset, and difficult to terminate. Although commoner in patients with clinical or subclinical cognitive dysfunction, emotional lability mostly occurs in people with clinically normal cognitive function, and this should be actively explained to the patient and family members for whom this symptom causes significant social morbidity.

Respiratory involvement may be an early or late feature of ALS, with a generally poor prognosis in the 1–2% of cases where it is the presenting feature [18]. For unexplained reasons most patients with respiratory-onset ALS are male. In a small minority of patients with respiratory-onset ALS, generalization of weakness to the limbs and bulbar muscles is delayed and the early and sustained use of non-invasive ventilation (NIV) can be very effective.

It has long been recognized that patients with ALS may exhibit cognitive impairments that have overlap with some forms of FTD [6]. Features of both behavioural variant and non-fluent aphasic FTD may be present, though notably few, if any, cases of true semantic dementia. Formal neuropsychological evaluation can reveal deficits in about 40% of ALS patients which are reflected in pathological changes (post-mortem and with neuroimaging *in vivo*). In most patients such deficits are usually mild. Whilst they generally then have no impact on the patient's formal capacity to make informed decisions, they frequently interfere with their ability to engage in care planning and can be a cause of significant anxiety in carers, especially spouses, who may report rigidity of thinking, irritability, apathy, or disinhibition with characteristically no patient insight. In less than 10% of cases, a more profound dementia is recognizable in ALS patients. Typically this presents early in the course of the motor degeneration and may even precede it by months. Behavioural change is often prominent and may include profound alteration in personality, ranging from extremes of either disinhibition or apathy. There may be a change in food preference with severe anorexia or over-indulgence in sweet foods.

The existence of isolated ALS as a paraneoplastic syndrome remains controversial. Two 'pure' motor neuronal clinical patterns have been described in the context of an underlying malignancy, but both are very rare. An UMN-predominant syndrome associated with anti-amphiphysin antibodies can occur in breast cancer [19], and an even rarer LMN-predominant syndrome has been occasionally associated with lymphoma [20].

Neurophysiology

Electromyography (EMG) can provide evidence of chronic denervation (long-duration, large-amplitude, polyphasic, unstable motor unit potentials) and acute denervation (positive sharp waves and fibrillation potentials). Neurophysiology is best viewed as a supportive paraclinical test and not as a diagnostic test for ALS. It should always be interpreted in the context of the clinical findings and, even in experienced hands, remains only 60% sensitive [21]. It is not uncommon, for example, to find patients with bulbar-onset symptoms and a visibly wasted tongue with no detectable denervation either in the tongue or limb muscles [22]. The diagnosis of ALS should still be confidently made on clinical grounds, avoiding delay in important interventions such as gastrostomy.

EMG and nerve conduction studies are important in providing support for the presence of non-clinically detectable denervation (i.e. LMN involvement), and in the exclusion of other LMN conditions such as pure motor inflammatory demyelinating neuropathies. Inclusion body myositis (see Chapter 32) can present as asymmetrical weakness and wasting and is well recognized to give a 'neurogenic' pattern on EMG, so can be a particular diagnostic challenge. There is no place for routine muscle biopsy in the diagnosis of typical ALS, however.

The Awaji-modified El Escorial criteria for the combined clinical and electrophysiological diagnosis of ALS rely on the presence of combined LMN and UMN features in four body regions (cranial, cervical, thoracic, and lumbar musculature). Broadly, as the number of such involved regions increases the terms 'possible' (one region), 'probable' (two regions), and 'definite' (three regions) ALS are used. However, this classification system has no prognostic value and many patients never pass beyond 'possible ALS' during their disease course, despite the diagnosis being obvious [23]. Use of these criteria should therefore be confined to a research or clinical trial setting.

Refined EMG-based techniques such as motor unit number estimation (MUNE) offer an alternative, quantitative assessment of LMN involvement [24]. Electrical impedance myography (EIM) exploits the change in muscle composition with progressive LMN denervation in ALS but is yet to be validated across multiple centres as a clinically useful surrogate marker [25].

Transcranial magnetic stimulation (TMS) is a non-invasive technique that can be used to explore the integrity of the corticospinal tract in ALS, reflected in the central motor conduction time. Other measures derived from paired-stimulation techniques can demonstrate cortical hyperexcitability as a key pathological feature in ALS patients [26], but this remains just a research tool at present.

Neuroimaging

Magnetic resonance imaging (MRI) is often necessary to exclude structural spinal pathology. However, coincident spondylotic disease is very common in the age group most likely to develop ALS and cervical myeloradiculopathy can present with a progressive pure motor syndrome without significant sensory or sphincter disturbance.

Studies show that up to 5% of patients subsequently diagnosed with ALS have had unnecessary spinal surgery. Therefore, careful clinical judgement is required in the selection of patients for surgery. A minority of patients (approximately 40%) have evidence of hyperintensity of the corticospinal tract on cerebral MRI [27]. The specificity of this finding is only 70% however (Fig. 4.3). Advanced MRI (including diffusion tensor imaging and resting-state functional MRI) has experimental potential as a future diagnostic tool for ALS [28].

Blood tests

Although usually clinically obvious, thyrotoxicosis may rarely be associated with proximal, usually lower limb, weakness with muscle wasting and should be excluded where relevant. The serum creatine phosphokinase (CPK) is frequently slightly elevated in ALS, reflecting muscle denervation, but this has very low diagnostic sensitivity and specificity. Levels above 1000 IU L^{-1} are unusual in ALS and should prompt diagnostic review, looking particularly for muscle disease.

Systematic studies in ALS patients from endemic areas have confirmed there is no link to Lyme disease [29], so that routine testing of *Borrelia* spp. serology is not appropriate. Similarly the clinical presentation of lead poisoning and porphyria have little overlap with ALS. Serum vitamin B_{12} and copper levels, plasma very long chain fatty acids, and human T-lymphotropic virus type 1 (HTLV-1) serology should be considered in cases of progressive myelopathy. Testing for HIV should be considered in those with appropriate risk factors and a progressive LMN-predominant syndrome.

Cerebrospinal fluid analysis

Lumbar puncture is not a mandatory investigation in typical ALS, unless there are credible grounds for considering an inflammatory or paraneoplastic syndrome. It is reasonable to examine the CSF in any patient with atypical clinical features. Modestly raised protein levels (<1 g L^{-1}) are frequently observed in ALS, and matched or even unmatched oligoclonal bands are well described [30]; but a raised leucocyte count (>5 mm^{-3}) strengthens the case for an alternative diagnosis.

Natural history, clinical variation, and prognosis

MND can be regarded as a syndrome in which the range of clinical manifestations reflects the pattern and progression of degeneration of upper and lower motor neurons but also the involvement of wider extramotor cortex and white matter. Typical ALS (with mixed upper and lower motor neuron signs) comprises at least 85% of cases, but the argument for considering the clinically heterogeneous spectrum of MND, including progressive muscular atrophy (PMA) and primary lateral sclerosis (PLS), as part of a common disease entity is supported by:

♦ the presence of common pathological features (e.g. ubiquitinated inclusions) in different clinical subtypes

♦ well-described families in which a single genetic mutation can produce any of the clinical subtypes of MND

♦ the ultimate progression of initially atypical presentations to a more generalized clinical picture of ALS.

Whilst the median survival from symptom onset is approximately 30 months, 5–10% of ALS patients survive for more than 10 years [31]. Many factors determine overall survival, and data about prognosis derived from large clinical case series may be difficult to apply to individual patients, particularly immediately after diagnosis. Statements about progression and prognosis are therefore generalizations, and each clinical pattern may be associated with rapidly or slowly progressive disease. In order to understand the pattern of progression in individuals and to guide management and prognostication, it is useful to consider the clinical pattern based on five levels of description:

1. age of onset
2. site of onset
3. the proportion of UMN versus LMN involvement
4. the degree of regional isolation versus generalized spread
5. the overall rate of functional decline.

The significance of age of onset

Although more than 50% of ALS patients are aged over 65 at presentation, 15–20% of patients are under 50 years. Even where the clinical pattern seems typical of classical ALS, there is a trend in this age group toward slower progression, with a lower incidence of disease onset in the bulbar territory. However, a broad range of patterns is still observed, and young-onset ALS is not a single condition [32]. Aggressive LMN-predominant ALS with onset between 15 and 25 years has been linked to mutations (in most cases *de novo*) of the fused-in-sarcoma (*FUS*) gene, characterized pathologically by basophilic intraneuronal inclusions [33]. However, most young-onset cases do not have a defined genetic aetiology. Rare juvenile forms of highly atypical ALS have been described, e.g. alsin (*ALS2*)- and senataxin (*ALS4*)-associated, but the relevance of these diseases to typical ALS remains uncertain [34].

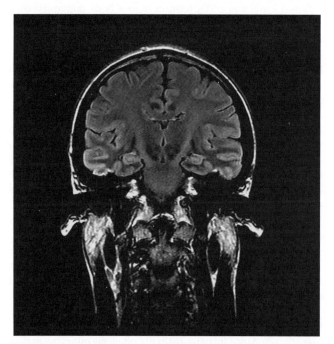

Fig. 4.3 Magnetic resonance imaging (MRI) fluid attenuation inversion recovery (FLAIR) coronal slice through the midbrain. Corticospinal tract hyperintensity is visible bilaterally. It is only 50% sensitive and insufficiently specific (70%) to have value as a single diagnostic test (this is an apparently healthy individual). Advanced MRI techniques may eventually offer improved accuracy.

The elderly (over 70 years) age group overall show more rapid disease progression and shorter survival. This is often attributed to the effect of comorbid medical conditions or simply the inherent frailty of old age. However, it is also possible that a neurodegenerative disease in which one of the primary triggers is aging simply runs a more aggressive course in an aged nervous system. There is an excess of elderly females among people with bulbar-onset ALS, many of whom display a progressive bulbar palsy phenotype (see the section Progressive bulbar palsy).

The clinical site of onset

Conventionally, ALS has been classified into 'spinal' or 'bulbar' onset. This dichotomy is unsatisfactory and fails to capture the full spectrum of clinical heterogeneity. However, as a broad generalization, patients with bulbar-onset symptoms, particularly middle-aged men, have a more aggressive disease course. The group of patients surviving for more than 10 years is predominantly composed of limb-onset cases. Generalized ALS appears to carry the same variation in prognosis regardless of whether it begins in the upper or lower limbs. Early weakness of the respiratory muscles is the feature most consistently associated with shorter survival.

UMN versus LMN involvement

At least 90% of post-mortem cases of MND show evidence of both UMN and LMN involvement pathologically. Relative involvement of these pathways is probably best considered as a continuous spectrum. 'UMN-predominant' and 'LMN-predominant' ALS are useful terms to describe patients who do not conform to the strict definitions of PMA and PLS but who still have a generally slower course than classical ALS (Fig. 4.4).

Progressive muscular atrophy

MND with only LMN signs is conventionally termed PMA. However, the clinical criteria for PMA have not been precisely defined, reflected in the widely varying incidence in different studies (7–20%). Absolutely pure LMN MND is probably rare, as many patients develop UMN signs at some point in the disease and autopsy studies also confirm involvement of the corticospinal tract in most cases. A more accurate term is therefore 'LMN-predominant ALS', but this encompasses a wide spectrum of patterns with different rates of progression.

The most characteristic form of PMA is the patient, usually male, who presents with asymmetrical weakness and wasting, often in the legs, which coalesces into four-limb LMN involvement. The degree of wasting is often out of proportion to the level of weakness, which has led to speculation that hypermetabolism may be present. Although there are very rapidly progressive cases, the overall survival is about 5 years, and there is an excess of long-term survivors (>10 years). The differential diagnosis includes conduction block neuropathy, X-linked spinobulbar muscular atrophy (Kennedy disease), and adult-onset spinal muscular atrophy (or hereditary motor neuropathy/axonal Charcot–Marie–Tooth disease), though these disorders are characteristically much more slowly progressive and less disabling. Hereditary motor neuropathies are a complex and diverse group of distal length-dependent neuropathies, and are characteristically symmetrical and slowly progressive. Onset is usually in the second or third decades. Only 20% of such cases have identifiable genetic mutations at present. Bulbar involvement is very rare, but vocal cord paresis is an occasional feature. These conditions are considered in more detail in Chapter 5.

Primary lateral sclerosis

UMN-only MND, termed PLS is rare and accounts for <3% of all MND [35]. Although it is a slowly progressive condition, consistent with survival for decades, the burden of disability in PLS is high. It is characterized by an ascending spastic tetraparesis with involvement of speech in the majority by 3 years. Urinary urgency is common. Marked cognitive involvement is the exception. Although there is a broad age of onset, the average is approximately 10 years younger than typical ALS. Some patients with apparent PLS develop wasting within 4 years and become reclassified as UMN-predominant ALS with a shorter survival than PLS, but still survive longer than typical ALS.

Primary progressive multiple sclerosis should be considered in the differential diagnosis of patients with apparent PLS, along with other causes of progressive myelopathy, including hereditary spastic paraplegia, adrenomyeloneuropathy, and vitamin B_{12} deficiency.

Regional isolation versus generalized spread

A striking and curious phenomenon in ALS is that functional impairment in some patients remains restricted to the region of onset for prolonged periods. Rapid generalization to involve more than one bodily region generally carries a poor prognosis. The explanation for this regional isolation is currently lacking.

Flail arm variant

The 'flail arm' variant of MND (known also as brachial diplegia, 'man-in-a-barrel', or Vulpian–Bernhardt syndrome) consists of bilateral weakness and wasting of the proximal upper limb which may only spread to other regions after a delay of a number of years [36]. A 'dropped head' is a frequent association (Fig. 4.5). Men appear to be affected much more frequently than women and it probably accounts for about 5–10% of all MND cases. Despite the proximity of the affected segments to the respiratory neurons, vital

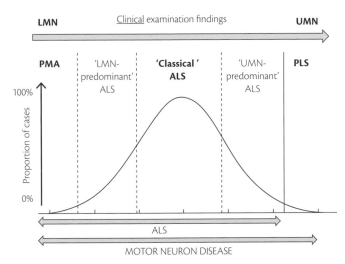

Fig. 4.4 The 'umbrella' term motor neuron disease encompasses amyotrophic lateral sclerosis (ALS, 85% of cases) with mixed upper (UMN) and lower motor neuron (LMN) signs on clinical examination, but also those much rarer cases with apparently 'pure' lower (progressive muscular atrophy, PMA) or upper (primary lateral sclerosis, PLS) motor neuron signs. Most PMA patients have subclinical corticospinal tract involvement, whereas PLS is more convincingly a distinct disorder and is consistently associated with survival into a second decade from symptom onset. At the margins cases may be termed lower or upper motor neuron-predominant ALS.

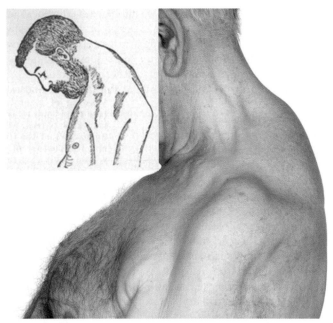

Fig. 4.5 Marked wasting of the anterior and posterior shoulder girdle muscles, with an inability to abduct the shoulders, results in a 'flail arm' syndrome. This presentation of amyotrophic lateral sclerosis was observed by Gowers. It is more common in males, and is associated with long disease survival. (Gowers WR. *A Manual of Diseases of the Nervous System.* London: J & A Churchill, 1886.)

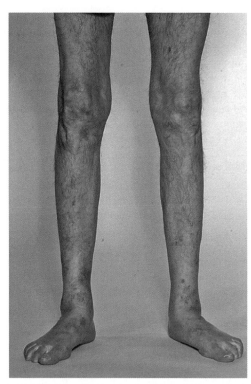

Fig. 4.6 The distal 'pseudopolyneuritic' presentation of amyotrophic lateral sclerosis is often difficult to diagnose, particularly in the early stages.

capacity may be unaffected until late in the disease and survival averages 5–7 years from symptom onset.

Lower limb-predominant MND

Distal lower limb-onset MND was often referred to in the past as 'the creeping paralysis' or the pseudopolyneuritic variant (Patrikios disease) [37] (Fig. 4.6). Spread beyond the leg of initial onset is more often to the contralateral leg (75%), otherwise to the ipsilateral arm (25%), but the pace is highly variable and hard to predict. Overall survival is 5–10 years.

Progressive bulbar palsy

The term 'progressive bulbar palsy' (PBP) has fallen out of fashion or is misused as a generic term for bulbar-onset ALS. However, PBP is a clinically useful distinction from typical 'bulbar-onset ALS' in which there is rapid generalization of weakness to the limbs and markedly reduced survival. People with PBP, more often women over the age of 65 years, typically retain normal limb strength despite progressing to complete anarthria within a year. PBP thus implies a period of relative regional isolation, although the pathological basis for this is unknown. UMN features (slow spastic tongue with a jaw jerk) usually predominate. The EMG is frequently normal, which should not prevent a diagnosis of ALS being made and supportive treatment with enteral feeding and communication aids being instituted as early as possible. The prognosis in PBP varies from 2 to 6 years and depends on the timing of respiratory and limb involvement.

Rate of change

Diagnostic latency, the time from symptom onset to firm diagnosis by a neurologist, remains one of the most robust indicators of prognosis in ALS. Early presentation to tertiary services is a surrogate marker for those cases with rapid progression. Decline in function

in ALS follows an approximately linear course, as measured by the ALS Functional Rating Scale (ALSFRS). The ALSFRS comprises 12 categories each scored from 0–4, thus with a maximum score of 48, with lower composite scores indicating greater disability. A progression rate can be estimated as:

$$(48 - \text{ALSFRS score at diagnosis}) \times \text{duration from onset of symptoms to diagnosis (months)}.$$

It is generally consistent for individuals over the central part of the disease course, and shows objective validity across groups of patients over the whole course [38].

Apparently abrupt changes in specific functions such as walking, standing, and transferring from bed to chair are best explained by muscle weakness exceeding a threshold of compensatory reserve, rather than by a sudden acceleration in disease activity. Thus, in an individual, a disease that is slowly progressive at the time of diagnosis is likely to remain so. A significant 'plateau' in the progression rate is exceptionally rare in ALS.

Timing of death in ALS is generally predictable, and occurs as a result of ventilatory insufficiency, the substrate for which is not simply diaphragmatic and intercostal muscle weakness but also involvement of brainstem respiratory patterning centres. Sudden unexpected death, usually during sleep, may be due to loss of these neurons but also to pulmonary embolism or cardiac dysrhythmia [39]. Occasionally patients may remain in the terminal phase for an unexpectedly long period of time, making care planning difficult.

Pathology of ALS

Autopsy studies of clinically well-characterized patients suggest that the pathological burden of disease is greatest in the area of the spinal cord related to the clinical site of onset, with UMN and LMN involvement spreading contiguously both in the vertical axis and across the midline [5]. Although there is also a cortical degenerative process apparent in nearly all cases cerebral atrophy is surprisingly rarely observed on MRI. The exact relationship of observable pathology in the spinal cord to downstream events at the neuromuscular junction or upstream cortical degeneration remains unclear, and the most appropriate model of ALS pathophysiology might be a combined corticomotorneuronal 'system' failure, rather than a 'dying back' or 'dying forward' process [40]. How this permits differential, even highly selective, involvement of UMN, LMN, and extramotor compartments is currently unknown.

As with other neurodegenerative diseases, the definitive diagnosis of ALS relies on post-mortem tissue findings (Fig. 4.7).

Key microstructural observations

TAR (transactive response) DNA-binding protein (TDP-43) is the major protein constituent of ubiquitinated inclusions present in the cell bodies of the spinal cord anterior horn motor neurons and those of the motor and frontotemporal cortices. It is considered the pathological hallmark of ALS/MND [41]. It is translocated from its normal position in the nucleus so that it accumulates in the cytoplasm in affected motor neurons in the spinal cord. Adjacent

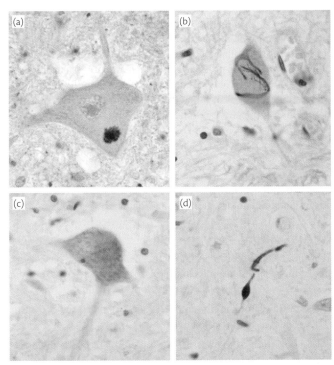

Fig. 4.7 Jean-Martin Charcot observed cellular 'debris' in his histopathological descriptions of amyotrophic lateral sclerosis (ALS). Mislocalized cytoplasmic inclusions of ubiquitinated protein (here stained with antibodies against p62) which contain TDP-43 are the pathological hallmark of nearly all cases of ALS (a), though not found in clinically identical cases associated with mutations in *SOD1*. Skein-like inclusions may also be seen (b). The Bunina body is highly specific for ALS but harder to spot (c, small brown inclusion). Dystrophic neurites are a more non-specific pathological observation (d). (Courtesy of Dr Olaf Ansorge, Department of Neuropathology, John Radcliffe Hospital, Oxford, UK). (See also figure in colour plate section)

oligodendroglia also stain positive for ubiquitin and TDP-43. Whether TDP-43 positive aggregates are damaging, protective, or irrelevant to the core mechanisms of motor neuron death is currently debated. There has been very little detailed pathological study of PLS patients, though TDP-43 has been reported in isolated case reports.

Bunina bodies are a characteristic form of ubiquitin inclusion, thought by some to be pathognomonic of sporadic ALS but only present in about 85% of cases. These small eosinophilic, paracrystalline inclusions are immunoreactive for the proteinase inhibitor cystatin C (a candidate biomarker in ALS, reduced in CSF and increased in serum compared with controls [42]).

Hyaline inclusions are less compact cytoplasmic inclusions, less frequent than ubiquitinated inclusions and immunoreactive for neurofilaments. These are particularly characteristic of some familial superoxide dismutase 1 (*SOD1*) mutation cases. Most ALS cases reporting a family history also have TDP-43 pathology. However, in the fifth of such cases that are associated with *SOD1* mutations, TDP-43 staining is absent by current staining methods [43]. The status of *SOD1*-related familial ALS as a model of the disease overall is therefore in doubt.

Basophilic neuronal inclusions immunoreactive for the FUS protein, and associated with *FUS* mutations, have been linked to aggressive ALS with onset typically in the late teens and early twenties [33].

ALS FTD cases with a hexanucleotide expansion mutation in the gene *C9orf72* show neuronal inclusions in the cerebellar cortex that are ubiquitin/p62 positive but TDP-43 negative [44]. Elsewhere, TDP-43/p62 positive inclusions are similar to non-mutation cases of ALS, but with a predilection for the hippocampus and frontal lobes.

Aetiology of ALS

The only unequivocal major risk factors for ALS are aging and a family history of the disease. The aetiology of ALS is therefore, in principle, a complex mixture of genetically determined susceptibility, associated with sequential age-dependent cellular 'hits'. Contributions from epigenetic and environmental determinants seem intuitively reasonable, though it has been difficult to date to determine what these might be [45]. An even more difficult aspect of neurodegeneration is the extent to which random biological events might trigger diseases like ALS on an appropriate genetic background.

Environment

The following factors argue that environmental influences either have a minor effect on ALS risk, or that there are many complex risk factors operating at the individual level with low explanatory power considered across the disease as a whole:

- a relative uniformity of the clinical spectrum and presentation of ALS in widely differing geographical areas
- no convincing examples of population clusters of typical ALS with TDP-43 pathology
- no increased risk in spouses
- an unvarying incidence of 2/100 000 per year in population studies [46]

◆ an absence of consistent associations between ALS and individual exposures (e.g. heavy metals, pesticides, physical trauma, etc.) in large case–control studies.

'Guamanian ALS' provides evidence that environmental factors may in principle have a major influence on the risk of neurodegeneration, but this disease is pathologically a 'tauopathy', and so very distinct from sporadic ALS.

Studies suggest that athleticism or leisure-time physical activity are associated with the risk of ALS [47,48], but data are inconsistent [49,50]. Reduced cardiovascular risk has also been noted among patients and their relatives [51]. An excess of sufferers among ex-service personnel [52], professional footballers [53], and among those employed in manual work [54] has also been observed. Whilst an abnormal response to physical exertion as a primary determinant of ALS pathogenesis remains a unifying possibility, it is equally the case that physical prowess in youth and the risk of getting ALS may have incidental shared genetic determinants.

Finally, a surrogate marker of higher intrauterine testosterone exposure (low index-to-ring finger length ratio) is commoner in ALS patients and raises the possibility that intrauterine factors, possibly involved in maturation of the motor system, might also have relevance to later risk [55].

Genetics

At least 5% of ALS patients have a history of a first-degree relative with ALS or FTD. Given the low incidence of the disease this is unlikely to occur by chance and is strong evidence that a gene of major effect, typically with autosomal dominant inheritance, is responsible. Similarly, a family in which the disease appears to skip a generation is more likely to indicate reduced penetrance of a familial form of ALS, rather than two sporadic cases in one family, although in this situation calculating the risk to other family members is much more difficult [56].

It is important to take a detailed family history in all patients with ALS, paying particular attention to any neurological disease and questioning labels such as 'multiple sclerosis', 'Alzheimer's' (which may in fact be FTD), and older terms for ALS like 'creeping paralysis' (which often appeared in the past on death certificates). The absence of a family history usually allows a confident diagnosis of sporadic ALS to be made. Although the relative risk to first-degree relatives in systematic studies is marginally higher than for the general population, the absolute risk remains low, so that reassurance that the disease is unlikely to be transmitted to children is appropriate. The recent finding of a common mutation (hexanucleotide expansions in C9orf72) in 10% of all ALS (40–50% of familial ALS and 7% of sporadic ALS) [57] suggests that it is not possible to apply a uniform approach to genetic counselling as a minority of the sporadic cases will be at higher risk.

Familial ALS

Familial ALS is clinically indistinguishable from sporadic disease in individual cases, but the median age of onset is about 10 years younger than for sporadic ALS. Interestingly all subtypes of ALS can be found in the familial ALS population which argues for significant overlap in pathophysiology between sporadic and familial ALS. The individual phenotypes of ALS, FTD, or their combination can occur in the same pedigree, notably in those with an intronic hexanucleotide repeat expansion in the C9orf72 gene, supporting the notion that both conditions are part of a clinicopathological spectrum.

The majority of familial ALS is now attributable to mutations in the followin   g genes [58]:

◆ a common hexanucleotide repeat expansion in C9orf72 (30–50%) [59,60]

◆ SOD1 (20%) [61]; over 120 different mutations have been described

◆ TARDPB (4%) [62]

◆ FUS (4%) mutations [63]

◆ Ubiquilin2 [64], angiogenin, optineurin (<1% each).

For each gene in which mutations have been identified as causing familial ALS, rare variants have also been described in a significant number of patients with apparently sporadic ALS. As these do not appear to occur in the non-ALS population, it is likely that they are relevant to the disease and act as rare risk alleles (in which the presence of a mutation confers a variable and individual risk in conjunction with other genetic and non-genetic factors). However, uncertainties about incomplete penetrance, and the lack of an effective treatment, mean that there is currently no place for the routine testing of patients with sporadic ALS or unaffected relatives of patients with familial ALS.

A number of other conditions have been labelled as forms of familial ALS (see Table 4.2) but are phenotypically quite different from the sporadic disease and cause young-onset, slowly progressive, atypical motor neuron degeneration. While understanding these conditions may provide insight into the general nature of motor neuron vulnerability, forms of familial ALS which are indistinguishable from sporadic ALS on clinical grounds are the main focus for current basic research in the molecular pathophysiology of MND.

Functional analysis of mutations in genes associated with familial ALS has implicated a number of pathways in the pathophysiology of motor neuron degeneration. Both cell culture and animal work indicate that there are a large number of potential interacting pathways which could serve as drug targets. However, it is unclear which, if any, of these diverse pathways are a primary part of the trigger to motor neuron degeneration, or simply part of the downstream phenomenology of motor neuron death.

Models of ALS

Therapeutic efforts using a SOD1 mouse model of ALS have generated some promising results but these have not translated into successful trials in humans. The reasons for this include:

◆ The initially poor methodology in animal studies which introduced biases and false positive results.

◆ The distortion of the normal pathophysiology of the disease by overexpressing transgenic protein in mice to high levels, which may recruit pathways which are responsive to treatment but are not part of the human disease, or at least are more reflective of end-stage pathology.

◆ The fact that animals are often treated at a much earlier stage than is currently possible in humans.

◆ The fact that clinical trials are probably being carried out in a heterogeneous patient population which contains people who have the disease for a large number of different reasons.

Table 4.2 Genetics of amyotrophic lateral sclerosis (ALS)

Gene	Proposed functions	Distinguishing features	Pathology	Frequency
Typical ALS				
C9orf72	Unknown	Worse survival, younger age of onset, variable penetrance, high rate of ALS/FTD	p62/TDP-43 positive aggregates; TDP-43 negative aggregates in cerebellum	About 40% of fALS, 7% of sALS, 10% of cases of pure FTD
SOD1	Free-radical scavenging	Typical ALS, but FTD not described. Recessive inheritance of D90A mutation in Scandinavia	Hyaline inclusions. TDP-43 negative intracellular aggregates	20% of fALS, occasional sALS
TDP-43	mRNA splicing	Typical ALS. Occasional cases of isolated FTD	TDP-43 positive ubiquitinated intraneuronal cytoplasmic inclusions	4–5% of fALS, occasional sALS, described in FTD rarely
FUS	mRNA splicing	Juvenile onset cases with P525L mutation.	FUS positive intraneuronal cytoplasmic inclusions	3–4% of fALS, occasional sALS, described in FTD
Valosin containing protein (*VCP*)	Protein turnover degradation	Spectrum of IBM–Paget disease-FTD, ALS or FTD	TDP-43 positive ubiquitinated intraneuronal cytoplasmic inclusions	1–2% of fALS
Optineurin (*OPTN*)	Ubiquitin and NF-kappa B binding	Recessive and occasional apparent heterozygous mutations. Generally slowly progressive. No FTD	OPTN-immunoreactive cytoplasmic inclusions	Very rare. A few Japanese families
Ubiquilin2	Ubiquitin binding	X-linked ALS and ALS/FTD. Dementia in 25% of mutation carriers	Ubiquilin2 stained skein-like inclusions	Rare, only a few families described
Angiogenin	Growth factor and other functions	Possible excess of bulbar cases, especially in Celtic populations	Rare reports, possible intranuclear inclusions	Rare variants in ALS and PD with low penetrance. Some rare families with segregation
Atypical forms of ALS				
Alsin (*ALS2*)		Juvenile-onset PLS	Unknown	Very rare, consanguineous pedigrees
Senataxin (*ALS4*)		Slowly progressive distal weakness and wasting with pyramidal signs. Juvenile onset	Unknown	Very rare
VAPB (*ALS8*)		Adult-onset proximal and distal SMA with some cases more typical of ALS	Unknown	Rare

fALS, familial ALS; sALS, sporadic ALS; FTD, frontotemporal dementia; IBM, inclusion body myositis; PD, Parkinson disease; PLS, primary lateral sclerosis; SMA, spinal muscular atrophy.

◆ Evidence that *SOD1* cases do not consistently demonstrate TDP-43 staining, currently considered to be the neuropathological 'signature' of ALS, raises doubts about the *SOD1* mouse model as a tool for translational research of general applicability.

Newer mouse models based on *TDP43, FUS,* and *C9orf72* mutations are in development and may provide important clues to the key pathways sensitive to therapeutic agents. In addition the recent exciting developments in the field of induced pluripotent stem cells, which can be derived from skin and other tissues and then induced to differentiate into motor neurons, provides for the first time an *in vitro* system for studying the primary cell of interest in this disease [65].

Management of ALS

Whilst a highly effective disease-modifying therapy is awaited, the cornerstone of management of ALS is regular individualized follow-up to maintain physical and psychological well-being and to maximize quality of life. In addition assessing the rate of change of the disease facilitates care planning and patient choice.

A multidisciplinary approach

Patients with ALS progressing at a typical rate should be seen about every 3 months. A multidisciplinary team approach has been shown to improve survival and enhance the quality of life in ALS [66]. Ideally the team should comprise the following members:

◆ A neurologist for diagnosis, assessment of disease progression, coordination of research, and management.

◆ A care coordinator, often a specialist nurse. This person can perform liaison between patients and clinical and paraclinical teams to ensure interventions are appropriate and timely, provide information and support to patients and carers, and education and outreach for allied healthcare professionals.

◆ A physiotherapist to assess motor dysfunction and provide ankle–foot orthoses, collars, and aids to walking. The physiotherapist can also teach exercises to prevent cramps and secondary disability, as well as techniques such as breath-stacking in the context of respiratory insufficiency.

◆ An occupational therapist—a specialist in posture management and assessment for wheelchairs and other mobility and posture aids.

◆ A speech and language therapist to give initial advice about how to avoid choking episodes and how to improve intelligibility. In selected patients with major communication problems the therapist can provide aids to communication such as the Lightwriter™

or voice synthesis software for use with tablet computers which can be critical in maintaining personal autonomy. In long-term survivors who lose all hand function, eye-tracking systems can be a helpful way of continuing to communicate and control the environment with computers.

- A dietician and enteral feeding specialist team who can initially advise about changes to the oral diet (softened and pureed food), then plan percutaneous endoscopic gastrostomy (PEG) or radiologically inserted gastrostomy (RIG) and subsequent follow-up.
- A respiratory team—a specialist nurse and physician for assessment of nocturnal sleep fragmentation with overnight oximetry and provision of non-invasive ventilation equipment.
- A psychologist to assess cognitive dysfunction, manage adjustment reactions, and support and counsel patients and relatives.

Riluzole

Over 100 drugs have been tried in the treatment of ALS. All have failed to significantly alter the primary end points, with the exception of riluzole, which is currently the only licensed disease-modifying therapy for ALS [67]. The original clinical trials used the El Escorial inclusion criteria for ALS, so whether other phenotypes of MND such as PLS or PMA might also benefit remains unclear, and prescribing practice for these forms is therefore variable.

Evidence for benefit comes from randomized trials which included around 1000 patients taking oral riluzole, 50 mg twice daily. Overall, the probability of survival at 1 year after starting the drug was about 10% greater than placebo, equating to approximately 3 months longer life expectancy over the course of the trial [68]. Importantly, however, there is no evidence of any effect of riluzole on quality of life, or improvement in specific symptoms.

Riluzole is well tolerated, with about 10% of patients stopping the drug because of nausea or lethargy. Baseline full blood count and liver function tests are required, repeated monthly for the first 3 months, 3-monthly for the first year, and annually thereafter. A small minority of patients exhibits a two- to three-fold rise in liver enzymes which may plateau, but if that continues the drug must be stopped. Bone marrow suppression is exceptional.

Nutrition

Weight loss in ALS is not just due to difficulty swallowing but also to a complex mixture of:

- reduced food intake due to dysphagia, fear of choking, and social embarrassment
- physical disability (e.g. upper limb weakness) leading to dependence on others for food preparation and feeding
- increased calorie requirements (hypermetabolism)
- muscle atrophy
- psychological factors (e.g. cognitive impairment)
- recurrent chest infections.

Nutritional status should be assessed at each clinic visit. A skilled multidisciplinary team will be able to anticipate which patients are likely to benefit from PEG feeding, and will support the patient in making a choice to have early PEG (or RIG) insertion before weight loss occurs. Late in the disease, the higher risks of gastrostomy may outweigh the shorter period of benefit.

Respiratory management

The provision of NIV for patients with ALS has been a major advance in symptom management and significantly extends life in selected patients [69]. It is best managed jointly between a neurologist and a respiratory team. However, the mode of death for the overwhelming majority of patients is still respiratory failure, and not all patients need symptom palliation. In some, often those with significant bulbar problems but also those with major upper limb weakness, NIV may be poorly tolerated.

A symptom enquiry should be carried out at each clinic visit specifically asking about breathlessness when lying flat and sleep fragmentation. Any change in sleep pattern, including new-onset nocturia, should be considered to be significant. Early morning clouding of thought processes, headache, nausea, daytime somnolence, and general fatigue may all indicate incipient respiratory insufficiency, and be amenable to improvement with NIV. Respiratory muscle weakness is most easily monitored by measuring forced vital capacity, as a percentage of predicted, based on height, age, gender, and race. A fall of 20% on lying flat indicates diaphragmatic weakness. Orthopnoea is a marker of patients who are likely to benefit from NIV. In patients with bulbar and corticobulbar involvement measurement of forced vital capacity is technically difficult and may be unreliable, in which case sniff nasal pressure is a good alternative. Overnight oximetry (which can easily be carried out in the patient's home) should be performed in all patients with symptoms. The presence of significant nocturnal desaturations and arousals is a marker of the need for NIV. A measurement of early morning arterial carbon dioxide level may be the most sensitive sign of significant respiratory compromise.

Specific symptom management [70]

Muscle symptoms

Spasticity (and the overlapping symptom of cramps) reflects UMN involvement and is particularly troublesome in PLS. Patients complain of stiff limbs, spasms and 'jumpiness' of limbs. This can lead to reduced dexterity, falls, and secondary contractures if untreated. Passive stretching exercises may need to be supplemented by antispasticity drugs such as baclofen, or low-dose benzodiazepines for particularly resistant localized spasticity phenomena such as jaw clamping. The use of botulinum toxin to reduce severe spasticity is occasionally indicated, but should be performed by a specialist, as significant doses may be required. Fasciculations generally fade with disease progression and rarely require treatment (beta blockers may be effective).

Bulbar symptoms

At least 80% of ALS patients, and a higher proportion of PLS patients, develop dysarthria and dysphagia. The degree of functional loss is variable, with many patients able to maintain adequate oral nutrition despite virtual anarthria. Choking as a mode of dying is not a feature of MND and patients value early reassurance over this common fear.

Reduced swallowing frequency and efficiency leads to sialorrhoea, but mouth-breathing and inadequate hydration may have the opposite result so that management of oral secretions becomes a balance between reducing the volume of saliva and avoiding exacerbating thick, tenacious secretions. Anticholinergic treatment (e.g. hyoscine patches, amitriptyline, or glycopyrrolate) achieves the former, whereas mucolytic enzymes in pineapple juice or carbocisteine, often supplemented by access to a suction device, may be effective for the latter.

The management of emotionality begins with explanation and reassurance, which can relieve the social embarrassment. Amitriptyline, if tolerated, can be effective in some patients, with selective serotonin reuptake inhibitors (SSRIs) less consistently useful. The use of dextromethorphan/quinidine is supported by recent clinical trial evidence [71]. Pathological yawning is a frequently observed associated feature. Laryngeal spasm is a particularly distressing, though relatively unusual, symptom of ALS. Paroxysmal attacks, accompanied by stridor, understandably lead to panic in patients and their carers. Reassurance that most episodes will self-terminate within 30 s may be sufficient, or judicious use of very low-dose lorazepam sublingually for clusters of attacks can be helpful.

Bladder and bowel symptoms

Sphincter dysfunction is not a primary symptom of MND but symptoms such as urgency and constipation often arise as a result of immobility (or dehydration in the case of the latter), and establishing a regular, predictable bowel habit is important. Bladder hypertonicity and detrusor instability are more common in PLS patients. Low-dose anticholinergic treatment may be helpful provided it does not provoke urinary tract infections. Involvement of a specialist bladder team is helpful.

Immobility-related symptoms

Musculoskeletal pain arising from secondary changes in posture and joint stability as a result of muscle atrophy is a common and often overlooked aspect of MND. Shoulder, hip, and back pain is particularly common. Use of regular paracetamol, supplemented by non-steroidal anti-inflammatory drugs where tolerated, may be adequate, though occasionally opiate-containing analgesics become necessary.

The skin of MND patients appears relatively resistant to pressure sores despite obvious risk factors. Dependent oedema is very common, and is often accompanied by significant discoloration of the feet in particular. Elevation of the legs or use of venous compression stockings is usually adequate. Diuretics should be avoided.

Psychological symptoms

Although the subject of ongoing debate, there is general consensus that the frequency of major depressive disorder is no greater than in the general population, and may even be lower. Whether this reflects the extramotor frontotemporal pathology of MND is not yet clear, but in general there is a surprising level of acceptance of the diagnosis among patients, so that routine use of antidepressant medication is not indicated. Although prominent in the media portrayal of MND, suicide is also exceptional in clinic-based populations.

Carers, by contrast, have very high rates of depression, and attention to this in the context of the multidisciplinary clinic is important. Behavioural changes in patients as part of the FTD-ALS spectrum may cause a particular strain in relationships and often need to be specifically explored by direct enquiry [72].

Conclusions

ALS represents a formidable challenge for patients, their carers and families, as well as for biomedical scientists in developing effective disease-modifying treatments. It is now clear that it is an aetiologically complex, multisystem neurodegenerative disease, overlapping with FTD, but without an overarching single cause. There has been a dramatic increase in knowledge of the genetic determinants of familial ALS, but defining the susceptible population who will go on to develop the commoner sporadic form of the disorder seems a distant prospect at present.

Despite the absence of reliable biomarkers, diagnosis is usually possible on the basis of careful history-taking and examination alone, with minimal investigations needed to exclude mimic disorders. The risk of diagnostic error in specialist settings is very low. Advances in multidisciplinary care, with access to enteral feeding and NIV, have improved quality of life and prolonged survival.

References

1. Kiernan MC, Vucic S, Cheah BC, et al. Amyotrophic lateral sclerosis. *Lancet* 2011; **377**: 942–55.
2. Turner MR, Bowser R, Bruijn L, et al. Mechanisms, models and biomarkers in amyotrophic lateral sclerosis. *Amyotroph Lateral Scler Frontotemporal Degener* 2013; **14**(Suppl. 1): 19–32.
3. Bäumer D, Ansorge O, Almeida M, Talbot K. The role of RNA processing in the pathogenesis of motor neuron degeneration. *Expert Rev Mol Med* 2010; **12**: e21.
4. Neumann M, Sampathu DM, Kwong LK, et al. Ubiquitinated TDP-43 in frontotemporal lobar degeneration and amyotrophic lateral sclerosis. *Science* 2006; **314**: 130–3.
5. Ravits JM, La Spada AR. ALS motor phenotype heterogeneity, focality, and spread: deconstructing motor neuron degeneration. *Neurology* 2009; **73**: 805–11.
6. Phukan J, Elamin M, Bede P, et al. The syndrome of cognitive impairment in amyotrophic lateral sclerosis: a population-based study. *J Neurol Neurosurg Psychiatry* 2012; **83**: 102–8.
7. Plato CC, Galasko D, Garruto RM, et al. ALS and PDC of Guam: forty-year follow-up. *Neurology* 2002; **58**: 765–73.
8. Johnston CA, Stanton BR, Turner MR, et al. Amyotrophic lateral sclerosis in an urban setting: a population based study of inner city London. *J Neurol* 2006; **253**: 1642–3.
9. Chio A, Mora G, Calvo A, Mazzini L, Bottacchi E, Mutani R. Epidemiology of ALS in Italy: a 10-year prospective population-based study. *Neurology* 2009; **72**: 725–31.
10. Talbot K. Familial versus sporadic amyotrophic lateral sclerosis—a false dichotomy? *Brain* 2011; **134**: 3429–31.
11. Turner MR, Kiernan MC, Leigh PN, Talbot K. Biomarkers in amyotrophic lateral sclerosis. *Lancet Neurol* 2009; **8**: 94–109.
12. Turner MR, Talbot K. Mimics and chameleons in motor neurone disease. *Pract Neurol* 2013; **13**: 153–64.
13. Traynor BJ, Codd MB, Corr B, Forde C, Frost E, Hardiman O. Amyotrophic lateral sclerosis mimic syndromes: a population-based study. *Arch Neurol* 2000; **57**: 109–13.
14. Mitchell JD, Callagher P, Gardham J, et al. Timelines in the diagnostic evaluation of people with suspected amyotrophic lateral sclerosis (ALS)/motor neuron disease (MND)—a 20-year review: Can we do better? *Amyotroph Lateral Scler* 2010; **11**: 537–41.
15. Eisen A, Kuwabara S. The split hand syndrome in amyotrophic lateral sclerosis. *J Neurol Neurosurg Psychiatry* 2012; **83**: 399–403.
16. Swash M. Why are upper motor neuron signs difficult to elicit in amyotrophic lateral sclerosis? *J Neurol Neurosurg Psychiatry* 2012; **83**: 659–62.
17. Turner MR, Scaber J, Goodfellow JA, Lord ME, Marsden R, Talbot K. The diagnostic pathway and prognosis in bulbar-onset amyotrophic lateral sclerosis. *J Neurol Sci* 2010; **294**: 81–5.
18. Shoesmith CL, Findlater K, Rowe A, Strong MJ. Prognosis of amyotrophic lateral sclerosis with respiratory onset. *J Neurol Neurosurg Psychiatry* 2007; **78**: 629–31.

19. Forsyth PA, Dalmau J, Graus F, Cwik V, Rosenblum MK, Posner JB. Motor neuron syndromes in cancer patients. *Ann Neurol* 1997; **41**: 722–30.

20. Younger DS, Rowland LP, Latov N, et al. Lymphoma, motor neuron diseases, and amyotrophic lateral sclerosis. *Ann Neurol* 1991; **29**: 78–86.

21. Douglass CP, Kandler RH, Shaw PJ, McDermott CJ. An evaluation of neurophysiological criteria used in the diagnosis of motor neuron disease. *J Neurol Neurosurg Psychiatry* 2010; **81**: 646–9.

22. Burrell JR, Vucic S, Kiernan MC. Isolated bulbar phenotype of amyotrophic lateral sclerosis. *Amyotroph Lateral Scler* 2011; **12**: 283–9.

23. Traynor BJ, Codd MB, Corr B, Forde C, Frost E, Hardiman OM. Clinical features of amyotrophic lateral sclerosis according to the El Escorial and Airlie House diagnostic criteria: a population-based study. *Arch Neurol* 2000; **57**: 1171–6.

24. Shefner JM, Cudkowicz ME, Zhang H, Schoenfeld D, Jillapalli D. The use of statistical MUNE in a multicenter clinical trial. *Muscle Nerve* 2004; **30**: 463–9.

25. Rutkove SB, Caress JB, Cartwright MS, et al. Electrical impedance myography as a biomarker to assess ALS progression. *Amyotroph Lateral Scler* 2012; **13**: 439–45.

26. Vucic S, Cheah BC, Yiannikas C, Kiernan MC. Cortical excitability distinguishes ALS from mimic disorders. *Clin Neurophysiol* 2011; **122**: 1860–6.

27. Peretti-Viton P, Azulay JP, Trefouret S, et al. MRI of the intracranial corticospinal tracts in amyotrophic and primary lateral sclerosis. *Neuroradiology* 1999; **41**: 744–9.

28. Turner MR, Agosta F, Bede P, Govind V, Lule D, Verstraete E. Neuroimaging in amyotrophic lateral sclerosis. *Biomark Med* 2012; **6**: 319–37.

29. Qureshi M, Bedlack RS, Cudkowicz ME. Lyme disease serology in amyotrophic lateral sclerosis. *Muscle Nerve* 2009; **40**: 626–8.

30. Apostolski S, Nikolic J, Bugarski-Prokopljevic C, Miletic V, Pavlovic S, Filipovic S. Serum and CSF immunological findings in ALS. *Acta Neurol Scand*. 1991; **83**: 96–8.

31. Turner MR, Parton MJ, Shaw CE, Leigh PN, Al-Chalabi A. Prolonged survival in motor neuron disease: a descriptive study of the King's database 1990–2002. *J Neurol Neurosurg Psychiatry* 2003; **74**: 995–7.

32. Chio A, Calvo A, Moglia C, Mazzini L, Mora G. Phenotypic heterogeneity of amyotrophic lateral sclerosis: a population based study. *J Neurol Neurosurg Psychiatry* 2011; **82**: 740–6.

33. Baumer D, Hilton D, Paine SM, et al. Juvenile ALS with basophilic inclusions is a FUS proteinopathy with FUS mutations. *Neurology* 2010; **75**: 611–18.

34. Al-Chalabi A, Jones A, Troakes C, King A, Al-Sarraj S, van den Berg LH. The genetics and neuropathology of amyotrophic lateral sclerosis. *Acta Neuropathol* 2012; **124**: 339–52.

35. Pringle CE, Hudson AJ, Munoz DG, Kiernan JA, Brown WF, Ebers GC. Primary lateral sclerosis. Clinical features, neuropathology and diagnostic criteria. *Brain* 1992; **115**: 495–520.

36. Hu MT, Ellis CM, Al Chalabi A, Leigh PN, Shaw CE. Flail arm syndrome: a distinctive variant of amyotrophic lateral sclerosis. *J Neurol Neurosurg Psychiatry* 1998; **65**: 950–1.

37. Cappellari A, Ciammola A, Silani V. The pseudopolyneuritic form of amyotrophic lateral sclerosis (Patrikios' disease). *Electromyogr Clin Neurophysiol* 2008; **48**: 75–81.

38. Kimura F, Fujimura C, Ishida S, et al. Progression rate of ALSFRS-R at time of diagnosis predicts survival time in ALS. *Neurology* 2006; **66**: 265–7.

39. Corcia P, Pradat PF, Salachas F, et al. Causes of death in a post-mortem series of ALS patients. *Amyotroph Lateral Scler* 2008; **9**: 59–62.

40. Eisen A, Kim S, Pant B. Amyotrophic lateral sclerosis (ALS): a phylogenetic disease of the corticomotoneuron? *Muscle Nerve* 1992; **15**: 219–24.

41. Geser F, Martinez-Lage M, Kwong LK, Lee VM, Trojanowski JQ. Amyotrophic lateral sclerosis, frontotemporal dementia and beyond: the TDP-43 diseases. *J Neurol* 2009; **256**: 1205–14.

42. Wilson ME, Boumaza I, Lacomis D, Bowser R. Cystatin C: a candidate biomarker for amyotrophic lateral sclerosis. *PLoS One* 2011; **5**(12): e15133.

43. Mackenzie IR, Bigio EH, Ince PG, et al. Pathological TDP-43 distinguishes sporadic amyotrophic lateral sclerosis from amyotrophic lateral sclerosis with SOD1 mutations. *Ann Neurol* 2007; **61**: 427–34.

44. Al-Sarraj S, King A, Troakes C, et al. p62 positive, TDP-43 negative, neuronal cytoplasmic and intranuclear inclusions in the cerebellum and hippocampus define the pathology of C9orf72-linked FTLD and MND/ALS. *Acta Neuropathol* 2011; **122**: 691–702.

45. Al-Chalabi A, Kwak S, Mehler M, et al. Genetic and epigenetic studies of amyotrophic lateral sclerosis. *Amyotroph Lateral Scler Frontotemporal Degener*. 2013; **44**(Suppl 1): 44–52.

46. Logroscino G, Traynor BJ, Hardiman O, et al. Incidence of amyotrophic lateral sclerosis in Europe. *J Neurol Neurosurg Psychiatry* 2010; **81**: 385–90.

47. Scarmeas N, Shih T, Stern Y, Ottman R, Rowland LP. Premorid weight, body mass, and varsity athletics in ALS. *Neurology* 2002; **59**: 773–5.

48. Huisman MH, Seelen M, De Jong SW, et al. Lifetime physical activity and the risk of amyotrophic lateral sclerosis. *J Neurol Neurosurg Psychiatry* 2013; **84**: 976–81.

49. Longstreth WT, McGuire V, Koepsell TD, Wang Y, van Belle G. Risk of amyotrophic lateral sclerosis and history of physical activity: a population-based case-control study. *Arch Neurol*. 1998; **55**: 201–6.

50. Turner MR. Increased premorbid physical activity and amyotrophic lateral sclerosis. Born to run rather than run to death, or a seductive myth? *J Neurol Neurosurg Psychiatry* 2013; **84**: 947.

51. Turner MR, Wotton C, Talbot K, Goldacre MJ. Cardiovascular fitness as a risk factor for amyotrophic lateral sclerosis: indirect evidence from record linkage study. *J Neurol Neurosurg Psychiatry* 2012; **83**: 395–8.

52. Weisskopf MG, O'Reilly EJ, McCullough ML, et al. Prospective study of military service and mortality from ALS. *Neurology* 2005; **64**: 32–7.

53. Chio A, Benzi G, Dossena M, Mutani R, Mora G. Severely increased risk of amyotrophic lateral sclerosis among Italian professional football players. *Brain* 2005; **128**: 472–6.

54. Beghi E, Logroscino G, Chio A, et al. Amyotrophic lateral sclerosis, physical exercise, trauma and sports: results of a population-based pilot case-control study. *Amyotroph Lateral Scler* 2010; **11**: 289–92.

55. Vivekananda U, Manjalay ZR, Ganesalingam J, et al. Low index-to-ring finger length ratio in sporadic ALS supports prenatally defined motor neuronal vulnerability. *J Neurol Neurosurg Psychiatry* 2011; **82**: 635–7.

56. Hanby MF, Scott KM, Scotton W, et al. The risk to relatives of patients with sporadic amyotrophic lateral sclerosis. *Brain* 2011; **134**: 3454–7.

57. Majounie E, Renton AE, Mok K, et al. Frequency of the C9orf72 hexanucleotide repeat expansion in patients with amyotrophic lateral sclerosis and frontotemporal dementia: a cross-sectional study. *Lancet Neurol* 2012; **11**: 323–30.

58. Andersen PM, Al-Chalabi A. Clinical genetics of amyotrophic lateral sclerosis: what do we really know? *Nat Rev Neurol* 2011; **7**: 603–15.

59. Renton AE, Majounie E, Waite A, et al. A hexanucleotide repeat expansion in C9ORF72 is the cause of chromosome 9p21-linked ALS-FTD. *Neuron* 2011; **72**: 257–68.

60. DeJesus-Hernandez M, Mackenzie IR, Boeve BF, et al. Expanded GGGGCC hexanucleotide repeat in noncoding region of C9ORF72 causes chromosome 9p-linked FTD and ALS. *Neuron* 2011; **72**: 245–56.

61. Rosen DR, Siddique T, Patterson D, et al. Mutations in Cu/Zn superoxide dismutase gene are associated with familial amyotrophic lateral sclerosis. *Nature* 1993; **362**(6415): 59–62.

62. Sreedharan J, Blair IP, Tripathi VB, et al. TDP-43 mutations in familial and sporadic amyotrophic lateral sclerosis. *Science* 2008; **319**: 1668–72.

63. Vance C, Rogelj B, Hortobagyi T, et al. Mutations in FUS, an RNA processing protein, cause familial amyotrophic lateral sclerosis type 6. *Science* 2009; **323**: 1208–11.

64. Deng HX, Chen W, Hong ST, et al. Mutations in UBQLN2 cause dominant X-linked juvenile and adult-onset ALS and ALS/dementia. *Nature* 2011; **477**: 211–15.

65. Bilican B, Serio A, Barmada SJ, et al. Mutant induced pluripotent stem cell lines recapitulate aspects of TDP-43 proteinopathies and reveal cell-specific vulnerability. *Proc Natl Acad Sci USA* 2012; **109**: 5803–8.

66. Andersen PM, Abrahams S, Borasio GD, et al. EFNS guidelines on the clinical management of amyotrophic lateral sclerosis (MALS)—revised report of an EFNS task force. *Eur J Neurol* 2012; **19**: 360–75.

67. Turner MR, Al-Chalabi A, Shaw CE, Leigh PN. Riluzole and motor neuron disease. *Pract Neurol* 2003; **3**: 160–70.

68. Bensimon G, Lacomblez L, Meininger V. A controlled trial of riluzole in amyotrophic lateral sclerosis. ALS/Riluzole Study Group. *N Engl J Med* 1994; **330**: 585–91.

69. Bourke SC, Tomlinson M, Williams TL, Bullock RE, Shaw PJ, Gibson GJ. Effects of non-invasive ventilation on survival and quality of life in patients with amyotrophic lateral sclerosis: a randomised controlled trial. *Lancet Neurol* 2006; **5**: 140–7.

70. Talbot K, Turner MR, Marsden R, Botell R. *Motor Neuron Disease: a Practical Manual*. Oxford: Oxford University Press, 2010.

71. Brooks BR, Thisted RA, Appel SH, et al. Treatment of pseudobulbar affect in ALS with dextromethorphan/quinidine: a randomized trial. *Neurology* 2004; **63**: 1364–70.

72. Oliver DJ, Turner MR. Some difficult decisions in ALS/MND. *Amyotroph Lateral Scler* 2010; **11**: 339–43.

CHAPTER 5

Spinal muscular atrophy and hereditary motor neuropathy

Dirk Bäumer and Kevin Talbot

Introduction

While the commonest motor neuron disease of adults is amyotrophic lateral sclerosis (ALS), neurologists working in neuromuscular clinics frequently encounter patients with a variety of other, individually rare, lower motor neuron-predominant disorders with overlapping presentations. While the distinction from ALS may occasionally be difficult and require long-term follow up, there are some general features that collectively point to a non-ALS aetiology, including:

- younger age of onset
- symmetrical involvement from the outset
- very slow progression of symptoms over years or decades
- the relatively rare involvement of bulbar and respiratory functions
- frequent restriction to specific anatomical territories, e.g. the lower limbs, for prolonged periods.

The pathology of these disorders, however, is poorly defined, and it is unclear if there is frank loss of motor neurons in the spinal cord. The terminology used to cover the spectrum of lower motor neuron disorders is not applied with consistency:

- 'Spinal muscular atrophy' (SMA) is used as an umbrella term for neurogenic weakness and muscle wasting, in which the pathology is presumed to be isolated loss of spinal motor neurons. More specifically it refers to the autosomal recessive lower motor neuron disease caused by mutations in the survival motor neuron (*SMN1*) gene.

- Confusingly, 'progressive spinal muscular atrophy' is sometimes used as a synonym for progressive muscular atrophy (PMA), in which there is a lack of overt clinical upper motor neuron features, but a neuropathology and natural history placing it in the same spectrum of degenerative motor neuron disease as ALS [1–3].

- 'Distal spinal muscular atrophy' (dSMA) and 'distal hereditary motor neuropathy' (dHMN) are synonyms to describe patients with a distal pattern of neurogenic weakness similar to Charcot–Marie–Tooth disease, without clinical sensory disturbance and with normal sensory nerve action potentials. This suggests a length-dependent, 'dying back', axonopathy. Forms of distal SMA are allelic with the axonal form of Charcot–Marie–Tooth disease (CMT2), indicating that they are essentially the same disease, but in which a minority of patients have detectable sensory

involvement (see Chapter 8). Notwithstanding the absence of a family history in many patients, the term dHMN probably most accurately captures the nature of the underlying pathological process in this group of patients.

- 'Motor neuronopathy' is sometimes used to imply that the disease process resides in the motor neuron cell body, though this is not easy to substantiate.

Further complexity arises in the classification of patients in which both the lower and upper motor neuron are involved, but who have a lower age of onset and far slower progression than ALS. Some of these disorders are now classified as 'distal HMN with pyramidal features', while others use the term 'atypical ALS' or 'juvenile ALS', without there necessarily being a logical underpinning to this distinction. For example, an autosomal dominant form of young-onset motor neuron disease was initially seen as a form of Charcot–Marie–Tooth disease [4] before being termed 'autosomal dominant juvenile ALS' or ALS4 when genetic linkage was established to chromosome 9 [5,6]. The same genetic disorder, caused by mutations in senataxin (*SETX*), was found in families diagnosed by others as 'dHMN' [7,8]. Likewise the term 'juvenile ALS' does not exclusively identify a homogeneous disease group with invariably slow progression. While this is true of motor neuron disorders linked to mutations in *ALSIN* (autosomal recessive, ALS2) [9], *SETX* (autosomal dominant, ALS4) and *SPATACSIN* (autosomal recessive, ALS5) [10], other forms of early onset motor neuron disease are rapidly progressive and fatal, and frequently display distinctive neuropathological features such as basophilic inclusions immunoreactive for FUS (fused-in-sarcoma) [11–13]. Therefore restricting the term ALS to degenerative motor neuron disorders with rapid progression would probably provide greater clarity.

In summary, the terms SMA, dHMN, and juvenile ALS are sometimes used interchangeably to describe a range of conditions with considerable genetic and clinical heterogeneity. As diagnostic labels, they therefore convey only limited information to the clinician with regards to the underlying pathology and prognosis. A reclassification of motor neuron disorders based on genetic criteria provides some clarity, but likewise will never be completely satisfactory. Many genetic disorders can have a wide range of clinical presentations, presumably due to environmental or genetic modifiers. As with ALS, sporadic phenocopies of genetic forms of hereditary motor neuropathies are common. Rather than replacing clinical diagnoses, genetic diagnosis is therefore one element of a multiaxial classification including age of onset, rate of progression, and, ultimately, underlying pathology. The diagnostic process necessarily starts with the clinical assessment. In the following sections we will outline the differential diagnosis of non-ALS motor neuron disease according to the main patterns of clinical presentation.

Proximal or generalized weakness

Depending on the rate of progression, the degree of wasting and fasciculation, and other clinical signs such as tendon reflexes it may first be necessary to exclude a myopathic process, myasthenia gravis, or chronic inflammatory demyelinating polyneuropathy, using blood tests [creatine kinase (CK) or anti-acetylcholine (anti-ACh) receptor antibodies, etc. as appropriate] and neurophysiology. Various forms of SMA enter the differential diagnosis of the patient with progressive proximal weakness (Table 5.1).

Autosomal recessive SMA

Autosomal recessive SMA is the commonest motor neuron disease of childhood, with an incidence of about 1/10 000 live births [14]. It is caused by disruption of the Survival Motor Neuron (*SMN1*) gene by deletion, gene conversion, or occasionally point mutation [15], with consequent severe reduction of SMN protein levels. The *SMN2* gene, a near identical paralogue of *SMN1* that has arisen from an evolutionary duplication event, produces small amounts of residual protein, obviating the inevitable lethality associated with complete loss of SMN protein. Disease severity is roughly proportional to residual SMN levels, which are a function of *SMN2* copy number, although other modifiers are likely to be important [16]. SMN has a critical role in the assembly of small nuclear ribonucleoproteins (snRNPs), which are essential for pre-mRNA splicing. However, the reason why reduction in SMN leads to specific degeneration of lower motor neurons is still unclear [17].

Table 5.1 Disorders presenting with proximal or generalized weakness

Disorder	Age of onset	Inheritance	Genetics	Other features
Progressive muscular atrophy (PMA)	Adulthood	Sporadic or familial	Genes associated with ALS	Overall rate of progression within the ALS spectrum; subclinical UMN involvement
Proximal spinal muscular atrophy (SMA)				
SMA Type I	Infantile	Autosomal recessive	Survival motor neuron (*SMN1*) gene deletion or conversion. Most have two copies of *SMN2*	Floppy infant. Never sits. Death from birth to age 2
SMA Type II	After 6 months	Autosomal recessive	Survival motor neuron (*SMN1*) gene deletion or conversion Most have three copies of *SMN2*	Never walks unaided
SMA Type III	Before 3 years (Type IIIa) or after 3 years (Type IIIb)	Autosomal recessive	Survival motor neuron (*SMN1*) gene deletion or conversion Most have three (Type IIIa) or four (Type IIIb) copies of *SMN2*	Achieves walking but majority lose ambulation (Type IIIa >>> Type IIIb). Prolonged survival
SMA Type IV	Adult onset (after 30 years)	Autosomal recessive, autosomal dominant, or sporadic	Only minority have survival motor neuron (*SMN1*) gene deletion or conversion	Normal survival
Proximal SMA, lower extremity dominant	Childhood, long survival	Autosomal dominant	*DYNC1H1* mutations	Quadriceps involvement
Proximal SMA	Adulthood	Autosomal dominant	*LMNA* mutations	Cardiac abnormalities
	Adulthood	Autosomal dominant	*VAPB* mutations	Allelic with ALS8
	Childhood or adulthood	Autosomal dominant	*SETX* mutations	Retained deep tendon reflexes
Scapuloperoneal spinal muscular atrophy	Childhood or adulthood	Heterogeneous, including sporadic	Autosomal dominant, autosomal recessive *TRPV4*, chromosome 17	Distal sensory loss. Allelic with CMT2
Spinal and bulbar muscular atrophy (Kennedy disease)	Adulthood	X-linked	Androgen receptor gene mutations. CAG repeat disorder	May present with proximal leg weakness
Infantile SMA with arthrogryposis	Infantile	X-linked	Ubiquitin-activating enzyme 1 (*UBE1*) missense mutations	
SMARD	Infantile	Autosomal recessive	*IGHMBP2* mutations	Diaphragm involvement. Distal weakness

SMA, spinal muscular atrophy; ALS, amyotrophic lateral sclerosis; UMN, upper motor neuron; CMT, Charcot–Marie–Tooth disease; SMARD, SMA with respiratory distress.

Patients present with variable degrees of symmetrical weakness, with a proximal lower limb predominance. The clinical classification outlined in the following list is based on the maximum motor milestones achieved [18]:

- Type I SMA presents before 6 months of age with generalized symmetrical muscle weakness leading to a 'floppy infant'. The onset in very severe cases is likely to be *in utero* (Type 0 SMA), and fetal hypotonia can lead to arthrogryposis. Severely affected children have an increased risk of congenital heart defects, indicating that other organ systems are vulnerable if SMN levels are low enough. Patients with Type I SMA are defined by never being able to sit unsupported. There may be tongue fasciculations. Although diaphragm function is relatively spared, death occurs before 2 years of age from respiratory failure. With assisted ventilation and enteral feeding, increasing numbers of children are surviving beyond the natural disease end point, but in a state of profound disability requiring complex care (reviewed in detail in [19]).

- Type II SMA is the intermediate form of SMA with onset after 6 months and survival beyond 2 years of age. Patients can sit (although this ability may be lost), but never walk. Kyphoscoliosis occurs in almost all patients who are non-ambulant. Patients with Type II SMA have varying degrees of bulbar involvement but invariably develop significant reduction in vital capacity. Prevention of infection with physiotherapy, cough assist devices, and non-invasive ventilation is the cornerstone of management.

- Type III SMA patients have a normal lifespan and are defined as initially able to walk. Disease onset is either before (Type IIIa) or after (Type IIIb) 3 years of age. Although there is a range of severity, half of patients with Type IIIa disease have lost ambulation by 14 years and a minority of patients are still ambulant by aged 40 years [20]. They may develop scoliosis and joint overuse symptoms.

- Type IV SMA is a milder form of the disease, with onset in adulthood and slowly progressive weakness (Fig. 5.1).

A major challenge for clinical trials in SMA is that, even in the more severe forms, there may be little discernible change in functional status from year to year. This clinical classification was developed before the cloning of the SMN genes, but has proved to have a remarkable overall congruence with *SMN2* copy number and overall protein levels, though exceptions occur [21]. In any patient with suspected proximal recessive SMA, genetic tests confirming the homozygous deletion of *SMN1* are readily available and have a sensitivity of approximately 95% in children and a specificity of 100%. If the patient retains one copy of *SMN1* by copy number analysis, the other allele should be sequenced for mutations. Genetic tests have made neurophysiology necessary in rare cases only, but if it is performed it shows normal sensory nerve action potentials (SNAPs), low-amplitude compound muscle action potentials, and EMG features of denervation including fibrillation potentials, positive sharp waves, and fasciculation potentials, as well as re-innervation with a decreased number of motor unit potentials of prolonged duration and amplitude.

Other forms of proximal SMA with survival into adulthood

SMA Type IV is genetically heterogeneous, with only approximately 50% of patients having SMN mutations [22]. Even before

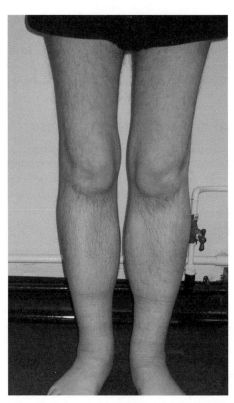

Fig. 5.1 Adult-onset autosomal recessive spinal muscular atrophy due to *SMN* deletions showing marked proximal symmetrical muscle wasting. Disease onset was aged 19 and the patient lost ambulation aged 45 years.

the identification of specific genetic defects, autosomal recessive, autosomal dominant, and X-linked patterns of inheritance were observed [23,24], as well as apparently sporadic cases [25–27]. Mutations in the *LMNA* gene, previously known to cause a variety of clinically diverse disorders classified as laminopathies, including myopathies, neuropathies, and cardiomyopathies, were found in two families with adult-onset proximal SMA [28]. These patients developed cardiac disease many years after onset of the neuromuscular problem. A single family with a senataxin (*SETX*) mutation and autosomal dominant proximal SMA with onset between 10 and 35 years of age has been described [29]. These patients had retained deep tendon reflexes, which is unusual in the classical SMAs and illustrates the difficulty in classifying this disorder as SMA rather than the atypical form of juvenile-onset ALS (ALS4) [7,8]. Similarly, mutations in the vesicle-associated membrane protein-associated protein gene *VAPB* show clinical heterogeneity with phenotypes ranging from typical amyotrophic lateral sclerosis (ALS8) to slowly progressive SMA without upper motor neuron signs [30].

A childhood-onset symmetrical proximal SMA with predominant leg weakness has recently been described and is due to mutations in the dynactin heavy chain gene (*DYNC1H1*) [31,32]. Patients showed prolonged survival well into adulthood with wasting and weakness particularly of the quadriceps muscles.

Other forms of infantile SMA

SMA with respiratory distress (SMARD) is an extremely rare autosomal recessive disorder presenting in infancy with distal muscle weakness and, unlike Type I SMA, marked diaphragmatic involvement, leading to death before 6 months in most cases. A large proportion of cases are accounted for by mutations in the immuno-globulin μ-binding protein gene (*IGHMBP2*) [33,34]. IGHMBP2 is a DNA/RNA helicase, and may have functions in mRNA splicing, but is also thought to associate with ribosomes in motor neuronal cytoplasm and the growth cone, suggesting various roles in RNA metabolism, similar to the SMN protein [35,36].

Another rare, severe infantile form of SMA with global weakness, anterior horn cell loss, arthrogryposis, bone fractures, and dysmorphic features, is similar to autosomal recessive SMA Type I but shows X-linked inheritance. It has been shown to be due to mutations in the gene *UBE1*, which codes for the ubiquitin-activating enzyme 1 [37].

Scapuloperoneal muscular atrophy (Davidenkow syndrome)

Proximal weakness, which may be asymmetrical and selective, paired with distal leg weakness, can be neurogenic in origin and has been described as a form of SMA, although distal sensory loss is involved in a number of cases, including in the first published series by Davidenkow [38]. Symptoms can start in childhood or adulthood, and sporadic as well as autosomal dominant and autosomal recessive cases have been described. Neurophysiology may show slowed sensory nerve conduction studies and delayed distal motor latencies, indicating a sensorimotor neuropathy rather than pure anterior horn cell disease [39]. In keeping with this, Harding and Thomas observed that the scapuloperoneal phenotype can occur in hereditary motor and sensory neuropathy Type I or hereditary neuropathy with liability to pressure palsies (HNPP) [40,41]. More recently, mutations in the gene encoding the transient receptor potential cation channel, subfamily V, member 4 (*TRPV4*) were identified in patients with scapuloperoneal SMA [42,43]. Mutations in *TRPV4* have been associated with a wide range of phenotypes with onset from childhood to late adulthood, in addition to scapuloperoneal SMA, including HMSN2c and a congenital form of dSMA. Vocal cord paralysis (vocal fold paresis) is a recognized complication of scapuloperoneal SMA in *TRPV4* mutations and can give rise to stridor and upper airway obstruction [44].

Distal weakness

Patients presenting with slowly progressive, symmetrical, distal muscle wasting and weakness (Table 5.2) fall under the clinical heading of peroneal muscular atrophy. In a prospective study of 262 patients,

Harding and Thomas classified 228 patients under hereditary motor and sensory neuropathy (HMSN), while 34 patients had no clinical sensory involvement, normal sensory nerve action potentials and motor conduction velocities, but EMG features of denervation [45]. Onset of weakness was mainly before the second decade, with mostly autosomal dominant, but also recessive, patterns of inheritance or sporadic occurrence. Pes cavus was frequent. To distinguish this disorder from HMSN, it was called 'hereditary distal SMA' [46], which as already outlined, is a term now used largely synonymously with dHMN. Eleven genes causing dHMN have been identified to date [47], but even when patients are systematically screened in specialist centres, up to 80% remain without a genetic diagnosis [48].

Causative genes have diverse physiological functions; they encode, amongst others, small heat shock proteins (*HSBP1*, *HSBP8*), tRNA synthetases (e.g. *GARS*), a DNA/RNA helicase (*SETX*), and an ion-channel (*TRPV4*) (see Chapter 8). Many genes have basic cellular functions and are ubiquitously expressed, and the basis for motor neuronal selectivity is not understood. It has also become clear that there is no categorical genotype–phenotype correlation, suggesting that there are genetic or environmental modifiers that determine, for example, whether patients with mutations in *HSBP1*/*HSBP8* develop CMT2 or dHMN. Even more striking is the range of phenotypes associated with even a single specific mutation in the *BSCL2* (Berardinelli-Seip congenital lipodystrophy type 2 (seipin)) gene. Carriers can present with dHMN starting in the legs, upper limb-onset dHMN, the Silver syndrome (wasted hands in the presence of a spastic paraparesis), or even the pure upper motor neuron phenotype of hereditary spastic paraplegia (HSP) [49,50]. Despite the clinical heterogeneity of these genetic disorders, narrowing down the clinical phenotype is helpful in reaching a genetic differential diagnosis. Some patients with presumed dHMN have fairly specific additional clinical features that help to focus the differential diagnosis, such as upper limb onset, bulbar or vocal cord involvement, or added upper motor neuron signs.

Lower limb-predominant distal weakness

Some patients present with symmetrical distal weakness in the legs and pes cavus, with subsequent involvement of the upper limbs, sometimes after a delay of years. There is no clinical sensory loss and sensory nerve conduction studies are normal. The age of onset is variable, and can be in childhood, adolescence, or less commonly adulthood. The rate of progression is generally slow. Patients with

Table 5.2 Disorders presenting with distal weakness

Presentation	Classification [46,47]	Inheritance	Genetics	Other features
Lower limb onset distal weakness	dHMN I	Autosomal dominant	*HSBP1*, *HSPB8*, *GARS*, *DYNC1H1*	Juvenile onset
	dHMN II	Autosomal dominant	*HSPB1*, *HSPB8*, *BSCL2*	Adult onset
	dHMN III	Autosomal recessive	11q13, *HSPB1*	
	X-linked dHMN	X-linked	*ATP7A*	Variable age of onset
Upper limb onset	dHMN V	Autosomal dominant	*GARS*, *BSCL2*	
Distal weakness and vocal cord paralysis	dHMN VII	Autosomal dominant	*TRPV4*, *DCTN1*	
Distal weakness and diaphragmatic weakness	dHMN VI, SMARD	Autosomal recessive	*IGHMBP2*	Infantile onset

dHMN, distal hereditary motor neuropathy; SMARD, spinal muscular atrophy with respiratory distress.

autosomal dominant inheritance and juvenile onset are classified as dHMN Type I [51]. Known causative genes are *HSPB1, HSPB8, GARS,* and *DYNC1H1.* Autosomal dominant disease with adult onset is classified as dHMN Type II, but the range of causative genes overlaps with Type 1 and includes *HSPB1, HSPB8,* and *BSCL2.* Autosomal recessive inheritance has been observed with *HSPB1* [52]. An X-linked form of distal lower limb-predominant HMN is due to mutations in the copper transporter gene *ATP7A,* which is also mutated in the severe infantile-onset neurodegenerative disorder Menke's disease. Mutations in X-linked distal HMN do not affect the region of the protein critical for copper homeostasis [53,54].

Upper limb-predominant distal weakness

Upper-limb-onset dHMN (or Type V in the Harding classification [45,46]), where weakness and wasting appear in the hands first, often most pronounced in the first dorsal interosseous and the thenar muscles, appears to be specifically associated with mutations in *GARS* [55] and *BSCL2* [49]. Lower limb involvement, again distally, can follow many years or even decades later. Indeed, detailed phenotypic analysis of patients with *GARS* mutations shows that lower limb onset is equally common and also demonstrates that there is a continuum between dHMN Type V and CMT2D, the latter showing clinical and neurophysiological sensory involvement and generally a more severe phenotype with more rapid progression [56].

Distal weakness with vocal cord paralysis

A highly distinctive phenotype is distal motor neuropathy with vocal cord paralysis (also referred to as vocal fold paresis). This is classified as dHMN Type VII. It is associated with mutations in *TRPV4* (which can also give rise to scapuloperoneal SMA with or without vocal cord paralysis, as described in the section Scapuloperoneal muscular atrophy (Davidenkow syndrome)) [43,44]. Stridor can be the presenting feature, though many patients develop distal weakness initially, which may begin in the hands or feet and be associated with pes cavus and hammer toes. Other abnormalities may be observed, including sensorineural hearing loss and urinary incontinence. Onset is usually in childhood. The other recognized genetic cause of dHMN Type VII is mutations in the p150 subunit of dynactin (*DCTN1*), in this case associated with adult onset and associated facial weakness [57,58].

Spinobulbar syndromes

The syndromes discussed here have more prominent bulbar involvement than the relatively isolated vocal cord paralysis seen in scapuloperoneal SMA and dHMN Type VII (see Table 5.3).

Brown–Vialetto–Van Laere and Fazio–Londe syndromes

Brown–Vialetto–Van Laere syndrome (BVVL) is the eponymous name for a progressive bulbar palsy with deafness that can occur sporadically or be inherited in a mainly autosomal recessive pattern [59]. It is rare, and a recent review only identified 58 cases in the literature [60]. Sensorineural deafness is a defining and often early feature, followed by a combination of lower cranial nerve palsies and lower motor neuron-predominant signs in the limbs. Onset is often in early childhood, but can be as late as the third decade. The disease course is variable but often prolonged. The clinical presentation of BVVL is very similar to what is called Madras-type motor neuron disease, prevalent in southern India and occurring more often sporadically than in a familial pattern [61,62]. A childhood-onset form of progressive bulbar palsy with upper and lower motor neuron signs that is indistinguishable from BVVL, except for the absence of hearing loss, is Fazio–Londe syndrome, and is even less common [63]. Genetic studies have confirmed the long-held view that the two disorders are the same entity.

Recent genetic studies in BVVL identified several mutations in the riboflavin transporter genes *SLC52A3* (formerly *C20orf54*) and *SLC52A2* [64]. In keeping with this genetic observation, several cases of both young-onset BVVL and Fazio–Londe syndrome were described which displayed a metabolic and biochemical profile suggestive of severe flavin deficiency and in which riboflavin supplementation appeared to result in clinical improvement [65,66]. Even though it is not clear that all cases of the BVVL spectrum are riboflavin related, the possibility of a successful treatment should lead to increased awareness of this rare disease and early consideration of riboflavin treatment. In fact, an open-label study of riboflavin in BVVL caused by *SLC52A2* mutations has reported significant clinical benefits in a cohort of 16 treated patients [66a]. Much more common than the BVVL-spectrum disorders is the adult-onset, X-linked spinal and bulbar muscular atrophy (SBMA) or Kennedy disease (see Chapter 6).

Facial-onset sensory and motor neuronopathy syndrome

The recently described facial-onset sensory and motor neuronopathy syndrome (FOSMN) occurs sporadically in the fourth decade [67]. It shares some clinical characteristics with SBMA, including bulbar dysfunction of the lower motor neuron type with dysarthria, dysphagia, and tongue fasciculations. Muscle weakness, wasting, and fasciculations occur in the upper limbs. The characteristic feature of this disorder, however, is the early occurrence of

Table 5.3 Spinobulbar syndromes

Diagnosis	Onset	Inheritance	Genetics	Other features
Brown–Vialetto–Van Laere syndrome	Infancy to third decade	Sporadic or recessive	*SLC52A3* (formerly *C20orf54*) and *SLC52A2* mutations	Sensorineural deafness. May respond to riboflavin therapy
Fazio–Londe syndrome	Childhood	Sporadic or recessive	*SLC52A3* (formerly *C20orf54*) mutations	No deafness. May respond to riboflavin therapy
SBMA (Kennedy disease)	Adulthood	X-linked	Androgen receptor gene mutations. CAG repeat disorder	Tongue fasciculations, jaw drop, proximal weakness
FOSMN	Adulthood	Sporadic		Facial sensory loss

SBMA, spinal and bulbar muscular atrophy; FOSMN, facial-onset sensory and motor neuronopathy syndrome.

Table 5.4 Asymmetrical and segmental weakness

Syndrome	Onset	Inheritance	Genetics	Other features
Davidenkow syndrome/ scapuloperoneal muscular atrophy	Childhood or adulthood	Sporadic, autosomal dominant or autosomal recessive	*TRPV4*	
Hirayama disease	Juvenile	Usually sporadic		Possibly ischaemic causation
Monomelic atrophy of the lower limb	Adulthood	Sporadic		
Progressive muscular atrophy	Adulthood	Sporadic or autosomal dominant		Variant of ALS

ALS, amyotrophic lateral sclerosis.

facial and oral sensory loss, in particular for pain and temperature, mimicking syringobulbia. The cause of FOSMN is unknown and it does not respond to immunosuppression. Disease duration ranges from 5–20 years and at autopsy there is widespread degeneration of sensory and motor neurons with no evidence of inflammation, amyloid deposition, or intraneuronal inclusions such as TDP-43, Bunina bodies, or ubiquitin inclusions [68].

Asymmetrical and segmental weakness

Asymmetrical onset of muscle weakness and wasting is typical of ALS, but some patients lack progression after initial disease onset and never develop upper motor neuron signs. Harding et al. described 18 patients with relatively young onset of asymmetrical lower motor neuron disease with lack of progression after 3 years and little EMG evidence of more widespread denervation, a condition they called 'chronic asymmetrical SMA' [69]. A variety of descriptive terms for similar presentations have been used, including benign focal amyotrophy and segmental SMA, but there is no overall satisfactory nosological classification and this is not a single clinicopathological entity (see Table 5.4). Multifocal motor neuropathy with conduction block needs to be considered in this group of patients.

Juvenile muscular atrophy of the distal upper extremity, or Hirayama disease

A distinct and puzzling condition, occurring almost exclusively in young men in their teens or early twenties, from Japan, China, and the Indian subcontinent, is characterized by distal asymmetrical upper limb weakness and wasting, often with retained reflexes but absent upper motor neuron or sensory signs [70]. Although the classical presentation is with weakness and wasting in the distribution of the C7–T1 myotomes (Fig. 5.2), more proximal involvement can occur clinically or neurophysiologically. Up to 20% of cases may be bilateral [71]. After initial progression over months the condition tends to plateau or to progress at an imperceptible rate [72,73]. Convincing cases of familial occurrence have not been described, though the striking restriction of the disorder to patients of Asian background surely suggests that genetic factors are relevant. Imaging studies and a few reported autopsies lend support to the view that Hirayama disease is a form ischaemic poliomyelopathy related to forward displacement of the posterior cervical dural sac and compressive flattening of the lower cervical cord during neck flexion rather than a primary neurodegenerative disorder (Fig. 5.3a,b) [74,75]. However, why this should result in primarily unilateral disease is unexplained. One autopsied case showed sparse

basophilic inclusions in addition to nerve cell loss and astrogliosis, but no hallmark features of ALS-like neurodegeneration [76].

It is likely that the syndrome of asymmetrical distal amyotrophy has heterogeneous causes. It is certainly the case that older male and female patients with similar patterns of monomelic amyotrophy, often labelled 'segmental distal SMA', are seen in neuromuscular clinics. The absence of the typical MRI changes described in Hirayama syndrome suggests the possibility of another disease mechanism [26].

Monomelic amyotrophy of the leg

Monomelic neurogenic atrophy of the lower limb is less common than the equivalent syndrome in the upper limb. Many case series come from the Indian subcontinent [77–79]. The majority of cases are sporadic, with male preponderance. The muscles involved can be distal, proximal, or both. Insidious onset is followed by slow progression and later stabilization in many cases, with absence of bulbar,

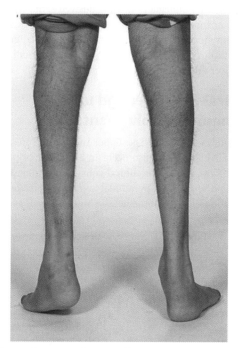

Fig. 5.2 Silver syndrome: mixed upper and lower motor neuron involvement due to the N88S mutation in the *BSCL2* gene. Note the peroneal wasting combined with tendon shortening due to spasticity. The patient had bilateral extensor plantar responses.

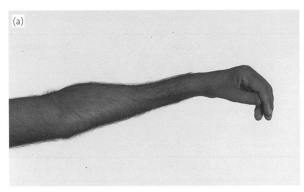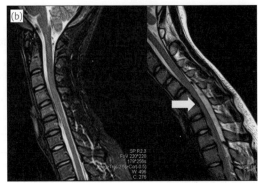

Fig. 5.3 (a) Muscle atrophy in Hirayama disease showing the characteristic atrophy of the flexor and extensor muscles in the forearm with sparing of brachioradialis. (b) T_2-weighted magnetic resonance imaging scan of the cervical spine in the neutral position (left) and then flexed (right), showing expansion of a posterior dural compartment with compression and flattening of the spinal cord in flexion (arrow).

pyramidal, or sensory involvement [80–82]. Despite the clinical involvement of one leg only, neurophysiology may demonstrate more widespread lower motor neuron involvement [83]. The aetiology of monomelic amyotrophy of a lower limb is obscure, and no unifying pathophysiological hypothesis such as that proposed in Hirayama disease has been put forward. Despite the relatively uniform description of cases, it is uncertain whether it is a single disease entity.

Other forms of asymmetrical or segmental lower motor neuron disease

Several acquired disorders of the lower motor neuron enter the differential diagnosis of asymmetrical or segmental SMA. Patients who only partially recovered from poliomyelitis with severe limb involvement may develop new or worsening symptoms after an interval of many years, the post-polio syndrome (see Chapter 7). HIV infection has been associated with a motor neuron disease, including brachial diplegia [84,85]. A delayed syndrome of denervation with normal sensory and motor nerve conduction can occur as a late complication of radiotherapy for pelvic malignancy [86]. Multifocal motor neuropathy is an important differential in asymmetrical lower motor neuron disorders (Chapter 16).

Disorders with lower and upper motor neuron involvement

The combination of lower and upper motor neuron signs is the hallmark of ALS, but can also occur in a number of other conditions that follow a different clinical course. This includes diseases classified as dHMN with pyramidal signs, complicated forms of HSP with added lower motor neuron signs, as well as conditions

termed 'atypical' or juvenile ALS. Growing understanding of the genetic basis of these conditions has shown that this distinction is at times arbitrary (Table 5.5).

Silver syndrome is the name given to an uncommon familial disorder with spastic paraparesis of variable severity together with bilateral wasting of the hands [87]. Affected patients have onset of symptoms between 8 years of age and the fourth decade, and very slow progression. Some family members have been ascertained in their 70s. Bulbar dysfunction does not occur. Mutations in the causative gene, *BSCL2*, give rise to clinically heterogeneous phenotypes including dHMN Type V, dHMN Type II, as well as spastic paraparesis with amyotrophy in the legs (SPG17) [49,50,88].

Several other HSPs show complex phenotypes that in addition to spasticity may include distal muscle wasting. SPG20, Troyer syndrome, is an autosomal recessive disorder initially found in the Old Order Amish [89,90]. Childhood-onset spasticity and wasting occur together with a corticobulbar palsy. It is caused by mutations in *SPG20*, encoding spartin [91]. A similar phenotype is caused by mutations in the neuropathy target esterase (*NTE*) gene [92].

Some familial young-onset motor neuron disorders with slow progression and prominent upper motor neuron involvement have been designated 'juvenile ALS'. An autosomal dominant pattern of inheritance is observed with ALS4, caused by mutations in *SETX* [8]. As already mentioned, this disorder is also called dHMN with pyramidal features, and is characterized by an early age of onset (average age 17 years), very slow progression, distal wasting and weakness in the arms and legs, added upper motor neuron signs, absence of sensory signs, and only the very rare occurrence of bulbar involvement [7].

Table 5.5 Disorders with upper and lower motor neuron involvement

Syndrome	Onset	Inheritance	Genetics	Other features
Silver syndrome, HSP17	Childhood or adulthood	Autosomal dominant	*BSCL2*	
Troyer syndrome	Childhood	Autosomal recessive	*SPG20* (spartin)	
ALS2	Juvenile	Autosomal recessive	*ALS2* (alsin)	Slowly progressive ALS. Juvenile PLS. HSP
ALS4	Juvenile	Autosomal dominant	*SETX*	Allelic with dHMN
ALS5	Juvenile	Autosomal recessive	*SPG11* (spatacsin)	Very slow progression

HSP, hereditary spastic paraplegia; ALS, amyotrophic lateral sclerosis; PLS, primary lateral sclerosis; dHMN, distal hereditary motor neuropathy.

Highly atypical, autosomal recessive forms of juvenile ALS occur with mutations in alsin (*ALS2*) and spatacsin. Alsin was found to be mutated in a previously described Tunisian kindred with a very slowly progressive pure motor disorder of childhood (mean age of onset 12) [93]. The phenotype was variable but comprised a bilateral pyramidal syndrome with additional limb wasting and bulbar involvement [94]. Other alsin-related motor neuron disorders include a young-onset pure upper motor neuron syndrome or 'juvenile primary lateral sclerosis' and a young-onset HSP [95,96].

ALS5, autosomal recessive juvenile ALS with linkage to chromosome 15q15-21 is caused by mutations in spatacsin (*SPG11*), a gene previously known to be associated with a complicated form of HSP with thin corpus callosum. All patients identified by Orlacchio et al. [10] came from consanguineous families and fulfilled the El Escorial criteria for ALS but had juvenile onset of symptoms at an average age of 16, and had very long disease courses of up to 40 years on ascertainment. Mixed upper and lower motor signs with bulbar involvement were present, with disability ranging from mild to wheelchair dependence. An autopsied case showed motor neuron loss and chromatolysis in remaining spinal motor neurons, but no skein-like inclusions or Bunina bodies as in typical adult-onset ALS.

Conclusions

With the increasing number of genes identified in motor neuron disorders comes a greater recognition of genetic and clinical heterogeneity. Perhaps the commonest clinical challenge in the adult neuromuscular clinic is that many patients have no family history and therefore do not easily fit into a genetic taxonomy. The distinction from slowly progressive, lower motor neuron-predominant forms of ALS may require prolonged follow-up. Where the history and clinical signs do not allow a firm diagnosis of slowly progressive motor neuron involvement, the first step is often to consider treatable mimic syndromes such as myasthenia gravis, inflammatory myopathies, or neuropathies such as chronic inflammatory demyelinating polyneuropathy and multifocal motor neuropathy.

Even when there is a characteristic clinical pattern and a family history, the yield from genetic testing may be low. This is likely to change dramatically with the advent of next-generation high-throughput gene sequencing. A precise molecular diagnosis may help estimate prognosis, genetic counselling, and ultimately facilitate clinical trials as disease-specific therapies become available. Finally, it is worth remembering that in the absence of a specific diagnosis, the rate of progression in the first few years of an illness is likely to be the most helpful indicator or future progression and overall prognosis. In a review of 49 cases of apparently sporadic lower motor neuron disease of more than 4 years' disease duration, Van den Berg-Vos and colleagues observed a good prognosis with prolonged survival [97], and in a later prospective study of 37 similar patients with more than 4 years' disease duration, only three patients subsequently developed ALS [98]. In contrast, 13 of 37 patients with a variety of lower motor neuron syndromes and a disease duration of less than 4 years progressed to ALS [2].

References

1. Geser F, Stein B, Partain M, et al. Motor neuron disease clinically limited to the lower motor neuron is a diffuse TDP-43 proteinopathy. *Acta Neuropathol* 2011; **121**: 509–17.

2. Visser J, Van den Berg-Vos RM, Franssen H, et al. Disease course and prognostic factors of progressive muscular atrophy. *Arch Neurol* 2007; **64**: 522–8.

3. Kim WK, Liu X, Sandner J, et al. Study of 962 patients indicates progressive muscular atrophy is a form of ALS. *Neurology* 2009; **73**: 1686–92.

4. Myrianthopoulos NC, Lane MH, Silberberg DH, Vincent BL. Nerve conduction and other studies in families with Charcot–Marie–Tooth disease. *Brain* 1964; **87**: 589–608.

5. Chance PF, Rabin BA, Ryan SG, et al. Linkage of the gene for an autosomal dominant form of juvenile amyotrophic lateral sclerosis to chromosome 9q34. *Am J Hum Genet* 1998; **62**: 633–40.

6. Rabin BA, Griffin JW, Crain BJ, Scavina M, Chance PF, Cornblath DR. Autosomal dominant juvenile amyotrophic lateral sclerosis. *Brain* 1999; **122**: 1539–50.

7. De Jonghe P, Auer-Grumbach M, Irobi J, et al. Autosomal dominant juvenile amyotrophic lateral sclerosis and distal hereditary motor neuronopathy with pyramidal tract signs: synonyms for the same disorder? *Brain* 2002; **125**: 1320–5.

8. Chen YZ, Bennett CL, Huynh HM, et al. DNA/RNA helicase gene mutations in a form of juvenile amyotrophic lateral sclerosis (ALS4). *Am J Hum Genet* 2004; **74**: 1128–35.

9. Hadano S, Hand CK, Osuga H, et al. A gene encoding a putative GTPase regulator is mutated in familial amyotrophic lateral sclerosis 2. *Nat Genet* 2001; **29**: 166–73.

10. Orlacchio A, Babalini C, Borreca A, et al. SPATACSIN mutations cause autosomal recessive juvenile amyotrophic lateral sclerosis. *Brain* 2010; **133**: 591–8.

11. Nelson JS, Prensky AL. Sporadic juvenile amyotrophic lateral sclerosis. A clinicopathological study of a case with neuronal cytoplasmic inclusions containing RNA. *Arch Neurol* 1972; **27**: 300–6.

12. Matsumoto S, Kusaka H, Murakami N, Hashizume Y, Okazaki H, Hirano A. Basophilic inclusions in sporadic juvenile amyotrophic lateral sclerosis: an immunocytochemical and ultrastructural study. *Acta Neuropathol* 1992; **83**: 579–83.

13. Baumer D, Hilton D, Paine SM, et al. Juvenile ALS with basophilic inclusions is a FUS proteinopathy with FUS mutations. *Neurology* 2010; **75**: 611–18.

14. Pearn J. Incidence, prevalence, and gene frequency studies of chronic childhood spinal muscular atrophy. *J Med Genet* 1978; **15**: 409–13.

15. Lefebvre S, Burglen L, Reboullet S, et al. Identification and characterization of a spinal muscular atrophy-determining gene. *Cell* 1995; **80**: 155–65.

16. Oprea GE, Krober S, McWhorter ML, et al. Plastin 3 is a protective modifier of autosomal recessive spinal muscular atrophy. *Science* 2008; **320**: 524–7.

17. Burghes AH, Beattie CE. Spinal muscular atrophy: why do low levels of SMN make motor neurons sick? *Nat Rev Neurosci* 2009; **10**: 597–609.

18. Munsat TL, Davies KE. International SMA consortium meeting. (26-28 June 1992, Bonn, Germany). *Neuromuscul Disord* 1992; **2**: 423–8.

19. Mercuri E, Bertini E, Iannaccone ST. Childhood spinal muscular atrophy: controversies and challenges. *Lancet Neurol* 2012; **11**: 443–52.

20. Zerres K, Rudnik-Schoneborn S. Natural history in proximal spinal muscular atrophy. Clinical analysis of 445 patients and suggestions for a modification of existing classifications. *Arch Neurol* 1995; **52**: 518–23.

21. Wirth B, Herz M, Wetter A, et al. Quantitative analysis of survival motor neuron copies: identification of subtle SMN1 mutations in patients with spinal muscular atrophy, genotype-phenotype correlation, and implications for genetic counseling. *Am J Hum Genet* 1999; **64**: 1340–56.

22. Zerres K, Wirth B, Rudnik-Schoneborn S. Spinal muscular atrophy—clinical and genetic correlations. *Neuromuscul Disord* 1997; **7**: 202–7.

23. Pearn JH, Hudgson P, Walton JN. A clinical and genetic study of spinal muscular atrophy of adult onset: the autosomal recessive form as a discrete disease entity. *Brain* 1978; **101**: 591–606.

24. Pearn JH, Hudgson P, Walton JN. A clinical and genetic study of spinal muscular atrophy of adult onset: the autosomal recessive form as a discrete disease entity. *Brain* 1978; **101**: 591–606.

25. Van Den Berg-Vos RM, Van Den Berg LH, Visser J, de Visser M, Franssen H, Wokke JH. The spectrum of lower motor neuron syndromes. *J Neurol* 2003; **250**: 1279–92.

26. Van den Berg-Vos RM, Visser J, Franssen H, et al. Sporadic lower motor neuron disease with adult onset: classification of subtypes. *Brain* 2003; **126**: 1036–47.

27. Van den Berg-Vos RM, Visser J, Kalmijn S, et al. A long-term prospective study of the natural course of sporadic adult-onset lower motor neuron syndromes. *Arch Neurol* 2009; **66**: 751–7.

28. Rudnik-Schoneborn S, Botzenhart E, Eggermann T, et al. Mutations of the LMNA gene can mimic autosomal dominant proximal spinal muscular atrophy. *Neurogenetics* 2007; **8**: 137–42.

29. Rudnik-Schoneborn S, Arning L, Epplen JT, Zerres K. SETX gene mutation in a family diagnosed autosomal dominant proximal spinal muscular atrophy. *Neuromuscul Disord* 2012; **22**: 258–62.

30. Nishimura AL, Mitne-Neto M, Silva HC, et al. A mutation in the vesicle-trafficking protein VAPB causes late-onset spinal muscular atrophy and amyotrophic lateral sclerosis. *Am J Hum Genet* 2004; **75**: 822–31.

31. Harms MB, Allred P, Gardner R, Jr, et al. Dominant spinal muscular atrophy with lower extremity predominance: linkage to 14q32. *Neurology* 2010; **75**: 539–46.

32. Harms MB, Ori-McKenney KM, Scoto M, et al. Mutations in the tail domain of DYNC1H1 cause dominant spinal muscular atrophy. *Neurology* 2012; **78**: 1714–20.

33. Grohmann K, Schuelke M, Diers A, et al. Mutations in the gene encoding immunoglobulin mu-binding protein 2 cause spinal muscular atrophy with respiratory distress type 1. *Nat Genet* 2001; **29**: 75–7.

34. Guenther UP, Varon R, Schlicke M, et al. Clinical and mutational profile in spinal muscular atrophy with respiratory distress (SMARD): defining novel phenotypes through hierarchical cluster analysis. *Hum Mutat* 2007; **28**: 808–15.

35. Grohmann K, Rossoll W, Kobsar I, et al. Characterization of Ighmbp2 in motor neurons and implications for the pathomechanism in a mouse model of human spinal muscular atrophy with respiratory distress type 1 (SMARD1). *Hum Mol Genet* 2004; **13**: 2031–42.

36. Guenther UP, Handoko L, Laggerbauer B, et al. IGHMBP2 is a ribosome-associated helicase inactive in the neuromuscular disorder distal SMA type 1 (DSMA1). *Hum Mol Genet* 2009; **18**: 1288–300.

37. Ramser J, Ahearn ME, Lenski C, et al. Rare missense and synonymous variants in UBE1 are associated with X-linked infantile spinal muscular atrophy. *Am J Hum Genet* 2008; **82**: 188–93.

38. Davidenkow S. Scapuloperoneal amyotrophy. *Arch Neurol Psychiatry* 1939; **41**: 694–701.

39. Schwartz MS, Swash M. Scapuloperoneal atrophy with sensory involvement: Davidenkow's syndrome. *J Neurol Neurosurg Psychiatry* 1975; **38**: 1063–7.

40. Harding AE, Thomas PK. Distal and scapuloperoneal distributions of muscle involvement occurring within a family with type I hereditary motor and sensory neuropathy. *J Neurol* 1980; **224**: 17–23.

41. Verma A. Neuropathic scapuloperoneal syndrome (Davidenkow's syndrome) with chromosome 17p11.2 deletion. *Muscle Nerve* 2005; **32**: 668–71.

42. Deng HX, Klein CJ, Yan J, et al. Scapuloperoneal spinal muscular atrophy and CMT2C are allelic disorders caused by alterations in TRPV4. *Nat Genet* 2010; **42**: 165–9.

43. Auer-Grumbach M, Olschewski A, Papic L, et al. Alterations in the ankyrin domain of TRPV4 cause congenital distal SMA, scapuloperoneal SMA and HMSN2C. *Nat Genet* 2010; **42**: 160–4.

44. Zimon M, Baets J, Auer-Grumbach M, et al. Dominant mutations in the cation channel gene transient receptor potential vanilloid 4 cause an unusual spectrum of neuropathies. *Brain* 2010; **133**: 1798–809.

45. Harding AE, Thomas PK. The clinical features of hereditary motor and sensory neuropathy types I and II. *Brain* 1980; **103**: 259–80.

46. Harding AE, Thomas PK. Hereditary distal spinal muscular atrophy. A report on 34 cases and a review of the literature. *J Neurol Sci* 1980; **45**: 337–48.

47. Rossor AM, Kalmar B, Greensmith L, Reilly MM. The distal hereditary motor neuropathies. *J Neurol Neurosurg Psychiatry* 2012; **83**: 6–14.

48. Dierick I, Baets J, Irobi J, et al. Relative contribution of mutations in genes for autosomal dominant distal hereditary motor neuropathies: a genotype-phenotype correlation study. *Brain* 2008; **131**: 1217–27.

49. Irobi J, Van den Bergh P, Merlini L, et al. The phenotype of motor neuropathies associated with BSCL2 mutations is broader than Silver syndrome and distal HMN type V. *Brain* 2004; **127**: 2124–30.

50. Auer-Grumbach M, Schlotter-Weigel B, Lochmuller H, et al. Phenotypes of the N88S Berardinelli-Seip congenital lipodystrophy 2 mutation. *Ann Neurol* 2005; **57**: 415–24.

51. Harding A. Inherited neuronal atrophy and degeneration predominantly of lower motor neurons. In: Dyck PJ, Thomas PK, Griffin JW, Low PA, Poduslo JF (ed) *Peripheral Neuropathy*, pp. 1051–64. Philadelphia: WB Saunders, 1993.

52. Houlden H, Laura M, Wavrant-De Vrieze F, Blake J, Wood N, Reilly MM. Mutations in the HSP27 (HSPB1) gene cause dominant, recessive, and sporadic distal HMN/CMT type 2. *Neurology* 2008; **71**: 1660–8.

53. Kennerson M, Nicholson G, Kowalski B, et al. X-linked distal hereditary motor neuropathy maps to the DSMAX locus on chromosome Xq13.1-q21. *Neurology* 2009; **72**: 246–52.

54. Kennerson ML, Nicholson GA, Kaler SG, et al. Missense mutations in the copper transporter gene ATP7A cause X-linked distal hereditary motor neuropathy. *Am J Hum Genet* 2010; **86**: 343–52.

55. Antonellis A, Ellsworth RE, Sambuughin N, et al. Glycyl tRNA synthetase mutations in Charcot–Marie–Tooth disease type 2D and distal spinal muscular atrophy type V. *Am J Hum Genet* 2003; **72**: 1293–9.

56. Sivakumar K, Kyriakides T, Puls I, et al. Phenotypic spectrum of disorders associated with glycyl-tRNA synthetase mutations. *Brain* 2005; **128**: 2304–14.

57. Puls I, Oh SJ, Sumner CJ, Wallace KE, et al. Distal spinal and bulbar muscular atrophy caused by dynactin mutation. *Ann Neurol* 2005; **57**: 687–94.

58. Puls I, Jonnakuty C, LaMonte BH, et al. Mutant dynactin in motor neuron disease. *Nat Genet* 2003; **33**: 455–6.

59. Megarbane A, Desguerres I, Rizkallah E, et al. Brown–Vialetto–Van Laere syndrome in a large inbred Lebanese family: confirmation of autosomal recessive inheritance? *Am J Med Genet* 2000; **92**: 117–21.

60. Sathasivam S. Brown–Vialetto–Van Laere syndrome. *Orphanet J Rare Dis* 2008; **3**: 9 doi: 10.1186/1750-1172-3-9.

61. Summers BA, Swash M, Schwartz MS, Ingram DA. Juvenile-onset bulbospinal muscular atrophy with deafness: Vialetto–van Laere syndrome or Madras-type motor neuron disease? *J Neurol* 1987; **234**: 440–2.

62. Nalini A, Thennarasu K, Yamini BK, Shivashankar D, Krishna N. Madras motor neuron disease (MMND): clinical description and survival pattern of 116 patients from southern India seen over 36 years (1971–2007). *J Neurol Sci* 2008; **269**: 65–73.

63. McShane MA, Boyd S, Harding B, Brett EM, Wilson J. Progressive bulbar paralysis of childhood. A reappraisal of Fazio–Londe disease. *Brain* 1992; **115**: 1889–900.

64. Green P, Wiseman M, Crow YJ, et al. Brown–Vialetto–Van Laere syndrome, a ponto-bulbar palsy with deafness, is caused by mutations in C20orf54. *Am J Hum Genet* 2010; **86**: 485–9.

65. Bosch AM, Abeling NG, Ijlst L, et al. Brown–Vialetto–Van Laere and Fazio Londe syndrome is associated with a riboflavin transporter defect mimicking mild MADD: a new inborn error of metabolism with potential treatment. *J Inherit Metab Dis* 2011; **34**: 159–64.

66. Anand G, Hasan N, Jayapal S, et al. Early use of high-dose riboflavin in a case of Brown–Vialetto–Van Laere syndrome. *Dev Med Child Neurol* 2012; **54**: 187–9.

66a. Foley AR, Menezes MP, Pandraud A, et al. Treatable childhood neuronopathy caused by mutations in riboflavin transporter RFVT2. *Brain* 2013; published online 19 November, doi: 10.1093/brain/awt315

67. Vucic S, Tian D, Chong PS, Cudkowicz ME, Hedley-Whyte ET, Cros D. Facial onset sensory and motor neuronopathy (FOSMN syndrome): a novel syndrome in neurology. *Brain* 2006; **129**: 3384–90.

68. Vucic S, Stein TD, Hedley-Whyte ET, et al. FOSMN syndrome: novel insight into disease pathophysiology. *Neurology* 2012; **79**: 73–9.

69. Harding AE, Bradbury PG, Murray NM. Chronic asymmetrical spinal muscular atrophy. *J Neurol Sci* 1983; **59**: 69–83.

70. Hirayama K, Tsubaki T, Toyokura Y, Okinaka S. Juvenile muscular atrophy of unilateral upper extremity. *Neurology* 1963; **13**: 373–80.

71. Pradhan S. Bilaterally symmetric form of Hirayama disease. *Neurology* 2009; **72**: 2083–9.

72. Sobue I, Saito N, Iida M, Ando K. Juvenile type of distal and segmental muscular atrophy of upper extremities. *Ann Neurol* 1978; **3**: 429–32.

73. Tashiro K, Kikuchi S, Itoyama Y, et al. Nationwide survey of juvenile muscular atrophy of distal upper extremity (Hirayama disease) in Japan. *Amyotroph Lateral Scler* 2006; **7**: 38–45.

74. Hirayama K. Juvenile muscular atrophy of distal upper extremity (Hirayama disease): focal cervical ischemic poliomyelopathy. *Neuropathology* 2000; **20** (Suppl): S91–S94.

75. Hirayama K, Tokumaru Y. Cervical dural sac and spinal cord in juvenile muscular atrophy of distal upper extremity. *Neurology* 2000; **54**: 1922–6.

76. Hirayama K, Tomonaga M, Kitano K, Yamada T, Kojima S, Arai K. Focal cervical poliopathy causing juvenile muscular atrophy of distal upper extremity: a pathological study. *J Neurol Neurosurg Psychiatry* 1987; **50**: 285–90.

77. Gourie-Devi M, Suresh TG, Shankar SK. Monomelic amyotrophy. *Arch Neurol* 1984; **41**: 388–94.

78. Prabhakar S, Chopra JS, Banerjee AK, Rana PV. Wasted leg syndrome: a clinical, electrophysiological and histopathological study. *Clin Neurol Neurosurg* 1981; **83**: 19–28.

79. Gourie-Devi M. Monomelic amyotrophy of upper or lower limbs. In: Wisen AA, Shaw PJ (ed) *Handbook of Clinical Neurology*, pp. 207–27. Amsterdam: Elsevier, 2007.

80. Di Muzio A, Delli Pizzi C, Lugaresi A, Ragno M, Uncini A. Benign monomelic amyotrophy of lower limb: a rare entity with a characteristic muscular CT. *J Neurol Sci* 1994; **126**: 153–61.

81. Uncini A, Servidei S, Delli Pizzi C, et al. Benign monomelic amyotrophy of lower limb: report of three cases. *Acta Neurol Scand* 1992; **85**: 397–400.

82. Felice KJ, Whitaker CH, Grunnet ML. Benign calf amyotrophy: clinicopathologic study of 8 patients. *Arch Neurol* 2003; **60**: 1415–20.

83. de Visser M, Ongerboer de Visser BW, Verbeeten B, Jr. Electromyographic and computed tomographic findings in five patients with monomelic spinal muscular atrophy. *Eur Neurol* 1988; **28**: 135–8.

84. Berger JR, Espinosa PS, Kissel J. Brachial amyotrophic diplegia in a patient with human immunodeficiency virus infection: widening the spectrum of motor neuron diseases occurring with the human immunodeficiency virus. *Arch Neurol* 2005; **62**: 817–23.

85. Rowland LP. HIV-related neuromuscular diseases: nemaline myopathy, amyotrophic lateral sclerosis and bibrachial amyotrophic diplegia. *Acta Myol* 2011; **30**: 29–31.

86. Bowen J, Gregory R, Squier M, Donaghy M. The post-irradiation lower motor neuron syndrome neuronopathy or radiculopathy? *Brain* 1996; **119**: 1429–39.

87. Silver JR. Familial spastic paraplegia with amyotrophy of the hands. *Ann Hum Genet* 1966; **30**: 69–75.

88. Windpassinger C, Auer-Grumbach M, Irobi J, et al. Heterozygous missense mutations in BSCL2 are associated with distal hereditary motor neuropathy and Silver syndrome. *Nat Genet* 2004; **36**: 271–6.

89. Cross HE, McKusick VA. The Troyer syndrome. A recessive form of spastic paraplegia with distal muscle wasting. *Arch Neurol* 1967; **16**: 473–85.

90. Proukakis C, Cross H, Patel H, Patton MA, Valentine A, Crosby AH. Troyer syndrome revisited. A clinical and radiological study of a complicated hereditary spastic paraplegia. *J Neurol* 2004; **251**: 1105–10.

91. Patel H, Cross H, Proukakis C, et al. SPG20 is mutated in Troyer syndrome, an hereditary spastic paraplegia. *Nat Genet* 2002; **31**: 347–8.

92. Rainier S, Bui M, Mark E, et al. Neuropathy target esterase gene mutations cause motor neuron disease. *Am J Hum Genet* 2008; **82**: 780–5.

93. Yang Y, Hentati A, Deng HX, et al. The gene encoding alsin, a protein with three guanine-nucleotide exchange factor domains, is mutated in a form of recessive amyotrophic lateral sclerosis. *Nat Genet* 2001; **29**: 160–5.

94. Ben Hamida M, Hentati F, Ben Hamida C. Hereditary motor system diseases (chronic juvenile amyotrophic lateral sclerosis). Conditions combining a bilateral pyramidal syndrome with limb and bulbar amyotrophy. *Brain* 1990; **113**: 347–63.

95. Panzeri C, De Palma C, Martinuzzi A, et al. The first ALS2 missense mutation associated with JPLS reveals new aspects of alsin biological function. *Brain* 2006; **129**: 1710–19.

96. Hadano S, Hand CK, Osuga H, et al. A gene encoding a putative GTPase regulator is mutated in familial amyotrophic lateral sclerosis 2. *Nat Genet* 2001; **29**: 166–73.

97. Visser J, Van den Berg-Vos RM, Franssen H, et al. Mimic syndromes in sporadic cases of progressive spinal muscular atrophy. *Neurology* 2002; **58**: 1593–6.

98. Van den Berg-Vos RM, Visser J, Kalmijn S, et al. A long-term prospective study of the natural course of sporadic adult-onset lower motor neuron syndromes. *Arch Neurol* 2009; **66**: 751–7.

CHAPTER 6

Kennedy disease

Christopher Grunseich and Kenneth Fischbeck

Background

Spinal and bulbar muscular atrophy (SBMA), also known as Kennedy disease [1], is caused by a trinucleotide (CAG) repeat expansion in the androgen receptor (AR) gene on the X chromosome [2], which results in an expanded polyglutamine tract and an androgen-dependent toxic gain of function in the mutant protein. The prevalence has been estimated to be about 1 in 40 000. Patients with SBMA have repeat lengths of between 40 and 62 CAGs [3,4], whereas normal individuals usually have between 11 and 32 CAGs [5–7]. The length of the CAG repeat correlates inversely with the age of disease onset, with longer repeats associated with earlier onset [5]. Affected males have a slowly progressive disease with weakness, atrophy, and fasciculations in the limb and bulbar muscles primarily due to lower motor neuron degeneration. There is currently no treatment available to alter the progression of this disease, and the precise mechanism by which the expansion results in the death of motor neurons remains to be determined.

Mechanism

The manifestations of SBMA occur because of a toxic gain of function of the AR protein that is dependent on androgens (testosterone and dihydrotestosterone). Loss of normal receptor function also contributes to the disease phenotype. The mutant protein is prone to aggregation and forms intracellular inclusions in susceptible cells [8,9]. The primary effect of the mutant AR protein is probably transcriptional dysregulation, with consequent alterations in cellular signal transduction, mitochondrial activity, and axonal transport [10–13]. While it is known that androgens have an important anabolic function in skeletal muscle, the relationship of this normal activity to the toxic effects of mutant AR protein on motor neurons and muscle is not well understood.

Clinical features

Several studies have helped to clarify the natural history of SBMA, which is important not only for characterizing the salient features of the disease but also for identifying outcome measures for clinical trials [3,4]. Neurological symptoms typically develop during the fourth or fifth decade of life, but the age of onset ranges from 18 to 64 years [4]. The most common presenting symptoms include muscle cramps, tremor, and weakness (Table 6.1). When weakness occurs, about half of patients report symptoms initially in the legs, and a third describe their first symptoms in the bulbar region [4]. Lower extremity weakness typically manifests as difficulty climbing stairs, standing, and walking long distances. The weakness affects both proximal and distal muscles of the upper and lower extremities, and the pattern is often somewhat asymmetric, with more involvement on the dominant side [4]. Eventually, gait impairment reduces overall mobility, and patients may become wheelchair dependent. Those with bulbar symptoms usually first notice dysarthria and nasal speech, which can progress to dysphagia and potentially predispose to aspiration pneumonia. Lower motor neuron signs are frequent, including decreased or absent deep tendon reflexes and fasciculations in the muscles of the extremities, chin (see Video 6.1), and tongue. Some patients also have distal sensory loss from degeneration of the dorsal root ganglia. Evidence of androgen insensitivity may manifest as gynaecomastia, reduced fertility, and erectile dysfunction.

Diagnostic studies

All affected individuals have a trinucleotide repeat expansion with at least 40 CAGs in the first exon of the AR gene [2]. Genetic testing is the definitive method of diagnosis. Creatine kinase is elevated in nearly 90% of patients, usually to the range of 900–1400 IU L^{-1}, although there is considerable variability [3,4]. Aspartate and aspartate aminotransferases are found to be mildly elevated above the reference range; however, this may not be the result of liver toxicity as gamma glutamyl transferase levels have been found to be normal. Patients with SBMA also often have elevation of low-density lipoprotein levels above reference control values and may have impaired glucose tolerance. The hormonal profile in subjects can also be abnormal, with elevations in average total testosterone, free testosterone, dihydrotestosterone, and estradiol, and reduced androstenedione. Although serum androgen levels are elevated on average in SBMA patients, a minority may have abnormally low levels of free testosterone and dihydrotestosterone [4].

On neurophysiological studies, more than 94% of SBMA patients have abnormally low sensory nerve amplitudes. Compound motor

Table 6.1 Common presenting symptoms in SBMA, in order of decreasing frequency

1. Muscle cramps
2. Tremor
3. Leg weakness
4. Arm weakness
5. Breast enlargement
6. Bulbar weakness

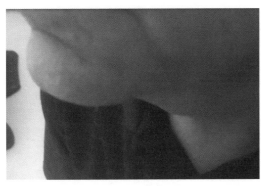

Video 6.1 Chin fasciculations in a patient with Kennedy disease.

action potentials may also be decreased [4]. Electromyography is usually consistent with diffuse denervation atrophy. Motor unit number estimation (MUNE) performed in the abductor pollicis brevis muscle has been found to be reduced to about half that of healthy control values. Recent work by Higashihara et al. [14] suggests that the clustering index method using surface electromyography may be a sensitive method for detecting subclinical motor unit loss in SBMA.

Muscle biopsy is usually not necessary to establish a diagnosis. The changes observed are generally consistent with neurogenic atrophy, as evidenced by angulated fibres, fibre type grouping, and clusters of small atrophied fibres [1,15]. Biopsies may also have myopathic features, including myofibrillar disorganization and central nuclei.

Family history

About two-thirds of SBMA patients have a positive family history [4]. As an X-linked disorder fully manifest only in males, SBMA may be transmitted through asymptomatic females, e.g. mothers, sisters, and daughters of affected patients. Children of affected patients are usually asymptomatic, with only a minority of female carriers experiencing symptoms of cramping [16]. The CAG repeat may change in length when passed on from one generation to the next, but it does not show as much instability as in other trinucleotide repeat expansion diseases [5]. Genetic counselling services should be offered to those who are carriers, or at risk of being carriers. Pre-implantation and prenatal genetic testing are available. Pre- and post-test genetic counselling is recommended when testing is being considered for at-risk, asymptomatic males, and such testing is usually only offered to adults. Before considering genetic testing, a genetic diagnosis should be established in an affected family member.

Prognosis

The disease progression is slow. In a recent clinical trial, muscle strength decreased in the placebo group by about 2% per year as measured by quantitative muscle assessment [17]. The median age at which subjects used a cane or wheelchair was about 60 [3]. Many patients have a normal life span; however, the average life expectancy may be reduced. In the study by Atsuta et al. of 223 patients [3], the median age of 15 subjects who died was 65 years. The cause of death in eight of these cases was aspiration pneumonia. The length of the CAG repeat in the *AR* gene does not correlate with the rate of

disease progression [3]. Contrary to what may be expected given the ligand-dependent toxic gain of function in the mutant AR protein, a cross-sectional study showed that patients with higher testosterone levels have better muscle strength and quality of life [4].

Management

There is currently no treatment known to reverse or stop the progression of the disease. Several interventions have been reported to be effective in transgenic mouse models, particularly androgen reduction therapy [18]. However, randomized, placebo-controlled, clinical trials of the androgen-reducing agents leuprorelin and dutasteride have not shown significant effects on primary outcome measures related to muscle strength and function and swallow function overall. Nonetheless, there were some indications of efficacy, e.g. on swallow function in subjects who had been symptomatic for less than 10 years [17,19,20].

The focus of management of SBMA at present is to prevent complications of the disease and enhance mobility so that function can be preserved. Evaluation for physical therapy is usually helpful to identify patients who may benefit from braces and assistive devices to improve ambulation. Speech and swallowing function should also be assessed, and pulmonary function testing performed if impairment is suspected. An exercise programme tailored to the patient's level of function could also help to maintain and improve mobility. The effect of exercise on progression of the disease remains uncertain, however. One study of eight subjects using moderate-intensity aerobic exercise found an increase in maximal work capacity, but an effect on maximal oxygen uptake and other measures was not detected [21]. It is possible that primary muscle involvement in SBMA attenuates the response to exercise. More studies are needed to assess whether functional exercise may be beneficial.

Differential diagnosis

The diagnosis of SBMA is relatively straightforward, given the characteristic clinical presentation and the availability of genetic testing. Accurate diagnosis is delayed for many patients however, in part due to a lack of general awareness of the disease. A recent cross-sectional study found an average time to diagnosis of 5.5 years from the onset of weakness and 3.5 years from first medical evaluation [4]. A third of patients were misdiagnosed with ALS. Both diseases cause weakness and denervation, but ALS unlike SBMA typically has upper motor neuron involvement resulting in spasticity and hyperreflexia, and it usually shows greater asymmetry and progresses much more rapidly. Speech involvement in SBMA is characteristically more nasal sounding, as opposed to the upper motor neuron pattern of dysarthria in ALS. In its early stages SBMA may also be confused with myasthenia gravis, chronic inflammatory neuropathy, polymyositis, and metabolic myopathy.

When to think of this disorder

A male patient, who may have gynaecomastia, with slowly progressive muscle wasting and fasciculations in the absence of upper motor neuron signs.

Conclusion

SBMA is caused by a CAG repeat expansion in the *AR* gene on the X chromosome and results in muscle cramps, weakness, atrophy, and fasciculations. Onset is in mid-adulthood, and progression is slow. There is currently no known effective treatments and management is symptomatic.

References

1. Kennedy WR, Alter M, Sung JH. Progressive proximal spinal and bulbar muscular atrophy of late onset: a sex-linked recessive trait. *Neurology* 1968; **18**: 671–80.

2. La Spada AR, Wilson EM, Lubahn DB, Harding AE, Fischbeck KH. Androgen receptor gene mutations in X-linked spinal and bulbar muscular atrophy. *Nature* 1991; **352**: 77–9.

3. Atsuta N, Watanabe H, Ito M, et al. Natural history of spinal and bulbar muscular atrophy (SBMA): a study of 223 Japanese patients. *Brain* 2006; **129**: 1446–55.

4. Rhodes LE, Freeman BK, Auh S, et al. Clinical features of spinal and bulbar muscular atrophy. *Brain* 2009; **132**: 3242–51.

5. La Spada AR, Roling D, Harding AE, et al. Meiotic stability and genotype-phenotype correlation of the trinucleotide repeat in X-linked spinal and bulbar muscular atrophy. *Nat Genet* 1992; **2**: 301–4.

6. Tanaka F, Doyu M, Ito Y, et al. Founder effect in spinal and bulbar muscular atrophy (SBMA). *Hum Molec Genet* 1996; **5**: 1253–7.

7. Edwards A, Hammond HA, Jin L, Caskey T, Chakraborty R. Genetic variation at five trimeric and tetrameric tandem repeat loci in four human population groups. *Genomics* 1992; **12**: 241–53.

8. Walcott JL, Merry DE. Ligand promotes intranuclear inclusions in a novel cell model of spinal and bulbar muscular atrophy. *J Biol Chem* 2002; **277**: 50855–9.

9. Li M, Miwa S, Kobayashi Y, et al. Nuclear inclusions of the androgen receptor protein in spinal and bulbar muscular atrophy. *Ann Neurol* 1998; **44**: 249–54.

10. McCampbell A, Taylor JP, Taye AA, et al. CREB-binding protein sequestration by expanded polyglutamine. *Hum Molec Genet* 2000; **9**: 2197–202.

11. Lieberman AP, Harmison G, Strand AD, Olson JM, Fischbeck KH. Altered transcriptional regulation in cells expressing the expanded polyglutamine androgen receptor. *Hum Molec Genet* 2002; **11**: 1967–76.

12. Ranganathan S, Harmison GG, Meyertholen K, Pennuto M, Burnett BG, Fischbeck KH. Mitochondrial abnormalities in spinal and bulbar muscular atrophy. *Hum Molec Genet* 2009; **18**: 27–42.

13. Katsuno M, Adachi H, Minamiyama M, et al. Reversible disruption of dynactin 1-mediated retrograde axonal transport in polyglutamine-induced motor neuron degeneration. *J Neurosci* 2006; **26**: 12106–17.

14. Higashihara M, Sonoo M, Yamamoto T, et al. Evaluation of spinal and bulbar muscular atrophy by the clustering index method. *Muscle Nerve* 2011; **44**: 539–46.

15. Soraru G, D'Ascenzo C, Polo A, et al. Spinal and bulbar muscular atrophy: skeletal muscle pathology in male patients and heterozygous females. *J Neurol Sci* 2008; **264**: 100–5.

16. Ishihara H, Kanda F, Nishio H, et al. Clinical features and skewed X-chromosome inactivation in female carriers of X-linked recessive spinal and bulbar muscular atrophy. *J Neurol* 2001; **248**: 856–60.

17. Fernández-Rhodes LE, Kokkinis AD, White MJ, et al. Efficacy and safety of dutasteride in patients with spinal and bulbar muscular atrophy: a randomised placebo-controlled trial. *Lancet Neurol* 2011; **10**: 140–7.

18. Katsuno M, Adachi H, Doyu M, et al. Leuprorelin rescues polyglutamine-dependent phenotypes in a transgenic mouse model of spinal and bulbar muscular atrophy. *Nature Med* 2003; **9**: 768–73.

19. Banno H, Katsuno M, Suzuki K, et al. Phase 2 trial of leuprorelin in patients with spinal and bulbar muscular atrophy. *Ann Neurol* 2009; **65**: 140–50.

20. Katsuno M, Banno H, Suzuki K, et al. Efficacy and safety of leuprorelin in patients with spinal and bulbar muscular atrophy (JASMITT study): a multicentre, randomised, double-blind, placebo-controlled trial. *Lancet Neurol* 2010; **9**: 875–84.

21. Preisler N, Andersen G, Thøgersen F, et al. Effect of aerobic training in patients with spinal and bulbar muscular atrophy (Kennedy disease). *Neurology* 2009; **72**: 317–23.

CHAPTER 7

Poliomyelitis

Robin S. Howard

Introduction

In the first half of the twentieth century poliomyelitis was common and widely feared across the world. It often struck without warning, was highly contagious, and usually affected young people, causing prolonged or permanent flaccid paralysis or death. There are arresting and disturbing accounts of the explosive nature of polio epidemics and the response of communities to these outbreaks [1]. It is probable that these epidemics were paradoxically due to improved sanitation. Polio was previously endemic in childhood and this had led to the development of widespread immunity and protection from maternal antibodies; however, as public health improved this immunity waned. Epidemics continued to occur until the widespread introduction of routine immunization with the Salk inactivated polio vaccine in 1956 and the Sabin oral live attenuated vaccine in 1962.

The effective control of poliomyelitis throughout most of the world has been a remarkable story of scientific and social progress. However, despite a global policy aimed at eradication, pockets of wild polio still exist in parts of sub-Saharan Africa and the Indian subcontinent and it continues to occur sporadically elsewhere. Furthermore there is a still a small incidence of vaccine-induced polio in infants and adults. Global eradication remains a goal of the World Health Organization (WHO) and public health policies throughout the world [2–6].

Aetiology

Poliomyelitis is caused by an enterovirus of high infectivity transmitted via orofaecal contact. The main route of infection is the human gastrointestinal tract but it may also be transmitted by pharyngeal spread. There are three subtypes, but before the introduction of polio vaccine Type 1 accounted for 85% of paralytic disease. The virus multiplies in the lymphatic tissue of the pharynx and intestine for 1 to 3 weeks before it is either contained by a local immune response or a viraemic phase occurs. The virus continues to be excreted in the saliva for 2 or 3 days and in the faeces for 2 to 3 weeks. The infection rate is extremely high, although it is probable that 95% of all infections are either asymptomatic or characterized by an abortive flu-like illness. Epidemics of polio occurred most commonly during the summer months in the temperate climates of the Northern Hemisphere and the incidence was greatest where children bathed together [7,8].

Acute illness

Following the minor, flu-like illness, a few patients develop a meningitic phase as the virus reaches the central nervous system (CNS); this is characterized by high fever with pharyngitis, myalgia, anorexia, nausea, vomiting, headache, and neck stiffness. The factors favouring the development of spinal poliomyelitis are unclear, but it has been suggested that physical activity and intramuscular injections during the minor illness may be an important predisposing factor. Spread may occur by direct passage across the blood–brain barrier or by retrograde axonal transport from muscle to spinal cord and brain. The onset of spinal poliomyelitis is associated with myalgia and severe muscle spasms, with the subsequent development of an asymmetrical, flaccid weakness which becomes maximal after 48 h. The lower limbs are affected more than the upper limbs and involvement tends to be proximal with loss of reflexes but normal sensation. A purely bulbar form with minimal limb involvement also occurs, particularly in children, and this was said to be more common in those whose tonsils and adenoids had been removed [9]. Bulbar poliomyelitis carries a particularly high mortality rate due to vasomotor disturbances such as hypertension, hypotension and circulatory collapse, autonomic dysfunction, dysphagia, dysphonia, and respiratory failure. Rarely poliomyelitis may cause brainstem encephalitis.

Diagnosis

The cerebrospinal fluid (CSF) shows increased protein content and pleocytosis with normal glucose. The virus is commonly isolated from the nasopharynx in the first week of the illness, or from the stool for several weeks. In the absence of a viral isolate serological diagnosis can be established by neutralization of sera against paired antigens of the three serotypes, which also allows differentiation of wild-type from vaccine-induced disease. Molecular diagnosis, using polymerase chain reaction (PCR) on CSF or blood, is now the technique of choice for serotypic identification of poliovirus and for differentiation of wild and vaccine-strain poliomyelitis [10].

Differential diagnosis

Acute flaccid paralysis (Table 7.1) is associated with infection by other enteroviruses, including Coxsackie virus A7 and Enterovirus 70 and 71, tick-borne encephalitis, and by flaviviruses including Japanese encephalitis and more recently West Nile virus. The differential diagnosis of asymmetric motor flaccid paralysis includes Guillain–Barré syndrome, acute intermittent porphyria, HIV neuropathy, diphtheria and *Borrelia bergdorferi* (Lyme disease) infections, and disorders at the neuromuscular junction such as myasthenia and botulism [11–14].

Prevention

The demonstration in 1949 that poliovirus could be successfully propagated to non-neuronal cell cultures led to the award of the Nobel Prize to Enders, Robbins, and Weller. This was the

Table 7.1 Causes of acute flaccid paralysis

Infection
  Viral
    Enterovirus
    Poliomyelitis (wild and vaccine-associated)
    Enterovirus 71, Coxsackie A
    Flavivirus
    Japanese encephalitis
    West Nile encephalitis
    Herpes virus
    Cytomegalovirus
    Epstein–Barr virus
    Varicella zoster virus
    Tick-borne encephalitis
    Human immunodeficiency virus-related (associated with opportunistic infections)
    Other neurotropic viruses
  Rabies
  Borrelia
  Mycoplasma
  Diphtheria
  Botulism

Neuropathy
    Acute inflammatory polyneuropathy
    Acute motor axonal neuropathy
    Critical illness neuropathy
    Lead poisoning
    Other heavy metals

Spinal cord
    Acute transverse myelitis
    Acute spinal cord compression
    Trauma
    Infarction

Neuromuscular junction
    Myasthenia gravis

Muscle
    Polymyositis
    Viral myositis
    Post-infectious myositis
    Critical illness myopathy

Functional

In currently or recently endemic countries every case of acute flaccid paralysis should be notified regardless of the likely aetiology. Two stool specimens should be collected within 14 days after the onset of paralysis, and virus isolation should be performed in a qualified laboratory.

catalyst for the development of effective immunization against poliomyelitis, initially by Jonas Salk and subsequently by Albert Sabin. The introduction in 1956 of the Salk trivalent inactivated polio vaccine (IPV) for routine immunization led to a reduction in the rate of polio in the United States of more than 90%. It is administered by injection and stimulates serum IgM, IgG, and IgA, but not secretory IgA, immunity being induced by antibody transuding into the oropharynx. Sabin trivalent oral live attenuated polio vaccine (OPV) replaced the Salk vaccine in 1962; this is composed of live attenuated strains of polioviruses I, II, and

III grown in cell culture. The advantages over the Salk vaccine were that it was cheap, could be administered orally, and caused an active attenuated infection of the oropharynx and intestinal endothelium stimulating local secretary IgA in addition to serum antibody production. Furthermore, the attenuated virus is excreted in the faeces leading to herd immunity. Complete immunization with OPV has, conventionally, included four doses routinely given at 2, 4, and 6–18 months with a booster at 4–6 years [15–18].

Following the introduction of mass vaccination programmes in the late 1950s and early 1960s the incidence of paralytic poliomyelitis was dramatically reduced; however, global vaccination was not possible. Furthermore, OPV vaccine-derived poliovirus is attenuated and may mutate and acquire properties similar to the wild type. This can result in vaccine-associated paralytic poliomyelitis (VAPP) occurring in recipients, particularly if they have B-cell immunodeficiency. Similarly vaccine-derived poliomyelitis (VDP) may occur in contacts, particularly in regions with low immunization rates. Once again the virus may mutate and it will then affect unimmunized direct contacts (e.g. those who change the nappies of infants who have recently received OPV) especially if they are immunosuppressed. In North America, Europe, Japan, Australia, and New Zealand, the ongoing occurrence of VAPP and VDP in the face of the elimination of wild-type polio has led to the increased use of IPV, culminating in the present recommendations of an all-IPV schedule [19–21].

Policies for global eradication

There have been no known cases of endemic wild-type polio in the West since 1991. Following the launch of the WHO global eradication initiative in 1988 there has been a dramatic reduction in the number of cases worldwide from 350 000 in 1988 to 900 cases in 2003. Six countries are considered to be polio endemic (Nigeria, India, Pakistan, Niger, Afghanistan, and Egypt) although imported wild disease occurs in seven other African countries with a recent, alarming epidemic in Nigeria. A case count register is available on the WHO website [22].

The present global eradication policy is based on a four-point strategy:

1. Routine immunization ensuring high infant coverage in the first year of life. Regions where eradication has been achieved must continue high levels of immunization to prevent the re-establishment of poliovirus if it is imported.

2. Mass immunization campaigns (mass immunization days) during which routine immunization is supplemented by the provision of two further doses of OPV to large numbers of children under the age of 5.

3. Continuous surveillance undertaken by national, regional, and global laboratories aims to identify all cases of acute flaccid paralysis regardless of the underlying cause, the diagnosis of polio being subsequently confirmed by the genomic sequencing of wild-type poliovirus.

4. Mopping-up campaigns are employed in countries where the final pockets of poliovirus transmission have been identified. These campaigns involve door-to-door immunization in high-risk districts where the virus is still known or suspected to be circulating. They are concentrated particularly where access

to healthcare is difficult and there is high population density and mobility, poor sanitation, and low routine immunization coverage [23].

Despite the success of this campaign, considerable difficulties remain and new outbreaks continue to occur due to importation even in previously polio-free countries like Angola, Chad, Congo, and Sudan. Even more recently outbreaks of wild-type polio virus I have occurred in Tajikistan, Chechnya, Kazakhstan, and Russia. It is difficult to provide adequate heat-stable OPV, to ensure adequate seroconversion in tropical populations, and to prevent the occurrence of VAPP and VDP. This has led to the suggestion, already mentioned, that OPV should be abandoned in favour of IPV. The cost of global eradication remains enormous and there are real concerns that the political determination to maintain eradication policies may be eroded by the success of the campaign. The WHO continues to warn of the increasing worldwide vulnerability to polio if the mass campaign is discontinued. This is a particular concern in areas of conflict such as the tribal areas between Pakistan and Afghanistan, and the difficulties may be made worse by mass migration and flooding. Therefore there remains a significant risk of reintroduction wild poliovirus because of the combination of international travel, poor healthcare, areas of low vaccine coverage, and delays in diagnosis of flaccid paralysis.

Management of the acute illness

All patients should be put on strict bed rest to prevent extension of the paralysis. Pain relief and frequent passive movements prevent contractures and joint ankylosis. Acute respiratory failure may develop rapidly, requiring intubation and intermittent positive pressure ventilation. If prolonged ventilation is needed, or there is coexisting bulbar weakness, tracheostomy may be necessary to protect the airway. Specific antiviral therapy using pleconaril may be helpful in treating Enterovirus infection.

During the first few weeks of mobilization, the main aim of management is to prevent deformity by stretching and splinting of affected limbs. Intensive physiotherapy is directed towards retraining affected muscles to regain strength and function and the provision of appropriate orthoses to compensate for loss of function, facilitate mobility, and prevent undue wear and tear. The older practices of splinting and casting led to severe disuse atrophy of muscles, whether or not they were affected by the disease. The early rehabilitation of polio was greatly influenced by the vision of Elizabeth Kenny, an Australian nurse practicing in the United States, who advocated the use of warm, moist heat, using wool packs, together with early mobilization of affected limbs. This work was given further impetus by the development of Warm Springs, Georgia, a rehabilitation centre supported by President Franklin D. Roosevelt following his own acute polio, where techniques of hydrotherapy and early mobilization with splinting and passive movements were developed to prevent contractures and joint ankylosis. Careful postural re-education and attention to activities of daily living were fundamental to successful early rehabilitation.

Later rehabilitation

Much of the late rehabilitation involved multiple orthopaedic procedures and the provision of appropriate orthoses. The orthopaedic management was aimed at maintaining stable mobility. Multiple surgical procedures were often undertaken to lengthen or shorten tendons, transfer muscles to affected limbs, fuse unstable joints, and correct other abnormalities.

Post-polio functional deterioration ('post-polio syndrome')

Following recovery from the acute illness and a period of rehabilitation, most people maintain stable function for many years. However, it has become increasingly clear that many patients with residual impairments develop new disabilities after a prolonged period of stability. These late functional changes were recognized and defined medically in terms of progressive muscular atrophy, weakness, pain, and fatigue [24,25].

Much has also been written about the illness of Franklin D. Roosevelt, who contracted polio at the age of 39. There is no doubt that, after a prolonged period of stability, his disabilities increased with age, and in his later years he even had difficulty lighting a cigarette, driving a car, and holding a cup of coffee [31–33].

Dalakas and colleagues [27–29] defined 'post-polio syndrome' as new neuromuscular symptoms that some patients develop 25–35 years after reaching maximum recovery from acute paralytic poliomyelitis; these symptoms are unrelated to any orthopaedic, neurological, psychiatric, or systemic medical illness. This definition included complaints such as muscle and joint pain, reduced exercise tolerance, impairment of activities of daily living, limb atrophy, cramps, and fatigue but specifically excluded musculoskeletal symptoms due to back injuries, radiculopathy, compression neuropathies, and other medical, neurological, orthopaedic, or psychiatric illnesses.

Most patients are aware of impairment of activities of daily living, mobility, upper limb function, and respiratory capacity [30–39]. They often describe an insidious onset of progressive impairment, but sometimes functional deterioration occurs as a consequence of a clear precipitating event such as a fall or intercurrent illness. Patients notice a lack of strength or endurance, which causes difficulty with normal activities such as walking to the shops or washing their hair. There may be prolonged fatigue following physical activity, or difficulty in recovering from periods of immobility. They often experience new musculoskeletal symptoms including cramps and fasciculations, increasing weakness of a limb or the trunk, unreliability in a previously stable joint (often in the upper limbs), pain in muscles and joints, and changes in the joint (often with a tendency to trip or fall). Weakness is most likely to be in a previously affected limb, but may also occur as a result of the extra load on an previously unaffected limb. Other prominent symptoms may be respiratory and swallowing difficulties and sleep disturbance. Respiratory symptoms due to weakness of the diaphragm and respiratory muscles may lead to breathlessness on exertion, orthopnoea, and progressive nocturnal hypoventilation. Nocturnal ventilatory impairment results in snoring, abnormal sleep movements, morning headache, daytime hypersomnolence, impaired intellectual function, irritability, and depression.

The nature of 'post-polio syndrome' remains controversial, with most definitions continuing to suggest that the new symptoms and signs should be unrelated to any orthopaedic, neurological, respiratory, or systemic medical illness. However, these criteria are somewhat inconsistent because most patients with post-polio functional deterioration have considerable pre-existing orthopaedic and neurological impairment, rendering them vulnerable to the development of new disabilities. Thus, new impairments may often occur as a consequence of prolonged stresses on skeletal deformity and previously weakened muscles, including entrapment neuropathy, radiculopathy, and orthopaedic problems.

Predisposing factors

The development of post-polio functional deterioration seems to depend on several factors (see Table 7.2). The extent of the original limb, trunk, respiratory, and bulbar weakness is an important factor in predisposing to the development of late functional deterioration, and the condition usually occurs in patients with significant residual disability. Some patients may be referred because of the development of disability even though the initial polio left no residual sequelae or in whom the original diagnosis was equivocal, but these patients generally have an alternative explanation for their symptoms [40,41]. The effects of growth are often significant. Polio developing before the growth spurt usually leads to progressive scoliosis because of the eccentric development of the spinal musculature. Furthermore, polio developing in the early years leads to limb shortening, which causes growth retardation during the adolescent growth spurt.

The use of callipers, crutches, or wheelchairs can lead to the development of compression neuropathies. Frequently there is progressive wasting and weakness in limbs already affected by poliomyelitis but this may also occur in the contralateral limb, i.e. secondary to weight bearing or distorted mechanics. Occasionally compensatory hypertrophy may occur in the contralateral limb for similar reasons [42]. Progressive joint contractures may lead to limb impairment, such as knee hyperextension, hip arthrosis, and scoliosis.

Pathophysiology

The aetiology of post-polio functional deterioration is uncertain but a number of theories have been proposed.

Table 7.2 Factors associated with the development of post-polio syndrome

Onset of functional deterioration after a prolonged period of stability
Young onset of acute polio
Severe limb, bulbar, or respiratory involvement during the acute polio
Incomplete recovery with residual disability
Greater physical activity during the intervening years
Development of new symptoms or impairment associated with intercurrent events

Development of symptoms including:
    Pain in joints, bones, and muscles
    Fatigue
    Cramps, fasciculation
    Wasting, weakness

Deterioration in functional abilities:
    Activities of daily living
    Mobility
    Upper limb function
    Respiratory function

The most likely cause is progressive degeneration of reinnervated motor units. In the acute illness loss of anterior horn cells and motor units leads to denervation. During the recovery period there is reinnervation of the muscle fibres and collateral sprouting, which results in motor unit enlargement. Over many years, the remaining healthy motor neurons become unable to maintain unstable new units and the process becomes overwhelmed, possibly as a consequence of increased metabolic demands, with a consequent loss of the vulnerable, collateral fibres. This is suggested by electrophysiological findings of active denervation, including spontaneous activity and increased fibre density with jitter and blocking on single-fibre studies. Certainly the most extensive reinnervated motor units are more likely to become unstable [43–46], excessive exercise or overuse predisposes to new weakness [41], and changes of denervation on muscle biopsy (small angulated fibres, group atrophy and fibre type grouping) become more apparent with time. However, similar changes are seen in both affected and unaffected muscle groups in surviving polio patients with and without 'post-polio syndrome', thus it remains uncertain whether these electrophysiological and biopsy changes are of clinical significance.

Progressive age-related loss of motor neurons may contribute to the progressive loss of motor units, but this is unlikely to be a major contributory factor because the condition is more dependent on latent period than age and new symptoms may start well before the age of 60. Furthermore, anterior horn cell dropout is not normally seen before the age of 70 years and very seldom do muscle biopsies show angulated fibres.

Alternative explanations have been proposed. The presence and reactivation of persistent neuronal poliovirus has been shown in tissue culture, and an early study did show the presence of an ongoing intrathecal antibody response and polio-sensitized cells in the CSF of patients with post-polio syndrome [47], although this finding has not been replicated subsequently [48,49].

An inflammatory or immune-mediated basis has been suggested by autopsy findings showing inflammatory change in the spinal cords of patients with post-polio syndrome [50]. This is supported by the observation of pro-inflammatory cytokines and abnormal activated peripheral blood T-lymphocyte subsets and ganglioside-specific IgG and IgM in the CSF and serum, and oligoclonal bands in the CSF [51].

It has been suggested that there is a geographical relationship between past notification rates of polio and current mortality from motor neuron disease in the UK [52,53]. However, this has not been confirmed. Indeed Armon [54] noted the relative paucity of classical motor neuron disease developing in survivors of paralytic poliomyelitis, and Swingler et al. [55] were unable to show any geographical association between past mortality from poliomyelitis and present morbidity and mortality from motor neuron disease in a Scottish population.

Causes and management of late functional deterioration

Orthopaedic complications

These are extremely common and reflect the prolonged abnormal stresses applied to joints due to skeletal deformation and muscle weakness. Abnormalities include fixed-flexion deformities, hyperextension, and lateral instability of the knee or hip. Other causes of deterioration include progressive instability of joints, fractures, osteoporosis, and osteoarthritis. Scoliosis frequently worsens over many years. Degenerative joint disease is most common in weight-bearing joints and weakened limbs. Cervical spondylosis is extremely common and causes neck pain and variable sensory radicular symptoms. Cord compression occurs in some patients and the diagnosis may be difficult if the limb is already affected by polio. Obesity frequently contributes to orthopaedic deterioration.

Specialized orthopaedic assessment is necessary in planning appropriate management, but a range of simple supports for the knee, ankle, and cervical spine, or correction of worn and damaged aids may provide considerable functional improvement. These include the provision of new callipers, braces, foot orthoses, knee and pelvic supports, shoe raises, collars, harnesses, and seating. Hip and knee deformities may be helped with physiotherapy, hydrotherapy, night splints, or foam supports.

Cervical decompression is usually indicated in the presence of severe established radiculopathy or myelopathy. If progressive scoliosis is contributing to respiratory insufficiency then spinal surgery may be undertaken or bracing without fusion may be attempted, but these are technically difficult procedures. With severe bilateral genu recurvatum causing posterior knee pain, if orthotic support fails bone block procedures using the patella have proved effective.

Respiratory insufficiency

Respiratory insufficiency due to respiratory muscle weakness leads to progressive nocturnal hypoventilation and this is exacerbated by chest wall deformity, progressive scoliosis, or other factors stressing critically compromised ventilation—respiratory tract infections, obstructive airways disease, obesity, pregnancy, and tracheostomy complications [56]. Sleep disturbance with resulting fatigue may be a clue to the development of respiratory insufficiency, although it is important to remember that it may also indicate the presence of an independent sleep disorder such as restless legs syndrome [57].

Some patients who were ventilated during the acute illness continue to require long-term intermittent or continuous support. Others were weaned after the acute illness but subsequently required intervention after developing ventilatory failure. In general those patients who received ventilation during the acute illness have residual respiratory muscle weakness and remain most at risk of respiratory compromise.

Negative-pressure ventilation using an iron lung or cuirass shell was the mainstay of respiratory support during the polio epidemics. Pressure changes applied to the trunk, but not the head, cause air to pass in and out of the lungs. The drawbacks to negative-pressure ventilation include lack of portability along with a physiological effect of increasing obstructive apnoeas during sleep, as negative pressure applied to the thorax leads to an increased tendency for the upper airway to collapse in the region of the velopharynx. In addition, negative-pressure ventilators may not lend themselves to use with patients who have major thoracic deformities. Its current use is confined to those patients who have been stable for many years and in whom negative-pressure ventilation was introduced before the availability of other convenient systems.

Positive-pressure ventilation is the most efficient form of assisted ventilation and was first applied in the polio epidemics. For continuous use (more than 16 h a day) a connection to the trachea via a cuffed endotracheal tube, or directly by tracheostomy, is required.

Non-invasive intermittent positive-pressure ventilation (NIV) requires a ventilator delivering a pre-determined pressure. It is usually used for night-time support although some patients use varying periods of ventilation during the daytime. The advantage lies in the patient being able to vary tidal volume on a breath-to-breath basis. These ventilators are leak compensating, which provides another advantage since intermittent speech is possible during the inspiratory stroke of the ventilator. They are particularly suitable for long-term domiciliary use in neurological disease and are usually simple and reliably constructed. NIV is applied via a tightly fitting nasal or facial mask or nasal 'pillows'. Interface design is constantly improving. With the range of masks now available, patient comfort with minimal leak can be achieved in all cases.

Cough and cough assist techniques

Whilst alveolar hypoventilation results from weakness of the inspiratory muscles, an effective cough is dependent on adequate inspiratory capacity, rapid contraction of the expiratory muscles, and sufficient bulbar control to allow an explosive expulsion of air. In polio-related respiratory muscle weakness and some neuromuscular diseases, early abdominal or bulbar muscle involvement may increase the risk of acute episodes of respiratory failure despite adequate nocturnal ventilation. In such individuals, improving cough by manually assisting spontaneous coughing effort with abdominal pressure may be important in preventing lower respiratory tract infection and possibly delaying the onset of respiratory failure. Another technique to improve clearance of secretions involves mechanical hyperinflation followed by the application of negative pressure, effectively sucking air out of the chest. There may be an important role for the use of a CoughAssist mechanical insufflator/exsufflator in the prevention of respiratory morbidity in post-polio respiratory muscle weakness.

Neurological complications

Neurological complications often reflect skeletal deformity, and the use of callipers, crutches, and wheelchairs predispose to the development of peripheral nerve entrapment. A small proportion of patients may develop worsening dysphagia, which is not usually associated with other evidence of bulbar weakness, but this rarely progresses to aspiration. Other neurological disturbances have been reported to coexist with previous polio (e.g. motor neuron disease, multiple sclerosis [58], syringomyelia, epilepsy, and meningioma), but there is no evidence to suggest these associations are anything but coincidental.

General medical disorders

General medical factors contributing to late deterioration have included chronic urinary disturbances, including renal or bladder calculi. Other important problems include the development of diabetes and hypertension [31,34].

Management

The effective management of post-polio functional deterioration requires a multidisciplinary approach involving both specific treatment of increasing impairment and a process of enabling the patient to cope with new disabilities. Physicians must recognize that patients may note changes in function that are not manifest by increasing weakness on neurological examination. What appears, on examination, to be a slight worsening of a severe disability, may have devastating functional consequences for the patient [59–65].

Polio survivors are often motivated and driven; they have conquered their disability, often by ignoring it completely, and have the most remarkable stories of achievement. Patients need to be reassured that the condition is not a form of motor neuron disease and nor is it likely to progress to severe impairment, although new functional disabilities are possible and must be appropriately managed.

Exercise

Many continue to deal with increasing disability by intensive exercise regimes to regain muscle mass, strength, and function. Although some forms of exercise are often helpful, this needs to be carefully assessed. The aim of management is to prevent overuse and subsequent deterioration; the key is to find the correct balance between activity and rest with careful prioritizing, planning, and pacing of activities, lifestyle modification, and the provision of assistive devices including orthoses, braces, and corsets. The importance of muscular training is supported by randomized controlled trials and a significant body of literature, as outlined in several reviews [59–61]. Graded exercise can improve symptoms of fatigue, weakness, and pain and non-swimming exercise in warm water is often helpful in conditioning to exercise, improving mobility, and reducing pain. However, there is uncontrolled and anecdotal evidence that regular graded exercise should be broken up by regularly spaced periods of rest.

Respiratory management

Patients with impaired respiratory function should be closely monitored and must be aware of the signs of a developing chest infection. They should have a prophylactic supply of antibiotics, receive influenza and pneumococcal immunization, and avoid smoking. It is essential that patients with known respiratory muscle weakness are monitored regularly with FVC measurements (erect and supine) and nocturnal oximetry.

Other aspects

Excess weight contributes to impaired mobility, the development of osteoarthrosis, and respiratory insufficiency because of hypoventilation and obstructive sleep apnoea. Weight loss is often very difficult because of the reduced mobility and a dietician is an extremely important member of the medical team. The most important factor, however, is the development of a graded exercise regime suited to the individual.

Pain management can be difficult as pain is often generalized, not localized to a joint or a limb. Simple physical measures such as warmth, cold, massage, or passive stretching may be of great value. Transcutaneous electrical nerve stimulation and acupuncture are also extremely helpful in some situations. Analgesics, particularly non-steroidal anti-inflammatory drugs, are required by some patients, particularly where there is an inflammatory component. In some patients a more holistic approach to long-term pain management will be provided by a pain clinic.

Fatigue is particularly difficult to treat. Many factors contribute to its development and exclusion of an underlying disorder is essential before effective management can be undertaken. The most important aspect of treating fatigue is the development of a graded exercise programme with clear and achievable goals. A variety of medications including pyridostigmine and modafanil have not proved helpful. Mild improvements have been reported with intravenous immunoglobulin, but the functional benefits remain doubtful [69,70].

These patients are particularly prone to depression, and coexisting anxiety is also common. Whilst treatment with antidepressants and anxiolytics is often helpful, there is no doubt that cognitive behavioural therapy is rapidly emerging as an extremely valuable tool in management.

A considerable burden falls on the carers, who have often been the only support for decades. They must be recognized, supported, and involved in ongoing rehabilitation and management.

The British Polio Society (<http://www.britishpolio.org>) provides a unique and invaluable resource for patients and their families. The society is unfailingly supportive and knowledgeable about the condition and the provision of rehabilitation, self-management, welfare benefits, disability equipment, housing, and holiday accommodation. Over many years this organization has undertaken much vociferous and highly effective lobbying on behalf of polio patients in particular, and the disabled in general.

Prognosis

Experience suggests that post-polio functional deterioration is not necessarily an on-going process. Fatigue and reduced mobility often may progress only slowly, or stabilize. The extent of functional deterioration also depends on the severity of the existing disability. The prognosis will also depend on the nature of any underlying cause for the functional deterioration.

Important websites

British Polio Society: <http://www.britishpolio.org>
Post-Polio Health International: <http://www.post-polio.org>. This is an important US organization providing regular information concerning research, aetiology, and management of post-polio disability.
www.ott.zynet.co.uk/polio/lincolnshire/—An extremely helpful resource centre established by a UK regional group with valuable and accurate links to relevant papers and clinical and research sites.
Global Polio Eradication Initiative: <http://www.polioeradication.org>. Outlines the history of poliomyelitis and the present global strategy for polio eradication.
www.who.int/vaccines/casecounts.cfm—Another WHO site containing detailed analysis of all world-wide reported cases of acute flaccid paralysis and acute poliomyelitis.

References

1. Gould T. *A Summer Plague—Polio and its Survivors*. New Haven, CT: Yale University Press, 1995.
2. Modlin JF. The bumpy road to polio eradication. *N Engl J Med* 2010; **362**: 2346–9.
3. Butcher J. Polio eradication nears the end game. *Lancet Neurol* 2008; **7**: 292–3.
4. Heymann DL, Aylward RB. Eradicating polio. *N Engl J Med* 2004; **351**: 1275–7.
5. *Geneva Declaration for the Eradication of Poliomyelitis*. Geneva: World Health Organization, 2004.
6. Lancet. Poliomyelitis-eradication initiative's wider lessons. *Lancet* 2004; **363**; 93.
7. Kidd D, Williams A, Howard RS. Classical diseases revisited—poliomyelitis. *Postgrad Med J* 1996; **72**: 641–7.
8. Russell WR. Paralytic poliomyelitis -the early symptoms and the effect of physical activity on the course of the disease. *Br Med J* 1949; **i**: 465–71.
9. Anderson GW, Rondeau SL. Absence of tonsils as a factor in the development of bulbar poliomyelitis. *J Am Med Assoc* 1954; **155**: 1123–30.
10. Kilpatrick DR, Nottay B, Yang C-F, et al. Group specific identification of poliovirus by PCR using primers containing mixed-base or

deoxyinosine residues at positions of codon degeneracy. *J Clin Microbiol* 1996; **34**: 2990–6.

11. Sejvar JJ. West Nile virus and 'poliomyelitis'. *Neurology* 2004; **63**: 206–7.
12. Solomon T, Willison HJ. Infectious causes of acute flaccid paralysis. *Curr Opin Infect Dis* 2003; **16**: 375–81.
13. Ooi MH, Wong SC, Lewthwaite P, et al. Clinical features, diagnosis, and management of enterovirus 71. *Lancet Neurol* 2010; **9**: 1097–105.
14. Marx A, Glass JD, Sutter RW. Differential diagnosis of acute flaccid paralysis and its role in poliomyelitis surveillance. *Epidemiol Rev* 2000; **22**: 298–316.
15. Rosen FS. Conquering polio: isolation of poliovirus—John Enders and the Nobel Prize. *N Engl J Med* 2004; **351**: 1481–3.
16. Lepow ML. Conquering polio: advances in virology—Weller and Robbins. *N Engl J Med* 2004; **351**: 1483–5.
17. Pearce JMS. Salk and Sabin: poliomyelitis immunisation. *J Neurol Neurosurg Psychiatry* 2004; **75**: 1552.
18. Katz SL. Conquering polio: from culture to vaccine—Salk and Sabin. *N Engl J Med* 2004; **351**: 1485–7.
19. Alexander LN, Seward JF, Santbanez TA, et al. Vaccine policy change and epidemiology of poliomyelitis in the United States. *J Am Med Assoc* 2004; **292**: 1696–701.
20. Kew OM, Wright PF, Agol VI, et al., Circulating vaccine-derived polioviruses; current state of knowledge. *Bull WHO* 2004; **82**: 16–23.
21. Jenkins HE, Aylward RB, Gasasira A, et al. Implications of a circulating vaccine-derived poliovirus in Nigeria. *N Engl J Med* 2010; **362**: 2360–9.
22. *Report of the WHO Consultation on Identification and Management of Vaccine-derived Polioviruses*. Geneva: World Health Organization (in press)
23. Fine PEM. Poliomyelitis: very small risks and very large risks. *Lancet Neurology* 2004; **3**: 703.
24. Graham JM. Post-polio deterioration. *Pract Neurol* 2004; **4**: 58–9.
25. Halstead LS. The lessons and legacies of polio. In: Halstead LS, Grimby G (ed), *Post-polio Syndrome*, pp. 199–214. Philadelphia, PA: Henley and Belfus, 1995.
26. Gallagher HG. Growing old with polio—a personal perspective. In: Halstead LS, Grimby G (ed), *Post-polio Syndrome*, pp. 215–22. Philadelphia, PA: Henley and Belfus, 1995.
27. Dalakas MC, Elder G, Hallett M, et al. A long-term follow-up study of patients with post-poliomyelitis neuromuscular symptoms. *N Engl J Med* 1986; **314**: 959–63.
28. Dalakas MC, Hallett M. The post polio syndrome. In: Plum F (ed) *Advances in Contemporary Neurology*, pp. 51–94. Philadelphia, PA: FA Davis, 1988.
29. Dalakas M. The post-polio syndrome as an evolved clinical entity. Definition and clinical description. *Ann NY Acad Sci* 1995; **753**: 68–80.
30. Trojan DA, Cashman NR. Post-poliomyelitis syndrome. *Muscle Nerve* 2005; **31**: 6–19.
31. Howard RS, Wiles CM, Spencer GT. The late sequelae of poliomyelitis. *Q J Med* 1988; **251**: 219–32.
32. Kidd D, Howard RS, Williams AJ, Heatley FW, Panayiotopoulos CP, Spencer GT. Late functional deterioration following paralytic poliomyelitis. *Q J Med* 1997; **90**: 189–96.
33. Windebank AI, Litchey WJ, Daub JR, Kurland LT, Codd MB, Iverson R. Late effects of paralytic poliomyelitis in Olmsted County Minnesota. *Neurology* 1991; **41**: 501–7.
34. Howard RS. Late post-polio functional deterioration. *Pract Neurol* 2003; **3**: 66–77.
35. Bridgens R, Sturman S, Davidson C on behalf of the British Polio Fellowship expert Panel. Post-polio syndrome—polio's legacy. *Clin Med* 2010; **10**: 213–14.
36. Editorial. Late sequelae of poliomyelitis. *Lancet* 1986; **ii**: 1195–6.
37. Halstead L, Wiechers D, Rossi D. Late effects of poliomyelitis: a national survey. In: Halstead L, Wiechers D (ed) *Late Effects of Poliomyelitis*, p. 11. Miami, FL: Symposia Foundation, 1985.
38. Jubelt B. Post-polio syndrome. *Curr Treat Options Neurol* 2004; **6**: 87–93.

39. Sorenson EJ, Daube JR, Windebank AJ. A 15 year follow-up of neuromuscular function in patients with prior poliomyelitis. *N Engl J Med* 2005; **64**: 1070–2.
40. Klingman J, Chui H, Corgiat M, Perry J. Functional recovery. A major risk factor for the development of postpoliomyelitis muscular atrophy. *Arch Neurol* 1988; **45**: 645–7.
41. Trojan DA, Cashman NR, Shapiro S, et al. Predictive factors for post-poliomyelitis syndrome. *Arch Phys Med Rehabil* 1994; **75**: 770–7.
42. Wilson H, Kidd D, Howard RS, Williams AJ. Calf hypertrophy following paralytic poliomyelitis. *Postgrad Med J* 2000; **76**: 179–81.
43. Emeryk B, Rowińska-Marcińska K, Ryniewicz B, Hausmanowa-Petrusewicz I. Disintegration of the motor unit in post-polio syndrome. Part II. Electrophysiological findings in patients with post-polio syndrome. *Electromyogr Clin Neurophysiol* 1990; **30**: 451–8.
44. Cashman NR, Maselli R, Wollmann RL, et al. Late denervation in patients with antecedent paralytic poliomyelitis. *N Engl J Med* 1987: **317**: 7–12.
45. Daube JR, Windebank AJ, Litchy WJ. Electrophysiologic changes in neuromuscular function over five years in polio survivors. *Ann NY Acad Sci* 1995; **753**: 120–8.
46. McComas AJ, Quartly C, Griggs RC. Early and late losses of motor units after poliomyelitis. *Brain* 1997; **120**: 1415–21.
47. Sharief MK, Hentges R, Ciardi M. Intrathecal immune response in patients with the post-polio syndrome. *N Engl J Med* 1991; **325**: 749–55.
48. Leon-Monzon ME, Dalakas MC. Detection of poliovirus antibodies and poliovirus genome in patients with the post-polio syndrome. *Ann NY Acad Sci* 1995; **753**: 208–18.
49. Muir P, Nicholson F, Spencer GT, et al. Enterovirus infection of the central nervous system of humans: lack of association with chronic neurological disease. *J Gen Virol* 1996; **77**: 1469–76.
50. Pezeshkpour GH, Dalakas MC. Long-term changes in the spinal cords of patients with old poliomyelitis. Signs of continuous disease activity. *Arch Neurol* 1988; **45**: 505–8.
51. Salazar-Grueso EF, Grimaldi LM, Roos RP, et al. Isoelectric focusing studies of serum and cerebrospinal fluid in patients with antecedent poliomyelitis. *Ann Neurol* 1989; **26**: 709–13.
52. Martyn CN, Barker DJP, Osmond C. Motoneurone disease and postpoliomyelitis in England and Wales. *Lancet* 1988; **i**: 1319–22.
53. Martyn CN. Poliovirus and motor neurone disease. *J Neurol* 1990; **237**: 336–8.
54. Armon C, Daube JR, Windebank AJ, Kurland LT. How frequently does classic amyotrophic lateral sclerosis develop in survivors of poliomyelitis? *Neurology* 1990; **40**: 172–4.
55. Swingler RJ, Frazer H, Warlow CP. Motor neurone disease and polio in Scotland. *J Neurol Neurosurg Psychiatry* 1992; **55**: 1116–20.
56. Howard RS, Davidson C. Long term ventilation in neurogenic respiratory failure. *J Neurol Neurosurg Psychiatry* 2003; **74** (Suppl III): iii24–iii30.
57. Steljes DG, Kryger MH, Kirk BW, Millar TW. Sleep in postpolio syndrome. *Chest* 1990; **98**: 133–40.
58. Chroni E, Howard RS, Panayiotopoulos CP, Spencer GT. Multiple sclerosis presenting as late functional deterioration after poliomyelitis. *Postgrad Med J* 1995; **71**: 52–4.
59. Farbu E, Gilhus NE, Barnes MP, et al. EFNS guideline on diagnosis and management of post-polio syndrome. Report of an EFNS task force. *Eur J Neurol* 2006; **13**: 795–801.
60. Jubelt B, Agre JC. Characteristics and management of post-polio syndrome. *J Am Med Assoc* 2000; **284**: 412–14.
61. Gonzalez H, Olsson T, Borg K. Management of postpolio syndrome. *Lancet Neurol* 2010; **9**; 634–42.
62. Chan KM, Amirjani N, Sumrain M, et al. Randomized controlled trial of strength training in post-polio patients. *Muscle Nerve* 2003; **27**: 332–8.

63. Waring WP, Maynard F, Grady W, et al. Influence of appropriate lower extremity orthotic management on ambulation, pain, and fatigue in a postpolio population. *Arch Phys Med Rehabil* 1989; **70**: 371–5.

64. Nollet F, de Visser M. Postpolio syndrome. *Arch Neurol* 2004; **61**: 1142–4.

65. Jubelt B. Post-polio syndrome. *Curr Treat Options Neurol* 2004; **6**: 87–93.

66. Horemans HL, Nollet F, Beelen A, et al. Pyridostigmine in postpolio syndrome: no decline in fatigue and limited functional improvement. *J Neurol Neurosurg Psychiatry* 2003; **74**: 1655–61.

67. Stein DP, Dambrosia JM, Dalakas MC. A double-blind, placebo-controlled trial of amantadine for the treatment of fatigue in patients with the post-polio syndrome. *Ann NY Acad Sci* 1995; **753**: 296–302.

68. Vasconcelos OM, Prokhorenko OA, Salajegheh MK, et al. Modafinil for treatment of fatigue in post-polio syndrome: a randomized controlled trial. *Neurology* 2007; **68**: 1680–6.

69. Farbu E, Rekand T, Vik-Mo E, et al. Post-polio syndrome patients treated with intravenous immunoglobulin: a double-blinded randomized controlled pilot study. *Eur J Neurol* 2007; **14**: 60–5.

70. Gonzalez H, Sunnerhagen KS, Sjöberg I et al. Intravenous immunoglobulin for post-polio syndrome: a randomised controlled trial. *Lancet Neurol* 2006; **5**: 493–500.

SECTION 3

Peripheral Nerve: Inherited

CHAPTER 8

Charcot–Marie–Tooth disease

Mary M. Reilly and Alexander M. Rossor

Introduction

In 1886, Jean-Martin Charcot and Pierre Marie in Paris and Howard Tooth in London independently published a series of patients with distal wasting and weakness. Whilst Charcot and Marie hypothesized that the pathology resided in the spinal cord, Tooth proposed that the disease was a peripheral nerve disorder. In recognition of their work, the disease they described is now referred to as Charcot–Marie–Tooth disease (CMT), a relatively common hereditary disease of the peripheral nerves with a prevalence of 1 in 2500 [1].

Following its original description it became apparent that CMT could be classified into autosomal dominant (AD), autosomal recessive (AR), and X-linked forms. Following the development of modern neurophysiology in the second half of the twentieth century, Dyck, Gilliatt, and Thomas further subclassified patients with CMT on the basis of their nerve conduction velocities into those with slow conduction and a presumed demyelinating pathology (CMT1) and those with normal or near normal velocities and a presumed primary axonal pathology (CMT2) [2].

The classification of CMT based on the mode of inheritance and neurophysiology further evolved in 1991 with the discovery of a duplication of part of chromosome 17 containing the gene peripheral myelin protein 22 (*PMP22*) as the cause of the commonest subtype of CMT, CMT1 [3]. Since then more than 40 genes have been identified, and as such CMT can be considered an encompassing term for a group of inherited peripheral neuropathies with a variety of aetiologies.

Terminology

CMT refers to a group of inherited neuropathies in which the neuropathy is the main or sole feature of the disease. This is in contrast to a host of inherited neurological and multisystem diseases in which the peripheral neuropathy forms only part of the disease (see Table 8.1). Within the broad category of CMT, those with a predominantly motor neuropathy are termed distal hereditary motor neuropathy (dHMN) or distal spinal muscular atrophy (dSMA; see Chapter 6) and those with a predominantly sensory picture, hereditary sensory neuropathy (HSN) (also called hereditary sensory and autonomic neuropathy/HSAN; see Chapter 9). Patients with an inherited mixed sensory and motor neuropathy are classified as having *bone fide* CMT, although in reality all patients have a mixed sensory and motor neuropathy, with those patients classified as having dHMN or HSN representing extremes of this spectrum. Hereditary neuropathy with liability to pressure palsies (HNPP) and hereditary neuralgic amyotrophy (HNA) may also be considered to be within the remit of CMT and will be covered in this chapter.

Classification

CMT has traditionally been subclassified into demyelinating (CMT1) and axonal (CMT2), based on the motor nerve conduction velocity of the median nerve [4]. Velocities below 38 m s^{-1} are classified as demyelinating and those above 38 m s^{-1} as axonal. Patients in whom the velocities are between 25 and 40 m s^{-1} may be termed 'intermediate' CMT, reflecting the difficulties with a diagnosis based on neurophysiology alone. AD CMT1 and CMT2 may also be referred to as the hereditary motor and sensory neuropathies (HMSN) Types 1 and 2. Autosomal recessive axonal neuropathies are termed ARCMT2 and, confusingly, autosomal recessive demyelinating neuropathies are termed CMT4. If the inheritance is X-linked it is termed CMT1X if demyelinating and CMT2X if axonal. X- linked genetic loci have also been added chronologically, so that the terms CMTX3, -X4, and -X5 also exist [5].

Dejerine–Sottas disease (DSD) and congenital hypomyelinating neuropathies (CHN) describe severe demyelinating neuropathies beginning in infancy. The disease was originally thought to be due to autosomal recessive mutations and was termed CMT3 or HMSN Type III. In UK and North American populations it is now known that such patients are more likely to have a *de novo* dominant mutation in one of the more common AD CMT1 genes, although autosomal recessive inheritance is occasionally seen [6]. The terms DSD and CHN may still be used, but it is clearer to refer to the phenotype as severe CMT1 in AD or *de novo* dominant cases, and CMT4 with infantile onset in the case of AR inheritance.

Approach to diagnosis

Is it hereditary?

Once it has been established that the patient has a peripheral neuropathy, the next step is to determine whether the neuropathy is likely to be genetic. If there is a positive family history, an affected parent or child of the index case makes AD or X-linked inheritance likely (clear evidence of male to male transmission rules out X-linked inheritance). Unaffected consanguineous parents of an affected patient and/or multiple affected siblings with unaffected parents make AR inheritance more likely. A family history, however, should not be taken at face value, and if possible other affected family members should be examined. It is important not to delay the diagnosis of a treatable acquired neuropathy on the basis of a history of a deceased parent or distant relative with difficulty walking in old age.

A number of patients with CMT, however, will not have a positive family history. Some of these apparently sporadic cases turn out to have a mildly affected parent, reflecting the phenotypic heterogeneity even for the same causative gene. Others turn out to

Table 8.1 A summary of inherited diseases in which neuropathy forms the sole part of the disease or is part of a more complex disorderi

Neuropathy as the main or sole feature of the disease
• Charcot–Marie–Tooth disease (CMT)
• Hereditary neuropathy with liability to pressure palsies (HNPP)
• Hereditary sensory and autonomic neuropathy (HSAN)
• Distal hereditary motor neuropathy (dHMN)
• Hereditary neuralgic amyotrophy (HNA)
Neuropathy as part of complex neurological or multi system disease
• Familial amyloid polyneuropathy
• Disturbances of lipid metabolism
• Leucodystrophies, e.g. adrenomyeloneuropathy
• Lipoprotein deficiencies, e.g. Tangier disease
• Peroxisomal storage diseases, e.g. Refsum disease
• α-Galactosidase deficiency, (Fabry disease)
• Cholestanolosis, e.g. cerebrotendinous xanthomatosis
• Porphyrias, e.g. acute intermittent porphyria
• Neuropathies associated with mitochondrial disease, e.g. neuropathy, ataxia and retinitis pigmentosa (NARP)
• Neuropathies associated with hereditary ataxias, e.g. Fredreich ataxia, ataxia with oculomotor apraxia (AOA2), autosomal recessive spinal cerebellar ataxia of Charlevoix Saguenay (ARSACS, demyelinating neuropathy), fragile X tremor ataxia syndrome, spinocerebellar ataxias.
• Disorders with defective DNA, e.g. ataxia telangiectasia, Cockayne syndrome, xeroderma pigmentosa

have either *de novo* dominant mutations in the common AD genes or a recessive mutation. In northern Europe and North America *de novo* mutations are probably more common, whereas in other parts of the world where consanguineous marriage is more prevalent, recessive mutations are a more likely cause.

Clues to the diagnosis in apparently sporadic cases include early onset and slow insidious progression. Poor performance in sport at school, frequent ankle sprains, and failed public service medicals may also point towards an inherited neuropathy. Clinical signs suggestive of CMT can be helpful but also misleading. The classic inverse champagne bottle leg (see Fig. 8.1) is observed in CMT and reflects a length-dependent neuropathy. This is not specific to CMT but can also be seen in some acquired, slowly progressive neuropathies. Similarly, a diagnosis of CMT should not be made solely on the basis of pes cavus without an appropriate history. Whilst some patients have obvious pes cavus, there is a group of patients who have high arches or wasting of the small muscles of the feet that give the appearance of pes cavus but simply reflect a variant of normal or an acquired and treatable neuropathy. A further clue in apparently sporadic cases is the relative absence of sensory symptoms compared to the degree of sensory loss on clinical and neurophysiological examination. Scoliosis and thickened peripheral nerves are also suggestive of CMT.

Genetic testing

Traditionally, genetic testing in CMT has involved a clinician requesting screening of a candidate gene based on the patient's phenotype and family history. The suggested approach in this scenario is to determine whether the neuropathy is demyelinating (<38 m s^{-1}) or axonal (>38 m s^{-1}) and to then request a specific gene test based on the mode of inheritance (see Fig. 8.2). Fortunately, about 60% of patients with genetically confirmed CMT will achieve a genetic diagnosis by screening for mutations in the four most common genes: *PMP22* (duplication/deletion/point mutation), *GJB1*, *MPZ*, and *MFN2* [7,8]. If the patient has AD CMT1 then the chance of achieving a genetic diagnosis approaches 100%. Unfortunately, each of the remaining identified genes (except *SH3TC2*) accounts for <1% of all cases of CMT. When one also considers that the causative genes for at least 40% of cases of CMT2 are unknown, then using a candidate gene approach can be costly and time-consuming. The diagnostic 'hit rate' for CMT2 can be improved by directing testing on the basis of phenotype and ethnic origin (see Table 8.1), although there is considerable phenotypic overlap between different genes.

The testing of individual genes has traditionally relied on 'Sanger sequencing', the same technology that was used to sequence the human genome for the first time. The advent of so-called 'next generation sequencing' allows the entire genome or exome (targeting only the protein-coding sequences of the human genome) to be sequenced at an increasingly affordable price and practical time scale. The challenge faced by this method is the exclusion of the many thousands of irrelevant polymorphisms and non-pathogenic variants in known CMT genes in the same individual. A vital role for the practising clinician in determining the mode of inheritance and phenotype of the patient is required to help exclude polymorphisms and identify the pathogenic variant. In addition to the requirement for complex bioinformatics it must also be appreciated that the genomic coverage from next generation technology is currently incomplete and may miss pathogenic mutations, copy number variations, long repeat sequences, and non-exonic variants.

Whilst the cost of these technologies continues to fall, for many the financial burden precludes its use in routine clinical diagnostics [9].

Methods for the detection of genomic rearrangements (insertions and deletions)

Genomic rearrangements (duplications and deletions of segments of DNA), often as a result of homologous recombination, are a recognized cause of CMT and include the most common cause of CMT, the 17p duplication. Importantly, large insertions and deletions may be missed using both Sanger and next generation sequencing technology. There are several methods employed to detect genomic rearrangements, the most commonly used of which is multiplex ligation-dependent probe amplification (MLPA) [10]. MLPA is now widely used in most diagnostic laboratories to detect rearrangements and can also detect small deletions that have been missed using PCR and microsatellite analysis. It may be necessary to request MLPA analysis of a gene when the clinical suspicion of a mutation is high but Sanger sequencing has failed to identify a mutation.

CMT genes

Table 8.2 gives a summary of the different subtypes of CMT including many of the known genes and loci.

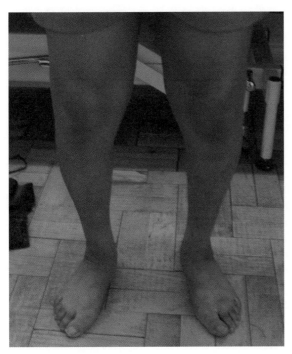

Fig. 8.1 Inverse champagne bottle legs.

CMT1

CMT1A

CMT1A is the commonest genetic subtype of CMT (see Fig. 8.3) accounting for 60–70% of all cases [11]. Patients usually present with lower limb motor symptoms including difficulty running, frequent trips, and ankle sprains and commonly have foot deformities such as pes cavus [12]. Of these patients, 75% develop symptoms in the first decade, 10% in the second decade, and 7% after the age of

20 years. On clinical examination there is often distal limb weakness, most evident in the lower limbs, with reduced or absent deep tendon reflexes. Sensory symptoms, however, are often minimal despite evidence of length-dependent sensory loss on examination [12]. Other clinical features include kyphoscoliosis, tremor, and thickened nerves [13]. Neurophysiology demonstrates slowing of the nerve conduction velocity in all carriers which is typically uniform across all peripheral nerves, with median motor nerve conduction velocities in the order of 20 m s^{-1} (range 7–33).

CMT1A is usually a slowly progressive disease with no effect on life expectancy [14]. It is very important to highlight this when delivering a new diagnosis of CMT1A. Most patients with CMT1A will remain ambulant but may require orthotic or other support with increasing disease duration [13]. Nerve biopsies show demyelination and remyelination with onion bulb formation [15]; however, widespread access to genetic testing has meant that nerve biopsy no longer plays a role in the diagnosis of CMT1A.

The vast majority of cases of CMT1A are due to a duplication of approximately 1.4 million base pairs on chromosome 17p11.1-012 [3]. This region is flanked by highly homologous repeat sequences predisposing it to unequal crossing over during meiosis and explaining the high prevalence of the duplication in the population [16]. The Peripheral Myelin Protein 22 (*PMP22*) gene is contained within the 1.4 million base pair region and is the gene responsible for the CMT1A phenotype [18–21]. CMT1A may therefore be considered a gene dosage disease, and in individuals with homozygous duplications (two-fold increase in *PMP22* expression), the disease severity is increased accordingly [17]. Intriguingly, deletions in the *PMP22* gene result in the disease HNPP, illustrating the delicate balance of *PMP22* expression in normal myelination and peripheral nerve function [18].

The mechanism by which overexpression of the PMP22 protein results in CMT1A is uncertain. It has been postulated that

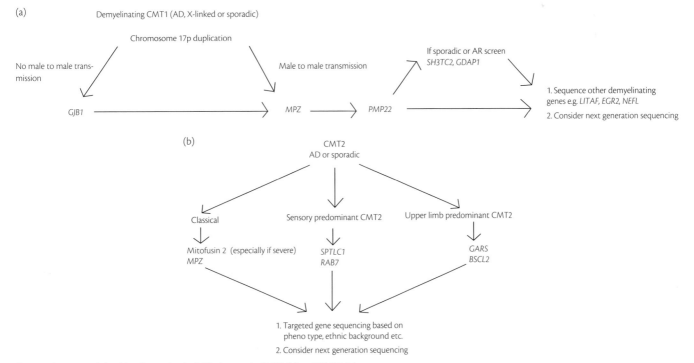

Fig. 8.2 A suggested algorithm for testing individual genes in CMT1 (a) and CMT2 (b).

Table 8.2 A summary of the different subtypes of Charcot–Marie–Tooth disease, including many of the known genes and loci

Type	Gene	Phenotype
Autosomal dominant CMT1 (AD CMT1)		
CMT1A	17p duplication (*PMP22*)	Classic CMT1
	PMP22 point mutation	Classic CMT1/DSD/CHN (rarely recessive)
CMT1B	*MPZ*	CMT1/DSD/CHN/CMT2 (rarely recessive)
CMT1C	*LITAF*	Classic CMT1
CMT1D	*EGR2*	Classic CMT1/DSD/CHN
CMT1F	*NEFL*	CMT2 but can have slow motor nerve conduction velocity in the CMT1 range
Hereditary neuropathy with liability to pressure palsies (HNPP)	Del 17p (*PMP22*)	Typical HNPP
	PMP22 (point mutation)	Typical HNPP
Autosomal recessive CMT1 (CMT4/ARCMT1)		
CMT4A	*GDAP1*	CMT1 or CMT2, usually severe early onset. Vocal cord and diaphragmatic paralysis described
CMT4B1	*MTMR2*	Severe CMT1/facial/bulbar/focally folded myelin
CMT4B2	*MTMR13*	Severe CMT1/glaucoma/focally folded myelin
CMT4C	*SH3TC2*	Severe CMT1/scoliosis/cytoplasmic inclusions
CMT4D (HMSNL)	*NDRG1*	Severe CMT1/gypsy/deafness/tongue atrophy
CMT4E	*EGR2*	CMT1/DSD/CHN phenotype
CMT4F	*PRX*	CMT1/more sensory/focally folded myelin
CMT4G (HMSN Russe)	*HK1*	Severe early onset CMT1/gypsy
CMT4H	*FGD4* (Frabin)	Classic CMT1
CMT4J	*FIG4*	CMT1/ predominantly motor/progressive
CCFDN	*CTDP1*	CMT1/gypsy/cataracts/dysmorphic features
Autosomal dominant CMT2 (AD CMT2)		
CMT2A	*MFN2*	CMT2/progressive/optic atrophy (rarely recessive)
CMT2B	*RAB7*	CMT2 with sensory complications (ulceromutilating)
CMT2C	*TRPV4*	CMT2/vocal cord paralysis
CMT2D	*GARS*	CMT2 with predominant hand wasting/dHMN Type V
dHMN Type V	*BSCL2*	dHMN Type V with predominant hand wasting/Silver syndrome, but can have sensory involvement like CMT2D
CMT2E	*NEFL*	CMT2 but can have nerve conduction velocity in the CMT1 range (rarely recessive CMT1)
CMT2F	*HSPB1*	Motor-predominant CMT2
CMT2G	12q12-q13.3	CMT2
CMT2I	*MPZ*	Late-onset CMT2
CMT2J	*MPZ*	CMT2 with hearing loss and pupillary abnormalities
CMT2K	*GDAP1*	Late-onset CMT2 (dominant)/severe CMT2 (recessive)
CMT2L	*HSPB8*	Motor-predominant CMT2
CMT2N	*AARS*	Classic CMT2
HMSN-P, Okinawa type	3q13.1	CMT2 with proximal involvement (optineurin spinal cord inclusions described)
CMT2P	*LRSAM1*	Mild sensory-predominant CMT2 (dominant and recessive)
SPG10	*KIF5A*	CMT2/hereditary spastic paraplegia
Autosomal recessive CMT2		
CMT2B1	*LMNA*	CMT2 rapid progression
CMT2B2	*MED25*	Classic CMT2

(continued)

Table 8.2 Continued

Type	Gene	Phenotype
X-linked CMT		
CMTX1	GJB1	Males CMT1 (patchy nerve conduction velocity)/females CMT2
CMTX2	Xp22.2	Intermediate CMT/infantile onset/learning disability
CMTX3	Xq26	Intermediate CMT
CMTX4 (Cowchock syndrome)	Xq24-26.1	CMT2/infantile onset/developmental delay/deafness/learning difficulties
CMTX5	PRPS1	CMT2/deafness/optic atrophy
Dominant intermediate CMT (CMTDI)		
CMTDIA	10q24.1-q25.1	Intermediate CMT
CMTDIB/CMT2M	DNM2	Intermediate CMT or CMT2/cataracts/ophthalmoplegia/ptosis
CMTDIC	YARS	Intermediate CMT
CMTDID	MPZ	Intermediate CMT
CMTDIE	IFN2	Intermediate CMT/focal segmental glomerulosclerosis/end-stage renal failure
Recessive intermediate CMT (RI-CMT)		
CMTRIA	GDAP1	Intermediate CMT
CMTRIB	KARS	Intermediate CMT/learning difficulty/vestibular schwannoma

CMT, Charcot–Marie–Tooth disease; DSD, Dejerine–Sottas disease; CHN, congenital hypomyelinating neuropathy; HMSN, hereditary motor and sensory neuropathy; dHMN, distal hereditary motor neuropathy.

its overexpression may lead to aberrant interaction with myelin protein zero (MPZ) [19,20] or may disrupt endosomal sorting of PMP22 to the cell membrane [21].

Point mutations in *PMP22* have also been reported to cause CMT1, but are a less common cause of CMT than the 17p duplication (1–5%), and may cause both CMT1A and HNPP, even within the same family [22]. The clinical phenotype of patients with point mutations in *PMP22* may vary and include more severe CMT1 than that seen with CMT1A. Occasionally the median motor nerve conduction velocities seen with *PMP22* point mutations are above 38 m s^{-1} [23,24].

CMT1B

CMT1B is the second commonest type of AD CMT and is due to mutations in *MPZ*, which encodes MPZ, a major myelin protein that is exclusively expressed in myelinating Schwann cells [25]. There is considerable phenotypic heterogeneity amongst patients with *MPZ* mutations, although most patients can be divided into one of three phenotypic categories: early onset, adult onset, and classical CMT [26].

Early onset

Patients in this category often present with delayed motor milestones and would previously have been described as having CHN or DSD. Whilst the disease can be severe, with 10% requiring a wheelchair in the third decade, life expectancy is usually unaffected [27,28]. Motor nerve conduction velocities in the upper limbs are often below 15 m s^{-1}.

Adult-onset neuropathy

Most patients with late-onset CMT1B develop symptoms in the fourth decade [26]. The severity and rate of progression is variable, with some patients requiring use of a wheelchair by 50 years of age and others remaining relatively mildly affected. Nerve conduction velocities are faster than the early onset group and in many are greater than 30 m s^{-1} in the upper limbs. Furthermore, a small group of patients with late-onset *MPZ* neuropathy may have nerve conduction velocities in the axonal range.

Classic phenotype

Patients in this subgroup present identically to CMT1A, developing symptoms and signs of a neuropathy in the second decade of life. Unlike CMT1A, however, nerve conduction velocities are often slower (<15 m s^{-1} in the upper limbs) [29].

CMT1C

Mutations in lipopolysaccharide induced transcription factor (*LITAF*) have been identified as the cause of CMT1C [30]. It is a rare form of CMT1 and presents almost identically to CMT1A with onset in the second decade of life and with nerve conduction velocities in the upper limb of approximately 25 m s^{-1} (range 15–35) [31].

CMT1D

The Early Growth Response 2 (*EGR2*) gene encodes a protein that serves as an essential transcription factor for peripheral nerve myelination and may cause both AD (CMT1D) and AR (CMT4E) demyelinating CMT [32,33]. Patients can be divided into those with a severe infantile-onset neuropathy (DSD/CHN) and those with an adolescent-onset, slowly progressive neuropathy [34].

Patients with infantile-onset disease may present with hypotonia and respiratory difficulties and have motor nerve conduction velocities as low as 8 m s^{-1} in the upper limbs [6]. Such patients may also demonstrate focally folded myelin on nerve biopsy. Patients with later-onset CMT1D typically develop symptoms in the first and second decade and have nerve conduction velocities similar to CMT1A (about 20 m s^{-1} in the upper limbs) [34]. Ocular cranial nerve palsies, scoliosis, vocal cord paralysis, and deafness have also been described [35].

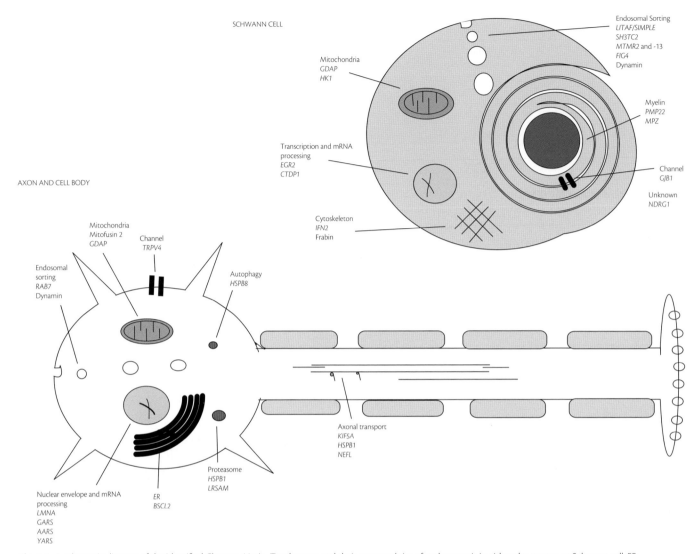

Fig. 8.3 A schematic diagram of the identified Charcot–Marie–Tooth genes and their proposed site of pathogenesis in either the neuron or Schwann cell. ER, endoplasmic reticulum.

CMT1F

CMT1F is unusual in that whilst it may be classified as a demyelinating neuropathy neurophysiologically, the underlying pathological defect is axonal. It is due to heterozygous mutations in the Neurofilament Light Chain (*NEFL*) gene, one of three neurofilaments (light, medium, and heavy chains; NEFL, NEFM, and NEFH) that form the most abundant intermediate cytoskeletal proteins in both central and peripheral nerve axons [36]. Patients may present from infancy to the second decade of life with features of a length-dependent neuropathy and nerve conduction velocities that can be classified as CMT1, CMT2, or intermediate CMT [37]. Deafness and global developmental delay are rare additional features and cases of AR CMT2 have also been described [37,38].

Autosomal recessive demyelinating CMT (CMT4)

CMT4A

Mutations in the ganglioside-induced differentiation-associated protein 1(*GDAP1*) gene, encoding a mitochondrial protein

expressed in the outer mitochondrial membrane [39], can cause both an AR axonal or demyelinating neuropathy and, rarely, an AD axonal neuropathy.

Recessive mutations in *GDAP1* lead to a severe infantile-onset neuropathy often associated with vocal cord and diaphragmatic paralysis [40]. AD axonal CMT (CMT2K) tends to follow a milder course, with a variable age of onset ranging from the first year of life to the fifth decade. The majority of patients with AD mutations remain ambulant, although some have been reported to require the use of a wheelchair in the seventh decade [41].

CMT4B1

Mutations in the Myotubularin-related protein 2 (*MTMR2*) gene result in a severe, early onset demyelinating neuropathy (CMT4B1) characterized by prominent facial weakness and the presence of 'myelin out-folding' on nerve biopsy [42]. It is an aggressive infantile-onset disease, often requiring non-invasive ventilation due to diaphragmatic involvement and with loss of ambulation by the third decade [43,44]. Motor nerve conduction velocities, when recordable, range from 9–20 m s^{-1}.

CMT4B2

Mutations in *MTMR13* have been described in families with AR demyelinating CMT4B2 from Turkey [45], Tunisia, Morocco, and Japan [46,47]. It is a milder disease than CMT4B1, often presenting before 5 years of age but with most carriers remaining ambulant into their third decade [45]. Cataracts are a common feature.

CMT4C

SH3TC2 encodes a 144 kDa protein with two N-terminal SH3 domains and five C-terminal TPR motifs. Mutations in this gene result in a form of AR demyelinating CMT (CMT4C) with early and prominent scoliosis. It is the commonest form of AR demyelinating neuropathy and should be considered in apparently sporadic cases of demyelinating CMT. Disease onset is in the first decade and progression is variable, with those most severely affected requiring a wheelchair by the third decade [48]. Median nerve conduction velocities can range from 4 to 37 m s^{-1} (mean 22 m s^{-1}) [42]. The presence of multiple Schwann cell cytoplasmic processes appears to be a distinguishing feature on nerve biopsy [49].

CMT4D

Mutations in N-myc downstream-regulated gene 1 (*NDRG1*) are responsible for CMT4D [50]. To date, mutations in *NDRG1* have only been described in Romani gypsies of Balkan descent. Disease onset is in the first decade of life. Additional clinical features include tongue hemiatrophy, deafness, and scoliosis.

CMT4F (periaxin)

Mutations in periaxin (*PRX*) have often been described as a cause of severe infantile onset neuropathy. Whilst the disease course can be severe, in many it is slowly progressive and dominated by distal sensory loss [51,52]. A useful clinical feature is the presence of very slow (<5 m s^{-1}) nerve conduction velocities.

CMT4G

Hereditary motor and sensory neuropathy Russe, or CMT4F, is an AR demyelinating neuropathy described in Bulgarian, Romanian, and Spanish gypsies [53,54]. The disease maps to chromosome 10q23 and is thought to be due to mutations in the gene Hexokinase 1 (*HK1*). Patients develop a severe disabling neuropathy beginning in the first and second decades of life. Interestingly, homozygous mutations in *HK1* are a cause of hereditary haemolytic anaemia [55].

CMT4H

CMT4H is due to mutations in *FGD4* encoding the Rho GDP/GTP exchange factor (frabin). The age of onset is in the first decade and may be associated with scoliosis and shortening of the neck [56]. Nerve conduction velocities may be as slow as 8 m s^{-1} in the upper limbs [57]. Myelin out-foldings have been observed in sural nerve biopsies [56].

CMT4J

CMT4J is caused by mutations in the gene *FIG4*. The disease is characterized by an aggressive and severe demyelinating neuropathy that can resemble the progressive muscular atrophy variant of motor neuron disease (MND; see Chapter 4). It is an AR disease in which all reported patients have been compound heterozygotes. The age of onset may vary from the first to the sixth decade, and whilst there is a distal predominance to the weakness, it is often asymmetric with prominent proximal involvement. The disease

course may be interrupted by random and rapid progression of weakness, such as the development of a flail limb on the background of a severe but predictable neuropathy. Respiratory involvement has been described but, unlike MND, bulbar involvement is not a common feature [58].

Like MND there are minimal sensory signs, although in the majority of patients the sural sensory action potential is unrecordable. Nerve conduction studies invariably demonstrate slowing of approximately 20 m s^{-1}, although a median nerve conduction velocity of 37 m s^{-1} has been described in a 15-year-old patient, indicating that conduction velocities may be in the axonal range in the first and second decades. The same individual progressed to the use of a wheelchair at the age of 20 [59].

CTDP1

Congenital cataract, facial dysmorphism and neuropathy syndrome is an autosomal recessive, multisystem disorder described in Bulgarian gypsies [60]. Affected individuals develop a distal demyelinating motor and sensory neuropathy accompanied by congenital cataracts and microcornea, facial dysmorphism, and delayed intellectual development. Mild non-progressive cognitive impairment, chorea, postural tremor, and ataxia have also been described. The disease is due to homozygous mutations in the gene, C-terminal-domain phosphatase of RNA polymerase II (*CTDP1*) [61].

Autosomal dominant axonal CMT (CMT2)

CMT2A

CMT2A, due to mutations in the gene Mitofusin 2 (*MFN2*), is the commonest known cause of AD CMT2 affecting between 11 and 30% of CMT2 patients [62]. It is an aggressive disease in comparison with other types of CMT2 with many patients requiring a wheelchair by the age of 20; it is sometimes associated with optic atrophy [63].

Screening for mutations in *MFN2* in patients with suspected or confirmed CMT2 can be arduous due to the high number of novel polymorphisms in this gene. A further matter of confusion is that mutations in *MFN2* have also been reported as a cause of AR CMT2 in which a point mutation in one allele is accompanied by a point mutation or a deletion in the other allele [64]. In this scenario, the deletion will only be detected if MLPA analysis is requested, having important ramifications for genetic counselling.

CMT2B

Mutations in the gene for the small GTPase late endosomal protein, *RAB7*, are a cause of CMT2B, which is very similar to cases of AD HSN. All patients develop distal weakness with moderate to severe sensory loss, and this has led to its classification as CMT2 as opposed to HSN. Despite being classified as CMT, almost all reported patients develop ulceration of the feet complicated by osteomyelitis, and in a significant proportion this may be complicated by amputation. The phenotype is very similar to that due to mutations in *SPTLC1*, the commonest cause of HSN Type I [65].

CMT2C

Dominant mutations in the transient receptor vallanoid 4 gene (*TRPV4*) have been linked to distal hereditary motor neuropathy (distal SMA), scapuloperoneal muscular atrophy (SPMA), congenital SMA and CMT2C [66–68]. The term CMT2C was originally coined by Dyck and colleagues to describe the phenotype of a family with distal wasting and weakness, a variable age of onset from the first to the sixth decade, and the distinguishing feature of vocal cord paralysis and diaphragmatic and intercostal muscle weakness [69]. Vocal cord palsy is present in over half of patients and is often unilateral and asymptomatic [70]. Sensory symptoms, if present, are mild.

CMT2D

CMT2D describes an upper limb, motor-predominant, axonal neuropathy and is linked to mutations in the gene Glycyl-tRNA synthetase (*GARS*), one of 37 nuclear-encoded amino acyl tRNA synthetases that function to attach amino acids onto their respective tRNAs for protein translation [71]. Disease onset is typically in the second decade of life, with the majority of patients functioning independently 40 years after disease onset [72]. The condition is allelic with dHMN Type V, a pure motor and upper limb-predominant neuropathy also due to mutations in *GARS*.

Heterozygous mutations in the gene Berardinelli-Seip congenital lipodystrophy type 2 (*BSCL2*) may also cause an upper limb, motor-predominant neuropathy (see Fig. 8.4), similar to CMT2D and a classic length-dependent neuropathy with brisk or preserved reflexes.

CMT2F

Mutations in the gene Heat Shock Protein B 1 (*HSPB1*), which encodes the ubiquitously expressed molecular chaperone protein HSP27, are the cause of CMT2F. CMT2F typically presents as a length-dependent motor neuropathy with minor or no sensory involvement. The average age of onset is 30 years and the rate of progression is slow, with only a minority of patients requiring a wheelchair in the seventh decade [73]. A useful clinical sign is the presence of ankle plantar flexion weakness either equal to or greater than ankle dorsiflexion weakness early in the disease course.

CMT2L

Mutations in *HSPB8* were first identified as a cause of dHMN in four separate families from the Czech Republic, Belgium, England, and Bulgaria [74], and subsequently in a Chinese family with CMT2 (now designated CMT2L) [75]. Like *HSPB1*, *HSPB8* is a member of the small heat shock family protein genes and codes for the chaperone protein HSP22 [76]. The phenotype of dHMN/CMT2L due to *HSPB8* mutations is indistinguishable from that due to mutations in *HSPB1* [77]. Mutations in *HSPB8* appear to be a much less common cause of neuropathy than in *HSPB1*.

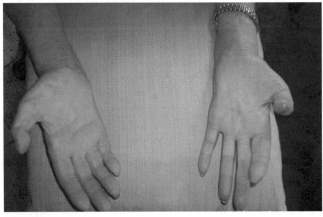

Fig. 8.4 Prominent wasting of the hands in CMT2D.

CMT2N

Mutations in Alanyl tRNA synthetase (*AARS*) have been identified as the cause of CMT2N in two unrelated French families. Symptom onset is typically in the third decade and is characterized by difficulty walking and distal weakness. In one patient there was marked asymmetric wasting of the legs [78].

CMT2P

Frame shift mutations in the gene Leucine-rich Repeat Sterile Alpha Motif-containing 1 (*LRSAM1*) have been identified as a cause of both AD and AR CMT2P in isolated Canadian and Dutch families, respectively. Patients develop symptoms of distal sensory loss in the third decade of life. Distal motor weakness is present but often functionally insignificant [79,80].

SPG10

Mutations in the gene kinesin motor protein *KIF5A* were first identified as a cause of spastic paraplegia type 10 (SPG10), an AD form of hereditary spastic paraplegia (HSP). Patients with SPG10 may present with a pure HSP or with additional features such as an axonal neuropathy, severe upper limb amyotrophy (similar to Silver syndrome), cognitive impairment, Parkinsonism, deafness, and retinitis pigmentosa [81]. Within the spectrum, a minority of patients have been described with pure CMT2 [81,82].

Autosomal recessive CMT2 (AR-CMT2)

CMT2B1

Homozygous mutations in the gene for the nuclear envelope protein lamin A/C (*LMNA*), have been described as a cause of AR CMT2 in families originating from north-west Africa [83–85]. Affected individuals develop an axonal, distal neuropathy with onset in the second decade. The rate of progression varies within families, with some developing proximal weakness early in the disease and others showing little progression [84]. Depending upon the functional domain affected, mutations in *LMNA* may also cause dilated cardiomyopathy, AD and AR Emery–Dreifuss muscular dystrophy, familial partial lipodystrophy, mandibuloacral dysplasia, progeria syndrome, Werner syndrome, and restrictive dermopathy. However, patients with CMT2 due to *LMNA* mutations do not develop audiological, ophthalmological, or cardiac anomalies, although a minority may develop scoliosis in adolescence [84].

CMT2B2

Homozygous mutations in the gene for mediator 25 (*MED25*) were identified in a large, consanguineous Costa Rican family of Spanish descent [86]. Affected individuals present with a length-dependent mixed motor and sensory neuropathy between the ages of 26 and 42 and remain ambulant in later life [87].

X-linked CMT

CMTX1

In 1889, not long after Charcot, Marie, and Tooth's original description of peroneal muscular atrophy, Herringham described a family with peripheral neuropathy in which men were more severely affected than women [88]. It is now known that the cause of the neuropathy in this family was a mutation in the Gap Junction B1 (*GJB1*) gene on the X chromosome, encoding the channel protein connexin 32.

CMT1X is the second most common cause of CMT accounting for 7–11% of all CMT cases [88]. The disease can be considered to be X-linked dominant, although it is usually more severe in men with symptom onset in the first and second decades of life. Positive sensory symptoms, including pain, appear to be relatively common as does the presence of the 'split hand' in which there is selective wasting and weakness of the thenar muscles of the hand with relative sparing of the interossei and hypothenar eminences, also commonly noted in MND [89].

Nerve conduction studies demonstrate a patchy demyelinating neuropathy, although nerve conduction velocities are often in the axonal range in affected females. Temporal dispersion and conduction block are well described and may lead to a misdiagnosis of chronic inflammatory demyelinating polyneuropathy and inappropriate immunosuppression [90,91].

Connexin 32 is also expressed in the central nervous system and it is perhaps not surprising that involvement of the central nervous system, although often asymptomatic, is described [88].

PRPS1 (CMTX5)

CMTX5 or the Rosenberg–Chutorian syndrome (RCS) is an X-linked disorder in which affected individuals develop sensory neuronal hearing loss and both peripheral and optic neuropathy without mental retardation [92]. The disorder is due to missense mutations in the gene Phosphoribosyl pyrophosphatase synthetase 1 (PRPS1), an essential enzyme in the biosynthesis of purines and pyrimidines.

Intermediate CMT

CMTDIB/CMT2M

Mutations in dynamin 2 (DNM2) are associated with both AD intermediate and axonal CMT [93], and also centronuclear myopathy (CNM) [94]. The age of onset may vary from the first to the sixth decade and it is often slowly progressive with no loss of ambulation [95]. Nerve conduction velocities may be in the intermediate ($29–38$ m s^{-1}) or the axonal range. Additional clinical features include neutropenia, cataracts, ptosis, and ophthalmoplegia [93,96].

CMTDIC

Heterozygous missense mutations in Tyrosyl tRNA synthetase (YARS) have been identified as the cause of dominant intermediate (DI) CMT in two unrelated families from Bulgaria and North America [97,98]. Affected individuals presented in the first and second decades of life (the oldest age of presentation being 59) with a motor-predominant length-dependent neuropathy. Nerve conduction velocities were between 30 and 40 m s^{-1} [37].

CMTDIC

Compound heterozygote mutations in lysyl tRNA synthetase (KARS) have been described in a single adopted patient with developmental delay, vestibular schwannoma, self-abusive behaviour, and a peripheral neuropathy with intermediate conduction velocities [99].

CMTDIE

Mutations in INF2 cause a unique syndrome of DI CMT and inherited focal segmental glomerulosclerosis (FSGS) [100]. Affected individuals developed features of a neuropathy in the 1st and 2 decade (range 5 -28 years) and end stage renal failure by 21 years of age (range 12 to 47). No mutations were identified in a cohort of 50 patients with uncomplicated CMT.

Hereditary neuropathy with liability to pressure palsies (HNPP)

HNPP is an autosomal dominant disorder that is most commonly due to a 1.4 Mb deletion of chromosome 17p12 but can also be caused by point mutations in the PMP22 gene. That duplication of the PMP22 gene causes CMT1A and a deletion HNPP, highlights the integral role of PMP22 gene dosage in demyelinating neuropathies. It is an episodic disorder characterised by recurrent, painless motor and sensory entrapment neuropathies often preceded by minimal trauma. It is a fully penetrant disease on neurophysiological examination with symptom onset beginning in adolescence. It is estimated to account for 5% of all cases of CMT which can be extrapolated to a population frequency of 1 in 40 000 [8].

The cardinal neurophysiological finding is the presence of a more generalized neuropathy outside of the clinically affected nerves. Mildly slowed motor and sensory nerve conduction velocities and conduction block at the sites of compression are seen [101]. Educating patients with HNPP on how to avoid pressure palsies is an essential aspect of management and includes the avoidance of excessive alcohol and meticulous intra-operative positioning for any planned surgery.

Hereditary neuralgic amyotrophy (HNA)

Neuralgic amyotrophy, also known as Parsonage–Turner syndrome, is an episodic peripheral nerve syndrome characterized by acute severe pain, wasting, and weakness of the upper limb muscles, that gradually recovers over months to years (see Chapter 15). Whilst the disease is most often idiopathic (INA), 10% of cases are estimated to be hereditary (HNA) and, of these, 55% are found to have either a missense mutation or deletion in the SEPT9 gene [102].

The disease most commonly involves the upper trunk of the brachial plexus leading to a winged scapular due to involvement of the long thoracic nerve and patchy sensory loss [102]. In 17% of patients with INA and 56% of patients with HNA, however, the neurological involvement extends outside of the brachial plexus, with the most common sites being the lumbosacral plexus, phrenic, and recurrent laryngeal nerves.

Distinguishing INA from HNA following a first acute attack is difficult. A history of severe recurrent attacks with poor recovery is more suggestive of HNA. Dysmorphic features such as short stature, epicanthic folds, hypotelorism, redundant cervical skin folds, and dysmorphic ears may suggest a diagnosis of HNA due to a mutation in SEPT9 [103,104].

Pathogenic mechanisms of CMT

Despite the majority of patents with CMT sharing a similar phenotype, the postulated pathogenic mechanisms of the genetic subtypes include many divergent cellular pathways. For example, demyelinating CMT may be due to altered myelin (CMT1A and CMT1B), Schwann cell endosomal trafficking (FIG4, MTMR2, etc.) integral cytoskeletal proteins (IFN2 and PRX) as well as impaired RNA processing (CTDP1).

The pathogenic mechanisms of axonal CMT are also divergent and include endosomal trafficking, altered cytoskeletal integrity, and impaired RNA processing. For other forms of CMT2, endoplasmic reticulum stress, mitochondrial dysfunction, altered axonal transport, and impaired protein degradation have all been proposed. Such divergent mechanisms have important therapeutic consequences for the management of patients with CMT and imply an era of individualized therapies based on the genetic subtype. This underlines the importance of achieving a genetic diagnosis in patients with CMT.

Management

CMT is a chronic disease and, although there is no current disease-modifying drug, much can be done to help symptomatically and functionally. Patients should be managed as part of a multidisciplinary team that includes a neurologist, neurophysiologist, nurse, physiotherapist, occupational therapist, podiatrist/orthotist, and, in selected cases, an orthopaedic surgeon. Whilst the management of CMT should be tailored to the individual needs of each patient, special consideration should be given to the delivery of the diagnosis and to managing the foot complications of CMT.

Genetic counselling

Genetic counselling in CMT includes three main categories: diagnostic testing, presymptomatic testing, and preconception counselling.

Whilst diagnostic testing in a patient with CMT may seem relatively straightforward, it is important to counsel the patient that such a test may have important implications for other family members. It is also important to convey to the patient the degree of certainty that any novel mutation is pathogenic.

Due to a lack of effective treatment presymptomatic testing of an individual at risk of developing CMT is not commonly requested, but if it is appropriate counselling about the gene being screened is necessary. Preconception counselling is an important aspect in the management of patients with CMT, and initially involves informing the patient of the most likely mode of inheritance and the risk that any offspring may be affected. When the pathogenic mutation is known, prenatal genetic testing for a CMT mutation can be performed, either by chorionic villous sampling (12 weeks' gestation) or amniocentesis (16 weeks' gestation). Both procedures carry a risk of miscarriage (about 1%) and as such only those patients contemplating a termination of pregnancy if the fetus has a pathogenic mutation should be offered testing. An alternative and increasingly requested option is pre-implantation genetic diagnosis (PGD). In this scenario, *in vitro* fertilization (IVF) is employed and genetic testing of the embryo is carried out at the eight-cell stage prior to implantation in the uterus. Whilst this option may seem attractive, it is associated with reduced rates of conception and is not universally available. All forms of prenatal testing should only be performed where there is strong evidence that the mutation being tested for is pathogenic.

Orthopaedic aspects of CMT

There are three main reasons for orthopaedic intervention in CMT: (1) scoliosis, (2) hip dysplasia, and (3) ankle–foot deformity [105], the latter being the most common indication. Scoliosis is reported to occur in 26–37% of patients with CMT, although it is often asymptomatic. The prevalence of hip dysplasia in CMT is less common (8.1%), and it may only be detected on radiological examination [106]. Nevertheless, any patient with CMT who presents with a significant deterioration in their gait, or hip pain, should have an X-ray to rule out acetabular dysplasia.

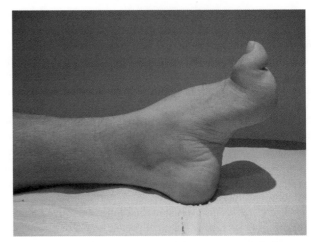

Fig. 8.5 Forefoot pes cavus in a patient with Charcot–Marie–Tooth disease.

Foot and ankle manifestations

There are three common foot deformities in CMT: claw toes, forefoot (pes) cavus, and hindfoot varus (ankle inversion deformity) (see Figs 8.5 and 8.6). Whilst there are many theories about the aetiology of pes cavus, the disorder is still incompletely understood. The most popular theory for its development is an imbalance between agonist and antagonist muscles.

Forefoot (pes) cavus

In CMT1A this is thought to occur due to the unopposed action of the relatively spared peroneus longus against the weakened tibialis anterior on the first ray of the foot, resulting in plantar flexion of the first metatarsal. This results in an increase in the height of the foot arch and tilting of the subtalar joint in to varus (resulting in ankle inversion). The raised arch is often accompanied by tightening of the plantar fascia.

Hindfoot (pes) cavus

Hindfoot pes cavus is due to an excessive pitch angle of the calcaneum. It is often seen in idiopathic pes cavus but was historically associated with poliomyelitis due to selective plantar flexion weakness.

Hindfoot varus (inversion)

Hindfoot varus refers to the inversion of the foot at the subtalar joint (ankle) in order to compensate for the plantar flexion of the

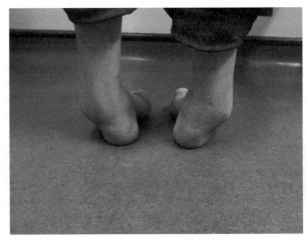

Fig. 8.6 Hindfoot varus in a patient with CMT1A.

first metatarsal causing forefoot (pes) cavus. The hindfoot varus deformity predisposes the patient to recurrent inversion injuries of the ankle.

Conservative management of foot deformity in CMT

The non-operative management of foot deformity in CMT includes gastrocnemius stretching exercises to prevent Achilles tendon tightening, and the provision of ankle–foot orthoses (AFOs). Whilst there is no evidence that custom designed AFOs prevent or slow the progression of foot deformities, they have been shown to reduce foot pain in patients with pes cavus and to improve ambulation when compared with sham AFOs [107]. A wide variety of AFOs exist offering different degrees of support and rigidity, and should be tailored to each individual's therapeutic needs.

Surgical management of foot deformity in CMT

Whilst many patients undergo surgery for foot deformity, there is no randomized evidence on when and how to operate. Nevertheless, the decision to operate is often determined by the age of the patient and the severity of the foot deformity and is aimed at preventing further deterioration.

There are three main types of foot operation for patients with CMT: soft tissue corrections, osteotomies, and fusions.

Soft tissue corrections

Soft tissue corrections are only likely to be effective in patients with 'supple' feet without fixed deformity. The most common soft tissue procedure is lengthening of the gastrocnemius complex for Achilles tendon tightness. Complete release of the plantar fascia may also be performed to correct the secondary contracture that forms in forefoot cavus deformity.

Transfer of the peroneus longus tendon to the peroneus brevis muscle may also be performed to correct forefoot cavus deformity. The procedure achieves two aims. Firstly, by severing the peroneus longus from the first ray, it reduces the plantar flexing forces on the first metatarsal causing the high arch. Secondly, the action of the stronger peroneus longus muscle on the everting peroneus brevis muscle insertion reduces the hindfoot varus (inversion) deformity.

Osteotomies

In patients with some rigid foot deformity osteotomies may be performed to increase the 'flexibility' of the foot and allow the correcting forces following tendon transfer to correct the forefoot cavus and hindfoot varus (see Fig. 8.7).

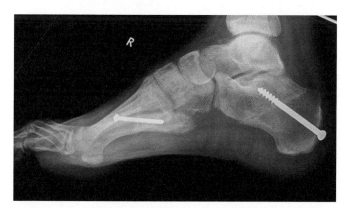

Fig. 8.7 A post-operative X-ray following osteotomies to the first metatarsal and calcaneum.

Fusions

Triple arthrodesis is the mainstay of treatment for a severely affected rigid cavovarus foot deformity. It is an option of last resort, however, and commonly results in accelerated arthritic change in the foot.

Future treatments

The development of mouse models of CMT has led to the identification of several potential therapies. Proposed therapeutic strategies have included ascorbic acid, curcumin, neurotrophin 3, progesterone antagonists, and histone deacetylase inhibitors.

Ascorbic acid

Ascorbic acid is thought to negatively regulate the transcription of *PMP22* and was therefore a promising candidate for CMT1A, in which there is overexpression. Treatment with ascorbic acid was shown to ameliorate the phenotype of a mouse model of CMT1A, paving the way for several large, double-blinded placebo-controlled randomized trials [108]. Unfortunately, all published trials have failed to identify a therapeutic effect of ascorbic acid, although this may in part be related to the slow progression of the disease and the limitations of current methods of monitoring disease progression [109–111].

Curcumin

Curcumin, derived from the spice turmeric, has been shown to be effective in a mouse model of CMT1A [112]. It is believed to act by promoting the translocation of misfolded proteins, such as mutant PMP22 and MPZ, from the endoplasmic reticulum to the plasma membrane, thereby suppressing the unfolded protein response and cell death [113].

Neurotrophin 3

Neurotrophin 3 (NT3), a neurotrophic factor that promotes axonal growth, has been shown to promote axonal regeneration in a mouse model and in a small randomized trial of six patients with CMT1A [114]. This study has not yet been performed in a larger patient population.

Progesterone antagonists

Progesterone increases PMP22 transcription and exacerbates the phenotype of murine CMT1A [115]. Treatment with the progesterone antagonist onapristone produces both a clinical and neuropathological improvement in CMT1A mice but is too toxic for use in humans [116]. Alternative progesterone antagonists are currently being evaluated.

Finally, histone deacetylase 6 inhibitors (HDAC6 inhibitors) have been shown to improve the phenotype of a murine model of CMT2F and represent the first potential therapeutic strategy in CMT2 [117].

Conclusion

Following its original description in 1886, CMT has evolved into a diverse group of conditions each with different modes of inheritance, severity, and causative mutations. Despite the advent of new genetic technologies, the cornerstone to making a diagnosis remains the history and the clinical examination. The subdivision of CMT into axonal and demyelinating forms is just as relevant today as it was 30 years ago, and provides a logical means of approaching a genetic diagnosis, either by targeted sequencing of known genes or using whole exome and genomic sequencing.

The modern-day management of a patient with CMT now entails effective physiotherapy, orthotic and orthopaedic assessment, and genetic counselling. Discussions around family planning, and the option of prenatal genetic testing, should be approached early so that patients have time to make an informed decision.

Whilst there are currently no effective treatments for CMT, this is a rapidly evolving area of research. Clinical trials for ascorbic acid in CMT1A have already been performed and, although negative, have paved the way for future treatment trials.

References

1. Reilly MM. Sorting out the inherited neuropathies. *Pract Neurol* 2007; **7**: 93–105.
2. Ouvrier R. What can we learn from the history of Charcot–Marie-Tooth disease? *Dev Med Child Neurol* 2010; **52**: 405–6.
3. Raeymaekers P, Timmerman V, Nelis E, et al. Duplication in chromosome 17p11.2 in Charcot–Marie–Tooth neuropathy type 1a (CMT 1a). The HMSN Collaborative Research Group. *Neuromusc Disord* 1991; **1**: 93–7.
4. Harding AE, Thomas PK. The clinical features of hereditary motor and sensory neuropathy types I and II. *Brain* 1980; **103**: 259–80.
5. Reilly MM, Murphy SM, Laura M. Charcot–Marie–Tooth disease. *J Peripheral Nervous Syst* 2011; **16**: 1–14.
6. Baets J, Deconinck T, De Vriendt E, et al. Genetic spectrum of hereditary neuropathies with onset in the first year of life. *Brain* 2011; **134**: 2664–76.
7. Saporta AS, Sottile SL, Miller LJ, et al. Charcot–Marie–Tooth disease subtypes and genetic testing strategies. *Ann Neurol* 2011; **69**: 22–33.
8. Murphy SM, Laura M, Fawcett K, et al. Charcot–Marie–Tooth disease: frequency of genetic subtypes and guidelines for genetic testing. *J Neurol Neurosurg Psychiatry* 2012; **83**: 706–10.
9. Metzker ML. Sequencing technologies—the next generation. *Nat Rev Genet* 2010; **11**: 31–46.
10. Schouten JP, McElgunn CJ, Waaijer R, et al. Relative quantification of 40 nucleic acid sequences by multiplex ligation-dependent probe amplification. *Nucleic Acids Res* 2002; **30**: e57.
11. Ionasescu VV. Charcot–Marie–Tooth neuropathies: from clinical description to molecular genetics. *Muscle Nerve* 1995; **18**(3): 267–75.
12. Thomas PK, Hoffbrand AV. Hereditary transcobalamin II deficiency: a 22 year follow up. *J Neurol Neurosurg Psychiatry* 1997; **62**: 197.
13. Birouk N, Gouider R, Le Guern E, et al. Charcot–Marie–Tooth disease type 1A with 17p11.2 duplication. Clinical and electrophysiological phenotype study and factors influencing disease severity in 119 cases. *Brain* 1997; **120**: 813–23.
14. Shy ME, Chen L, Swan ER, et al. Neuropathy progression in Charcot–Marie–Tooth disease type 1A. *Neurology* 2008; **70**: 378–83.
15. Gabreels-Festen AA, Bolhuis PA, Hoogendijk JE, et al. Charcot–Marie–Tooth disease type 1A: morphological phenotype of the 17p duplication versus PMP22 point mutations. *Acta Neuropathol* 1995; **90**: 645–9.
16. Palau F, Lofgren A, De Jonghe P, et al. Origin of the de novo duplication in Charcot–Marie–Tooth disease type 1A: unequal nonsister chromatid exchange during spermatogenesis. *Hum Mol Genet* 1993; **2**: 2031–5.
17. Lupski JR, de Oca-Luna RM, Slaugenhaupt S, et al. DNA duplication associated with Charcot–Marie–Tooth disease type 1A. *Cell* 1991; **66**: 219–32.
18. Chance PF, Alderson MK, Leppig KA, et al. DNA deletion associated with hereditary neuropathy with liability to pressure palsies. *Cell* 1993; **72**: 143–51.
19. D'Urso D, Ehrhardt P, Muller HW. Peripheral myelin protein 22 and protein zero: a novel association in peripheral nervous system myelin. *J Neurosci* 1999; **19**: 3396–403.
20. Hasse B, Bosse F, Hanenberg H, et al. Peripheral myelin protein 22 kDa and protein zero: domain specific trans-interactions. *Molec Cell Neurosci* 2004; **27**: 370–8.
21. Chies R, Nobbio L, Edomi P, et al. Alterations in the Arf6-regulated plasma membrane endosomal recycling pathway in cells overexpressing the tetraspan protein Gas3/PMP22. *J Cell Sci* 2003; **116**: 987–99.
22. Russo M, Laura M, Polke JM, et al. Variable phenotypes are associated with PMP22 missense mutations. *Neuromusc Disord* 2011; **21**: 106–14.
23. Shy ME, Scavina MT, Clark A, et al. T118M PMP22 mutation causes partial loss of function and HNPP-like neuropathy. *Ann Neurol* 2006; **59**: 358–64.
24. Gess B, Jeibmann A, Schirmacher A, et al. Report of a novel mutation in the PMP22 gene causing an axonal neuropathy. *Muscle Nerve* 2011; **43**: 605–9.
25. Ikegami T, Ikeda H, Mitsui T, et al. Novel mutation of the myelin Po gene in a pedigree with Charcot–Marie–Tooth disease type 1B. *Am J Med Genet* 1997; **71**: 246–8.
26. Shy ME. Peripheral neuropathies caused by mutations in the myelin protein zero. *J Neurol Sci* 2006; **242**: 55–66.
27. Gabreels-Festen AA, Hoogendijk JE, Meijerink PH, et al. Two divergent types of nerve pathology in patients with different P0 mutations in Charcot–Marie–Tooth disease. *Neurology* 1996; **47**: 761–5.
28. Meijerink PH, Hoogendijk JE, Gabreels-Festen AA, et al. Clinically distinct codon 69 mutations in major myelin protein zero in demyelinating neuropathies. *Ann Neurol* 1996; **40**: 672–5.
29. Young P, Grote K, Kuhlenbaumer G, et al. Mutation analysis in Chariot-Marie Tooth disease type 1: point mutations in the *MPZ* gene and the *GJB1* gene cause comparable phenotypic heterogeneity. *J Neurol* 2001; **248**: 410–15.
30. Street VA, Bennett CL, Goldy JD, et al. Mutation of a putative protein degradation gene LITAF/SIMPLE in Charcot–Marie–Tooth disease 1C. *Neurology* 2003; **60**: 22–6.
31. Latour P, Gonnaud PM, Ollagnon E, et al. SIMPLE mutation analysis in dominant demyelinating Charcot–Marie–Tooth disease: three novel mutations. *J Periph Nervous Syst* 2006; **11**: 148–55.
32. Jessen KR, Mirsky R. Signals that determine Schwann cell identity. *J Anat* 2002; **200**: 367–76.
33. Warner LE, Mancias P, Butler IJ, et al. Mutations in the early growth response 2 (*EGR2*) gene are associated with hereditary myelinopathies. *Nat Genet* 1998; **18**: 382–4.
34. Chung KW, Sunwoo IN, Kim SM, et al. Two missense mutations of *EGR2* R359W and *GJB1* V136A in a Charcot–Marie–Tooth disease family. *Neurogenetics* 2005; **6**: 159–63.
35. Pareyson D, Taroni F, Botti S, et al. Cranial nerve involvement in CMT disease type 1 due to early growth response 2 gene mutation. *Neurology* 2000; **54**: 1696–8.
36. Gentil BJ, Minotti S, Beange M, et al. Normal role of the low-molecular-weight neurofilament protein in mitochondrial dynamics and disruption in Charcot–Marie–Tooth disease. *FASEB J* 2011; **26**: 1194–203.
37. Jordanova A, De Jonghe P, Boerkoel CF, et al. Mutations in the neurofilament light chain gene (NEFL) cause early onset severe Charcot–Marie–Tooth disease. *Brain* 2003; **126**: 590–7.
38. Yum SW, Zhang J, Mo K, et al. A novel recessive *Nefl* mutation causes a severe, early-onset axonal neuropathy. *Ann Neurol* 2009; **66**: 759–70.
39. Noack R, Frede S, Albrecht P, et al. Charcot–Marie–Tooth disease CMT4A: GDAP1 increases cellular glutathione and the mitochondrial membrane potential. *Hum Molec Genet* 2012; **21**: 150–62.
40. Nelis E, Erdem S, Van Den Bergh PY, et al. Mutations in *GDAP1*: autosomal recessive CMT with demyelination and axonopathy. *Neurology* 2002; **59**: 1865–72.
41. Zimon M, Baets J, Fabrizi GM, et al. Dominant GDAP1 mutations cause predominantly mild CMT phenotypes. *Neurology* 2011; **77**: 540–8.

42. Dubourg O, Azzedine H, Verny C, et al. Autosomal-recessive forms of demyelinating Charcot–Marie–Tooth disease. *Neuromolec Med* 2006; **8**: 75–86.

43. Houlden H, King RH, Wood NW, et al. Mutations in the 5′ region of the myotubularin-related protein 2 (*MTMR2*) gene in autosomal recessive hereditary neuropathy with focally folded myelin. *Brain* 2001; **124**: 907–15.

44. Quattrone A, Gambardella A, Bono F, et al. Autosomal recessive hereditary motor and sensory neuropathy with focally folded myelin sheaths: clinical, electrophysiologic, and genetic aspects of a large family. *Neurology* 1996; **46**: 1318–24.

45. Senderek J, Bergmann C, Weber S, et al. Mutation of the SBF2 gene, encoding a novel member of the myotubularin family, in Charcot–Marie–Tooth neuropathy type 4B2/11p15. *Hum Molec Genet* 2003; **12**: 349–56.

46. Azzedine H, Bolino A, Taieb T, et al. Mutations in MTMR13, a new pseudophosphatase homologue of MTMR2 and Sbf1, in two families with an autosomal recessive demyelinating form of Charcot–Marie–Tooth disease associated with early-onset glaucoma. *Am J Hum Genet* 2003; **72**: 1141–53.

47. Hirano R, Takashima H, Umehara F, et al. SET binding factor 2 (*SBF2*) mutation causes CMT4B with juvenile onset glaucoma. *Neurology* 2004; **63**: 577–80.

48. Houlden H, Laura M, Ginsberg L, et al. The phenotype of Charcot–Marie–Tooth disease type 4C due to *SH3TC2* mutations and possible predisposition to an inflammatory neuropathy. *Neuromusc Disord* 2009; **19**: 264–9.

49. Gabreels-Festen A, van Beersum S, Eshuis L, et al. Study on the gene and phenotypic characterisation of autosomal recessive demyelinating motor and sensory neuropathy (Charcot–Marie–Tooth disease) with a gene locus on chromosome 5q23-q33. *J Neurol Neurosurg Psychiatry* 1999; **66**: 569–74.

50. Kalaydjieva L, Hallmayer J, Chandler D, et al. Gene mapping in Gypsies identifies a novel demyelinating neuropathy on chromosome 8q24. *Nat Genet* 1996; **14**: 214–17.

51. Takashima H, Boerkoel CF, De Jonghe P, et al. Periaxin mutations cause a broad spectrum of demyelinating neuropathies. *Ann Neurol* 2002; **51**: 709–15.

52. Kijima K, Numakura C, Shirahata E, et al. Periaxin mutation causes early-onset but slow-progressive Charcot–Marie–Tooth disease. *J Hum Genet* 2004; **49**: 376–9.

53. Thomas PK, Kalaydjieva L, Youl B, et al. Hereditary motor and sensory neuropathy-russe: new autosomal recessive neuropathy in Balkan Gypsies. *Ann Neurol* 2001; **50**: 452–7.

54. Rogers T, Chandler D, Angelicheva D, et al. A novel locus for autosomal recessive peripheral neuropathy in the EGR2 region on 10q23. *Am J Hum Genet* 2000; **67**: 664–71.

55. Bianchi M, Magnani M. Hexokinase mutations that produce nonspherocytic hemolytic anemia. *Blood Cells Molecules Dis* 1995; **21**: 2–8.

56. De Sandre-Giovannoli A, Delague V, Hamadouche T, et al. Homozygosity mapping of autosomal recessive demyelinating Charcot–Marie–Tooth neuropathy (CMT4H) to a novel locus on chromosome 12p11.21-q13.11. *J Med Genet* 2005; **42**: 260–5.

57. Houlden H, Hammans S, Katifi H, et al. A novel Frabin (*FGD4*) nonsense mutation p.R275X associated with phenotypic variability in CMT4H. *Neurology* 2009; **72**: 617–20.

58. Zhang X, Chow CY, Sahenk Z, et al. Mutation of *FIG4* causes a rapidly progressive, asymmetric neuronal degeneration. *Brain* 2008; **131**: 1990–2001.

59. Nicholson G, Lenk GM, Reddel SW, et al. Distinctive genetic and clinical features of CMT4J: a severe neuropathy caused by mutations in the PI(3,5)P phosphatase FIG4. *Brain* 2011; **134**: 1959–71.

60. Tournev I, King RH, Workman J, et al. Peripheral nerve abnormalities in the congenital cataracts facial dysmorphism neuropathy (CCFDN) syndrome. *Acta Neuropathol* 1999; **98**: 165–70.

61. Varon R, Gooding R, Steglich C, et al. Partial deficiency of the C-terminal-domain phosphatase of RNA polymerase II is associated with congenital cataracts facial dysmorphism neuropathy syndrome. *Nat Genet* 2003; **35**: 185–9.

62. Verhoeven K, Claeys KG, Zuchner S, et al. MFN2 mutation distribution and genotype/phenotype correlation in Charcot–Marie–Tooth type 2. *Brain* 2006; **129**: 2093–102.

63. Zuchner S, Mersiyanova IV, Muglia M, et al. Mutations in the mitochondrial GTPase mitofusin 2 cause Charcot–Marie–Tooth neuropathy type 2A. *Nat Genet* 2004; **36**: 449–51.

64. Polke JM, Laura M, Pareyson D, et al. Recessive axonal Charcot–Marie–Tooth disease due to compound heterozygous mitofusin 2 mutations. *Neurology* 2011; **77**: 168–73.

65. Rotthier A, Baets J, De Vriendt E, et al. Genes for hereditary sensory and autonomic neuropathies: a genotype-phenotype correlation. *Brain* 2009; **132**: 2699–711.

66. Auer-Grumbach M, Olschewski A, Papic L, et al. Alterations in the ankyrin domain of TRPV4 cause congenital distal SMA, scapuloperoneal SMA and HMSN2C. *Nat Genet* 2010; **42**: 160–4.

67. Deng HX, Klein CJ, Yan J, et al. Scapuloperoneal spinal muscular atrophy and CMT2C are allelic disorders caused by alterations in TRPV4. *Nat Genet* 2010; **42**: 165–9.

68. Landoure G, Zdebik AA, Martinez TL, et al. Mutations in TRPV4 cause Charcot–Marie–Tooth disease type 2C. *Nat Genet* 2010; **42**: 170–4.

69. Dyck PJ, Litchy WJ, Minnerath S, et al. Hereditary motor and sensory neuropathy with diaphragm and vocal cord paresis. *Ann Neurol* 1994; **35**: 608–15.

70. Zimon M, Baets J, Auer-Grumbach M, et al. Dominant mutations in the cation channel gene transient receptor potential vanilloid 4 cause an unusual spectrum of neuropathies. *Brain* 2010; **133**: 1798–809.

71. Ibba M, Soll D. Aminoacyl-tRNAs: setting the limits of the genetic code. *Genes Dev* 2004; **18**: 731–8.

72. Sivakumar K, Kyriakides T, Puls I, et al. Phenotypic spectrum of disorders associated with glycyl-tRNA synthetase mutations. *Brain* 2005; **128**: 2304–14.

73. Houlden H, Laura M, Wavrant-De Vrieze F, et al. Mutations in the HSP27 (HSPB1) gene cause dominant, recessive, and sporadic distal HMN/CMT type 2. *Neurology* 2008; **71**: 1660–8.

74. Irobi J, Van Impe K, Seeman P, et al. Hot-spot residue in small heat-shock protein 22 causes distal motor neuropathy. *Nat Genet* 2004; **36**: 597–601.

75. Tang BS, Zhao GH, Luo W, et al. Small heat-shock protein 22 mutated in autosomal dominant Charcot–Marie–Tooth disease type 2L. *Hum Genet* 2005; **116**: 222–4.

76. Kappe G, Franck E, Verschuure P, et al. The human genome encodes 10 alpha-crystallin-related small heat shock proteins: HspB1-10. *Cell Stress Chaperones* 2003; **8**: 53–61.

77. Tang BS, Luo W, Xia K, et al. A new locus for autosomal dominant Charcot–Marie–Tooth disease type 2 (CMT2L) maps to chromosome 12q24. *Hum Genet* 2004; **114**: 527–33.

78. Latour P, Thauvin-Robinet C, Baudelet-Mery C, et al. A major determinant for binding and aminoacylation of tRNA(Ala) in cytoplasmic Alanyl-tRNA synthetase is mutated in dominant axonal Charcot–Marie–Tooth disease. *Am J Hum Genet* 2010; **86**: 77–82.

79. Guernsey DL, Jiang H, Bedard K, et al. Mutation in the gene encoding ubiquitin ligase LRSAM1 in patients with Charcot–Marie–Tooth disease. *PLoS Genet* 2010; **6**(8): e1001081. doi:10.1371/journal.pgen.1001081.

80. Weterman MA, Sorrentino V, Kasher PR, et al. A frameshift mutation in LRSAM1 is responsible for a dominant hereditary polyneuropathy. *Hum Molec Genet* 2012; **21**: 358–70.

81. Goizet C, Boukhris A, Mundwiller E, et al. Complicated forms of autosomal dominant hereditary spastic paraplegia are frequent in SPG10. *Hum Mutat* 2009; **30**: E376–E385.

82. Crimella C, Baschirotto C, Arnoldi A, et al. Mutations in the motor and stalk domains of KIF5A in spastic paraplegia type 10 and in axonal Charcot–Marie–Tooth type 2. *Clin Genet* 2012; **82**: 157–64.

83. De Sandre-Giovannoli A, Chaouch M, Kozlov S, et al. Homozygous defects in LMNA, encoding lamin A/C nuclear-envelope proteins, cause autosomal recessive axonal neuropathy in human (Charcot–Marie–Tooth disorder type 2) and mouse. *Am J Hum Genet* 2002; **70**: 726–36.

84. Tazir M, Azzedine H, Assami S, et al. Phenotypic variability in autosomal recessive axonal Charcot–Marie–Tooth disease due to the R298C mutation in lamin A/C. *Brain* 2004; **127**: 154–63.

85. Bouhouche A, Birouk N, Azzedine H, et al. Autosomal recessive axonal Charcot–Marie–Tooth disease (ARCMT2): phenotype-genotype correlations in 13 Moroccan families. *Brain* 2007; **130**: 1062–75.

86. Leal A, Huehne K, Bauer F, et al. Identification of the variant Ala335Val of MED25 as responsible for CMT2B2: molecular data, functional studies of the SH3 recognition motif and correlation between wild-type MED25 and PMP22 RNA levels in CMT1A animal models. *Neurogenetics* 2009; **10**: 275–87.

87. Berghoff C, Berghoff M, Leal A, et al. Clinical and electrophysiological characteristics of autosomal recessive axonal Charcot–Marie–Tooth disease (ARCMT2B) that maps to chromosome 19q13.3. *Neuromusc Disord* 2004; **14**: 301–6.

88. Kleopa KA, Scherer SS. Molecular genetics of X-linked Charcot–Marie–Tooth disease. *Neuromolec Med* 2006; **8**: 107–22.

89. Eisen A, Kuwabara S. The split hand syndrome in amyotrophic lateral sclerosis. *J Neurol Neurosurg Psychiatry* 2012; **83**: 399–403.

90. Tabaraud F, Lagrange E, Sindou P, et al. Demyelinating X-linked Charcot–Marie–Tooth disease: unusual electrophysiological findings. *Muscle Nerve* 1999; **22**: 1442–7.

91. Gutierrez A, England JD, Sumner AJ, et al. Unusual electrophysiological findings in X-linked dominant Charcot–Marie–Tooth disease. *Muscle Nerve* 2000; **23**: 182–8.

92. Kim HJ, Sohn KM, Shy ME, et al. Mutations in PRPS1, which encodes the phosphoribosyl pyrophosphate synthetase enzyme critical for nucleotide biosynthesis, cause hereditary peripheral neuropathy with hearing loss and optic neuropathy (cmtx5). *Am J Hum Genet* 2007; **81**: 552–8.

93. Zuchner S, Noureddine M, Kennerson M, et al. Mutations in the pleckstrin homology domain of dynamin 2 cause dominant intermediate Charcot–Marie–Tooth disease. *Nat Genet* 2005; **37**: 289–94.

94. Bitoun M, Maugenre S, Jeannet PY, et al. Mutations in dynamin 2 cause dominant centronuclear myopathy. *Nat Genet* 2005; **37**: 1207–9.

95. Haberlova J, Mazanec R, Ridzon P, et al. Phenotypic variability in a large Czech family with a Dynamin 2-associated Charcot–Marie–Tooth neuropathy. *J Neurogenet* 2011; **25**: 182–8.

96. Bitoun M, Stojkovic T, Prudhon B, et al. A novel mutation in the dynamin 2 gene in a Charcot–Marie–Tooth type 2 patient: clinical and pathological findings. *Neuromusc Disord* 2008; **18**: 334–8.

97. Jordanova A, Thomas FP, Guergueltcheva V, et al. Dominant intermediate Charcot–Marie–Tooth type C maps to chromosome 1p34-p35. *Am J Hum Genet* 2003; **73**: 1423–30.

98. Jordanova A, Irobi J, Thomas FP, et al. Disrupted function and axonal distribution of mutant tyrosyl-tRNA synthetase in dominant intermediate Charcot–Marie–Tooth neuropathy. *Nat Genet* 2006; **38**: 197–202.

99. McLaughlin HM, Sakaguchi R, Liu C, et al. Compound heterozygosity for loss-of-function lysyl-tRNA synthetase mutations in a patient with peripheral neuropathy. *Am J Hum Genet* 2010; **87**: 560–6.

100. Boyer O, Nevo F, Plaisier E, et al. INF2 mutations in Charcot–Marie–Tooth disease with glomerulopathy. *N Engl J Med* 2011; **365**: 2377–88.

101. Chance PF. Inherited focal, episodic neuropathies: hereditary neuropathy with liability to pressure palsies and hereditary neuralgic amyotrophy. *Neuromolec Med* 2006; **8**: 159–74.

102. van Alfen N. Clinical and pathophysiological concepts of neuralgic amyotrophy. *Nat Rev Neurol* 2011; **7**: 315–22.

103. Laccone F, Hannibal MC, Neesen J, et al. Dysmorphic syndrome of hereditary neuralgic amyotrophy associated with a SEPT9 gene mutation--a family study. *Clin Genet* 2008; **74**: 279–83.

104. Ueda M, Kawamura N, Tateishi T, et al. Phenotypic spectrum of hereditary neuralgic amyotrophy caused by the SEPT9 R88W mutation. *J Neurol Neurosurg Psychiatry* 2010; **81**: 94–6.

105. Yagerman SE, Cross MB, Green DW, et al. Pediatric orthopedic conditions in Charcot–Marie–Tooth disease: a literature review. *Curr Opin Pediatr* 2012; **24**: 50–6.

106. Walker JL, Nelson KR, Heavilon JA, et al. Hip abnormalities in children with Charcot–Marie–Tooth disease. *J Pediatr Orthop* 1994; **14**: 54–9.

107. Burns J, Crosbie J, Ouvrier R, et al. Effective orthotic therapy for the painful cavus foot: a randomized controlled trial. *J Am Podiatr Med Assoc* 2006; **96**: 205–11.

108. Passage E, Norreel JC, Noack-Fraissignes P, et al. Ascorbic acid treatment corrects the phenotype of a mouse model of Charcot–Marie–Tooth disease. *Nat Med* 2004; **10**: 396–401.

109. Burns J, Ouvrier RA, Yiu EM, et al. Ascorbic acid for Charcot–Marie–Tooth disease type 1A in children: a randomised, double-blind, placebo-controlled, safety and efficacy trial. *Lancet Neurol* 2009; **8**: 537–44.

110. Micallef J, Attarian S, Dubourg O, et al. Effect of ascorbic acid in patients with Charcot–Marie–Tooth disease type 1A: a multicentre, randomised, double-blind, placebo-controlled trial. *Lancet Neurol* 2009; **8**: 1103–10.

111. Pareyson D, Reilly MM, Schenone A, et al. Ascorbic acid in Charcot–Marie–Tooth disease type 1A (CMT-TRIAAL and CMT-TRAUK): a double-blind randomised trial. *Lancet Neurol* 2011; **10**: 320–8.

112. Khajavi M, Shiga K, Wiszniewski W, et al. Oral curcumin mitigates the clinical and neuropathologic phenotype of the Trembler-J mouse: a potential therapy for inherited neuropathy. *Am J Hum Genet* 2007; **81**: 438–53.

113. Khajavi M, Inoue K, Wiszniewski W, et al. Curcumin treatment abrogates endoplasmic reticulum retention and aggregation-induced apoptosis associated with neuropathy-causing myelin protein zero-truncating mutants. *Am J Hum Genet* 2005; **77**: 841–50.

114. Sahenk Z, Nagaraja HN, McCracken BS, et al. NT-3 promotes nerve regeneration and sensory improvement in CMT1A mouse models and in patients. *Neurology* 2005; **65**: 681–9.

115. Sereda MW, Meyer zu Horste G, Suter U, et al. Therapeutic administration of progesterone antagonist in a model of Charcot–Marie–Tooth disease (CMT-1A). *Nat Medi* 2003; **9**: 1533–7.

116. Meyer zu Horste G, Prukop T, Liebetanz D, et al. Antiprogesterone therapy uncouples axonal loss from demyelination in a transgenic rat model of CMT1A neuropathy. *Ann Neurol* 2007; **61**: 61–72.

117. d'Ydewalle C, Krishnan J, Chiheb DM, et al. HDAC6 inhibitors reverse axonal loss in a mouse model of mutant HSPB1-induced Charcot–Marie–Tooth disease. *Nat Med* 2011; **17**: 968–74.

CHAPTER 9

Hereditary sensory and autonomic neuropathies

Michaela Auer-Grumbach

Introduction

The hereditary sensory neuropathies (HSNs) are a clinically and genetically heterogeneous group of disorders that are characterized by exclusive or predominant axonal atrophy and degeneration of the sensory neurons [1]. Hallmark features comprise progressive distal sensory loss, nail changes, painless injuries, and chronic skin ulcers which are frequently complicated by spontaneous fractures and neuropathic arthropathy that often lead to amputations of distal or even proximal parts of the limbs. The term hereditary sensory and autonomic neuropathy (HSAN) is used when autonomic features represent a predominant sign of the disease [1].

The classification of HSN/HSAN is still based on the clinical presentation, the genetic background, and the age of disease onset, which may range from congenital and juvenile to adulthood onset [1–3]. The mode of inheritance may be autosomal dominant (HSN I, HSAN I; HSAN VII) or autosomal recessive (HSN, HSAN II–VI). In HSN I additional distal muscle weakness and wasting is common, and HSN I therefore sometimes mimics a hereditary motor and sensory neuropathy (HSMN) phenotype [i.e. Charcot–Marie–Tooth (CMT) disease] [4–6]. Occasionally, additional features such as deafness, dementia, upper motor neuron signs, and cough and gastro-oesophageal reflux may be observed [4,7–9].

In the past two decades mutations in 15 genes have been indentified: seven genes for autosomal dominant HSN/HSAN (*SPTLC1*, *SPTLC2*, *RAB7A*, *ATL1*, *DNMT1*, *SCN11A*, *ATL3*) [5,8–11] and eight genes for autosomal recessive forms of HSN/HSAN (*WNK1/HSN2*, *FAM134B*, *KIF1A*, *IKBKAP*, *NTRK1*, *NGFB*, *CCT5*, *DST*) [12–19] (see Table 9.1). The identification of these genes has provided insights into the pathogenesis of HSN/HSAN and is a basis for developing therapies in the future. Still, in the majority of HSN/HSAN patients the genetic background remains to be elucidated and further genetic heterogeneity has to be expected [20]. This chapter reviews the HSN/HSAN genes that we know to date and their corresponding phenotypes.

Genes involved in autosomal dominantly inherited HSN/HSAN

Serine-palmitoyltransferase, long chain base subunit 1 (*SPTLC1*)

Mutations in *SPTLC1*, encoding serine palmitoyltransferase (SPT), long chain base subunit 1, are associated with the typical HSN I phenotype. Disease onset is usually between the second and fourth decades of life or sometimes later. Initial signs comprise distal loss of pain and temperature sensation in the lower limbs that lead to painless injuries and foot ulcerations. Positive sensory phenomena such as numbness, paraesthesia, burning, and shooting pains usually occur with progression of the disease. Interestingly, vibration sense remains preserved for a long time [6]. If sensory loss is unheeded, chronic ulcerations are followed by osteomyelitis, and subsequently often require amputations. Neuropathic joints are common. Distal muscle wasting and weakness may be pronounced as well. Upper limbs subsequently become involved [4,21]. Sensorineural hearing loss is variably present, and if so starts in middle to late adulthood. Tendon reflexes may be preserved or brisk and then indicate some upper motor neuron involvement [4]. Nerve conduction studies (NCS) are compatible with a sensory axonal neuropathy [4]. Neuropathological studies show a distal axonal degeneration with loss of unmyelinated, small myelinated, and large myelinated fibres but are not diagnostic and are therefore only recommended for differential diagnostic purposes [21,22].

Only a few mutations in *SPTLC1* (C133Y, C133W, V144D, S331F, S331Y, and A352V) have been reported so far as the underlying cause of HSN I [10,20,23,24,25a,25b]. The C133W mutation has been identified in families from both Australia and England and has been shown to have a common British founder [21,25]. *De novo* mutations at S331 have been reported in four unrelated patients and displayed an unusually severe syndromic phenotype characterized by congenital onset with severe growth retardation, hand tremor, hypotonia, juvenile cataracts and vocal cord paralysis [20,25a,25b].

SPT is located at the outer membrane of the endoplasmic reticulum (ER), where it catalyses the pyridoxal-5′-phosphate (PLP)-dependent condensation of L-serine with palmitoyl-CoA. This is the first and rate-limiting step in the *de novo* biosynthesis of sphingolipids [11,26]. It has been shown that the mutant forms of the enzyme show a shift from their canonical substrate L-serine to the alternative substrate L-alanin. This shift leads to increased formation of neurotoxic desoxysphingolipids (dSLs). Notably, dSLs were found to be highly elevated not only in cells expressing the mutant forms of SPT but also in plasma of HSN I patients carrying *SPTLC1* mutations and in mice bearing a transgene expressing mutant *SPTLC1* [27,28]. A subsequent study examined whether, *in vivo*, specific amino acid substrate supplementation might influence dSL levels and disease severity in HSN I patients. Indeed, in a pilot study of 14 patients with HSN I, L-serine supplementation reduced dSL levels, therefore raising the prospect of L-serine supplementation as a first treatment option for this disorder [29].

Table 9.1 Summary of hereditary sensory neuropathy (HSN)/hereditary sensory and autonomic neuropathy (HSAN) genes, gene locations, and Online Mendelian Inheritance in Man (OMIM) links

Type/inheritance	Gene locus	Gene	Age at onset	OMIM no.
Autosomal dominant HSN/HSAN				
HSAN IA/HSN IA	9q22.31	SPTLC1	Teens to adulthood	162400
HSN/HMSN IIB	3q21.3	RAB7A	Teens to adulthood	600882
HSAN IC/HSN IC	14q24.3	SPTLC2	Adulthood	613640
HSAN ID/HSN ID	14q22.1	ATL1	Adulthood	613708
HSAN IE/HSN IE	19p13.2	DNMT1	Adulthood	614116
HSN with cough and gastro-oesophageal reflux	3p22-p24	Unknown	Adulthood	608088
HSAN VII	3p22.2	SCN11A	Birth/congenital	604385
HSN I	11q13.1	ATL3	Teens to adulthood	
Autosomal recessive HSN/HSAN				
HSAN IIA/HSN IIA	12p13.33	WNK1/HSN2	Infancy/childhood	201300
HSAN IIB/HSN IIB	5p15.1	FAM134B	Infancy/childhood	613115
HSAN IIC/HSN IIC	2q37.3	KIF1A	Infancy/childhood	614213
HSAN III/HSN III	9q31.3	IKBKAP	Birth/congenital	223900
HSAN IV/HSN IV	1q23.1	NTRK1	Birth/congenital	256800
HSAN II/HSN II + spasticity	5p15.2	CCT5	Infancy	256840
HSAN V/HSN V	1p13.2	NGFB	Birth/congenital	608654
HSAN VI	6p12.1	DST	Birth/congenital	614653
Related disorders				
Congenital inability to experience pain	2q24.3	SCN9A	Birth/congenital	243000

Serine-palmitoyltransferase, long chain base subunit 2 (SPTLC2)

Despite negative results when screening a series of HSN/HSAN patients for mutations in SPTLC2 [30], three heterozygous missense mutations (G382V, V359M, I504F) were identified in four index patients in a later study [11]. Individuals carrying the G382V and V359M mutations, respectively, presented with a phenotype indistinguishable from HSN I due to SPTLC1 mutations. The I504F mutation occurred *de novo* in a patient presenting with an early onset sensorimotor neuropathy, complicated by ulcerations and osteomyelitis. Functional studies suggested that the three SPTLC2 mutations change the enzymatic properties of SPT, resulting in a partial to complete loss of SPT activity and causing the formation of the neurotoxic sphingoid metabolite 1-deoxysphinganine. While the G382V mutation loses the ability to generate SPT activity, the two other mutations retain partial activity. Structurally, the G382 residue is located in the putative interface between SPTLC1 and SPTLC2. The two other mutations (V359M and I504F) are located on the surface of the protein. This possibly explains their differential effect on SPT activity [11].

Ras-related protein (RAB7A)

RAB7A belongs to the large superfamily of small GTPases. It binds to subdomains of early endosomes, escorts proteins via late endosomes to lysosomes, and it is involved in the endocytosis and transport of glycosphingolipids from the plasma membrane to the Golgi [31]. To date it remains unclear how mutations in this ubiquitously expressed gene lead to a HSN phenotype. The first symptoms occur in the second or third decades. The clinical phenotype is characterized by severe sensory disturbances affecting all senses, foot ulcers, and amputations (Fig. 9.1), but also a usually prominent distal motor neuropathy [3,32–36]. Therefore, the disease was originally denoted CMT2B [32,33].

Variability within a family varies widely, and subclinically affected mutation carriers have also been reported [35]. Because only a few missense mutations in RAB7A have been reported (L129F, K157N, N161T, V162M) to date, and no mutations were identified in a large series of HSN patients examined, it has been suggested that RAB7A mutations are a rare cause of familial and idiopathic sensory neuropathy [37].

Atlastin 1 (ATL1)

Mutations in atlastin 1 (ATL1), a gene that encodes the large dynamin-related GTPase atlastin-1 have been reported as a frequent cause of early onset spastic paraplegia (SPG3a) [38]. In 2010, Guelly et al. [8] carried out a genome-wide scan in a HSN I family which was excluded for mutations in the known HSN I genes. Massive parallel exon sequencing of the 14.3 Mb disease interval

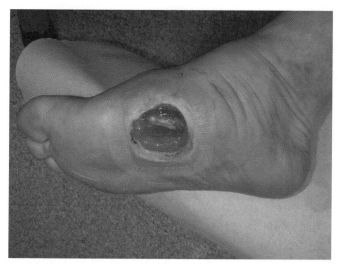

Fig. 9.1 Deep plantar foot ulceration in a patient with hereditary sensory neuropathy carrying a mutation in *RAB7A*.

on chromosome 14q detected a novel missense mutation (N355K) in *ATL1*. Patients of this family exhibited a severe distal sensory neuropathy in the lower limbs affecting all senses, foot ulcers, and amputations up to the knees. Prominent distal muscle weakness and wasting were not observed, and NCS revealed a prominent motor and sensory axonal neuropathy. In contrast to patients with typical HSN I, upper motor neuron signs consisting of variable spasticity and/or brisk tendon reflexes in the lower limbs were a common finding. The mutant protein exhibited reduced GTPase activity and prominently disrupted ER network morphology when expressed in COS-7 cells. An expanded screen in 115 additional HSN I patients identified two additional dominant *ATL1* mutations (E66Q; V326WfsX8) [8].

DNA methyltransferase 1 (*DNMT1*)

DNA methyltransferase 1 (DNMT1) is crucial for maintenance of methylation, gene regulation, and chromatin stability. *DNMT1* mutations (Y495C, D490E, P491Y) have been identified by exome sequencing in families with HSAN I, dementia, and hearing loss. The mutations in *DNMT1* were shown to cause both central and peripheral neurodegeneration. Functional studies revealed premature degradation of mutant proteins, reduced methyltransferase activity, and impaired heterochromatin binding during the G_2 cell cycle phase leading to global hypomethylation and site-specific hypermethylation, and indicated that *DNMT1* mutations cause the aberrant methylation implicated in complex pathogenesis [9].

Sodium channel, voltage-gated, type XI, alpha subunit (*SCN11A*)

SCN11A is a newly identified gene for dominant HSAN and was first reported in 2013 by Leipold et al. [38a]. In two unrelated patients from Germany and Sweden, they identified the same *de novo* heterozygous missense mutation in the *SCN11A* gene (L811P). SCN11A encodes Nav1.9, a voltage-gated sodium ion channel that is primarily expressed in nociceptors, which function as key relay stations for the electrical transmission of pain signals from the periphery to the central nervous system. Both patients presented with congenital inability to experience pain since birth, resulting

in severe mutilations. Wound healing was delayed and painless fractures occured frequently. There was no intellectual impairment, but both affected individuals had mild muscle weakness. Nerve conduction studies showed slightly reduced motor and sensory nerve conduction velocities but normal amplitudes. Hyperhidrosis and gastrointestinal dysfunction were observed in both, suggesting autonomic involvement. Heterozygous knock-in mice carrying the orthologous mutation showed reduced sensitivity to pain and self-inflicted tissue lesions, recapitulating aspects of the human phenotype. Mutant Nav1.9 channels displayed excessive activity at resting voltages, causing sustained depolarization of nociceptors, impaired generation of action potentials, and aberrant synaptic transmission. The gain-of-function mechanism that underlies this channelopathy suggested an alternative way to modulate pain perception. This novel HSAN subtype has also been classified as HSAN VII. In addition, two further heterozygous mutations (R225C) and (A808G) in *SCN11A* have been reported in two large Chinese families presenting with autosomal-dominant episodic pain [38b]. Expressing the two *SCN11A* mutations in mouse dorsal root ganglion neurons showed that both mutations enhanced the channel's electrical activities and induced hyperexcitablity of dorsal root ganglion neurons.

Atlastin 3 (*ATL3*)

In a family with autosomal dominant sensory neuropathy, loss of pain perception, and destruction of the pedal skeleton whole exome sequencing identified a missense mutation in a highly conserved amino acid residue of atlastin GTPase 3 (ATL3), an endoplasmic reticulum-shaping GTPase. Screening a large cohort of 115 patients detected the same mutation (Y192C) in a second family exhibiting a similar phenotype with distal sensory loss in the lower limbs, reduced tendon reflexes, and acromutilations. Functional studies showed that mutant ATL3-Y192C fails to localize to branch points, but instead disrupts the structure of the tubular endoplasmic reticulum, suggesting that the mutation exerts a dominant negative effect [38c].

HSN I with cough and gastro-oesophageal reflux linked to chromosome 3p

In two Australian families with an autosomal dominant adult-onset distal sensory loss, a sensory axonal neuropathy and paroxysmal cough and gastro-oesophageal reflux, the disease was linked to chromosome 3p22-p24 [7,39]. Additional features included throat clearing, hoarse voice, cough syncope, and sensorineural hearing loss. Mutation analysis of genes in the candidate region has not yet identified the disease-causing gene [7].

Genes involved in autosomal recessively inherited HSN/HSAN

WNK lysine deficient protein kinase 1 (*WNK1/HSN2*)

The first mutation in the *WNK1/HSN2* gene was identified in isolated Canadian populations [12]. Since the original description several additional—mainly frameshift or nonsense—mutations in the *WNK1* gene have been identified in many further HSN II patients and families exhibiting a typical phenotype with a disease onset in infancy or early childhood. HSN II patients usually complain of distal numbness in the upper and lower limbs and a glove and

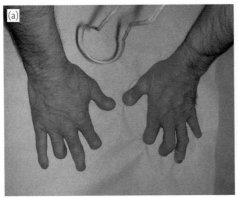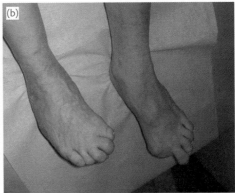

Fig. 9.2 Acromutilations and amputations of fingers (a) and toes (b) in a patient carry a mutation in the *WNK1/HSN2* gene.

stocking like sensory loss. Later on patients develop impairment of pain, temperature, and touch sensation, sometimes involving the trunk as well [12,40]. Other characteristics include loss of tendon reflexes, plantar and finger ulcers, and amputations after injuries or even spontaneous amputations (Fig. 9.2). In contrast to HSN I, muscle weakness and wasting is usually absent or only mild [12]. Autonomic dysfunction may be minimal and can include hyperhidrosis, tonic pupils, and urinary incontinence in cases with more advanced disease [40–43]

Family with sequence similarity 134, member B (*FAM134B*)

In 2009, a loss-of function mutation (S309X) in a further gene, *FAM134B*, encoding a newly identified *cis*-Golgi protein located on chromosome 5p15.1, was identified in a consanguineous Saudi Arabian family with a typical HSN II phenotype as described in the Introduction [13]. Further mutations (P7GfsX133, Q145X), including a mutation in the splice-donor consensus site of intron 7 (c.873+2T>C), were identified in the same gene. The mutations in *FAM134B* lead to severe protein truncation and/or nonsense-mediated mRNA decay compatible with loss of function and were shown to result in structural alterations of the *cis*-Golgi compartment and induce apoptosis in some primary dorsal root ganglion neurons, implicating *FAM134B* as critical for long-term survival of nociceptive and autonomic ganglion neurons [13].

Kinesin family member 1A (*KIF1A*)

KIF1A is an axonal transporter of synaptic vesicles and interacts with the domain encoded by the *HSN2* exon. A genome-wide homozygosity mapping in a consanguineous HSN II Afghan family identified a unique region of homozygosity located on chromosome 2q37.3 and revealed a truncating *KIF1A* mutation in this family segregating with the disease phenotype. Subsequent sequencing of *KIF1A* in a series of 112 unrelated patients detected truncating mutations in three additional families, thus indicating that mutations in *KIF1A* are a rare cause of HSN II [14].

Inhibitor of kappa light polypeptide gene enhancer in B-cells, kinase complex-associated protein (*IKBKAP*)

Mutations in the *IKBKAP* gene are the cause of HSAN III, also known as familial dysautonomia or Riley–Day syndrome, which

is a developmental disorder affecting small myelinated and unmyelinated neurons. Familial dysautonomia is characterized by a distinct phenotype consisting of a variety of symptoms which are present from birth with the earliest signs being poor suck and hypotonia. Clinical diagnostic criteria include absent lachrymation, absent deep-tendon reflexes, and absent lingual fungiform papillae. Autonomic dysfunction also results in periodic vomiting crises comprising nausea, retching, hypersalivation, and cardiovascular lability with postural hypotension and episodic hypertension. Sensory dysfunction affects pain and temperature perception, but is less profound as that in HSAN IV [44]. Only a few different *IKBKAP* mutations have been described [15,16,45,46] but 99.5 % of all patients with familial dysautonomia carry the same splice site mutation in intron 20 (c.2204+6T>C) [15]. A high frequency has been shown among the Ashkenazi Jews [45]. The mutation causes a decrease of the splicing efficiency with sporadic skipping of exon 20, thereby reducing the level of wild-type IKBKAP mRNA in a patient's cells [15].

Neurotrophic tyrosine kinase, receptor, type 1 (*NTRK1/TRKA*)

Mutations in the *NTRK1* gene lead to HSAN IV which is also known as congenital insensitivity to pain and anhidrosis (CIPA). CIPA starts at birth and is associated with a distinct phenotype due to prominent autonomic disturbances. Patients show congenital profound sensory loss affecting the perception of pain and temperature and absence of sweating (anhidrosis), which may lead to episodic fever and recurrent hyperpyrexia because of poor thermoregulation. Anhidrosis is also responsible for the thick and calloused appearance of the skin with lichenification of the palms, areas of hypotrichinosis on the scalp, and dystrophic nail changes [44]. Secondary consequences of reduced pain perception include oral self-mutilation like biting of the tongue, lips, and buccal mucosa, fingertip biting as well as repeated bone fractures and joint trauma, thermal injuries, and severe mutilations of the hands and feet. Learning problems, hyperactivity, and emotional lability are common. Deep tendon reflexes are usually preserved [47]. Histopathological findings consist of decreased numbers of unmyelinated and small myelinated fibres in sensory nerves, including the sural nerve and the cutaneous branch of the radial nerve [48–50]. Several different missense, nonsense, and frameshift, as well as splice site, mutations, have been described in CIPA families and patients in most ethnic groups but with a relatively high prevalence in Israeli-Bedouin Arabs [51–55].

The TRKA protein is a receptor tyrosine kinase, which is phosphorylated in response to nerve growth factor (NGF). NGF supports the survival of sympathetic ganglion neurons and nociceptive sensory neurons in the dorsal root ganglia [56]. Indo et al. [17] also suggested that the NGF–NTRK system has a crucial role in the development and function of the nociceptive reception system, as well as establishment of thermal regulation via sweating in humans.

Nerve growth factor, beta (NGFB)

Mutations in the *NGFB* gene are a rare cause of HSAN V which is separated from HSAN IV based on the pattern of nerve fibre loss [57]. Another important difference is the greater severity of anhidrosis in HSAN IV and the normal intelligence in patients with HSAN V. In HSAN V there is a selective loss of pain perception but normal response to tactile, vibratory, and thermal stimuli. Neurological examination is otherwise normal [44]. In 2001, Houlden et al. [58] observed a *NTRK1* mutation in a HSAN V patient, suggesting that HSAN V and HSAN IV might be allelic. However, in 2004 a homozygous mutation in the coding region of the *NGFB* gene was identified in a large multigenerational consanguineous family from northern Sweden classified as HSAN V [18].

Chaperonin containing TCP1, subunit 5 (epsilon) (CCT5)

Mutations in *CCT5* have been identified in a consanguineous Moroccan family with four affected sibs who had a severe mutilating sensory neuropathy but additional spastic paraplegia [19]. Autosomal recessive ulcero-mutilating neuropathy with spastic paraplegia has been described in only a few families so far [19,59,60]. Age at onset ranges from 1 to 5 years. Affected individuals present with distal sensory loss for all modalities in upper and lower limbs, pronounced in the feet, lower limb spasticity, hyperreflexia with clonus, and positive Babinski sign. Mild distal amyotrophy may be present but motor function is normal. Progression of spasticity is slow but the sensory neuropathy may be progressive and severe.

Dystonin (DST)

In a large consanguineous family of Ashkenazi Jewish descent three infants and a fetus with a severe and lethal form of sensory and autonomic neuropathy and joint contractures were reported. Some features like alacrima, absent corneal reflexes, and decreased fungiform papillae amongst others were similar to those seen in patients with familial dysautonomia. All patients had neonatal hypotonia with poor feeding and poor respiratory effort with apnoeic spells necessitating artificial ventilation. Mild dysmorphic features, including low-set ears, high-arched palate, and small chin were seen in one of the infants. MRI of the brain was normal in all three patients. The use of homozygosity mapping followed by exome sequencing enabled the identification of a deleterious homozygous 1-bp deletion (14865delA) in the *DST* gene, resulting in a frameshift that starts at glu4955 and a premature termination predicted to lead to the loss of the C-terminal 502 amino acids. The mutation affected only the neuronal- and muscle-specific DST isoforms [60a]. *DST* encodes dystonin, a cytoskeleton linker protein.

Interestingly, dystonin is significantly more abundant in cells of familial dysautonomia patients with the IKBKAP (I-κ-B kinase complex-associated protein) mutation compared with fibroblasts of controls, suggesting that upregulation of dystonin is responsible for the milder course in familial dysautonomia.

Related disorders

Congenital inability to experience pain caused by mutations in the voltage-gated sodium channel gene due to mutations in SCN9A

Mutations in the *SCN9A* gene, encoding the alpha-subunit of the voltage-gated sodium channel, which is strongly expressed in nociceptive neurons, are associated with an extraordinary phenotype of a congenital inability to perceive any form of pain with all other sensory modalities preserved and the peripheral and central nervous systems apparently otherwise intact [61]. Patients never feel any pain, at any time, in any part of their body. Complications include frequent bruises, cuts, fractures or osteomyelitis, and injuries of lips or tongue. Intelligence is normal. Additional patients carrying mutations in *SCN9A* have been reported since the original description [62–66]. In particular, this disease has to be considered as a differential diagnosis of CIPA.

Management and treatment

At present treatment of HSN/HSAN remains symptomatic in most cases. It has to be oriented to prevention of self-mutilation and orthopaedic complications. Early and appropriate counselling and training of patients and parents of affected children is necessary to avoid complications. Careful daily inspection of the hands and feet for early signs of unrecognized injuries is important and shoes must always fit well. If injuries, wounds, or other complications are already present, these must be treated immediately by specialists. Antiseptic treatment to eradicate infections may help to prevent osteomyelitis and amputations. In HSAN IV control of hyperthermia is required. High fever responds to use of acetaminophen and/or ibuprofen or direct cooling in a bath or cooling blanket. Early diagnosis and specific dental care for patients with HSAN IV can help prevent the fingertip biting and orofacial manifestations. Ophthalmological examination must be performed to detect keratoconjunctivitis [67]. Neuropathic pain, which is often a feature in HSN I, may be treated symptomatically by using gabapentin, pregabalin, carbamazepine, or amitriptyline, or a combination of an antiepileptic and an antidepressant [4]. Gene therapy is currently not available for any of the known HSN/HSAN genetic subtypes. Clinical evaluation, genetic counselling, and molecular genetic testing should be offered to HSN/HSAN patients and family members at risk. Promising progress for future treatment of HSN I patients carrying mutations in *SPTLC1* has been described in the section Serine-palmitoyltransferase, long chain base subunit 1 (*SPTLC1*) [29].

References

1. Dyck PJ. Neuronal atrophy and degeneration predominantly affecting peripheral sensory and autonomic neurons, In: Dyck PJ, Thomas PK, Griffin JW, Low PA, Poduslo JF (ed) *Peripheral Neuropathy*, 3rd edn, pp. 1065–93. Philadelphia, PA: WB Saunders Company, 1993.

2. Verhoeven K, Timmerman V, Mauko B, et al. Recent advances in hereditary sensory and autonomic neuropathies. *Curr Opin Neurol* 2006; **19**: 474–80.

3. Houlden H, King RH, Muddle J, et al. A novel RAB7 mutation associated with ulcero-mutilating neuropathy. *Ann Neurol* 2004; **56**: 586–90.

4. Nicholson GA. Hereditary sensory neuropathy type IA. In: Pagon RA, Bird TC, Dolan CR, Stephens K (ed), *GeneReviews* [Internet]. Seattle, WA: University of Washington, Seattle, 2002. Updated July 2010 and March 2013. Available at: <http://www.ncbi.nlm.nih.gov/books/NBK1390/>.

5. Verhoeven K, De Jonghe P, Coen K, et al. Mutations in the small GTP-ase late endosomal protein RAB7 cause Charcot–Marie–Tooth type 2B neuropathy. *Am J Hum Genet* 2003; **72**: 722–7.

6. Auer-Grumbach M, De Jonghe P, Verhoeven K, et al. Autosomal dominant inherited neuropathies with prominent sensory loss and mutilations: a review. *Arch Neurol* 2003; **60**: 329–34.

7. Kok C, Kennerson ML, Spring PJ, et al. A locus for hereditary sensory neuropathy with cough and gastroesophageal reflux on chromosome 3q22-p24. *Am J Hum Genet* 2003; **73**: 632–7.

8. Guelly C, Zhu PP, Leonardis L, et al. Targeted high-throughput sequencing identifies mutations in atlastin-1 as a cause of hereditary sensory neuropathy type I. *Am J Hum Genet* 2011; **88**: 99–105.

9. Klein CJ, Botuyan MV, Wu Y, et al. Mutations in DNMT1 cause hereditary sensory neuropathy with dementia and hearing loss. *Nat Genet* 2011; **43**: 595–600.

10. Dawkins JL, Hulme DJ, Brahmbhatt SB, et al. Mutations in SPTLC1, encoding serine palmitoyltransferase, long chain base subunit-1, cause hereditary sensory neuropathy type I. *Nat Genet* 2001; **27**: 309–12.

11. Rotthier A, Auer-Grumbach M, Janssens K, et al. Mutations in the SPTLC2 subunit of serine palmitoyltransferase cause hereditary sensory and autonomic neuropathy type I. *Am J Hum. Genet* 2010; **87**: 513–22.

12. Lafrenière RG, MacDonald ML, Dube MP, et al. Identification of a novel gene (HSN2) causing hereditary sensory and autonomic neuropathy type II through the Study of Canadian Genetic Isolates. *Am J Hum Genet* 2004; **74**: 1064–73.

13. Kurth I, Pamminger T, Hennings JC, et al. Mutations in FAM134B, encoding a newly identified Golgi protein, cause severe sensory and autonomic neuropathy. *Nat Genet* 2009; **41**: 1179–81.

14. Rivière JB, Ramalingam S, Lavastre V, et al. KIF1A, an axonal transporter of synaptic vesicles, is mutated in hereditary sensory and autonomic neuropathy type 2. *Am J Hum Genet* 2011; **89**: 219–30.

15. Slaugenhaupt SA, Blumenfeld A, Gill SP, et al. Tissue-specific expression of a splicing mutation in the IKBKAP gene causes familial dysautonomia. *Am J Hum Genet* 2001; **68**: 598–605.

16. Anderson SL, Coli R, Daly IW, et al. Familial dysautonomia is caused by mutations of the IKAP gene. *Am J Hum Genet* 2001; **68**: 753–8.

17. Indo Y, Tsuruta M, Hayashida Y, et al. Mutations in the TRKA/NGF receptor gene in patients with congenital insensitivity to pain with anhidrosis. *Nat Genet* 1996; **13**: 485–8.

18. Einarsdottir E, Carlsson A, Minde J, et al. A mutation in the nerve growth factor beta gene (NGFB) causes loss of pain perception. *Hum Mol Genet* 2004; **13**: 799–805.

19. Bouhouche A, Benomar A, Bouslam N, et al. Mutation in the epsilon subunit of the cytosolic chaperonin-containing t-complex peptide-1 (Cct5) gene causes autosomal recessive mutilating sensory neuropathy with spastic paraplegia. *J Med Genet* 2006; **43**: 441–3.

20. Rotthier A, Baets J, De Vriendt E, et al. Genes for hereditary sensory and autonomic neuropathies: a genotype-phenotype correlation. *Brain* 2009; **132**: 2699–711.

21. Houlden H, King R, Blake J, et al. Clinical, pathological and genetic characterization of hereditary sensory and autonomic neuropathy type 1 (HSAN I). *Brain* 2006; **129**: 411–25.

22. Thomas PK. Hereditary sensory neuropathies. *Brain Pathol* 1993; **3**: 157–63.

23. Bejaoui K, Wu C, Scheffler MD, et al. SPTLC1 is mutated in hereditary sensory neuropathy, type 1. *Nat Genet* 2001; **27**: 261–2.

24. Geraldes R, de Carvalho M, Santos-Bento M, et al. Hereditary sensory neuropathy type 1 in a Portuguese family-electrodiagnostic and autonomic nervous system studies. *J Neurol Sci* 2004; **227**: 35–8.

25. Nicholson GA, Dawkins JL, Blair IP, et al. Hereditary sensory neuropathy type I: haplotype analysis shows founders in southern England and Europe. *Am J Hum Genet* 2001; **69**: 655–9.

25a. Suh BC, Hong YB, Nakhro K, et al. Early-onset severe hereditary sensory and autonomic neuropathy type 1 with S331F SPTLC1 mutation. *Mol Med Rep* 2014; **9**: 481–6.

25b. Auer-Grumbach M, Bode H, Pieber TR, et al. Mutations at Ser331 in the HSN type I gene SPTLC1 are associated with a distinct syndromic phenotype. *Eur J Med Genet* 2013; **56**: 266–9.

26. Hanada K. Serine palmitoyltransferase, a key enzyme of sphingolipid metabolism. *Biochim Biophys Acta* 2003; 1632: 16–30.

27. Eichler FS, Hornemann T, McCampbell A, et al. Overexpression of the wild-type SPT1 subunit lowers desoxysphingolipid levels and rescues the phenotype of HSAN I. *J Neurosci* 2009; **29**: 14646–51.

28. Penno A, Reilly MM, Houlden H, et al. Hereditary sensory neuropathy type 1 is caused by the accumulation of two neurotoxic sphingolipids. *J Biol Chem* 2010; **285**: 11178–87.

29. Garofalo K, Penno A, Schmidt BP, et al. Oral l-serine supplementation reduces production of neurotoxic desoysphingolipids in mice and humans with hereditary sensory autonomic neuropathy type 1. *J Clin Invest* 2011; **121**: 4735–45.

30. Dawkins JL, Brahmbhatt S, Auer-Grumbach M, et al. Exclusion of serine palmitoyltransferase long chain base subunit 2 (SPTLC2) as common cause for hereditary sensory neuropathy. *Neuromusc Disord* 2002; **12**: 656–8.

31. Vonderheit A, Helenius A Rab7 associates with early endosomes to mediate sorting and transport of semliki forest virus to late endosomes. *PLoS Biol* 2005; **3**: 1225–38.

32. Kwon JM, Elliott JL, Yee WC, et al. Assignment of a second Charcot-Marie-Tooth type II locus to chromosome 3q. *Am J Hum Genet* 1995; **57**: 853–8.

33. Elliott JL, Kwon JM, Goodfellow PJ, et al. Hereditary motor and sensory neuropathy IIB: clinical and electrodiagnostic characteristics. *Neurology* 1997; **48**: 23–8.

34. De Jonghe P, Timmerman V, FitzPatrick D, et al. Mutilating neuropathic ulcerations in a chromosome 3q13-q22 linked Charcot–Marie–Tooth disease type 2B family. *J Neurol Neurosurg Psychiatry* 1997; **62**: 570–3.

35. Auer-Grumbach M, De Jonghe P, Wagner K, et al. Phenotype-genotype correlations in a CMT2B family with refined 3q13-q22 locus. *Neurology* 2000; **55**: 1552–7.

36. Meggouh F, Bienfait HM, Weterman MA, et al. Charcot–Marie–Tooth disease due to a de novo mutation of the RAB7 gene. *Neurology* 2006; **67**: 1476–8.

37. Klein CJ, Wu Y, Kruckeberg KE, et al. SPTLC1 and RAB7 mutation analysis in dominantly inherited and idiopathic sensory neuropathies. *J Neurol Neurosurg Psychiatry* 2005; **76**: 1022–4.

38. Namekawa M, Ribai P, Nelson I, et al. SPG3A is the most frequent cause of hereditary spastic paraplegia with onset before age 10 years. *Neurology* 2006; **66**: 112–14.

38a. Leipold E, Liebmann L, Korenke GC, et al. A de novo gain-of-function mutation in SCN11A causes loss of pain perception. *Nat Genet* 2013; **45**: 1399–404.

38b. Zhang XY, Wen J, Yang W, et al. Gain-of-function mutations in SCN11A cause familial episodic pain. *Am J Hum Genet* 2013; **93**: 957–66.

38c. Kornak U, Mademan I, Schinke M, et al. Sensory neuropathy with bone destruction due to a mutation in the membrane-shaping atlastin GTPase 3. *Brain* 2014; doi: 10.1093/brain/awt357.

39. Spring PJ, Kok C, Nicholson GA, et al. Autosomal dominant hereditary sensory neuropathy with chronic cough and gastro-oesophageal

reflux: clinical features in two families linked to chromosome 3p22-p24. *Brain* 2005; **128**: 2797–810.

40. Kurth I. Hereditary sensory and autonomic neuropathy type II. In: Pagon RA, Bird TC, Dolan CR, Stephens K (ed), *GeneReviews* [Internet]. Seattle, WA: University of Washington, Seattle, 2010. Updated November 2011. Available at: <http://www.ncbi.nlm.nih.gov/books/NBK49247/>.

41. Rivière JB, Verlaan DJ, Shekarabi M, et al. A mutation in the HSN2 gene causes sensory neuropathy type II in a Lebanese family. *Ann Neurol* 2004; **56**: 572–5.

42. Roddier K, Thomas T, Marleau G, et al. Two mutations in the HSN2 gene explain the high prevalence of HSAN2 in French Canadians. *Neurology* 2005; **64**: 1762–7.

43. Coen K, Pareyson D, Auer-Grumbach M, et al. Novel mutations in the HSN2 gene causing hereditary sensory and autonomic neuropathy type II. *Neurology* 2006; **66**: 748–51.

44. Axelrod FB, Gold-von Simson G, Oddoux C. Hereditary sensory and autonomic neuropathy IV. In: Pagon RA, Bird TC, Dolan CR, Stephens K (ed), *GeneReviews* [Internet]. Seattle, WA: University of Washington, 2008. Updated November 2009. Available at: <http://www.ncbi.nlm.nih.gov/books/NBK1769/>.

45. Leyne M. Identification of the first non-Jewish mutation in familial dysautonomia. *Am J Med Genet* 2003; **118A**: 305–8.

46. Sugarman E Familial dysautonomia mutation frequency: clinical testing of greater than 2700 specimens confirms high frequency in Ashkenazi Jews. *Am J Hum Genet* 2002; **71**(Suppl.): 387.

47. Axelrod FB, Hilz MJ. Inherited autonomic neuropathies. *Semin Neurol* 2003; **23**: 381–90.

48. Swanson AG, Buchan GC, Alvord EC. Anatomic changes in congenital insensitivity to pain. *Arch Neurol* 1965; **12**: 12–18.

49. Goebel HH, Veit S, Dyck PJ. Confirmation of virtual unmyelinated fiber absence in hereditary sensory neuropathy type IV. *J Neuropathol Exp Neurol* 1980; **39**: 670–5.

50. Itoh Y, Yagishita S, Nakajima S, et al. Congenital insensitivity to pain with anhidrosis: morphological and morphometrical studies on the skin and peripheral nerves. *Neuropediatrics* 1986; **17**: 103–10.

51. Shatzky S, Moses S, Levy J, et al. Congenital insensitivity to pain with anhidrosis (CIPA) in Israeli-Bedouins: genetic heterogeneity, novel mutations in the TRKA/NGF receptor gene, clinical findings, and results of nerve conduction studies. *Am J Med Genet* 2000; **92**: 353–60.

52. Lee ST, Lee J, Lee M, et al. Clinical and genetic analysis of Korean patients with congenital insensitivity to pain with anhidrosis. *Muscle Nerve* 2009; **40**: 855–9.

53. Lin YP, Su YN, Weng WC, et al. Novel neurotrophic tyrosine kinase receptor type 1 gene mutation associated with congenital insensitivity to pain with anhidrosis. *J Child Neurol* 2010; **25**: 1548–51.

54. Mardy S, Miura Y, Endo F, et al. Congenital insensitivity to pain with anhidrosis: novel mutations in the TRKA (NTRK1) gene encoding a high-affinity receptor for nerve growth factor. *Am J Hum Genet* 1999; **64**: 1570–9.

55. Mardy S, Miura Y, Endo F, et al. Congenital insensitivity to pain with anhidrosis (CIPA): effect of TRKA (NTRK1) missense mutations on autophosphorylation of the receptor tyrosine kinase for nerve growth factor. *Hum Mol Genet* 2001; **10**: 179–88.

56. Levi-Montalcini R The nerve growth factor 35 years later. *Science* 1987; **237**: 1154–62.

57. Minde J, Toolanen G, Andersson T, et al. Familial insensitivity to pain (HSAN V) and a mutation in the NGFB gene. A neurophysiological and pathological study. *Muscle Nerve* 2004; **30**: 752–60.

58. Houlden H, King RH, Hashemi-Nejad A, et al. A novel TRK A (NTRK1) mutation associated with hereditary sensory and autonomic neuropathy type V. *Ann Neurol* 2001; **49**: 521–5.

59. Cavanagh NPC, Eames RA, Galvin RJ, et al. Hereditary sensory neuropathy with spastic paraplegia. *Brain* 1979; **102**: 79–94.

60. Thomas PK., Misra VP, King RHM, et al. Autosomal recessive hereditary sensory neuropathy with spastic paraplegia. *Brain* 1994; **117**: 651–9.

60a. Edvardson S, Cinnamon Y, Jalas C, et al. Hereditary sensory autonomic neuropathy caused by a mutation in dystonin. *Ann Neurol* 2012; **71**: 569–72.

61. Cox JJ, Reimann F, Nicholas AK, et al. An SCN9A channelopathy causes congenital inability to experience pain. *Nature* 2006; **444**: 894–8.

62. Ahmad S, Dahllund L, Eriksson AB, et al. A stop codon mutation in SCN9A causes lack of pain sensation. *Hum Mol Genet* 2007; **16**: 2114–21.

63. Nilsen KB, Nicholas AK, Woods CG, et al. Two novel SCN9A mutations causing insensitivity to pain. *Pain* 2009; **143**: 155–8.

64. Kurban M, Wajid M, Shimomura Y, et al. A nonsense mutation in the SCN9A gene in congenital insensitivity to pain. *Dermatology* 2010; **221**: 179–83.

65. Staud R, Price DD, Janicke D, et al. Two novel mutations of SCN9A (Nav1.7) are associated with partial congenital insensitivity to pain. *Eur J Pain* 2011; **15**: 223–30.

66. Cox JJ, Sheynin J, Shorer Z, et al. Congenital insensitivity to pain: novel SCN9A missense and in-frame deletion mutations. *Hum Mutat* 2010; **31**: E1670–E1686.

67. Bodner L, Woldenberg Y, Pinsk V, et al. Orofacial manifestations of congenital insensitivity to pain with anhidrosis: a report of 24 cases. *ASDC J Dent Child* 2002; **69**: 292–6.

CHAPTER 10

Familial amyloid polyneuropathy

Violaine Planté-Bordeneuve

Introduction

The term familial amyloid polyneuropathy (FAP) refers to multi-system disorders transmitted as an autosomal dominant trait and involving nerve lesions induced by deposits of amyloid fibrils. Most cases are related to mutations of the transthyretin gene (*TTR*). TTR-FAP has a devastating course leading to death within 10 years. Mutant apolipoprotein A1 or gelsolin are rarer precursors of amyloidosis.

TTR amyloidosis

Clinical aspects

Sensorimotor polyneuropathy

The characteristic fibre length-dependent sensorimotor neuropathy is related to early and predominant involvement of unmyelinated and small myelinated fibres [1]. In Portugal, where the disease was originally described [2], symptoms start in the third to fifth decade of life. Inaugural manifestations include numbness and pain in the feet. Pain and temperature sensations are impaired over the distal lower limbs, while light touch and position sense remain preserved. Sensory deficit progresses towards the proximal part of the lower limbs; the upper extremities become involved when sensory loss has reached mid-thigh level. The anterior trunk is then affected, with sensory loss extending upwards and laterally towards the spine. This progression of sensory loss suggests a fibre length-dependent degenerative process with subsequent involvement of large sensory and motor fibres. After a few years the patient is markedly disabled by bilateral foot drop, hand muscle atrophy, and associated autonomic dysfunction. Ultimately the patient is bedbound by a flaccid paralysis that affect all four limbs. Apart from Portugal and Brazil, where the average age of onset of symptoms is 30 years, a later age of onset is observed beyond 60 years in many other countries. In such cases, due to low penetrance of *TTR* mutations, TTR-FAP often presents sporadically [3,4].

Focal nerve lesions

Amyloid deposits may accumulate locally and occasionally induce focal deficit of a cranial nerve, a nerve trunk, or a plexus. Carpal tunnel syndrome is a common and early but non-specific manifestation of FAP, yet median nerve lesions are more severe in FAP than in non-amyloid cases [5].

Autonomic dysfunction

Association of a length-dependent polyneuropathy with autonomic dysfunction is the hallmark of early onset FAP. Cardiocirculatory dysautonomia is responsible for orthostatic hypotension, which may induce blurred vision or dizziness or even syncope when standing up, or remain asymptomatic and be detected only by a fall in blood pressure of more than 30 mmHg upon standing without acceleration of heart rate. Diarrhoea, gastroparesis, and post-prandial vomiting may cause dehydration and increase postural hypotension and progressive loss of weight. In men, erectile dysfunction is an early and nearly constant feature that may precede sensory symptoms of neuropathy. Autonomic dysfunction seems less prominent in late-onset FAP.

Extraneurological manifestations

Cardiac manifestations

Cardiomyopathy seems more common among men with a non-Val30Met mutation and a late onset [6,7]. Progressive amyloid deposition in the myocardium leads to restrictive cardiomyopathy. Alteration of the electrical conduction system is responsible for unpredictable episodes of arrhythmia, severe conduction disorders responsible for syncope or even sudden death. Atrioventricular block and bundle branch blocks often require implantation of a pacemaker.

Other extraneurological manifestations

Ocular abnormalities, which include vitreous and corneal opacities, or glaucoma are observed in 10% of patients. Progressive renal failure with proteinuria seems relatively common in Portugal. End-stage cachexia results from gastrointestinal symptoms, dysautonomia, and muscle atrophy from denervation and infection. Patients become bedridden and exposed to bedsores, venous thrombosis, and pulmonary embolism.

Neurobiology and genetics

Most TTR is synthesized in the liver and a minor proportion in the choroid plexus and epithelial cells of the retina. TTR circulates in soluble form. Pathogenic mutations decrease the stability of TTR tetramers and enhance their dissociation into monomers. The *TTR* gene (18q11.2-12) contains four exons. More than 100 variants of the *TTR* gene have been identified: Val30Met is the most frequent substitution, and is virtually the only variant detected in Portugal, Brazil, and Sweden.

In the United States, the most common pathogenic variant is Val122Ile. It is detected in up to 3–4% of the African-American population. Its main clinical expression is a hypertrophic restrictive cardiomyopathy with mild or no neurological symptoms [8].

TTR-FAP has an important genotypic heterogeneity. At the age of 50 years, penetrance of Val30Met FAP is 80% in Portuguese families whereas it is only 18% and 11% in French and Swedish families, respectively [9,10].

Thanks to DNA testing, genetic information can be delivered to at-risk family members. DNA testing offers the possibility of presymptomatic predictive diagnosis. Other predictive approaches such as prenatal diagnosis or pre-implantation diagnosis can be offered on request to affected families with an early age of onset. Cases of TTR-FAP without a family history are termed sporadic and represent up to half of FAP patients in non-endemic areas. Diagnosis can be difficult in this setting, with an average delay of 4 years [4].

Pathology

Amyloid deposits are found in virtually every tissue at post-mortem examination. In nerve specimens taken by biopsy or at post-mortem examination, amyloid deposits are characteristically found in the endoneurium and around nerve blood vessels [1,11] (see Fig. 10.1) The density of myelinated fibres is markedly decreased with a mixture of demyelination and axonal degeneration. At post-mortem examination amyloid is found in the choroid plexuses, the leptomeninges, and around blood vessels that penetrated the central nervous system, in the Virchow–Robin spaces.

Diagnosis

The diagnosis of FAP rests on the association of a sensorimotor and autonomic polyneuropathy with a family history of neuropathy. In some patients, however, cardiac manifestations predominate. In patients with a known family history, TTR-FAP is considered early. In sporadic cases, TTR-FAP should be considered in patients with a progressive small-fibre polyneuropathy, especially when associated with autonomic dysfunction, cardiac manifestation, or carpal tunnel syndrome. Amyloid deposits can be visualized in nerve biopsy specimens, salivary glands, or abdominal fat. Negative biopsy findings do not rule out amyloidosis.

Congo red tinctorial affinity or thioflavin T along with a characteristic yellow-green birefringence under polarized light confirm the amyloid nature of the deposit. Electron microscopy shows its specific fibrillar aspect, made up of unbranched fibrils of 10 nm diameter with parallel dense borders. Mass spectroscopy-based proteomic analysis can be used to identify the amyloid type. Immunolabelling with anti-TTR antibody favours the genetic origin of the disease. However, false positive or false negative results may occur and DNA testing remains mandatory.

When a patient does not have a family history of FAP, a diagnosis of chronic inflammatory demyelinating polyneuropathy (CIDP) is often considered first. In such cases, a nerve biopsy is useful. After detection of amyloid in biopsy specimens, the diagnosis of light-chain amyloidosis is often considered because of the high incidence of monoclonal gammopathies in the elderly and immunolabelling can be misleading. DNA testing remains necessary in all cases.

Treatment of TTR-FAP

Treatment of symptoms

Useful treatments for neuropathic pains include gabapentin, pregabalin, or duloxetine. Tricyclic antidepressants may increase orthostatic hypotension. Carpal tunnel syndrome will be partially alleviated by surgical decompression. Patients with FAP need advice about foot care and footwear and about the protection of hyposensitive areas and pressure points, to prevent the occurrence of painless ulcers. Orthostatic hypotension may require treatment with midodrine and/or 9-α-fluorohydrocortisone. Implantation of a permanent cardiac pacemaker is often needed.

Liver transplantation

Liver transplantation aims to prevent the formation of additional amyloid deposits. By replacing the liver with part or all of one carrying a normal *TTR* gene, the circulating levels of mutant TTR can be dramatically reduced, which slows or even prevent the progression of the sensorimotor and autonomic neuropathy, particularly in Val30Met early onset patients. It does not prevent the development of cardiac manifestations however.

Medical treatment

Tafamidis is the only approved drug for treatment of patients at early stage of TTR-FAP in Europe [12]. It binds specifically to the TTR tetramers increasing their stability. In premarketing studies tafamidis decreased the rate of deterioration of the neuropathy and quality of life. It seems now reasonable to start treatment with tafamidis early in symptomatic patients and perform liver transplantation when there is disease progression. Gene therapy of TTR-FAP is currently being explored.

Apolipoprotein A1 amyloidosis

The disease predominantly affects the kidney, liver, and gastrointestinal tract in the fourth decade of life. A length-dependent polyneuropathy is not prominent. Sixteen mutations of the apolipoprotein A1 (*ApoA1*) gene are associated with hereditary amyloidosis [13]. The neuropathic pattern is associated with the Gly26Arg mutation, which has also been found in non-neuropathic forms. There is no specific treatment for ApoA1 FAP (see review in Planté-Bordeneuve and Said [14]).

Gelsolin amyloidosis

Hereditary gelsolin amyloidosis (HGA) is an autosomal dominant systemic amyloidosis, first described in Finland in 1969 by

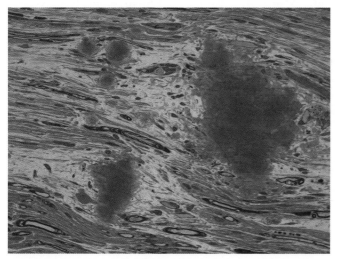

Fig. 10.1 Superficial peroneal nerve biopsy specimen to show massive endoneurial amyloid deposits from a patient with the Tyr77 mutation. One micron thick plastic section with thionin staining. With acknowledgement to Professor Said. (See also figure in colour plate section)

Meretoja [15]. HGA is characterized by adult onset of a slowly progressive neuropathy, corneal lattice dystrophy, cranial neuropathy, and cutis laxa. The amyloid fibrils are composed of fragments of gelsolin generating gelsolin amyloid (or A-Gel), caused by a mutation of the gelsolin gene. Most cases are clustered in Finland, where all patients carry the single base mutation at nucleotide 654A in the gelsolin gene on chromosome 9 [16]. This disease does not significantly shorten the life expectancy of affected individuals but greatly impairs their quality of life.

Conclusion

The most common form of FAP is related to mutations in the *TTR* gene. TTR being mainly secreted by the liver, early liver transplantation is now recommended in patients with symptomatic neuropathy related to the Val30Met mutation. Tafamidis, a recently introduced TTR stabilizer, seems to favourably influence the course of the disease. The gelsolin FAP (HGA) is virtually only observed in Finland. This disease does not significantly shorten life expectancy of affected individuals but greatly impairs quality of life. The ApoA1 FAP is dominated by life-threatening multisystem manifestations with only occasional neuropathy.

References

1. Said G, Ropert A, Faux N. Length dependent degeneration of fibres in Portuguese amyloid polyneuropathy. A clinicopathological study. *Neurology* 1984; **34**: 1025–32.
2. Andrade C. A peculiar form of peripheral neuropathy: familial atypical generalized amyloidosis with special involvement of the peripheral nerves. *Brain* 1952; **75**: 408–27.
3. Ikeda S, Nakazato M, Ando Y, et al. Familial transthyretin-type amyloid polyneuropathy in Japan: clinical and genetic heterogeneity. *Neurology* 2002; **58**: 1001–7.
4. Plante-Bordeneuve V, Ferreira A, Lalu T, et al. Diagnostic pitfalls in sporadic transthyretin familial amyloid polyneuropathy (TTR-FAP). *Neurology* 2007; **69**: 693–8.
5. Koike H, Morozumi S, Kawagashira Y, et al. The significance of carpal tunnel syndrome in transthyretin Val30Met familial amyloid polyneuropathy. *Amyloid* 2009; **16**: 142–8.
6. Suhr OB, Lindqvist P, Olofsson BO, et al. Myocardial hypertrophy and function are related to age at onset in familial amyloidotic polyneuropathy. *Amyloid* 2006; **13**: 154–9.
7. Hörnsten R, Pennlert J, Wiklund U, et al. Heart complications in familial transthyretin amyloidosis: impact of age and gender. *Amyloid* 2010; **17**: 63–8.
8. Jacobson DR, Pastore RD, Yaghoubian R, et al. Variant-sequence transthyretin (isoleucine 122) in late-onset cardiac amyloidosis in black Americans. *N Engl J Med* 1997; **336**: 466–73.
9. Hellman U, Alarcon F, Lundgren HE, et al. Heterogeneity of penetrance in familial amyloid polyneuropathy, ATTR Val30Met, in the Swedish population. *Amyloid* 2008; **15**: 181–6.
10. Planté-Bordeneuve V, Carayol J, Ferreira A, et al. Genetic study of transthyretin amyloid neuropathies: carrier risks among French and Portuguese families. *J Med Genet* 2003; **40**: e120 2003.
11. Said G, Plante-Bordeneuve V. Familial amyloid polyneuropathy: a clinico-pathologic study. *J Neurol Sci* 2009; **284**: 149–54.
12. Said G, Grippon S, Kirkpatrick P. Tafamidis. *Nat Rev Drug Discov* 2012; **11**:185–6.
13. Raimondi S, Guglielmi F, Giorgetti S, et al. Effects of the known pathogenic mutations on the aggregation pathway of the amyloidogenic peptide of apolipoprotein A-I. *J Mol Biol* 2011; **407**: 465–76.
14. Planté-Bordeneuve V, Said G. Familial amyloid polyneuropathy. *Lancet Neurol.* 2011; **10**: 1086–97.
15. Meretoja J. Familial systemic paramyloidosis with lattice dystrophy of the cornea, progressive cranial neuropathy, skin changes and various internal symptoms: A previously unrecognized heritable syndrome. *Ann Clin Res* 1969; **1**: 314–24.
16. Kiuru S. Review: gelsolin-related familial amyloidosis, Finnish type (FAF), and its variants found worldwide. *Amyloid* 1998; **5**: 55–66.

CHAPTER 11

Inherited metabolic neuropathies

Lionel Ginsberg

Introduction

It is conventional to divide the inherited neuropathies into those in which the neuropathy is the sole or predominant clinical manifestation and those that also have major central nervous system (CNS) and/or systemic features (Table 11.1). The latter group is largely synonymous with diseases where the neuropathy arises from a specific inborn error of intermediary metabolism, but the distinction between these two categories of inherited neuropathy is becoming increasingly blurred, for two reasons. First, paralleling the advent of DNA analysis for many of the genes responsible for Charcot–Marie–Tooth disease (CMT), hereditary sensory neuropathies (HSNs), and allied conditions, their phenotypes have become better defined and have broadened, in some instances to include CNS features. For example, X-linked CMT, caused by mutations of the *GJB1* gene, commonly involves the CNS [1]. Secondly, with the identification of many of these genes, it has become possible to elucidate pathogenetic mechanisms in some cases, and these mechanisms sometimes involve metabolic defects. Thus, HSN Type I is usually caused by mutations of the *SPTLC1* gene, encoding an enzyme which, when mutated, catalyses the production of neurotoxic sphingolipids [2]. Bearing these caveats in mind, this chapter will focus on selected examples of diseases in the right-hand column of Table 11.1, classifying them according to the primary organellar localization of the metabolic defect.

Lysosomal storage disorders

Lysosomal storage disorders (LSDs) comprise a group of more than 40 diseases in which mutations of genes encoding lysosomal degradative enzymes (or, in some cases, their cofactors) cause a block in a catabolic pathway, resulting in accumulation and tissue deposition of the substrate for the enzyme in question. The clinical features of LSDs often consist of a combination of severe neurodevelopmental manifestations, skeletal deformity, and visceromegaly. Peripheral neuropathy, if present, may be masked by CNS involvement, but can be a prominent aspect, particularly in some of the sphingolipidoses (Fig. 11.1). Among these, Fabry disease is the archetypal condition in which neuropathy is a dominant feature.

Fabry disease

Fabry disease (FD) is caused by mutations of the *GLA* gene on chromosome Xq22.1 [3]. This gene encodes the enzyme α-galactosidase A, and in FD there is storage of its substrate(s), predominantly globotriaosylceramide (Gb3), in many tissues including neurons and blood vessels. This tissue distribution and other incompletely understood factors give FD a rather atypical phenotype for a LSD. Non-neurological features include a characteristic skin rash (angiokeratoma corporis diffusum) favouring the 'bathing trunk' area (groin, buttocks, upper thighs), ocular changes (cornea verticillata, cataract, retinal and conjunctival vascular tortuosity), gastrointestinal symptoms, hypohidrosis, and ultimately life-threatening nephropathy and cardiac manifestations (cardiomyopathy, valvulopathy, arrhythmias, and ischaemic heart disease). In the CNS, the dominant complication is an increased risk of stroke, with an early age of onset [4]. Magnetic resonance imaging (MRI) may also reveal asymptomatic CNS lesions in FD. Despite the X-chromosomal mode of inheritance, females are not

Table 11.1 Inherited neuropathies

Predominant neuropathy	Neuropathy with systemic and/or CNS features
Charcot–Marie–Tooth diseases	Lysosomal storage disorders, e.g. Fabry disease
Hereditary neuropathy with liability to pressure palsies	Peroxisomal defects, e.g. Refsum disease
Hereditary brachial plexus neuropathy	Mitochondrial diseases, e.g. MNGIE
Hereditary sensory (and autonomic) neuropathies	Other conditions, e.g. porphyrias, Tangier disease
Distal hereditary motor neuropathies	
Familial amyloid polyneuropathies	
Giant axonal neuropathy	

CNS, central nervous system; MNGIE, mitochondrial neurogastrointestinal encephalomyopathy.

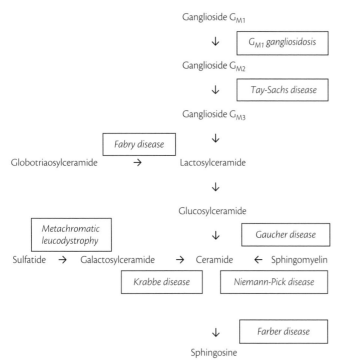

Fig. 11.1 Metabolic interrelationships in the sphingolipidoses. The diseases associated with metabolic blocks at several of the enzymatic steps are shown in the boxes.

merely carriers and may express the disease fully, though not usually as severely or as early as males [5]. The birth frequency of FD has been quoted as lying between 1 in 40 000 and 1 in 117 000, but may be much higher if milder mutations and later-onset forms are included. Either way, it is one of the commoner LSDs.

The peripheral neuropathy of FD affects most patients, and is largely (but not exclusively) a length-dependent, painful, small-fibre, sensory process. Patients present typically in childhood (hemizygous males) or later (heterozygous females) with acroparaesthesiae, but these symptoms may persist into adolescence and adulthood. Fabry crises may be triggered by infection, exercise, or other stressors. In these attacks, patients experience severe pain, not necessarily confined to the extremities, lasting for hours, days, or even weeks. There may be fever and a rise in the erythrocyte sedimentation rate, potentially leading to diagnostic errors if the patient is not yet known to have FD. Neurological signs of FD neuropathy are sparse—usually restricted to some distal loss of nociception, with preservation of the ankle reflexes, though Charcot joints may occur. Likewise, large-fibre nerve conduction studies are usually normal, but small-fibre abnormalities are detectable on thermal threshold testing [6,7]. The pattern of these abnormalities, with greater loss of cold than warm sensitivity, suggests predominant involvement of small myelinated fibres. This conclusion is supported by morphometric studies of nerve biopsies from FD patients, where selective injury of the small myelinated fibre population was also seen [8,9]. Although there is glycolipid deposition in peripheral nerves, mainly in the perineurium and blood vessels, the primary site of the neuropathic lesion in FD is thought to be at dorsal root ganglion level, where lipid has been identified in perikarya [10].

In the absence of a family history, the diagnosis of FD may be difficult and delayed because of the variable multisystem manifestations [11], and despite the importance of reaching a diagnosis as soon as possible now that specific treatment is available. FD should be suspected in young patients with a painful, small-fibre neuropathy, once commoner causes such as diabetes have been excluded. In males, the diagnosis may be made by measuring plasma and/or white cell enzyme activity. This is not possible in females, as the enzyme activity in heterozygotes may overlap the normal range, hence DNA analysis is required.

Supportive management of painful neuropathy in FD includes the use of conventional antiepileptic and antidepressant agents. Specific treatment has been revolutionized by the availability of enzyme replacement therapy (ERT). There are two products—agalsidase alfa and agalsidase beta—both administered every 2 weeks intravenously, and both very expensive and subject to manufacturing shortages. To date, ERT has been shown to benefit many non-neurological manifestations of FD [12,13] and some neurological features, including peripheral nerve function [14,15], although its impact on intra-epidermal nerve fibre density has been less convincing [16,17]. ERT is far from curative for FD, and newer specific treatments are being developed, including substrate reduction, molecular chaperones, and gene therapy. Their role, either as monotherapy or in combination with ERT, is currently under investigation.

Other LSDs

As already noted, peripheral neuropathy in most sphingolipidoses and other LSDs, if present, is masked by the CNS features. This is usually the case in the infantile and juvenile forms of metachromatic leucodystrophy, an autosomal recessive disease caused by aryl sulfatase A deficiency. Occasional patients with this condition present in adolescence or adult life, however [18], and these individuals may have clinical or electrical evidence of a demyelinating neuropathy in combination with cognitive or behavioural disorder. Similarly, late-onset presentations of Krabbe leucodystrophy, another autosomal recessive inborn error (Fig. 11.1), may include a demyelinating neuropathy among the clinical and paraclinical features. In a minority of patients with Type I Gaucher disease, neuropathy is the only neurological feature [19], the clinical presentation being dominated by complications of visceral and skeletal involvement (though there is a risk of parkinsonism in older patients). In the other types of Gaucher disease, CNS manifestations are predominant. Polyneuropathy is not generally an aspect of the mucopolysaccharidoses, another class of LSD, but these patients may have symptomatic entrapment mononeuropathies, notably carpal tunnel syndrome, presumably as a consequence of substrate deposition in connective tissues. All these LSDs were once considered untreatable, but ERT is now available for Type I Gaucher disease and for some of the mucopolysaccharidoses, and selected patients with leucodystrophies have been treated by bone marrow transplantation as an alternative means of enzyme replacement.

Peroxisomal defects

Peroxisomal defects are caused by mutations in genes encoding enzymes or other proteins which localize to the peroxisome. Some of these disorders can bear a superficial clinical resemblance to LSDs, and neuropathy is an important feature of at least two—Refsum disease and adrenomyeloneuropathy.

Table 11.2 Mitochondrial diseases with polyneuropathy as a prominent clinical feature*

Disease	Major features	Other features
Mitochondrial neurogastrointestinal encephalomyopathy (MNGIE)	Gastrointestinal dysmotility, cachexia, polyneuropathy, progressive external ophthalmoplegia, leucoencephalopathy on magnetic resonance imaging	Hearing loss, pigmentary retinopathy
Neuropathy, ataxia, and retinitis pigmentosa (NARP)	Neurogenic muscle weakness, gait and limb ataxia, retinitis pigmentosa	Developmental delay, seizures, dementia, optic atrophy, sensory neuropathy
Sensory ataxic neuropathy, dysarthria, and ophthalmoparesis (SANDO)	Sensory ataxic neuropathy, progressive external ophthalmoplegia, dysarthria	Migraine, depression

*Occasional patients with other mitochondrial diseases, such as Kearns–Sayre syndrome, myoclonic epilepsy with ragged red fibres (MERRF), Twinkle gene mutations and the
   3243A>G mutation, have a significant neuropathy, but these conditions are more usually associated with mild or subclinical involvement of the peripheral nerves.
This table is reproduced with permission from Ginsberg et al. [26].

Refsum disease

Refsum disease is an autosomal recessive condition caused by phytanoyl CoA hydroxylase (PHYH) deficiency [20]. Its clinical features include retinitis pigmentosa, leading to night-blindness in childhood and ultimately progressing to visual field defects. Other neurological aspects comprise anosmia, deafness, and ataxia in addition to the neuropathy. Non-neurological manifestations affect the skin (ichthyosis), eyes (cataract, glaucoma, lens subluxation), heart (arrhythmias, heart failure), and skeleton (deformities, especially of the toes). These features may vary in the extent to which they are expressed clinically, hence the diagnosis is not always straightforward, particularly as the onset of the disease may be well into adult life. The neuropathy of Refsum disease is a sensorimotor demyelinating process which may be acutely relapsing and remitting or chronically progressive, and which may be associated with a markedly elevated cerebrospinal fluid protein concentration. The diagnosis of Refsum disease is confirmed by the measurement of elevated plasma phytanic acid levels. In a biochemically related and clinically similar condition raised pristanic acid levels are diagnostic. The recognition that these branched-chain fatty acids are exclusively of dietary origin forms the theoretical basis for dietary manipulation as the mainstay of treatment of Refsum disease. Diets low in phytanic acid involve the avoidance of dairy products and ruminant meats. Plasmapheresis is also occasionally used in the acute management of the condition.

Adrenomyeloneuropathy

Adrenomyeloneuropathy (AMN) is one of the modes of presentation of X-linked adrenoleucodystrophy (ALD) [21]. Though clinically milder than the childhood cerebral form, patients with AMN (usually male, but occasionally manifesting females) may become significantly disabled, over years or decades from early adulthood onwards, by a slowly progressive spastic paraparesis (eventually with sensory and sphincter involvement), which may or may not be accompanied by adrenal failure. The neuropathy is often masked by the myelopathy, but examination may show absent ankle reflexes in combination with upgoing plantar responses, and nerve conduction studies may confirm a neuropathy, which is usually axonal or mixed axonal and demyelinating. The diagnosis is made by finding elevated plasma levels of very long chain fatty acids (VLCFAs). The underlying molecular defect is not in an enzyme directly concerned with VLCFA metabolism, but is rather a mutation in a gene for a peroxisomal membrane protein belonging to the ATP-binding cassette (ABC) superfamily [22]. Unfortunately, unlike the situation in Refsum disease, VLCFAs are produced endogenously rather than entering the metabolome from an exclusively exogenous source. Hence, attempts to treat AMN, and ALD generally, with diet or with exogenous lipids ('Lorenzo's oil') have proved unsuccessful clinically, albeit partially reversing the biochemical defect. Selected patients with the more severe forms of ALD have been treated by bone marrow transplantation, with the aim of correcting the molecular defect before irreversible CNS damage has occurred [23]. This approach is not currently recommended for AMN patients.

Mitochondrial diseases

Peripheral neuropathy is not usually a prominent feature of mitochondrial disease, with certain exceptions (Table 11.2). Of these, one will be described in more detail, as an archetypal example.

Mitochondrial neurogastrointestinal encephalomyopathy

Mitochondrial neurogastrointestinal encephalomyopathy (MNGIE) is an example of a nuclear gene defect which leads to secondary mitochondrial DNA (mtDNA) damage. It is an autosomal recessive disease, caused by mutations in the gene encoding thymidine phosphorylase (TYMP) [24]. The clinical features develop between the first and fifth decades, and comprise peripheral neuropathy in combination with gastrointestinal dysmotility, cachexia, ptosis, and other manifestations of mitochondrial myopathy, and asymptomatic cerebral white matter lesions. Although the presentation is relatively homogeneous, regardless of the type or position of the mutation, the diagnosis is often delayed and difficult, partly because of the rarity of the condition and partly because the neuropathic and gastrointestinal aspects can mimic other commoner diseases. Thus, children and adolescents with loss of appetite and weight have been misdiagnosed as having anorexia nervosa. Patients presenting with peripheral neuropathy have been wrongly labelled as having chronic inflammatory demyelinating polyneuropathy (CIDP) because nerve conduction studies in MNGIE can suggest a patchy demyelinating process [25]. More acute neuropathic presentations may even resemble Guillain–Barré syndrome [26].

The *TYMP* gene, also known as *ECGF1* (for platelet-derived endothelial cell growth factor) encodes a 482-amino-acid protein, which ultimately functions as a homodimeric cytosolic enzyme, responsible for the degradation of thymidine and deoxyuridine, and hence the homeostasis of nucleotide pools (Fig. 11.2). The

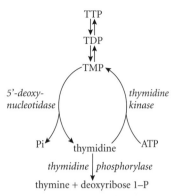

Fig. 11.2 The pyrimidine salvage pathway. Key enzymes are shown in italics: TTP, thymidine triphosphate; TDP, thymidine diphosphate; TMP, thymidine monophosphate.

location of this enzyme in a pathway concerned with pyrimidine salvage helps explain the mitochondrial impact of the disease. In dividing cells, defects in this salvage pathway are compensated by a *de novo* biosynthetic pathway. In non-dividing cells, as found in nerve and muscle tissue, however, failure of the salvage pathway is uncompensated, but nuclear DNA synthesis is not occurring, by definition. Hence, the consequences of the biochemical defect are only manifested as mtDNA instability—deletions, depletion, and point mutations—in these cells, which are highly dependent on oxidative phosphorylation for their energy requirements. A mitochondrial phenotype results, with clinical and histological evidence of neuropathy and myopathy. Interestingly, and paradoxically, TYMP is not expressed in skeletal muscle. Presumably, increased extracellular thymidine pools consequent on TYMP deficiency in other tissues could lead to myopathy in MNGIE by driving incorporation of the nucleoside into muscle cells to toxic concentrations.

The diagnosis of MNGIE rests on detecting grossly elevated levels of thymidine and deoxyuridine in plasma, along with minimal or absent TYMP enzyme activity in platelets (one of the richest sources of the enzyme) or white cells. Indeed, the definition of MNGIE demands this molecular basis, with underlying *TYMP* mutations. However, occasional patients have been identified with MNGIE-like phenotypes caused by other enzyme deficiencies, including POLG (mtDNA polymerase gamma) [27], and RIR2B, a ribonucleoside reductase subunit [28]. Previously considered progressive and lethal, there are now treatments for MNGIE, all based on the principles of substrate reduction or enzyme replacement. These therapeutic approaches include peritoneal dialysis [29], platelet infusion [30], allogeneic stem cell transplantation [31], and administration of stabilized, active TYMP enzyme, encapsulated in red cell ghosts [32].

Other conditions

Porphyria

The porphyrias are caused by genetic defects of haem biosynthesis—a cascade of cytosolic and mitochondrial enzymes [33]. Three are particularly associated with episodic neurological features—acute intermittent porphyria, variegate porphyria, and hereditary coproporphyria, known collectively as the hepatic porphyrias. The last two also have cutaneous manifestations (photosensitivity, hyperpigmentation, hypertrichosis, skin fragility). All three conditions are inherited in an autosomal dominant fashion with incomplete penetrance. Episodes of porphyria start after puberty and may be triggered by drugs (Table 11.3), hormones, infection, or low carbohydrate intake. Abdominal symptoms herald the onset of an attack—pain, nausea, vomiting, and constipation. A minority of patients then develop neurological and psychiatric complications—depression, psychosis, seizures, delirium, coma. The onset of weakness is typically acute and severe, mimicking Guillain–Barré syndrome. The neuropathy is predominantly motor; weakness may be proximal and asymmetrical. Tendon reflexes are usually reduced or absent, but the ankle jerks may be retained paradoxically. Cranial nerves are commonly involved as is the cardiovascular autonomic nervous system. Sensory symptoms and signs are generally mild, but some patients have distal or proximal sensory loss and neuropathic pain. Nerve conduction studies indicate predominantly axonal damage.

The common biochemical mechanism unifying the triggers for porphyria is that they are all enzyme inducers for δ-aminolaevulinic acid synthase, which is the rate-limiting step in haem biosynthesis. With porphyrin metabolism blocked downstream by the genetic defect, δ-aminolaevulinic acid and porphobilinogen then accumulate and may be directly neurotoxic. Certainly, the presence of these metabolites in urine during a neurovisceral attack of porphyria is important diagnostically.

The treatment of acute porphyria comprises supportive care and elimination of potential triggers—treating infection and discontinuing relevant drugs (Table 11.3). Hepatic δ-aminolaevulinic acid synthase can be inhibited by high carbohydrate intake and haem, given as haem arginate. Once the diagnosis of porphyria has been established, most patients do well provided exposure to unsafe drugs is prevented and good carbohydrate intake is maintained, but a minority have chronic recurring attacks and some patients have persistent disability from a neuropathic episode.

Tangier disease

Tangier disease is a very rare autosomal recessive condition in which there is severe deficiency or absence of plasma high-density lipoprotein and hence apolipoprotein A1, with resulting hypocholesterolaemia and hypertriglyceridaemia. The age of onset ranges from childhood to late adult life. Lipid is deposited in lymphoreticular tissue leading to lymphadenopathy, hepatosplenomegaly, and a characteristic appearance of enlarged yellow-orange tonsils. Other non-neurological manifestations include consequences of splenomegaly—thrombocytopenia and reticulocytosis. Patients are also at increased risk of coronary artery disease. Like ALD, the gene for Tangier disease encodes a protein belonging to the ABC superfamily, but, in this case, the location of the transporter, ABCA1, is at the cell surface rather than the peroxisomal membrane, where the protein is involved in lipid trafficking [34–37].

Up to 50% of patients with Tangier disease have a slowly progressive predominantly sensory neuropathy [38]. Several patterns are recognized: younger patients with relapsing multiple mononeuropathies [39], a rare distal symmetrical sensorimotor polyneuropathy [40], and a striking pseudo-syringomyelic syndrome [41]. In the last of these patterns, patients lose nociceptive sensation over the trunk, face, and arms with relative preservation of joint position and vibration sense. There is wasting and weakness of the hands, bilateral facial weakness, and shooting pain in the arms. Nerve conduction

Table 11.3 Safe and unsafe drugs in porphyria

Drug class	Probably safe	Unsafe
Antiepileptic	Diazepam, lorazepam, magnesium sulphate, gabapentin	Barbiturates, phenytoin, carbamazepine, sodium valproate, ethosuximide, clonazepam
Psychiatric	Chlorpromazine, lithium, fluoxetine	Tricyclic antidepressants, sulpiride, monoamine oxidase inhibitors, thioridazine
Endocrine	Insulin	Oestrogens, progestogens, danazol, tamoxifen, anabolic steroids, sulphonylureas
Analgesic	Aspirin, codeine, morphine, ibuprofen	Oxycodone, pentazocine
Antimicrobial	Penicillin, aminoglycosides	Sulphonamides, trimethoprim, erythromycin, nitrofurantoin, isoniazid, pyrazinamide, dapsone, griseofulvin
Other	Allopurinol, furosemide (frusemide), warfarin	Ergot derivatives, statins, amiodarone, baclofen, chlorambucil, hydralazine, ranitidine, nifedipine, verapamil

studies show mixed axonal and demyelinating features. The pathogenesis of the neuropathy in Tangier disease is incompletely understood, though lipid is deposited in peripheral nerves, particularly in Schwann cells [42]. Treatment of the neuropathy is symptomatic.

Other lipid and lipoprotein disorders

Abetalipoproteinaemia (Bassen–Kornzweig syndrome) and familial hypobetalipoproteinaemia have distinct genetic bases but similar clinical and paraclinical features—acanthocytosis, apolipoprotein B deficiency, retinopathy, and progressive neurological dysfunction. The lipoprotein deficiency leads to low plasma cholesterol and triglyceride concentrations. The neurological manifestations resemble Friedreich ataxia and include an axonal large-fibre sensory neuropathy in addition to cerebellar disturbance. Both the retinopathy and the neurological aspects are consequences of vitamin E deficiency, a lipid-soluble vitamin which requires normal lipoprotein levels and function for its absorption and transport. Treatment is therefore with high-dose vitamin E, which can prevent, stabilize, and perhaps even reverse neurological damage.

Cerebrotendinous xanthomatosis is a rare autosomal recessive disease caused by mutations in the gene encoding sterol 27-hydroxylase. The metabolic defect results in absent bile chenodeoxycholic acid and increased blood cholestanol, which is also deposited in tissues including tendons and neurons. Neurological features typically develop in late childhood or early adulthood and include dementia, spasticity, ataxia, and neuropathy; systemic aspects are tendon xanthomas, cataract, osteoporosis, and premature atherosclerosis. Early recognition and diagnosis are important as effective treatment is available in the form of chenodeoxycholic acid, which can lower blood cholestanol concentration and arrest disease progression [43].

Conclusion

The inherited metabolic neuropathies are individually rare but collectively constitute a significant source of morbidity and mortality. They may be classified according to the subcellular, organellar localization of the causative metabolic defect, e.g. lysosomal, peroxisomal, mitochondrial. The clinical features of the resulting neuropathies are highly heterogeneous and their presentations are rendered even more distinctive by coexistent systemic and CNS manifestations. Unlike some other genetic neuropathies, there are specific treatments, or at least preventative measures, for many of these conditions, often based on the principles of enzyme replacement or substrate reduction.

References

1. Scherer SS, Kleopa KA. X-linked Charcot–Marie–Tooth disease. In: Dyck PJ, Thomas PK (ed) *Peripheral Neuropathy*, 4th edn, Vol. 2, pp. 1791–804. Philadelphia, PA: Elsevier Saunders, 2005.
2. Penno A, Reilly MM, Houlden H, et al. Hereditary sensory neuropathy type 1 is caused by the accumulation of two neurotoxic sphingolipids. *J Biol Chem* 2010; **285**: 11178–87.
3. Desnick RJ, Ioannou YA, Eng CM. α-Galactosidase A deficiency: Fabry disease. In: Scriver CR, Beaudet AL, Sly WS, Valle D (ed) *The Metabolic and Molecular Bases of Inherited Disease*, 8th edn, Vol. 2, pp. 3733–74. New York, NY: McGraw-Hill, 2001.
4. Ginsberg L. Monogenic disorder: Fabry disease. In Sharma P, Meschia JF (ed) *Stroke Genetics*, pp. 97–106. London: Springer, 2012.
5. Deegan PB, Baehner AF, Barba Romero MA, Hughes DA, Kampmann C, Beck M; for the European FOS Investigators. Natural history of Fabry disease in females in the Fabry Outcome Survey. *J Med Genet* 2006; **43**: 347–52.
6. Morgan SH, Rudge P, Smith SJ, et al. The neurological complications of Anderson–Fabry disease (alpha-galactosidase A deficiency)—investigation of symptomatic and presymptomatic patients. *Q J Med* 1990; **75**: 491–507.
7. Luciano CA, Russell JW, Banerjee TK, et al. Physiological characterization of neuropathy in Fabry's disease. *Muscle Nerve* 2002; **26**: 622–9.
8. Kocen RS, Thomas PK. Peripheral nerve involvement in Fabry's disease. *Arch Neurol* 1970; **22**: 81–8.
9. Ginsberg L. Specific painful neuropathies. In: Cervero F, Jensen TS (ed) *Handbook of Clinical Neurology*, Vol. 81, pp. 635–52. Edinburgh: Elsevier, 2006.
10. Onishi A, Dyck PJ. Loss of small peripheral sensory neurons in Fabry disease. Histologic and morphometric evaluation of cutaneous nerves, spinal ganglia and posterior columns. *Arch Neurol* 1974; **31**: 120–7.
11. Mehta A, Ricci R, Widmer U, et al. Fabry disease defined: baseline clinical manifestations of 366 patients in the Fabry Outcome Survey. *Eur J Clin Invest* 2004; **34**: 236–42.
12. Schiffmann R, Kopp JB, Austin HA, 3rd, et al. Enzyme replacement therapy in Fabry disease: a randomized controlled trial. *J Am Med Assoc* 2001; **285**: 2743–9.
13. Eng CM, Guffon N, Wilcox WR, et al., for the International Collaborative Fabry Disease Study Group. Safety and efficacy of recombinant human alpha-galactosidase A replacement therapy in Fabry's disease. *N Engl J Med* 2001; **345**: 9–16.
14. Schiffmann R, Floeter MK, Dambrosia JM, et al. Enzyme replacement therapy improves peripheral nerve and sweat function in Fabry disease. *Muscle Nerve* 2003; **28**: 703–10.

15. Hilz MJ, Brys M, Marthol H, Stemper B, Dütsch M. Enzyme replacement therapy improves function of C-, A delta-, and A beta-nerve fibers in Fabry neuropathy. *Neurology* 2004; **62**: 1066–72.

16. Schiffmann R, Hauer P, Freeman B, et al. Enzyme replacement therapy and intraepidermal innervation density in Fabry disease. *Muscle Nerve* 2006; **34**: 53–6.

17. Üçeyler N, He L, Schönfeld D, et al. Small fibers in Fabry disease: baseline and follow-up data under enzyme replacement therapy. *J Peripher Nerv Syst* 2011; **16**: 304–14.

18. Ginsberg L. Inherited metabolic storage diseases. In: Scolding N (ed) *Contemporary Treatments in Neurology*, pp. 249–63. Oxford: Butterworth Heinemann, 2001.

19. Biegstraaten M, Mengel E, Maródi L, et al. Peripheral neuropathy in adult type 1 Gaucher disease: a 2-year prospective observational study. *Brain* 2010; **133**: 2909–19.

20. Jansen GA, Wanders RJA, Watkins PA, Mihalik SJ. Phytanoyl-coenzyme A hydroxylase deficiency—the enzyme defect in Refsum's disease. *N Engl J Med* 1997; **337**: 133–4.

21. Moser HW. Adrenoleukodystrophy: phenotype, genetics, pathogenesis and therapy. *Brain* 1997; **120**: 1485–508.

22. Mosser J, Douar AM, Sarde CO, et al. Putative X-linked adrenoleukodystrophy gene shares unexpected homology with ABC transporters. *Nature* 1993; **361**: 726–30.

23. Aubourg P, Blanche S, Jambaqué I, et al. Reversal of early neurologic and neuroradiologic manifestations of X-linked adrenoleukodystrophy by bone marrow transplantation. *N Engl J Med* 1990; **322**: 1860–6.

24. Nishino I, Spinazzola A, Hirano M. Thymidine phosphorylase gene mutations in MNGIE, a human mitochondrial disorder. *Science* 1999; **283**: 689–92.

25. Bedlack RS, Vu T, Hammans S, et al. MNGIE neuropathy: five cases mimicking chronic inflammatory demyelinating polyneuropathy. *Muscle Nerve* 2004; **29**: 364–8.

26. Ginsberg L, Schapira AHV, Taanman J-W. Grand round: relapsing neuropathy in an 18-year-old woman. *Lancet Neurol* 2007; **6**: 192–8.

27. Van Goethem G, Schwartz M, Löfgren A, Dermaut B, Van Broeckhoven C, Vissing J. Novel POLG mutations in progressive external ophthalmoplegia mimicking mitochondrial neurogastrointestinal encephalomyopathy. *Eur J Hum Genet* 2003; **11**: 547–9.

28. Shaibani A, Shchelochkov OA, Zhang S, et al. Mitochondrial neurogastrointestinal encephalopathy due to mutations in RRM2B. *Arch Neurol* 2009; **66**: 1028–32.

29. Yavuz H, Ozel A, Christensen M, et al. Treatment of mitochondrial neurogastrointestinal encephalomyopathy with dialysis. *Arch Neurol* 2007; **64**: 435–8.

30. Lara MC, Weiss B, Illa I, et al. Infusion of platelets transiently reduces nucleoside overload in MNGIE. *Neurology* 2006; **67**: 1461–3.

31. Hirano M, Martí R, Casali C, et al. Allogeneic stem cell transplantation corrects biochemical derangements in MNGIE. *Neurology* 2006; **67**: 1458–60.

32. Moran NF, Bain MD, Muqit MM, Bax BE. Carrier erythrocyte entrapped thymidine phosphorylase therapy for MNGIE. *Neurology* 2008; **71**: 686–8.

33. Anderson KE, Sassa S, Bishop DF, Desnick RJ. Disorders of heme biosynthesis: X-linked sideroblastic anemia and the porphyrias. In: Scriver CR, Beaudet AL, Sly WS, Valle D (ed) *The Metabolic and Molecular Bases of Inherited Disease*, 8th edn, Vol. 2, pp. 2991–3062. New York, NY: McGraw-Hill, 2001.

34. Bodzioch M, Orso E, Klucken J, et al. The gene encoding ATP-binding cassette transporter 1 is mutated in Tangier disease. *Nat Genet* 1999; **22**: 347–51.

35. Brooks-Wilson A, Marcil M, Clee SM, et al. Mutations in ABC1 in Tangier disease and familial high-density lipoprotein deficiency. *Nat Genet* 1999; **22**: 336–45.

36. Rust S, Rosier M, Funke H, et al. Tangier disease is caused by mutations in the gene encoding ATP-binding cassette transporter 1. *Nat Genet* 1999; **22**: 352–5.

37. Lawn RM, Wade DP, Garvin MR, et al. The Tangier disease gene product ABC1 controls the cellular apolipoprotein-mediated lipid removal pathway. *J Clin Invest* 1999; **104**: R25–R31.

38. Assmann G, Von Eckardstein A, Brewer HB, Jr. Familial analphalipoproteinemia: Tangier disease. In: Scriver CR, Beaudet AL, Sly WS, Valle D (ed) *The Metabolic and Molecular Bases of Inherited Disease*, 8th edn, Vol. 2, pp. 2937–60. New York, NY: McGraw-Hill, 2001.

39. Engel WK, Dorman JD, Levy RI, Fredrickson DS. Neuropathy in Tangier disease. Alpha-lipoprotein deficiency manifesting as familial recurrent neuropathy and intestinal lipid storage. *Arch Neurol* 1967; **17**: 1–9.

40. Marbini A, Gemignani F, Ferrarini G, et al. Tangier disease. A case with sensorimotor distal polyneuropathy and lipid accumulation in striated muscle and vasa nervorum. *Acta Neuropathol* 1985; **67**: 121–7.

41. Gibbels E, Schaefer HE, Runne U, Schröder JM, Haupt WF, Assmann G. Severe polyneuropathy in Tangier disease mimicking syringomyelia or leprosy. Clinical, biochemical, electrophysiological, and morphological evaluation, including electron microscopy of nerve, muscle, and skin biopsies. *J Neurol* 1985; **232**: 283–94.

42. Dyck PJ, Ellefson RD, Yao JK, Herbert PN. Adult onset of Tangier disease: I. Morphometric and pathologic studies suggesting delayed degradation of neutral lipids after fiber degeneration. *J Neuropathol Exp Neurol* 1978; **37**: 119–37.

43. Kuriyama M, Tokimura Y, Fujiyama J, Utatsu Y, Osame M. Treatment of cerebrotendinous xanthomatosis: effects of chenodeoxycholic acid, pravastatin, and combined use. *J Neurol Sci* 1994; **125**: 22–8.

SECTION 4

Peripheral Nerve: Acquired

CHAPTER 12

Mononeuropathy

Neil G. Simon and Matthew C. Kiernan

Pathogenesis and diagnosis of mononeuropathy

Introduction

Mononeuropathy reflects an insult or injury to a single peripheral nerve, which may be isolated (mononeuropathy simplex) or alternatively may be mechanistically linked with other peripheral nerve lesions (mononeuropathy multiplex). Mononeuropathy represents a common problem in clinical neurological practice, with peripheral nerve lesions accounting for 10% of the caseload of British neurologists [1] and over 40% of all clinical neurophysiology referrals.

Mononeuropathy may masquerade as alternative pathology, such as radiculopathy, and an accurate initial diagnosis will avoid unnecessary investigation and treatment. Conversely, multifocal or generalized processes may initially present with a mononeuropathy, particularly the inflammatory neuropathies. In such cases, careful attention to the patterns of clinical involvement, with a thorough and complete knowledge of the underlying anatomy, will help to avoid misdiagnosis.

Clinical assessment and appropriate investigation must be considered carefully, as variations from the typical occur, particularly with incomplete lesions. However, a detailed history and directed examination should confirm the diagnosis in the majority, with subsequent support provided by electrodiagnostic and other investigations as necessary, including structural imaging.

In the present chapter, the principles of pathogenesis and the varied clinical presentations of peripheral nerve injury will be reviewed, incorporating detailed description of the underlying anatomy, to facilitate the diagnosis and management of the clinical mononeuropathies.

Mechanisms of nerve injury

Entrapment and compression

Most mononeuropathies are caused by compressive nerve injury (see Table 12.1). Much of the understanding of the pathophysiology of compressive nerve injury was derived from experimental animal studies which demonstrated that application of localized compression to the nerve resulted in secondary changes to the myelin sheath, with early changes at the edge of the compressed area. Displacement of the axoplasm caused traction at the node of Ranvier, with invagination of the myelin sheath. Subsequently, localized myelin loss occurred, producing conduction block, generally within 1 week of injury. The changes were most prominent in the large myelinated fibres, sparing small myelinated and unmyelinated fibres with distal segments of the nerve unaffected. With maintained pressure, axonal injury occurred, and

Wallerian degeneration ensued, with degeneration of axons and Schwann cells, initially most marked in distal portions of the nerve.

It has been suggested that a proximal compressive lesion may exacerbate a distal process, e.g. cervical radiculopathy coexisting with carpal tunnel syndrome (CTS). To explain this 'double-crush' concept, it was suggested that a proximal compressive lesion may impair axoplasmic flow and hence render distal segments of the axon more susceptible to compressive injury. While this theory continues to receive support, particularly in the surgical literature, it has been vigorously critiqued [2], and the validity of the 'double-crush syndrome' remains controversial.

The effects of compression may also precipitate underlying genetic abnormality. Specifically, hereditary neuropathy with liability to pressure palsy (HNPP) is a dominantly inherited condition, characterized by recurrent focal pressure neuropathies and the development of a mild peripheral polyneuropathy. The causative genetic abnormality has been identified as a deletion or mutation of *PMP22* on chromosome 17p11.2. Nerve biopsy in this condition has identified dysmyelination with tomaculous thickening of the myelin sheath, underlying the sensitivity to the effects of pressure.

Separate to the above mechanisms, isolated nerve trauma may be induced by penetrating injury or traction, the latter being a common complication of orthopaedic injuries such as fracture or joint dislocation.

Anatomical considerations of nerve injury and repair

The extent of nerve injury is important when considering subsequent mechanisms of nerve regeneration. The most commonly used classification system divided nerve injuries into 'neuropraxia', 'axonotmesis', and 'neurotmesis' [3].

The mildest form of injury, neuropraxia, typically involves focal demyelination following a compressive injury. In the absence of ongoing injury, regeneration and complete functional recovery is relatively rapid (over 2–12 weeks) with restoration of the myelin sheath and abolition of conduction block.

Axonotmesis involves disruption of the axon and myelin sheath with preservation of the connective tissue elements of the nerve. The process of nerve regeneration begins within days of injury. Initially, inflammatory cells clear myelin debris [4]. Schwann cells form bands of Büngner, which act as guides for the regenerating nerve fibres [5]. Collateral sprouts arise from the nodes of Ranvier in the proximal stump and grow at a rate of approximately 1 mm a day. Distal regeneration also occurs in incomplete nerve lesions and is the dominant process in milder axonal injuries. Sprouts from remaining axons within partially denervated muscle extend to

Table 12.1 Disease processes and mechanisms of injury associated with mononeuropathy

Mechanisms of focal nerve injury	
Trauma:	Viral infection:
• Entrapment and compression	• Human immunodeficiency virus-1
• Laceration	• Epstein–Barr virus
• Crush	• Cytomegalovirus
• Traction	• Varicella zoster virus
• Electrical injury	• Hepatitis B virus
• Radiotherapy	• Hepatitis C virus
Metabolic and endocrine disorders:	Bacterial infection:
• Diabetes mellitus	• Lyme disease
• Uraemia	• Leprosy
• Hypothyroidism	Mass lesions:
• Acromegaly	• Primary nerve sheath tumours:
Inflammatory disorders:	• Schwannoma
• Neuralgic amyotrophy	• Neurofibroma
• Vasculitic mononeuritis	• Neurofibrosarcoma
• Isolated peripheral nerve vasculitis	• Metastatic tumours
• Cryoglobulinaemia	• Intraneural ganglion cyst
• Polyarteritis nodosa	Paraneoplastic mononeuritis:
• Wegener granulomatosis	• Small cell lung cancer
• Giant cell arteritis	• Lung adenocarcinoma
• Sarcoidosis	• Hairy cell leukaemia
• Sensory perineuritis	• Prostate cancer
Connective tissue diseases:	• Endometrial adenocarcinoma
• Systemic lupus erythematosis	• Renal cell carcinoma
• Rheumatoid arthritis	Drugs and toxins:
• Sjögren syndrome	• Lead poisoning
• Systemic sclerosis	• Amphetamine
• Mixed connective tissue disease	• Cocaine
Infiltrative disorders:	• Heroin
• Neurolymphomatosis	• Vincristine
• Amyloidosis	Hereditary disorders:
• Waldenström macroglobulinaemia	• Hereditary neuropathy with liability to pressure palsies
Ischaemia	• Hereditary neuralgic amyotrophy

denervated endplates along Schwann cell processes. Axonotmesis injuries generally demonstrate significant or complete clinical recovery.

More severe injuries, termed neurotmesis, involve damage to connective tissue elements of the nerve (endoneurium, perineurium, epineurium) and are seen in severe crush injuries, transection, or ischaemic injury of the nerve. Regeneration depends on the integrity of residual connective tissue elements and the distance between proximal and distal portions of the nerve. Motor nerve regeneration may take up to 24 months to complete, but after this time muscles become fibrotic. Regeneration of sensory fibres may occur over longer periods. Surgical apposition of the proximal and distal segments after nerve transection may be required to promote regeneration.

Clinical features of the mononeuropathies

Upper limb mononeuropathy

Anatomical considerations

The brachial plexus is formed from the anterior primary rami of the C5 to T1 nerve roots. The typical organization of the brachial plexus is depicted in Fig. 12.1, although there may also be additional contribution of C4 or T2 segments. Whilst there is some variation in anatomy between individuals, the plexus can be divided into trunks, divisions, cords, and major branches.

Spinal nerve roots pass between the scalene muscles to enter the posterior triangle of the neck where they form the upper, middle, and lower trunks. Each trunk splits into an anterior and posterior division. The three posterior divisions coalesce to form the posterior cord, which divides into the radial and axillary nerves. The anterior divisions of the superior and middle trunks join to form the lateral cord, whilst the anterior division of the lower trunk continues as the medial cord. The medial cord divides to form the ulnar nerve and a contribution to the median nerve. The lateral cord splits into the musculocutaneous nerve, with a contribution to the median nerve.

The trunks of the brachial plexus lie in close approximation to the subclavian artery in the interscalene triangle at the base of the neck. Anomalous structures, such as fibrous bands, cervical ribs, and anomalous muscles, may impinge upon the brachial plexus at this point, forming the basis of neurogenic thoracic outlet syndrome. The brachial plexus passes through the costoclavicular triangle with the subclavian vessels, before entering the axilla with its cords and branches surrounding the axillary artery.

Median neuropathy (Table 12.2)

Carpal tunnel syndrome

Carpal tunnel syndrome is the most common human entrapment neuropathy, with estimates of prevalence between 1 and 8% of the population [6,7]. The condition is more common in women, and with advancing age. The median nerve becomes entrapped and compressed as it passes through the carpal tunnel at the wrist, deep to the flexor retinaculum and superficial to the tendons of the finger flexors and flexor pollicis longus (FPL) (Fig. 12.2). Entrapment may be precipitated by thickening of the flexor retinaculum and flexor tendons, or encroachment on the space by degenerative disease involving the carpal bones and joints.

A number of predisposing factors have been associated with an increased incidence of symptomatic CTS. Constitutional features, such as a small hand, predispose to CTS [8,9]. There is a higher rate of CTS in workers whose occupations involve significant hand-transmitted vibration or repeated forceful movements of the hand and wrist [10], although employment considerations remain controversial. Comorbid medical conditions, such as diabetes mellitus (DM), renal failure, tenosynovitis, rheumatoid arthritis, hypothyroidism, acromegaly, and amyloidosis have all been associated with a higher incidence of CTS.

Pregnancy may be a common precipitant of CTS, with up to 60% of pregnant women experiencing symptoms at some stage and up to 40% meeting neurophysiological criteria for the diagnosis of CTS [11]. Hormonal factors in pregnancy promoting fluid retention may result in oedema of the contents of the carpal tunnel, although symptoms may persist for 3 or more years after

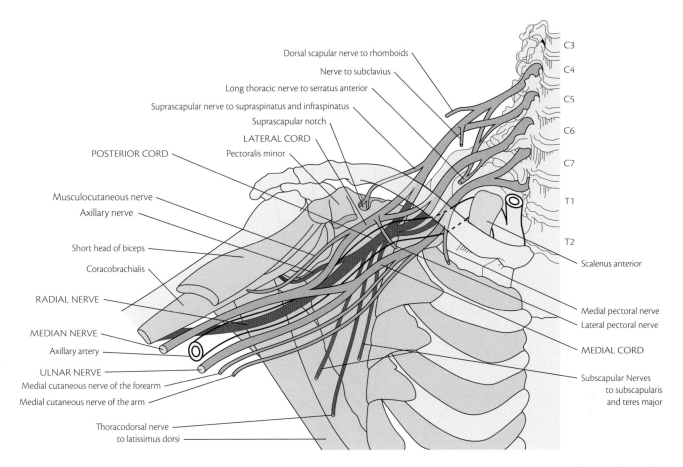

Fig. 12.1 Anatomy of the brachial plexus. (Adapted from O'Brien MD (2000). *Aids to the Examination of the Peripheral Nervous System*, 4th edn. Elsevier, Oxford, with kind permission of Elsevier). (See also figure in colour plate section)

Table 12.2 Median nerve anatomy and common sites of injury

Median nerve
Spinal nerve roots: C6–T1
Brachial plexus: upper, middle, and lower trunks > medial and lateral cords

Major branches	Innervated structures	Sites of injury
Proximal median nerve	Motor: Palmaris longus Pronator teres Flexor carpi radialis Flexor digitorum superficialis	Ligament of Struthers Pronator teres syndrome
Anterior interosseous nerve	Motor: Flexor pollicis longus Flexor digitorum profundus (digits 2 and 3) Pronator quadratus	Forearm
Palmar cutaneous branch	Sensory: Thenar eminence	Wrist (e.g. division of flexor retinaculum)
Terminal sensory branch	Sensory: Palmar surface lateral 3 ½ digits	Carpal tunnel syndrome
Terminal motor branch	Motor: Abductor pollicis brevis Flexor pollicis brevis (with ulnar nerve) Opponens pollicis Lumbricals 1 and 2	Carpal tunnel syndrome 'Thenar motor neuropathy'

delivery [12]. Obesity is a risk factor for CTS, especially in younger patients [13]. However, this relationship is not straightforward, as rapid weight loss after treatment for obesity is also associated with higher rates of CTS than expected [14].

The characteristic clinical presentation of CTS is nocturnal paraesthesiae affecting the dominant hand. Pain may also be reported involving the hand, forearm, elbow, or shoulder, mimicking cervical radiculopathy in some cases. Patients often report shaking their hand to ease the symptoms during a nocturnal episode, or sleep with the hand hanging over the edge of the bed. The symptoms may also be precipitated by persistent wrist flexion or extension, such as when driving, with these positions of the wrist resulting in a reduction in the cross-sectional area of the carpal tunnel [15,16].

While sensory disturbance commonly affects digits 1 to 3 and the radial half of digit 4, alterations of this pattern are frequent, and patients may complain of sensory disturbance in all digits, one digit, or even rarely only ulnar-innervated digits. Sensation over the palm is typically spared as the palmar branch of the median nerve crosses the wrist outside the carpal tunnel. Tinel and Phalen signs may be noted, with the latter test being of higher sensitivity and specificity [17,18], but these are not specific for CTS and may be found in many cases of tenosynovitis [19].

Subjectively reduced grip strength and a tendency to drop objects may be reported by some patients. Severe, chronic nerve compression may result in numbness of median innervated digits and weakness and wasting of thenar muscles, particularly abductor pollicis brevis (APB) (Fig. 12.3a). The appearance of a 'simian hand' (Fig. 12.3c) may be noted with severe APB weakness, with

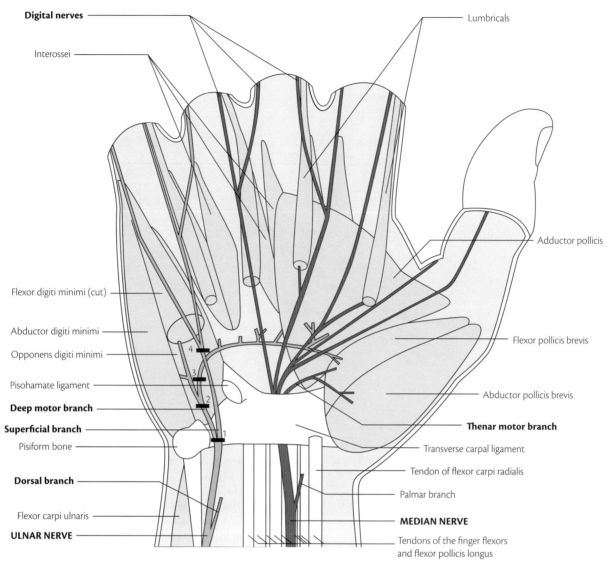

Fig. 12.2 The median and ulnar nerves in the wrist and hand. Patterns of ulnar nerve injury are indicated by numbers: (1) deep and superficial branches; (2) deep branch proximal to the origin of branches to the hypothenar muscles; (3) deep branch distal to the origin of branches to the hypothenar muscles; (4) superficial branch only. (See also figure in colour plate section)

recession of the thumb to the plane of the hand due to unopposed action of the extensor pollicis longus (EPL) and adductor pollicis. Predominant or isolated motor involvement, or 'thenar motor neuropathy', may be observed in the dominant hand of manual workers [20].

Proximal median neuropathy

Damage to the median nerve in the axilla and upper arm may be caused by orthopaedic trauma, penetrating injuries, or use of inappropriately fitted crutches [21]. The median nerve may be injured above the elbow by brachial artery catheterization [22,23], arterial or venous aneurysm [24,25], and other vascular anomalies [26].

An anomalous supracondylar process exists in 1% of the population [27], which lies approximately 5 cm above the medial epicondyle on the anteromedial humerus. The ligament of Struthers connects the supracondylar process to the medial epicondyle. The median nerve and brachial artery (and rarely the ulnar nerve) pass underneath the ligament, and this anatomical variant is generally asymptomatic. Rarely, entrapment of the nerve and artery results in elbow pain and median nerve deficits, and may produce characteristic reduction of the radial pulse on elbow flexion [28].

Complete proximal median neuropathies above the elbow produce weakness and wasting of all muscles supplied by the median nerve, as motor branches generally arise distal to the elbow. A characteristic posture of the hand is noted on making a fist with extension of digit 2 and incomplete flexion of digit 3 ('benediction hand'). Sensory loss may be noted over the palm and digits. Involvement of autonomic fibres may produce vasomotor abnormalities (Fig. 12.3).

Pronator teres syndrome

The median nerve may become entrapped as it passes between the two heads of the pronator teres (PT) and under the tendinous arch of the flexor digitorum superficialis (FDS). This is most common in the dominant arm and in the context of occupations requiring recurrent, forceful pronation and finger flexion, producing PT

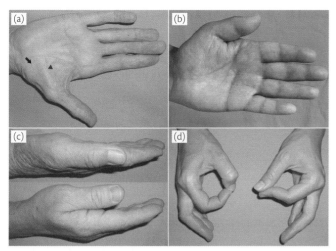

Fig. 12.3 Clinical signs associated with injury to the median nerve and its branches. (a) Wasting of the thenar eminence in severe carpal tunnel syndrome. Note the marked wasting of abductor pollicis brevis (APB, arrow) and relative sparing of flexor pollicis brevis (arrowhead), with dual median and ulnar innervation. (b) Vasomotor changes in median innervated digits and palm, seen after an acute proximal median neuropathy. (c) The 'simian hand' depicted in the upper image (normal hand depicted below), caused by severe APB weakness and unopposed action of the extensor pollicis longus and adductor pollicis. (d) 'Pinch attitude' seen in anterior interosseous neuropathy and due to weakness of flexor pollicis longus and flexor digitorum profundus.

Table 12.3 Ulnar nerve anatomy and common sites of injury

Ulnar nerve Spinal nerve roots: C8–T1 Brachial plexus: lower trunk > medial cord		
Major branches	**Innervated structures**	**Sites of injury**
Proximal ulnar nerve	Motor: Flexor carpi ulnaris Flexor digitorum profundus (digits 4 and 5)	Cubital tunnel
Dorsal branch	Sensory: Dorsal ulnar hand	Wrist
Superficial branch	Sensory: Hypothenar eminence Digit 5, medial half digit 4	Guyon canal
Deep branch	Motor: Abductor digiti minimi Opponens digiti minimi Flexor digiti minimi Adductor pollicis Flexor pollicis brevis (with median nerve) Lumbricals 3 and 4 Interossei	Guyon canal

hypertrophy [29]. Clinically, pain and tenderness may develop with weakness of the thenar muscles, FPL, and the lateral two heads of flexor digitorum profundus (FDP), and sensory disturbance in the median nerve distribution. Relative sparing of PT, FDS, and flexor carpi radialis (FCR) may be observed, as branches to these muscles arise proximal to PT.

Anterior interosseous neuropathy

The anterior interosseous nerve (AIN) arises from the median nerve in the cubital fossa and runs in the forearm in front of the interosseous membrane. Isolated involvement of muscles supplied by the AIN has been reported in association with trauma [30,31], surgery [32], and venous catheterization [33]. Most commonly, however, no clear trigger is identified [34] and focal neuritis, including neuralgic amyotrophy, may be the underlying mechanism [35,36].

Injury to the AIN presents with weakness of FPL, FDP (digits 2 and 3), and mild weakness of forearm pronation from involvement of the pronator quadratus (PQ). A characteristic 'pinch attitude' is observed when the patient attempts to flex the distal thumb and index finger joints (Fig. 12.3d). Pain in the shoulder or forearm may precede the onset of weakness [37], but sensory loss is not expected. A pseudo-AIN syndrome has been described, with predominant involvement of muscles innervated by AIN but with a lesion more proximal to the origin of the nerve, owing to involvement of the fascicles destined to become the AIN [38].

Ulnar neuropathy (Table 12.3)
Ulnar neuropathy at the elbow

Ulnar neuropathy at the elbow is the second most common human entrapment neuropathy, with the most common site of injury at the elbow, within the cubital tunnel. This region is formed by a retinaculum connecting the medial epicondyle and the olecranon, and the fascia of the flexor carpi ulnaris (FCU). Hypertrophy of the

aponeurotic arch, abnormalities of the elbow joint and ligaments, or an anomalous anconeus epitrochlearis muscle may cause compression of the nerve. The incidence of cubital tunnel syndrome is increased with repetitive flexion of the elbow (e.g. baseball pitchers) [39], is commonly seen in patients receiving haemodialysis for end-stage renal failure [40], and may be seen after surgery under general anaesthesia [41].

A complete ulnar nerve lesion above the elbow produces weakness and wasting of ulnar innervated muscles and sensory loss involving digits 4–5. Lesions at the cubital tunnel may spare FCU due to a proximal take off of this motor branch [42]. An ulnar claw hand may be present with severe ulnar motor lesions, due to paresis of lumbricals 3 and 4 and interossei. More proximal ulnar motor lesions produce less severe clawing than distal ulnar neuropathies ('the ulnar paradox') due to sparing of the FDP and increased flexion of the distal interphalangeal joints of digits 4–5 (Fig. 12.4).

Thickening and tenderness of the nerve at the elbow and the Tinel phenomenon are useful indicators of cubital tunnel syndrome. Characteristic symptoms may also be reproduced with the elbow flexion test, in which the patient's upper limb is positioned with the shoulder externally rotated, the elbow fully flexed, the forearm supinated, and the wrist fully extended.

Distal ulnar neuropathy

The ulnar nerve is susceptible to compression as it enters the hand in the Guyon canal, which is bordered medially by the pisiform bone and laterally by the hook of hamate (Fig. 12.2). Nerve injury may be secondary to pressure from a ganglion [43], ulnar artery thrombosis, vascular malformation [44–46], fracture [47],

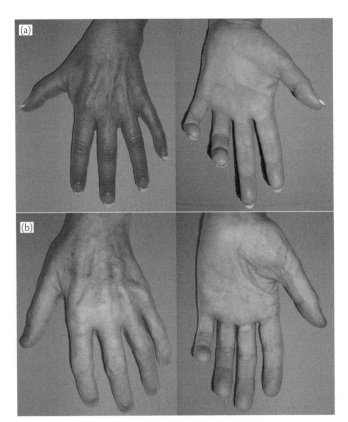

Fig. 12.4 The ulnar claw hand and ulnar paradox. Chronic distal ulnar neuropathy (a) produced more marked clawing than chronic ulnar neuropathy at the elbow (b) due to sparing of flexor digitorum profundus.

Table 12.4 Radial nerve anatomy and common sites of injury

Radial nerve
Spinal nerve roots: C5–C8
Brachial plexus: upper, middle, and lower trunks > posterior cord

Major branches	Innervated structures	Sites of injury
Proximal radial nerve	Motor:	Spiral groove
	Triceps	
	Anconeus	
	Brachioradialis	
	Extensor carpi radialis longus	
Posterior cutaneous nerve of the arm	Sensory:	
	Posterior arm	
Posterior cutaneous nerve of the forearm	Sensory:	
	Extensor surface of forearm	
Superficial radial nerve	Sensory:	Distal forearm
	Radial aspect dorsal hand	
	Dorsum of thumb	
	Dorsal aspect digits 2, 3,	
	Lateral half digit 4	
Posterior interosseous nerve	Motor:	Radial tunnel
	Supinator	
	Extensor digitorum	
	Extensor indicis	
	Extensor carpi radialis brevis	
	Extensor digiti minimi	
	Extensor carpi ulnaris	
	Abductor pollicis longus	
	Extensor pollicis longus	
	Extensor pollicis brevis	

or rheumatoid arthritis [48]. The ulnar nerve is also susceptible to injury by extrinsic compression, such as the use of crutches [49], cycling ('handlebar palsy') [50], and repetitive trauma to the hand ('pizza cutter's palsy') [51,52].

The clinical presentation of distal ulnar neuropathy depends on the location of nerve injury, and may be divided into groups (Fig. 12.2):

1. Compression of the ulnar nerve as it enters the hand, with weakness of all ulnar-innervated hand muscles and sensory loss of the palmar aspect of the medial hand and digits 4–5, due to involvement of both superficial and deep branches of the ulnar nerve.

2. Compression of the deep branch within the Guyon canal, with weakness of all ulnar-innervated hand muscles but without sensory loss.

3. Compression of the distal deep motor branch with sparing of the hypothenar muscles.

4. Isolated compression of the superficial branch with lesions at the distal end of the Guyon canal. Sensation in the distribution of the dorsal cutaneous branch is spared with an ulnar neuropathy distal to the wrist.

Radial neuropathy (Table 12.4)
Proximal radial neuropathy
The radial nerve is susceptible to injury as it winds around the posterior aspect of the humerus in the spiral groove, with injury secondary to humeral fracture or extrinsic compression. A patient may classically describe waking with a wrist drop after a night of heavy drinking ('Saturday night palsy'), due to deep sleep with the arm hanging over a chair. Other mechanisms of proximal radial nerve injury include compression from crutches or a tourniquet [53], shoulder dislocation, and the underarm action of softball pitching [54].

Radial neuropathy above the spiral groove presents with weakness of wrist and finger flexion, supination, elbow extension, and loss of the triceps and brachioradialis reflex. Sensory loss develops over the posterior aspect of the arm and forearm and the dorsum of the hand. Lesions in the spiral groove spare triceps and the posterior cutaneous nerve of the arm, and may spare the posterior cutaneous nerve of the forearm.

Radial tunnel syndrome and posterior interosseous neuropathy
More distal radial nerve compression may occur in the radial tunnel, a potential space between the radiohumeral joint and distal edge of the supinator muscle (Fig. 12.5). Through this space, the radial nerve and posterior interosseous nerve (PIN) are crossed by a number of structures including fibrous bands, arterial branches, and the arcade of Frohse, which is the fibrous proximal edge of the supinator. Compression of the nerve by one of these structures may

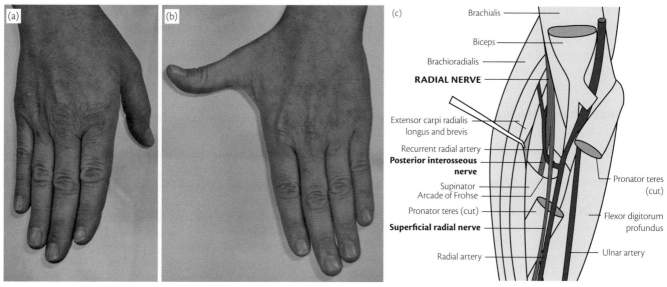

Fig. 12.5 The radial tunnel syndrome. Right posterior interosseous neuropathy resulted in weakness of thumb extension (a) when compared with the unaffected hand (b). The anatomy of the radial tunnel is illustrated (c), demonstrating the relationship of the posterior interosseous nerve to supinator. (See also figure in colour plate section)

result in the 'radial tunnel syndrome', a rare entity characterized by pain in the forearm and weakness of the muscles supplied by the PIN (Fig. 12.5, Box 12.1). It may be precipitated by activities requiring repetitive supination and pronation of the forearm [55,56] or prolonged position of the arm with hyperpronation of the forearm, wrist extension, and elbow flexion ('knapsack palsy') [57]. Some authors have ascribed persistent lateral forearm pain and tenderness, without weakness, to radial nerve compression within the radial tunnel]58]. However, this entity has been debated [59], with clear clinical overlap with lateral epicondylitis.

The PIN may be injured by trauma or surgery, and by compressive masses at the proximal forearm or elbow. Isolated PIN injury associated with pain may also be seen in neuralgic amyotrophy [59]. Clinically, patients have weakness of finger and thumb extension, without sensory loss. Sparing of the extensor carpi radialis longus (ECRL) may cause radial deviation during extension of the wrist, and the supinator is generally spared.

Superficial radial neuropathy

Lesions of the superficial branch of the radial nerve may develop after fracture of the radius or with compression from handcuffs, a tight wristwatch band, or bracelet. Sensory loss and paraesthesia may be present over the dorsal aspect of the hand and lateral 3½ digits, although objective findings may be limited to a small area of skin at the base of the thumb.

Musculocutaneous neuropathy

The musculocutaneous nerve is a mixed nerve that supplies motor fibres to biceps brachii, corachobrachialis, and brachialis. It terminates as the lateral cutaneous nerve of the forearm, supplying sensation to skin of the lateral forearm.

Isolated injury to the musculocutaneous nerve, producing weakness of elbow flexion and sensory disturbance over the lateral aspect of the forearm, is most commonly seen in the context of repetitive lifting or throwing, such as baseball pitching [60,61], rowing [62], or football [63]. It may also be seen after strenuous exercise or weight-lifting [64–66], in occupations with recurrent

Box 12.1 Illustrative case history

A 38-year-old female chef developed forearm pain and right hand weakness after an unusually prolonged session of whisking. Clinical examination, 5 days after onset, demonstrated severe weakness of finger and thumb extension without sensory abnormality (Fig 12.5). Posterior interosseous neuropathy was suspected, and NCS 1 week later confirmed block of radial nerve motor conduction to extensor indicis with stimulation above the lateral epicondyle. Minimal improvement was noted after 8 weeks of treatment with rest and splinting of the limb and repeat NCS demonstrated persistent conduction block. Surgical exploration demonstrated a thickened fibrous band at the proximal edge of the supinator, compressing the posterior interosseous nerve. Following resection of the band and external neurolysis, clinical improvement and resolution of the neurophysiological abnormalities was observed.

pressure to the upper arm ('carpet carrier's palsy') [67], and after surgery [68].

The lateral cutaneous nerve of the forearm may be injured in the cubital fossa producing isolated sensory involvement, e.g. after venepuncture [69]. A painful entrapment of the lateral cutaneous nerve of the forearm by the biceps tendon or aponeurosis has also been described [70,71].

Axillary neuropathy

The axillary nerve gives off motor fibres to the deltoid and teres minor and terminates as the superior lateral brachial cutaneous nerve, which supplies sensation to the skin overlying the lateral shoulder.

Injury to the axillary nerve is most common following direct trauma, anterior dislocation, or fracture dislocation of the shoulder [72–74], with traction on the nerve as it courses around the humeral neck. Traumatic axillary nerve injury may be in isolation or associated with injuries to the suprascapular, radial, and musculocutaneous nerves, or more extensive involvement of the brachial plexus. Injury to the axillary nerve has been reported after shoulder surgery, such as joint stabilization procedures [75,76]. Weakness of shoulder abduction and sensory disturbance over the deltoid ('regimental badge area') is expected on clinical examination.

Mononeuropathies of the brachial plexus

Suprascapular neuropathy

The suprascapular nerve passes through the suprascapular notch before branching to supply the supraspinatus muscle. The branch to infraspinatus travels around the spine of the scapula through the spinoglenoid notch before entering the muscle. The suprascapular nerve provides sensory innervation to the shoulder joint, and may contribute to sensory innervation of the overlying skin [77].

Traction or impingement of the suprascapular nerve as it passes through the suprascapular or spinoglenoid notches of the scapula may be caused by activities involving repetitive overhead movement, such as volleyball [78,79]. Entrapment of the nerve may also be caused by hypertrophy or ossification of the suprascapular ligament [80], spinoglenoid ligament hypertrophy [81], or a ganglion at the suprascapular or spinoglenoid notch [82–84]. Acute injury may be seen after orthopaedic injuries, such as large rotator cuff tears [85], scapular fracture [86], and anterior dislocation of the shoulder [87].

Lesions at the suprascapular notch are associated with weakness and atrophy of supraspinatus and infraspinatus. There is also generally deep shoulder pain with lesions at this level, due to involvement of sensory fibres from the shoulder joint. Injury at the spinoglenoid notch causes isolated infraspinatus involvement, and is generally painless due to the absence of sensory fibres in the distal portion of the nerve [88].

Pectoral neuropathies

The lateral pectoral nerve supplies the clavicular head of pectoralis major. The medial pectoral nerve, along with branches from a loop connecting it with the lateral pectoral nerve, supplies the sternal head of pectoralis major and pectoralis minor. Focal involvement of the pectoral nerves is rarely encountered. Bilateral medial pectoral neuropathy, producing wasting of the inferior sternal divisions of pectoralis major, has been reported in a weightlifter [89], and attributed to compression of the nerve during its course through a hypertrophied pectoralis minor muscle. The lateral pectoral nerve does not pass through pectoralis minor; however, isolated injury of the nerve has been reported as a result of seatbelt injury [90].

Subscapular neuropathy

The upper and lower subscapular nerves supply subscapularis and teres major respectively. Clinical weakness may develop with lesions of the posterior cord of the brachial plexus. Isolated subscapular neuropathies are rarely encountered, with reports in the context of gunshot wounds [91].

Thoracodorsal neuropathy

The thoracodorsal nerve travels along the posterior wall of the axilla to innervate latissimus dorsi. The nerve is liable to injury during a posterolateral thoracotomy [92] and isolated involvement may be seen in bodybuilders [93]. Latissimus dorsi weakness rarely produces major functional deficits, although wasting may be evident in muscular individuals.

Medial cutaneous neuropathies

The medial cutaneous nerves supply sensation to the skin over the medial and anterior aspects of the forearm and arm. The nerves may rarely be injured during surgical procedures to the arm, such as resection of excessive skin (brachioplasty) following massive weight loss [94].

Mononeuropathy proximal to the brachial plexus

Dorsal scapular neuropathy

Isolated dorsal scapular neuropathy is rare, and may develop in association with hypertrophy of the scalenus medius muscle [95], through which the nerve passes, or enlargement of the C7 transverse process [96]. Dorsal scapular neuropathy has been reported in bodybuilders [93] or in patients whose occupations involve extended overhead work [97].

Dorsal scapular neuropathy presents with pain in the neck or shoulder region. Lateral displacement and rotation of the medial border of the scapula, due to weakness of the rhomboids, may be evident on clinical examination, although atrophy of the muscle is not generally evident.

Long thoracic neuropathy

Long thoracic neuropathy may develop in the context of acute or repetitive trauma to the neck and shoulder [98], such as carrying a heavy backpack [99]. It has also been described after general anaesthesia, some cases being associated with prolonged elevation of the arm during the procedure [100,101], rib resection, mastectomy, axillary dissection, other thoracic surgical procedures [100], apical lung tumour [102], radiation therapy after breast cancer [103], and familial brachial plexus neuropathy [104].

Long thoracic neuropathy commonly presents with pain in the shoulder. The patient may also complain of weakness or easy fatigue of the shoulder when the arm is raised above the head. On examination, paresis of the serratus anterior produces winging of the scapula when the patient pushes forward with outstretched arms.

Lower limb mononeuropathy

Anatomical considerations

The lumbar plexus (Fig. 12.6) is formed from the anterior primary rami of L1 to L4 nerve roots, anterior to the transverse processes of the lumbar vertebrae, within the psoas muscle, which is supplied by branches of the roots as they enter the muscle (predominantly L2 and L3).

Branches from L1 form the iliohypogastric and ilioinguinal nerves, which supply the internal oblique and transversus abdominis muscles and sensation to the skin over the outer buttock and hip (iliohypogastric) and medial inguinal and pubic regions (ilioinguinal). The inferior branch of L1 joins the superior branch of L2 to form the genitofemoral nerve, which supplies the cremaster muscle and sensation to the skin of the scrotum or labia majoris and lateral inguinal region. The inferior branches of L2, L3, and L4 divide into anterior and posterior parts. The anterior parts coalesce to form the obturator nerve and the posterior parts combine to form the femoral nerve. The posterior parts of L2 and L3 give off branches that form the lateral femoral cutaneous nerve (LFCN).

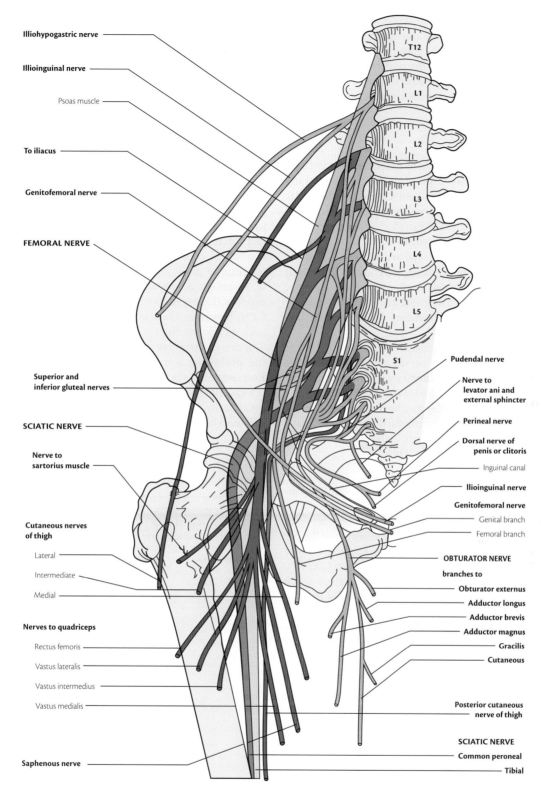

Fig. 12.6 The anatomy of the lumbosacral plexus. (Adapted from O'Brien MD (2000). *Aids to the Examination of the Peripheral Nervous System*, 4th edn. Elsevier, Oxford, with kind permission of Elsevier). (See also figure in colour plate section)

The sacral plexus is formed by the anterior primary rami of the L4 to S4 nerve roots, and lies on the dorsal wall of the pelvis in proximity to the internal iliac vessels and ureter. The L4 to S2 roots divide into anterior and posterior parts. The posterior parts contribute to the peroneal division of the sciatic nerve. In addition, the posterior parts give off branches to form the superior and inferior gluteal nerves.

The anterior parts of L4 to S2 roots combine with a contribution from S3 to produce the tibial division of the sciatic nerve, which lies medial and bound to the common peroneal division. In addition to the tibial division, branches arise to supply quadratus femoris and inferior gemellus (L4–S1), obturator internus and superior gemellus (L5–S2), and the posterior cutaneous nerve of the thigh (S1–S3), which supplies sensation to the posterior thigh and buttock. A contribution from S4 joins the anterior parts of S2 and S3 to form the pudendal nerve, which supplies sensation to the external genitalia.

Sciatic neuropathy (Table 12.5)

Proximal sciatic neuropathy

High sciatic nerve lesions are occasionally encountered in the context of nerve trauma after dislocation of the hip [105], total hip replacement surgery [106], or misplaced gluteal intramuscular injection [107,108]. Traction of the nerve may occur after prolonged positioning with the hip flexed and abducted, such as surgery in the lithotomy position [109], or the lotus yoga position [110]. Extrinsic compression may occur, for example, due to a bulky wallet carried in the back pocket [111] or after a prolonged period on a toilet seat [112]. Involvement of the intrapelvic portion of the nerve may be encountered in the context of pelvic malignancy, irradiation, or surgery [113–116], and severe endometriosis has been reported to produce cyclical symptoms [117,118].

High sciatic lesions produce weakness in muscles supplied by the sciatic, common peroneal, and tibial nerves, with loss of the ankle jerk, and altered sensation over the lateral leg and the whole of the foot (excluding the medial malleolus). Pain radiating down the posterior thigh and leg (sciatica) may also be noted. Partial lesions are frequently encountered, with the peroneal division of the sciatic nerve more commonly involved due to its lateral position, and this may be reflected in the clinical findings [119].

Piriformis syndrome

The piriformis syndrome denotes sciatic nerve irritation or compression by a hypertrophied or inflamed piriformis muscle after it passes through the greater sciatic foramen. Commonly reported clinical features include buttock pain that increases when the hip is flexed, adducted, and internally rotated, with tenderness over the sciatic notch, and symptoms on the straight leg raise test [120].

There is no diagnostic test for the piriformis syndrome and it remains a controversial entity [121,122]. Abnormalities of the piriformis muscle and sciatic nerve have been identified on MRI and magnetic resonance neurography [123–125]. Prolongation of the tibial H-reflex latency with the hip flexed, adducted, and internally rotated (the FAIR test) has been reported to be of high sensitivity and specificity [120,126], but methodological issues have been highlighted

[122]. Diagnosis of the piriformis syndrome hinges on the presence of a response to treatment, such as corticosteroid, local anaesthetic, or botulinum toxin injection into the piriformis muscle. However, a number of other local non-neuropathic conditions are also ameliorated by these treatment modalities [122], and hence a treatment response is not definitive evidence of sciatic nerve involvement.

Common peroneal neuropathy (Table 12.6)

Injury at the fibular head

Common peroneal neuropathy (CPN) is the most common lower limb mononeuropathy. The nerve is susceptible to injury as it passes around the fibular neck through the fibular tunnel, a musculoaponeurotic arch formed from the peroneus longus and soleus muscles. A number of mechanisms have been implicated in injury, with local trauma, perioperative injury, and external compression most common [127]. Weight loss as a result of anorexia nervosa, obesity surgery, or malignancy is common prior to the onset of CPN, and has led to the title of 'slimmer's neuropathy' [14,128–131]. Habitual leg crossing exposes the nerve to repeated trauma and may predispose to CPN; however, it is a ubiquitous habit, and additional factors such as concomitant weight loss are usually observed [127]. Traction of the nerve has been associated with activities involving prolonged squatting ('strawberry picker's palsy') [132]. Entrapment of the nerve by a fibrous band at the fibular tunnel is a rare phenomenon [133].

Clinically, CPN presents as foot drop, with acute or subacute weakness of ankle dorsiflexion and foot eversion and preservation

Table 12.6 Common peroneal nerve anatomy and common sites of injury

Common peroneal nerve Spinal nerve roots: L4–S2 Sacral plexus > sciatic nerve		
Major branches	**Innervated structures**	**Sites of injury**
Common peroneal nerve	Motor: Biceps femoris (short head)	Fibular tunnel
Deep peroneal nerve	Motor: Tibialis anterior Peroneus tertius Extensor hallucis longus Extensor digitorum longus Extensor digitorum brevis Sensory: First web space	Fibular tunnel Anterior compartment syndrome
Superficial peroneal nerve	Motor: Peroneus longus Peroneus brevis Sensory: Distal anterolateral leg Dorsal foot	Fibular tunnel Ankle
Lateral sural cutaneous nerve	Sensory: Posterolateral leg Contribution to sural nerve	Posterior leg

Table 12.5 Sciatic nerve anatomy and common sites of injury

Sciatic nerve Spinal nerve roots: L4–S3 Sacral plexus		
Major branches	**Innervated structures**	**Sites of injury**
Proximal sciatic nerve	Motor: Semitendinosus Semimembranosus Biceps femoris (long head) Adductor magnus (with obturator nerve)	Pelvis Buttock Piriformis syndrome

of power in foot inversion. Apparent foot inversion weakness may develop in the context of severe foot drop, as inversion is normally strongest with the foot held in slight dorsiflexion [134]. The deep peroneal component is more often affected than the superficial peroneal component, due to proximity to bone at the fibular head. Thus, weakness of ankle dorsiflexion is often more marked than eversion weakness. Additionally, while sensory symptoms are present in the majority of patients, these are generally minor, and sensory examination usually demonstrates mild patchy sensory loss over the dorsum of the foot. In terms of differential diagnoses, L5 radiculopathy is the most likely, and can be distinguished by the presence of foot inversion weakness. In the appropriate clinical setting, partial sciatic neuropathy involving only peroneal fibres may be considered.

Tibial neuropathy (Table 12.7)
Proximal tibial neuropathy

Proximal lesions of the tibial nerve are uncommon. Trauma is the most common cause of injury, including tibial fracture and penetrating injury [135]. Abnormalities may develop as a complication

of knee surgery, compartment syndrome, involvement with tumour, entrapment by a tendinous arch in the popliteal fossa, or after rupture of a Baker cyst [135–137]. Clinical features include sensory disturbance involving the plantar and lateral aspects of the foot and weakness of plantar flexion, toe flexion, and inversion, often with reduction of the ankle jerk [135,137].

Tarsal tunnel syndrome

The tarsal tunnel syndrome (TTS) is an over-diagnosed syndrome, in which the tibial nerve becomes compressed as it passes between the talus and navicular bones medially, and the overlying fibrous flexor retinaculum. The nerve may be compressed in the tarsal tunnel by disorders of the tarsal bones and joints, such as tumours, ganglion cysts, fractures, and tenosynovitis [138–144], or regional muscular or vascular anomalies [145,146]. Idiopathic TTS is a more controversial entity, but may be seen in the context of underlying anatomical susceptibilities, such as talocalcaneal coalition and pes planus, and exacerbated by regular vigorous physical activity [147,148].

Clinical features of TTS are vague, and this adds to the diagnostic difficulties. The predominant symptom is usually unilateral pain in the heel or foot, which may have a burning quality, and is characteristically exacerbated during weight-bearing activities or at night. Less commonly, there may be paraesthesiae or numbness over the plantar aspect of the foot, and the Tinel sign may be positive at the ankle.

Sural neuropathy

Isolated sural neuropathy is uncommon and is usually associated with trauma or surgery to the ankle. Vasculitis, connective tissue disease, and diabetes mellitus have also been associated with idiopathic sural neuropathy [149]. Sural neuropathy presents with pain, numbness, or paraesthesiae over the lateral surface of the foot and ankle.

Femoral neuropathy (Table 12.8)
Proximal femoral neuropathy

Femoral neuropathy is often iatrogenic, e.g. caused by self-retaining retractors used during abdominal surgery [150], prolonged positioning in the lithotomy position [151], total hip arthroplasty [152],

Table 12.7 Tibial nerve anatomy and common sites of injury

Tibial nerve Spinal nerve roots: L4–S3 Sacral plexus > sciatic nerve		
Major branches	**Innervated structures**	**Sites of injury**
Tibial nerve	Motor: Popliteus Gastrocnemius Soleus Plantaris Tibialis posterior Flexor hallucis longus Flexor digitorum longus	Popliteal fossa
Medial sural cutaneous nerve	Sensory: Posterior leg Contributes to sural nerve	Posterior leg
Medial plantar nerve	Motor: Abductor hallucis Flexor digitorum brevis Flexor hallucis brevis Lumbrical 1 Sensory: Medial plantar foot	Tarsal tunnel, ankle
Lateral plantar nerve	Motor: Quadratus plantae Interossei Lumbricals Abductor digiti quinti brevis Sensory: Lateral plantar foot	Tarsal tunnel, ankle
Medial calcaneal nerve	Sensory: Medial and posterior heel	Tarsal tunnel, ankle

Table 12.8 Femoral nerve anatomy and common sites of injury

Femoral nerve Spinal nerve roots: L2–L4 Lumbar plexus		
Major branches	**Innervated structures**	**Sites of injury**
Femoral nerve	Motor: Sartorius Pectineus Quadriceps	Psoas muscle Iliopsoas groove Inguinal ligament
Medial femoral cutaneous nerve	Sensory: Anteromedial thigh	Anterior superior iliac spine/inguinal ligament
Saphenous nerve	Sensory: Medial aspect of leg Medial dorsal foot	Adductor canal

renal transplantation [153], femoral nerve block for orthopaedic surgery [154], or instrumentation of the femoral artery [155]. Other causes include psoas haematoma or abscess, or invasion by tumour such as colorectal carcinoma [156]. Painful femoral neuropathy may be the dominant feature of proximal diabetic neuropathy [157], although this is usually in the context of plexopathy or polyradiculopathy. Repeated activity may cause femoral neuropathy in dancers [158,159], and prolonged hyperextension of the hip, such as with the legs hanging over the edge of a bed, has also been implicated [160].

Femoral neuropathies present with weakness of knee extension and reduction of the knee jerk. Minor weakness of hip extension may be present, with weakness of rectus femoris and sartorius, although weakness of hip adduction or significant weakness of hip flexion suggests a more proximal lesion. Variable sensory loss in the anteromedial thigh may be described.

Saphenous neuropathy

The saphenous nerve is most commonly injured during trauma [161], vascular procedures involving the femoral artery or saphenous vein [162,163], or knee surgery, such as arthroscopy [164]. Recurrent pressure to the nerve with the knees pressed together or against a firm object may be seen in surfers [165], or while working in a kneeling position. Sensory loss and paraesthesiae in the distribution of the saphenous nerve may develop, associated with neuropathic pain.

Obturator neuropathy (Table 12.9)

Isolated obturator neuropathy is uncommon, caused by disease involving the pelvis or pelvic cavity such as pelvic fracture [166], malignancy, endometriosis, or retroperitoneal haemorrhage. The nerve may be compressed during childbirth or by an obturator hernia. Pelvic or hip surgery may damage the nerve due to direct injury or traction [167–169].

Clinically, obturator neuropathy is dominated by sensory symptoms, and there may be associated medial thigh or groin pain. Weakness of hip adduction is less common [170], dependent on the severity of the nerve lesion.

Lateral femoral cutaneous neuropathy

The LFCN exits the psoas muscle and crosses the iliacus before entering the thigh medial to the anterior superior iliac spine

Table 12.9 Obturator nerve anatomy and common sites of injury

Obturator nerve Spinal nerve roots: L2–L4 Lumbar plexus		
Major branches	**Innervated structures**	**Sites of injury**
Anterior branch	Motor:	Pelvis
	Adductor longus	Obturator foramen
	Adductor brevis	
	Gracilis	
Posterior branch	Obturator externus	Pelvis
	Adductor magnus (with sciatic nerve)	Obturator foramen
Cutaneous branch	Sensory:	Pelvis
	Medial thigh	Obturator foramen

and below the inguinal ligament. It supplies sensation to the anterolateral thigh.

Injury to the LFCN may be spontaneous or iatrogenic, and is associated with numbness and paraesthesiae (meralgia paraesthetica) of the anterolateral thigh. Spontaneous injury is associated with increased intra-abdominal pressure, such as seen in obesity, pregnancy, or large pelvic tumours [171–173]. Extrinsic compression is noted in some cases and may be associated with tight-fitting garments ('supermodel syndrome'), belts, or implements worn around the waist such as tools or a gun [174–176]. Diabetics may develop a spontaneous lesion [177]. Iatrogenic injury is associated with iliac crest bone harvesting, retroperitoneal dissection, and spinal surgery [178].

Principles of diagnosis

In addition to the clinical history and examination findings, nerve conduction studies (NCS) remain critically important in the diagnosis of mononeuropathy, enabling localization and quantification of nerve injury, assessment of the contribution of axonal loss and focal demyelination to the pathogenesis of the nerve injury, monitoring of recovery, and determining prognosis.

Axonal changes

Focal axonal injury manifests as reduction in amplitude of the sensory action potential (SAP) or compound muscle action potential (CMAP). Following nerve section, motor amplitudes reduce over days and are generally unobtainable 4–12 days afterwards [179,180]. After complete nerve transection, responses with stimulation proximal to the lesion are absent immediately. With partial axonal lesions, small potentials are obtainable above and below the lesion. Conduction velocities tend to remain similar at both points.

Demyelination

Neuropraxic injury may induce focal demyelination with characteristic neurophysiological changes.

Pathological temporal dispersion may develop when focal demyelination slows impulses through a segment of the nerve. This results in increased duration of the potential above the focal lesion. Phase-cancellation of individual potentials may produce reduction of the peak amplitude, and a complex CMAP with an increased number of turns (Fig. 12.7).

Focal demyelination tends to result in slowing across the point of nerve injury. Inching studies may be employed to identify the exact position of nerve injury. Demyelination of distal nerve segments will be evident as prolongation of the terminal latency (TL).

Distal conduction slowing needs to be interpreted with caution, particularly as limb temperature has a significant bearing on TL and conduction velocity [181]. Specifically, nerve conduction is slower at cooler temperatures, of particular importance in a superficial distal nerve or a wasted limb. Ideally the limb should be warmed to 32°C prior to testing to eliminate this potentially confounding factor.

Significant reduction in the CMAP amplitude with proximal stimulation implies block of a proportion of the nerve fibres (Fig. 12.7). However, marked reduction of proximally elicited CMAP with preserved distal CMAP may also develop within the first days after partial or complete axonotmesis or neurotmesis of a nerve. Apparent (pseudo-) conduction block may also be seen early

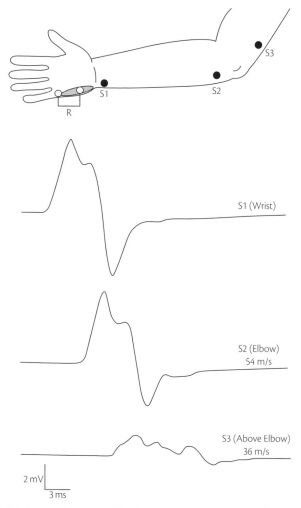

Fig. 12.7 Nerve conduction studies of the ulnar nerve, stimulating at the wrist (S1), below (S2), and above the elbow (S3), and recording from abductor digiti minimi (R). Conduction block and relative slowing of the conduction velocity is noted with stimulation proximal to the elbow, consistent with cubital tunnel syndrome.

in the course of vasculitic mononeuritis due to ischaemic axonal conduction failure [182].

Electromyography

Electromyography (EMG) is useful for establishing the pattern of nerve involvement in focal neuropathies, to exclude myopathic causes of weakness (Fig. 12.8) and to guide assessment of prognosis, particularly after axonal injury. Spontaneous activity (increased insertional activity, fibrillation potentials, positive sharp waves) provides evidence of acute axonal loss. Spontaneous activity develops within 2 to 6 weeks of axonal injury and may persist for several months despite clinical and neurophysiological improvement. A progress study 3–6 months after injury is generally recommended to assess for recovery. The absence of reinnervation at this stage suggests a poorer prognosis for complete recovery, and may suggest the need for surgical intervention.

Ultrasonography

Ultrasound of muscle and nerve is gaining utility as an adjunct to clinical neurophysiology in the diagnosis of neuromuscular diseases, including focal neuropathies. In chronic compressive neuropathies, enlargement of the nerve at the site of compression may be detected with high-resolution ultrasound [183]. Nerve enlargement may be associated with a reduction in the echogenicity of the nerve [184], or increase in the intraneurial blood flow [185].

Ultrasound has also been used to evaluate muscle in neuromuscular disease. Disturbance of the normal muscle histology is evident as increased muscle echogenicity and possible obscuration of bone edge definition [186,187], although this does not easily distinguish between neurogenic and myopathic processes, besides some qualitative differences in the homogeneity of the changes. Fasciculations within a muscle can also be detected on ultrasound [188], which may be useful when assessing muscles that are deep or difficult to access with a standard needle electrode.

Whilst there may be advantages of ultrasound in diagnosis of compressive neuropathies, e.g. in patients with coexistent severe peripheral neuropathy, standard electrodiagnostic assessments remain the gold standard. However, neuromuscular ultrasound may become a useful adjunct to electrodiagnostic studies with further advances in technology and understanding of the findings in normal and disease states.

Magnetic resonance imaging

Structural imaging with MRI remains an invaluable tool in neuromuscular diagnosis, particularly in the assessment of spinal and spinal root pathology. In addition, advances in imaging techniques have enabled the detection of peripheral nerve and muscle abnormalities (Fig. 12.9). The sensitivity of MRI diagnosis for some compressive neuropathies, such as cubital tunnel syndrome, may be increased when NCS alone have not localized the lesion [189]. MRI of muscle may not distinguish between neurogenic and myopathic processes, hence limiting the discriminative value of the technique, while there also remain issues with cost and availability.

Illustrative electrodiagnosis of selected mononeuropathies

Carpal tunnel syndrome

Approximately 90% of patients with a clinical diagnosis of CTS demonstrate one or more diagnostic abnormalities on NCS [190]. Slowing of median nerve conduction across the palm to wrist segment, with normal conduction in other segments, is consistent with a diagnosis of CTS. A number of neurophysiological techniques are used to identify selective slowing of the median nerve at the wrist compared with nerves that do not traverse the carpal tunnel. Comparisons include digit 4 median and ulnar sensory latencies [191], digit 1 median and superficial radial sensory latencies [192], palm-to-wrist median and ulnar mixed nerve latencies [193,194], median and ulnar motor latencies to lumbrical and interosseous muscles [195], and median sensory short segment stimulation across the wrist [196]. It may be necessary to perform multiple comparison studies in the context of equivocal results. Rarely, slowing of median motor conduction across the wrist may be the only abnormality found [197]. Additionally, median to ulnar communications in the forearm (Martin–Grüber anastomosis) are common and may confound the results of motor studies [18].

In severe CTS, where median sensory and motor responses are absent, EMG may be required to confirm neurogenic changes confined to muscles innervated by the median nerve distal to the carpal

ANATOMY　　　　**ELECTROMYOGRAPHY**

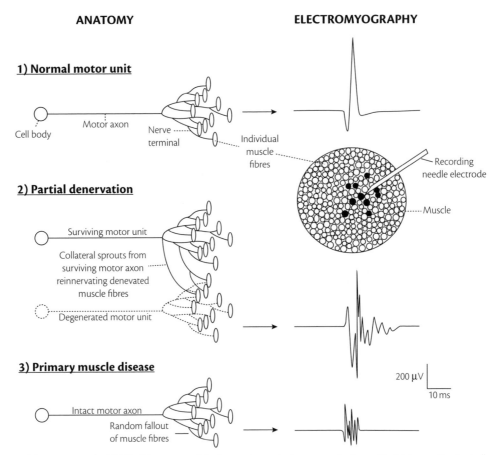

Fig. 12.8 The anatomy and electromyography (EMG) of the motor unit in denervation and primary muscle disease. Partial denervation typically results in polyphasic motor units of prolonged duration on EMG, while small and polyphasic motor units of short duration are characteristically observed in primary muscle disease.

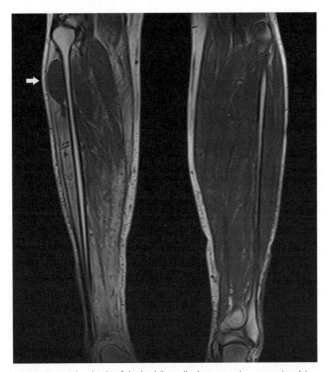

Fig. 12.9 T_1-weighted MRI of the leg bilaterally demonstrating a mass involving the common peroneal nerve (arrow). Muscle atrophy is evident in the anterior and posterior compartments suggesting involvement proximal to the common peroneal nerve.

tunnel. In this instance, the latency to PQ may be useful to exclude a more proximal median neuropathy.

Ulnar neuropathy at the elbow

Standard NCS may localize an ulnar neuropathy in 65–80% [189,198], demonstrating conduction block or slowing of conduction with stimulation proximal to the elbow (Fig. 12.7). Short segment stimulation (inching studies) of the ulnar nerve around the elbow increases the likelihood of localizing an ulnar neuropathy [199], as does recording from both abductor digiti minimi (ADM) and first dorsal interosseous (FDI) [200]. Prolongation of the latency to FCU may be helpful to localize ulnar nerve injury to the elbow when the motor amplitude to ADM is markedly reduced [201]. In addition, NCS of the medial cutaneous nerve of the forearm may also be useful to assess for a lower brachial plexus injury [202].

Diagnostic considerations

Inflammatory mononeuropathy

Vasculitic involvement of the peripheral nervous system (discussed in Chapter 14) characteristically produces an asymmetric peripheral neuropathy or mononeuritis multiplex; however, mononeuritis simplex is possible early in the course of the disease.

Sarcoidosis has protean neurological manifestations, and peripheral nerve involvement may occur rarely in isolation or, more commonly, in association with systemic disease. Facial neuropathy is the most common mononeuropathy seen in sarcoidosis [203], often caused by granulomatous involvement of the parotid gland,

and may form part of the uveoparotid fever or Heerfordt syndrome. Sarcoidosis may also manifest as other mononeuropathies, mononeuritis multiplex, polyradiculopathy, or peripheral neuropathy.

Of the inflammatory disorders, neuralgic amyotrophy commonly affects the upper limb, and the clinical and neurophysiological findings may be isolated to single peripheral upper limb nerves, commonly the median or anterior interosseous nerves [35]. It is characterized by severe shoulder or forearm pain followed by monophasic weakness of the shoulder girdle and upper limb. Whilst the pathogenesis has not been fully elucidated, an inflammatory mechanism has been proposed [204], perhaps triggered by trauma, and an autosomal dominant hereditary form has also been recognized.

Diabetes mellitus

Patients with DM may develop isolated cranial or peripheral mononeuritis in the setting of mild or well-controlled diabetes [205]. DM also predisposes to entrapment neuropathy, and there is a higher rate of CTS in patients with DM than is expected from population-based estimates [206]. Diabetic neuropathies are discussed in detail in Chapter 17.

Infiltrative lesions

Tumours such as neurofibromas and schwannomas may arise along the course of a peripheral nerve. Intraneural ganglion cysts, are most common in the common peroneal nerve [207], and arise from an articular branch to a degenerative joint [208]. They may be progressive and invade or compress the nerve, resulting in focal neuropathy [209].

Neurolymphomatosis may manifest as polyradiculoneuropathy, polyneuropathy, cranial neuropathy, or peripheral mononeuropathy [210], and may be difficult to diagnose antemortem. Computed tomography–positron emission tomography and MRI studies are the most sensitive means of diagnosis [211]. Negative cerebrospinal fluid cytology does not exclude neurolymphomatosis. Nerve biopsy is frequently helpful, but may be limited by involvement of inaccessible nerves or when there is an unacceptable risk of neurological morbidity as a consequence of the biopsy, e.g. with involvement of a large motor nerve. The prognosis of neurolymphomatosis is generally poor with a median survival of 10 months despite treatment [210].

Infection

Human Immunodeficiency Virus Type 1 (HIV-1) is uncommonly associated with transient unilateral or bilateral facial neuropathy during seroconversion [212] or mononeuropathy (most commonly mononeuropathy multiplex) in late stages of the infection [213]. Other viruses, such as Varicella Zoster virus, Epstein–Barr virus, Cytomegalovirus, Hepatitis B virus and Hepatitis C virus have also been associated with peripheral mononeuropathies.

Bacterial infections are uncommon causes of mononeuropathy. Lyme disease (*Borrelia burgdorferi*), endemic to parts of Europe, Asia, and North America, most commonly causes central nervous system manifestations or polyradiculopathy, but may also rarely cause isolated peripheral or facial mononeuropathy. Tuberculoid leprosy (*Mycobacterium leprae*) is a common cause of peripheral neuropathy worldwide, particularly in developing countries. The predilection of the organism for Schwann cells and cooler tissue temperatures results in localized infections of the skin and subcutaneous nerves. Larger superficial nerves such as the digital, sural, superficial radial, ulnar, and peroneal nerves may become involved in the infection, producing localized nerve thickening and appropriate focal neurological deficits.

Ischaemia

Chronic ischaemia of a limb may result in neuropathy, e.g. in patients with severe peripheral vascular disease. Histopathological changes of nerves are widespread and show segmental demyelination and remyelination, with a lesser degree of axonal degeneration, and clinical features are consistent with a distal peripheral neuropathy [214]. Ischaemic monomelic neuropathy may be precipitated acutely by the placement of a brachiocephalic arteriovenous fistula in the forearm or thromboembolic occlusion of a major proximal limb artery [215]. Hypoperfusion of the vasa nervorum results in distal axonal infarction in multiple nerves, with sensory nerve fibres more sensitive than motor fibres, producing sensory disturbance and weakness, often in association with significant pain.

Unusual causes

Wartenberg's migrant sensory neuritis is characterized by numbness in the distribution of one or more cutaneous nerves, which is often preceded by pain in the same distribution. Nerves of the limbs are most frequently affected, although cranial or thoracic nerves may also be involved. Motor nerve function remains unaffected. The course is typically mild and symptoms generally stabilize or remit without progression to confluent sensory loss [216]. Sensory NCS commonly demonstrate reduction of one or more sensory amplitudes.

Sensory perineuritis has a similar clinical presentation to that of Wartenberg syndrome, with patchy numbness and pain involving the limbs. Whilst nerve biopsy in Wartenberg syndrome may show a variety of pathologies, sensory perineuritis is characterized by chronic inflammation and perineurial fibrosis of some fascicles of involved nerves [217]. Immune-based therapies, such as corticosteroids or plasma exchange, may provide benefit in more severe cases [218].

Localized hypertrophic mononeuropathy is a poorly understood condition in which progressive perineurial cellular proliferation occurs focally within a peripheral nerve. Static or progressive neurological deficits may ensue [219].

Principles of management

Principles of management may be applied across the range of mononeuropathies. Specifically, core management strategies consist of prevention of recurrent nerve injury, monitoring for clinical and electromyographic evidence of recovery (or progression), rehabilitation of focal neurological deficits, and treatment of associated symptoms such as neuropathic pain. In selected cases, surgical intervention and local corticosteroid injection may also be considered.

Conservative therapies

Many mononeuropathies recover spontaneously, and hence clinical observation may be sufficient. Neuropraxic injuries may be expected to resolve over an 8–12 week period. The original severity of the lesion has an important bearing on clinical outcome after nerve injury. For example, 90% of mild ulnar neuropathies at the elbow resolve or improve without specific intervention [220].

Prevention of further injury is an integral component of early management. Education about the pathogenic mechanism of nerve injury and modification of activity should be considered. In some instances a splint is applied for symptomatic relief or minimization of ongoing injury. Nocturnal splinting is sometimes employed for the management of ulnar neuropathy at the elbow, but it may not add to education alone [221]. Extension wrist splinting or ankle–foot orthosis may be required after radial or peroneal neuropathies, respectively.

Splinting of the wrist in CTS warrants particular consideration. The cross-sectional area of the carpal tunnel is reduced, and carpal tunnel pressure is increased, with flexion and extension of the wrist [16,222,223]. The use of a wrist splint at night, which holds the wrist in a neutral position, provides symptomatic benefit for patients with predominantly nocturnal symptoms [224]. Neurophysiological parameters may also improve with wrist splinting [225]. Discomfort when wearing the splint is a major limitation of therapy.

Metabolic factors

Weight loss has been implicated in the pathogenesis of compressive neuropathies, particularly common peroneal neuropathy at the fibular head. Neuropathy characteristically develops after rapid weight loss, which may be associated with a catabolic state, for example from metastatic malignancy [131], or deliberate weight loss, such as after obesity surgery [14]. In these instances, loss of subcutaneous fat predisposes the nerve to compression, although nerve excitability data have identified metabolic sensitivity of nerves at common sites of compression [226,227]. Of relevance, there is a higher rate of other compressive neuropathies, in particular CTS, following rapid weight loss [14], which would not be expected as a result of alterations in subcutaneous fat alone. Hence, compressive neuropathy following rapid weight loss may be a consequence of relative metabolic deficiency within the nerve exposing anatomic susceptibility or pre-existing subclinical nerve injury.

Patients diagnosed with mononeuropathy in the context of weight loss should have special attention given to the adequacy of their nutritional intake. Additional efforts should be undertaken to avoid nerve compression, e.g. appropriate pressure care during surgical procedures or when the patient is confined to bed.

Nutritional deficiencies should also be assessed and corrected in the context of peripheral nerve injuries. Vitamin deficiencies may develop in isolation, with a malabsorption state, or accompanying marked weight loss. Vitamin B_{12} and folate, pyridoxine (B_6), vitamin E, and thiamine have all been implicated in the pathogenesis of peripheral neuropathy [228]. While a specific association with focal mononeuropathy has not been identified, it is recommended that adequate replacement be given if deficiencies are detected on investigation of otherwise unexplained mononeuropathy.

Corticosteroid injection

Local corticosteroid injection is commonly used as a bridging therapy in the treatment of compressive neuropathies, to improve symptoms during recovery or treat exacerbations of a chronic entrapment neuropathy. This treatment is most commonly used after failed conservative therapies for CTS; however, it may be of benefit in a wide range of compressive neuropathies.

In patients with CTS, local injection of corticosteroid commonly provides symptomatic improvement and may improve neurophysiological parameters up to 6 months after treatment [229,230].

Occasionally, patients experience longer periods of symptom remission after local corticosteroid injection, usually in patients with milder neurophysiological deficits [231].

Surgical considerations

Surgical management of peripheral nerve injuries is conceptually divided into two groups. First, acute nerve trauma may require surgical management where there is transection of a nerve or significant crush injury. The second group that may benefit from surgical intervention are patients with chronic compressive neuropathies, unresponsive to conservative or other forms of therapy.

Surgical management of acute nerve trauma
Timing of surgical repair

The mechanism of traumatic injury determines the time course of surgical management. Immediate surgical repair, within 72 h of injury, is optimal in the context of sharp transection of a nerve, such as a knife or glass wound. In the presence of coexistent wound contamination or tissue ischaemia, e.g. with concomitant compartment syndrome, nerve repair is typically deferred until those issues are resolved.

A delay of several days or weeks is usually considered in the context of blunt transection or avulsion of a nerve in order for the degree of injury to the nerve stumps to be adequately demarcated. However, it is common practice for the stumps to be sutured to surrounding tissues acutely to prevent retraction and subsequent difficulty reuniting them.

Delayed nerve reconstruction is considered after blunt nerve trauma, stretch or contusion injuries, when the nerve is continuous but the completeness of axonal injury remains uncertain. In this instance, delays of up to 6 months may be permitted in order to assess evidence of clinical or electromyographic recovery, as incomplete lesions commonly achieve satisfactory clinical recovery without surgery [232] or may require less extensive surgical intervention than complete lesions [233]. The optimum timing for surgical intervention needs to be carefully considered, however, as earlier nerve reconstruction yields better functional results [234].

Surgical techniques

The nature and extent of the nerve injury determines the choice of surgical repair. Focal transections and short segment injuries are repaired using end-to-end neurorrhaphy, where nerve stumps are aligned and joined. Excessive tension on the nerve repair, or residual scarring of the nerve stump, compromises the clinical outcome. In general, direct neurorrhaphy produces clinical improvement in up to 70% of cases. The best clinical outcomes after neurorrhaphy are generally observed in younger patients and injuries associated with less extensive tissue damage [235].

When there is a large defect in the nerve, or when end-to-end neurorrhaphy is associated with excessive tension, a graft may be required to prevent scar tissue from forming between the nerve stumps and to allow a conduit for axonal regeneration. Autologous, non-critical, sensory nerve grafts, such as from the sural or forearm cutaneous nerves, are most commonly utilized. Grafting produces fewer satisfactory outcomes than direct suture repair of the nerve, and longer graft lengths are associated with poor neurological recovery [236].

Neurotization procedures may be performed when there is a long segment of nerve injury without transection, or when preganglionic injury prevents grafting. Neurotization involves the transfer of intact nerves to the distal end of an injured nerve, and is most frequently performed after traumatic brachial plexus injury, primarily to restore elbow flexion and shoulder abduction movements. Side-to-side anastomosis of an intact nerve to a damaged nerve has also been undertaken in this setting [237]. Intra-operative nerve conduction studies may be undertaken to confirm failure of conduction of a nerve action potential across an injured segment prior to surgical repair. Motor nerves are most commonly used, such as the thoracic intercostal nerves [238], or branches from the pectoral or distal spinal accessory nerves [239,240]. Extensive postoperative rehabilitation and retraining may be required after neurotization.

Surgical management of compressive neuropathies

The ideal timing and choice of surgical management for chronic compressive neuropathies remains less clear. Of the mononeuropathies, surgical decompression is most frequently performed for CTS, ulnar neuropathy at the elbow, and peroneal neuropathy at the fibular head. Neurolyisis procedures are common, which involve surgical dissection of epineurial or perifascicular scar tissue at the site of nerve injury.

There is clear evidence that surgical division of the flexor retinaculum at the wrist improves symptoms in patients with CTS [241,242]. However, patient selection and the timing of surgery remain areas of controversy. While surgical decompression produces superior outcomes to splinting, it is unclear whether surgery is superior to local corticosteroid injection alone [243]. The role of surgery in patients with severe CTS, associated with absent median motor and sensory potentials on electrodiagnostic testing, is also debated. However, surgical treatment in this group of patients may still result in improvement of symptoms and neurophysiological measures over the long term [244]. Accordingly, surgical treatment of CTS is recommended for patients with symptoms refractory to other measures or if severe or progressive neurophysiological changes are identified.

The evidence for surgical treatment of other compressive neuropathies is less clear. There are many surgical series reporting favourable results on a wide range of entrapment and compressive neuropathies. However, spontaneous recovery after nerve injury hampers interpretation of the findings as surgical outcomes are rarely compared with natural history controls. In general, surgical decompression should be considered in a patient with a severe or progressive nerve lesion that has not responded to a trial of more conservative therapy.

Conclusion

Mononeuropathy is a common problem in clinical neurological practice. Diagnosis requires careful clinical assessment to exclude alternative pathology, such as radiculopathy and multifocal or systemic processes, and may be confirmed using neurophysiological testing and other investigations. Many mononeuropathies recover with conservative therapy alone, although splinting and injection of corticosteroid are required in some instances. Surgical therapy may be useful when there is progressive nerve injury or when clinical recovery is not observed with conservative and other therapies.

References

1. Hopkins A, Menken M, DeFriese G. A record of patient encounters in neurological practice in the United Kingdom. *J Neurol Neurosurg Psychiatry* 1989; **52**: 436–8.

2. Wilbourn AJ, Gilliatt RW. Double-crush syndrome: a critical analysis. *Neurology* 1997; **49**: 21–9.

3. Seddon HJ. Three types of nerve injury. *Brain* 1943; **66**: 237–88.

4. Stoll G, Jander S, Myers RR. Degeneration and regeneration of the peripheral nervous system: from Augustus Waller's observations to neuroinflammation. *J Peripher Nerv Syst* 2002; **7**: 13–27.

5. Stoll G, Griffin JW, Li CY, Trapp BD. Wallerian degeneration of the peripheral nervous system: participation of both Schwann cells and macrophages in myelin degradation. *J Neurocytol* 1989; **18**: 671–83.

6. de Krom MC, Knipschild PG, Kester AD, Thijs C, Boekkooi PF, Spaaris F. Carpal tunnel syndrome: prevalence in the general population. *J Clin Epidemiol* 1992; **45**: 373–6.

7. Reading I, Walker-Bone K, Palmer KT, Cooper C, Coggon D. Anatomic distribution of sensory symptoms in the hand and their relation to neck pain, psychosocial variables and occupational activities. *Am J Epidemiol* 2003; **157**: 524–30.

8. Nakamichi K, Tachibana S. Small hand as a risk factor for carpal tunnel syndrome. *Muscle Nerve* 1995; **18**: 664–6.

9. Bleeker ML, Bohlman M, Moreland R, Tipton A. Carpal tunnel syndrome: role of carpal canal size. *Neurology* 1985; **35**: 1599–604.

10. Palmer KT. Carpal tunnel syndrome: the role of occupational factors. *Best Pract Res Clin Rheumatol* 2011; **25**: 15–29.

11. Padua L, di Pasquale A, Pazzaglia C, Liotta GA, Librante A, Mondelli M. Systematic review of pregnancy-related carpal tunnel syndrome. *Muscle Nerve* 2010; **42**: 697–702.

12. Mondelli M, Rossi S, Monti E, et al. Long term follow-up of carpal tunnel syndrome during pregnancy: a cohort study and review of the literature. *Electromyogr Clin Neurophysiol* 2007; **47**: 259–71.

13. Bland JD. The relationship of obesity, age, and carpal tunnel syndrome: more complex than was thought? *Muscle Nerve* 2005; **32**: 527–32.

14. Thaisetthawatkul P, Collazo-Clavell ML, Sarr MG, et al. A controlled study of peripheral neuropathy after bariatric surgery. *Neurology* 2004; **63**: 1462–70.

15. Skie M, Zeiss J, Ebraheim NA, Jackson WT. Carpal tunnel changes during wrist flexion and extension seen by magnetic resonance imaging. *J Hand Surg* 1990; **15A**: 934–9.

16. Kiernan MC, Mogyoros I, Burke D. Conduction block in carpal tunnel syndrome. *Brain* 1999; **122**: 933–41.

17. Kuschner SH, Ebramzadeh E, Johnson D, Brien WW, Sherman R. Tinel's sign and Phalen's test in carpal tunnel syndrome. *Orthopedics* 1992; **15**: 1297–302.

18. Boland RA, Kiernan MC. Assessing the accuracy of a combination of clinical tests for identifying carpal tunnel syndrome. *J Clin Neurosci* 2009; **16**: 929–33.

19. El Miedany Y, Ashour S, Youssef S, Mehanna A, Meky FA. Clinical diagnosis of carpal tunnel syndrome: old test-new concepts. *Joint Bone Spine* 2008; **75**: 451–7.

20. Mondelli M, Aretini A, Ginanneschi F, Padua L. Thenar motor neuropathy electrophysiological study of 28 cases. *J Clin Neurophysiol* 2010; **27**: 344–9.

21. Subramony SH. Electrophysiological findings in crutch palsy. *Electromyogr Clin Neurophysiol* 1989; **29**: 281–5.

22. Lázaro-Blázquez D, Soto O. Combined median and medial antebrachial cutaneous neuropathies: an upper-arm neurovascular syndrome. *Electromyog Clin Neurophysiol* 2004; **44**: 187–91.

23. Watson ME. Median nerve damage from brachial artery puncture: a case report. *Respir Care* 1995; **40**: 1141–3.

24. Marquardt G, Angles SM, Leheta FD, Seifert V. Median nerve compression caused by a venous aneurysm. *J Neurosurg* 2001; **94**: 624–6.

25. Heberman ET, Cabot WD. Median nerve compression secondary to false aneurysm of the brachial artery. *Bull Hosp Joint Dis* 1974; **35**: 158–61.

26. Bilecenoglu B, Uz A, Karalezi N. Possible anatomic structures causing entrapment neuropathies of the median nerve. *Acta Orthop Belg* 2005; **71**: 169–76.

27. Bernard JB, McCoy SM. The supracondyloid process of the humerus. *J Bone Joint Surg (Am)* 1946; **28**: 845–50.

28. Bilge T, Yalaman O, Bilge S, Çokneşeli MD, Barut S. Entrapment neuropathy of the median nerve at the level of the ligament of Struthers. *Neurosurgery* 1990; **27**: 787–9.

29. Morris HH, Peters BH. Pronator syndrome: clinical and electrophysiological features in seven cases. *J Neurol Neurosurg Psychiatry* 1976; **39**: 461–4.

30. Mirovsky Y, Hendel D, Halperin N. Anterior interosseous nerve palsy following closed fracture of the proximal ulna. A case report and review of the literature. *Arch Orthop Trauma Surg* 1988; **107**: 61–4.

31. Stahl S, Freiman S, Volpin G. Anterior interosseous nerve palsy associated with Galeazzi fracture. *J Pediatr Orthop B* 2000; **9**: 45–6.

32. Keogh P, Khan H, Cooke E, McCoy G. Loss of flexor pollicis longus function after plating of the radius. Report of six cases. *J Hand Surg Br* 1997; **22**: 375–6.

33. Puhaindran ME, Wong HP. A case of anterior interosseous nerve syndrome after peripherally inserted central catheter (PICC) line insertion. *Singapore Med J* 2003; **44**: 653–5.

34. Ulrich D, Piatkowski A, Pallua N. Anterior interosseous nerve syndrome: retrospective analysis of 14 patients. *Arch Orthop Trauma Surg* 2011: **131**: 1561–5.

35. England JD, Sumner AJ. Neuralgic amyotrophy: an increasingly diverse entity. *Muscle Nerve* 1987; **10**: 60–8.

36. Kiloh LG, Nevin S. Isolated neuritis of the anterior interosseous nerve. *Br Med J* 1952; **1**: 850–1.

37. Seki M, Nakamura H, Kono H. Neurolysis is not required for young patients with a spontaneous palsy of the anterior interosseous nerve: retrospective analysis of cases managed non-operatively. *J Bone Joint Surg Br* 2006; **88**: 1606–9.

38. Wertsch JJ, Sanger JR, Matloub HS. Pseudo-anterior interosseous nerve syndrome. *Muscle Nerve* 1985; **8**: 68–70.

39. Aoki M, Kanaya K, Aiki H, Wada T, Yamashita T, Ogiwara N. Cubital tunnel syndrome in adolescent baseball players: a report of six cases with 3- to 5-year follow-up. *Arthroscopy* 2005; **21**: 758.

40. Nardin R, Chapman KM, Raynor EM. Prevalence of ulnar neuropathy in patients receiving hemodialysis. *Arch Neurol* 2005; **62**: 271–5.

41. Miller RG, Camp PE. Postoperative ulnar neuropathy. *J Am Med Assoc* 1979; **242**: 1636–9.

42. Campbell WW, Pridgeon RM, Riaz G, Astruc J, Leahy M, Crostic EG. Sparing of the flexor carpi ulnaris in ulnar neuropathy at the elbow. *Muscle Nerve* 1989; **12**: 965–7.

43. Papathanasiou ES, Loizides A, Panayiotou P, Papacostas SS, Kleopa KA. Ulnar neuropathy at Guyon's canal: electrophysiological and surgical findings. *Electromyogr Clin Neurophysiol* 2005; **45**: 87–92.

44. Monacelli G, Rizzo MI, Spagnoli AM, Monarca C, Scuderi N. Ulnar artery thrombosis and nerve entrapment at Guyon's canal: our diagnostic and therapeutic algorithm. *In Vivo* 2010; **24**: 779–82.

45. Yoshii S, Ikeda K, Murakami H. Ulnar nerve compression secondary to ulnar artery true aneurysm at Guyon's canal. *J Neurosurg Sci* 1999; **43**: 295–7.

46. Kim SS, Kim JH, Kang HI, Lee SJ. Ulnar nerve compression at Guyon's canal by an arteriovenous malformation. *J Korean Neurosurg Soc* 2009; **45**: 57–9.

47. Teissier J, Escare P, Asencio G, Gomis R, Allieu Y. Rupture of the flexor tendons of the little finger in fractures of the hook of the hamate bone. Report of two cases. *Ann Chir Main* 1983; **2**: 319–27.

48. Dell PC. Compression of the ulnar nerve at the wrist secondary to a rheumatoid synovial cyst: case report and review of the literature. *J Hand Surg Am* 1979; **4**: 468–73.

49. Ginanneschi F, Filippou G, Milani P, Biasella A, Rossi A. Ulnar nerve compression neuropathy at Guyon's canal caused by crutch walking: case report with ultrasonographic nerve imaging. *Arch Phys Med Rehabil* 2009; **90**: 522–4.

50. Capitani D, Beer S. Handlebar palsy—a compression syndrome of the deep terminal (motor) branch of the ulnar nerve in biking. *J Neurol* 2002; **249**: 1441–5.

51. Krishnan AV, Fulham MJ, Kiernan MC. Another cause of occupational entrapment neuropathy: la main du cuisinier (the chef's hand). *J Clin Neurophysiol* 2009; **26**: 129–31.

52. Jones HR. Pizza cutter's palsy. *N Engl J Med* 1988; **319**: 450.

53. On AY, Ozdemir O, Aksit R. Tourniquet paralysis after primary nerve repair. *Am J Phys Med Rehabil* 2000; **79**: 298–300.

54. Sinson G, Zager EL, Kline DG. Windmill pitcher's radial neuropathy. *Neurosurgery* 1994; **34**: 1087–9; discussion 1089–90.

55. Kaplan PE. Posterior interosseous neuropathies: natural history. *Arch Phys Med Rehabil* 1984; **65**: 399–400.

56. Wilson SM, Devarj V, Gardner-Thorpe C. Upholsterer's PIN. *J Neurol Neurosurg Psychiatry* 2001; **70**: 706–7.

57. Pringle CE, Guberman AH, Jacob P. Another kind of knapsack palsy. *Neurology* 1996; **46**: 585.

58. Roles NC, Maudsley RH. Radial tunnel syndrome. Resistant tennis elbow as a nerve entrapment. *J Bone Joint Surg* 1972; **54B**: 499–508.

59. Rosenbaum R. Disputed radial tunnel syndrome. *Muscle Nerve* 1999; **22**: 960–7.

60. Henry D, Bonthius DJ. Isolated musculocutaneous neuropathy in an adolescent baseball pitcher. *J Child Neurol* 2011; **26**: 1567–70.

61. Hsu JC, Paletta GA, Gambardella RA, Jobe FW. Musculocutaneous nerve injury in major league baseball pitchers: a report of two cases. *Am J Sports Med* 2007; **35**: 1003–6.

62. Mastaglia FL. Musculocutaneous neuropathy after strenuous physical activity. *Med J Aust* 1986; **145**: 153–4.

63. Kim SM, Goodrich JA. Isolated musculocutaneous nerve palsy: a case report. *Arch Phys Med Rehabil* 1984; **65**: 735–6.

64. Braddom RL, Wolfe C. Musculocutaneous nerve injury after heavy exercise. *Arch Phys Med Rehabil* 1978; **59**: 290–3.

65. Swain R. Musculocutaneous nerve entrapment: a case report. *Clin J Sports Med* 1995; **5**: 196–8.

66. Cisneros C, Geiringer S, Loewenson R. Isolated musculocutaneous nerve injury: a case report. *Int J Occup Environ Health* 1995; **1**: 257–9.

67. Sander HW, Quinto CM, Elinzano H, Chokroverty S. Carpet carrier's palsy: musculocutaneous neuropathy. *Neurology* 1997; **48**: 1731–2.

68. Dundore DE, DeLisa JA. Musculocutaneous nerve palsy: an isolated complication of surgery. *Arch Phys Med Rehabil* 1979; **60**: 130–3.

69. Berry PR, Wallis WE. Venepuncture nerve injuries. *Lancet* 1977; **1**: 1236–7.

70. Naam NH, Massoud HA. Painful entrapment of the lateral antebrachial cutaneous nerve at the elbow. *J Hand Surg Am* 2004; **29**: 1148–53.

71. Davidson JJ, Bassett FHI, Nunley JAJ. Musculocutaneous nerve entrapment revisited. *J Shoulder Elbow Surg* 1998; **7**: 250–5.

72. Liveson JA. Nerve lesions associated with shoulder dislocation; an electrodiagnostic study of 11 cases. *J Neurol Neurosurg Psychiatry* 1984; **47**: 742–4.

73. Kline DG, Kim DH. Axillary nerve repair in 99 patients with 101 stretch injuries. *J Neurosurg* 2003; **99**: 630–6.

74. Bonnard C, Anastakis DJ, van Melle G, Narakas AO. Isolated and combined lesions of the axillary nerve. A review of 146 cases. *J Bone Joint Surg Br* 1999; **81**: 212–17.

75. Bryan WJ, Schauder K, Tullos HS. The axillary nerve and its relationship to common sports medicine shoulder procedures. *Am J Sports Med* 1986; **14**: 113–16.

76. Loomer R, Graham B. Anatomy of the axillary nerve and its relation to inferior capsular shift. *Clin Orthop Relat Res* 1989; **243**: 100–5.

77. Horiguchi M. The cutaneous branch of some human suprascapular nerves. *J Anat* 1980; **130**: 191–5.

78. Ferretti A, De Carli A, Fontana M. Injury of the suprascapular nerve at the spinoglenoid notch. The natural history of infraspinatus atrophy in volleyball players. *Am J Sports Med* 1998; **26**: 759–63.

79. Holzgraefe M, Kukowski B, Eggert S. Prevalence of latent and manifest suprascapular neuropathy in high-performance volleyball players. *Br J Sports Med* 1994; **28**: 177–9.

80. Garcia G, McQueen D. Bilateral suprascapular nerve entrapment syndrome; case report and review of the literature. *J Bone Joint Surg (Am)* 1981; **63A**: 491–2.

81. Aiello I, Serra G, Traina GC, Tugnochi V. Entrapment of the suprascapular nerve at the spinoglenoid notch. *Ann Neurol.* 1982; **12**: 314–16.

82. Hirayama T, Takemitsu Y. Compression of the suprascapular nerve by a ganglion at the suprascapular notch. *Clin Orthop* 1981; **155**: 95–6.

83. Ganzhorn RW, Hocker JT, Horowitz M. Suprascapular nerve entrapment; a case report. *J Bone Joint Surg (Am)* 1981; **63A**: 492–4.

84. Thompson RCJ, Schneider W, Kennedy T. Entrapment neuropathy of the inferior branch of the suprascapular nerve by ganglia. *Clin Orthop* 1982; **166**: 185–7.

85. Vad VB, Southern D, Warren RF, Altchek DW, Dines D. Prevalence of peripheral neurologic injuries in rotator cuff tears with atrophy. *J Shoulder Elbow Surg* 2003; **12**: 333–6.

86. Ederland HG, Zachrisson BE. Fracture of the scapular notch associated with lesion of the suprascapular nerve. *Acta Orthop Scand* 1975; **46**: 758–63.

87. Zoltan JD. Injury to the suprascapular nerve associated with anterior dislocation of the shoulder: case report and review of the literature. *J Trauma* 1979; **19**: 203–6.

88. Liveson JA, Bronson MJ, Pollack MA. Suprascapular nerve lesions at the spinoglenoid notch: report of three cases and review of the literature. *J Neurol Neurosurg Psychiatry* 1991; **54**: 241–3.

89. Rossi F, Triggs WJ, Gonzalez R, Shafer SJ. Bilateral medial pectoral neuropathy in a weight lifter. *Muscle Nerve* 1999; **22**: 1597–9.

90. Marrero JL, Goldfine LJ. Isolated lateral pectoral nerve injury: trauma from a seat belt. *Arch Phys Med Rehabil* 1989; **70**: 239–40.

91. Secer HI, Daneyemez M, Tehli O, Gonul E, Izci Y. The clinical, electrophysiologic, and surgical characteristics of peripheral nerve injury caused by gunshot wounds in adults: a 40-year experience. *Surg Neurol* 2008; **69**: 143–52.

92. Nguyen HV, Nguyen H. Anatomical basis of modern thoracotomies: the latissimus dorsi and the 'serratus anterior-rhomboid' complex. *Surg Radiol Anat* 1987; **9**: 85–93.

93. Mondelli M, Cioni R, Federico A. Rare mononeuropathies of the upper limb in bodybuilders. *Muscle Nerve* 1998; **21**: 809–12.

94. Knoetgen JI, Moran SL. Long-term outcomes and complications associated with brachioplasty: a retrospective review and cadaveric study. *Plast Reconstr Surg* 2006; **117**: 2219–23.

95. Nakano KK. The entrapment neuropathies. *Muscle Nerve* 1978; **1**: 264–79.

96. Wood VE, Twito RS, Verska JM. Thoracic outlet syndrome: the results of first rib resection in 100 patients. *Orthop Clin North Am* 1988; **19**: 131–46.

97. Akgun K, Aktas I, Terzi Y. Winged scapula caused by a dorsal scapular nerve lesion: a case report. *Arch Phys Med Rehabil* 2008; **89**: 2017–20.

98. Johnson JTH, Kendall HO. Isolated paralysis of the serratus anterior muscle. *J Bone Joint Surg Am* 1955; **37A**: 567–74.

99. Mäkelä JP, Ramstad R, Mattila V, Pihlajamäki H. Brachial plexus lesions after backpack carriage in young adults. *Clin Orthop Relat Res* 2006; **452**: 205–9.

100. Kaupilla LI, Vastamäki M. Iatrogenic serratus anterior paralysis: long-term outcome in 26 patients. *Chest* 1996; **109**: 31–4.

101. Martin JT. Postoperative isolated dysfunction of the long thoracic nerve: a rare entity of uncertain etiology. *Anesth Analg* 1989; **69**: 614–19.

102. Toshkezi G, Dejesus J, Jabre JF, Hohler A, Davies K. Long thoracic neuropathy caused by an apical pulmonary tumour. *J Neurosurg* 2009; **110**: 754–7.

103. Pugliese GN, Green RF, Antonacci A. Radiation-induced long thoracic nerve palsy. *Cancer* 1987; **60**: 1247–8.

104. Phillips LH, 2nd. Familial long thoracic nerve palsy: a manifestation of brachial plexus neuropathy. *Neurology* 1986; **36**: 1251–3.

105. Cornwall R, Radomisli TE. Nerve injury in traumatic dislocation of the hip. *Clin Orthop Relat Res* 2000; **377**: 84–91.

106. Weale AE, Newman P, Ferguson IT, Bannister GC. Nerve injury after posterior and direct lateral approaches for hip replacement. A clinical and electrophysiological study. *J Bone Joint Surg Br* 1996; **78**: 899–902.

107. Villarejo FJ, Pascual AM. Injection injury of the sciatic nerve (370 cases). *Childs Nerv Syst* 1993; **9**: 229–32.

108. Akyuz M, Turhan N. Post injection sciatic neuropathy in adults. *Clin Neurophysiol* 2006; **117**: 1633–5.

109. Batres F, Barclay DL. Sciatic nerve injury during gynecologic procedures using the lithotomy position. *Obstet Gynecol* 1983; **62**(3 Suppl): 92s–94s.

110. Vogel CM, Albin R, Alberts JW. Lotus footdrop: sciatic neuropathy in the thigh. *Neurology* 1991; **41**: 605–6.

111. Lutz EG. Credit-card-wallet sciatica. *J Am Med Assoc* 1978; **240**: 738.

112. Holland NR, Schwartz-Williams L, Blotzer JW. 'Toilet seat' sciatic neuropathy. *Arch Neurol* 1999; **56**: 116.

113. Lefevre JH, Parc Y, Lewin M, Bennis M, Tiret E, Parc R. Radiofrequency ablation for recurrent pelvic cancer. *Colorectal Dis* 2008; **10**: 781–4.

114. McMillan HJ, Srinivasan J, Darras BT, et al. Pediatric sciatic neuropathy associated with neoplasms. *Muscle Nerve* 2011; **43**: 183–8.

115. Gikas PD, Hanna SA, Aston W, et al. Post-radiation sciatic neuropathy: a case report and review of the literature. *World J Surg Oncol* 2008; **6**: 130.

116. Pradat PF, Bouche P, Delanian S. Sciatic nerve mononeuropathy: an unusual late effect of radiotherapy. *Muscle Nerve* 2009; **40**: 872–4.

117. Mannan K, Altaf F, Maniar S, Tirabosco R, Sinisi M, Carlstedt T. Cyclical sciatica: endometriosis of the sciatic nerve. *J Bone Joint Surg Br* 2008; **90**: 98–101.

118. Salazar-Grueso E, Roos R. Sciatic endometriosis: a treatable sensorimotor mononeuropathy. *Neurology* 1986; **36**: 1360–3.

119. Yuen EC, Olney RK, So YT. Sciatic neuropathy: clinical and prognostic features in 73 patients. *Neurology* 1994; **44**: 1669–74.

120. Fishman LM, Dombi GW, Michaelsen C, et al. Piriformis syndrome: diagnosis, treatment, and outcome—a 10-year study. *Arch Phys Med Rehabil* 2002; **83**: 295–301.

121. Halpin RJ, Ganju A. Piriformis syndrome: a real pain in the buttock? *Neurosurgery* 2009; **65** (4 Suppl): A197–A202.

122. Stewart JD. The piriformis syndrome is overdiagnosed. *Muscle Nerve* 2003; **28**: 644–6.

123. Filler AG, Haynes J, Jordan SE, et al. Sciatica of nondisc origin and piriformis syndrome: diagnosis by magnetic resonance neurography and interventional magnetic resonance imaging with outcome study of resulting treatment. *J Neurosurg Spine* 2005; **2**: 99–115.

124. Jankiewicz JJ, Hennrikus WL, Houkom JA. The appearance of the piriformis muscle syndrome in computed tomography and magnetic resonance imaging. A case report and review of the literature. *Clin Orthop Relat Res* 1991; **262**: 205–9.

125. Beauchesne RP, Schutzer SF. Myositis ossificans of the piriformis muscle: an unusual cause of piriformis syndrome. A case report. *J Bone Joint Surg Am* 1997; **79**: 906–10.

126. Fishman LM, Zybert PA. Electrophysiologic evidence of piriformis syndrome. *Arch Phys Med Rehabil* 1992; **73**: 359–64.

127. Katirji MB, Wilbourn AJ. Common peroneal mononeuropathy: a clinical and electrophysiological study of 116 lesions. *Neurology* 1988; **38**: 1723–8.

128. Lutte I, Rhys C, Hubert C, et al. Peroneal nerve palsy in anorexia nervosa. *Acta Neurol Belg* 1997; **97**: 251–4.

129. Rubin DI, Kimmel DW, Cascino TL. Outcome of peroneal neuropathies in patients with systemic malignant disease. *Cancer* 1998; **83**: 1602–6.

130. Sotaniemi K. Slimmer's paralysis—peroneal neuropathy during weight reduction. *J Neurol Neurosurg Psychiatry* 1984; **47**: 564–6.

131. Simon NG, Kiernan MC. Common peroneal neuropathy and cancer. *Intern Med J* 2012; **42**: 837–40.

132. Koller RL, Blank NK. Strawberry pickers' palsy. *Arch Neurol* 1980; **37**: 320.

133. Thoma A, Fawcett S, Ginty M, Veltri K. Decompression of the common peroneal nerve: experience with 20 consecutive cases. *Plast Reconstr Surg* 2001; **107**: 1183–9.

134. Katirji B. Peroneal neuropathy. *Neurol Clin* 1999; **17**: 567–91.

135. Drees C, Wilbourn AJ, Stevens GH. Main trunk tibial neuropathies. *Neurology* 2002; **59**: 1082–4.

136. Ji JH, Shafi M, Kim WY, Park SH, Cheon JO. Compressive neuropathy of the tibial nerve and peroneal nerve by a Baker's cyst: case report. *Knee* 2007; **14**: 249–52.

137. Mastaglia FL. Tibial nerve entrapment in the popliteal fossa. *Muscle Nerve* 2000; **23**: 1883–6.

138. Pho RW, Rasjid C. A ganglion causing the tarsal tunnel syndrome: report of a case. *Aust NZ J Surg* 1978; **48**: 96–8.

139. Edwards WG, Lincoln CR, Bassett FH, 3rd, Goldner JL. The tarsal tunnel syndrome. Diagnosis and treatment. *J Am Med Assoc* 1969; **207**: 716–20.

140. Cetinkal A, Topuz K, Kaya S, Colak A, Demircan MN. Anterior tarsal tunnel syndrome secondary to missed talus fracture: a case report. *Turk Neurosurg* 2011; **21**: 259–63.

141. Stefko RM, Lauerman WC, Heckman JD. Tarsal tunnel syndrome caused by an unrecognized fracture of the posterior process of the talus (Cedell fracture). A case report. *J Bone Joint Surg Am* 1994; **76**: 116–18.

142. Olivieri I, Gemignani G, Siciliano G, Gremignai G, Pasero G. Tarsal tunnel syndrome in seronegative spondyloarthropathy. *Br J Rheumatol* 1989; **28**: 537–9.

143. Miranpuri S, Snook E, Vang D, Yong RM, Chagares WE. Neurilemoma of the posterior tibial nerve and tarsal tunnel syndrome. *J Am Podiatr Med Assoc* 2007; **97**: 148–50.

144. Jaffe KA, Wade JD, Chivers FS, Siegal GP. Extraskeletal osteosarcoma: an unusual presentation as tarsal tunnel syndrome. *Foot Ankle Int* 1995; **16**: 796–9.

145. Gould N, Alvarez R. Bilateral tarsal tunnel syndrome caused by variscosities. *Foot Ankle* 1983; **3**: 290–2.

146. Kinoshita M, Okuda R, Morikawa J, Abe M. Tarsal tunnel syndrome associated with an accessory muscle. *Foot Ankle Int* 2003; **24**: 132–6.

147. Kinoshita M, Okuda R, Yasuda T, Abe M. Tarsal tunnel syndrome in athletes. *Am J Sports Med* 2006; **34**: 1307–12.

148. Baxter DE, Thigpen CM. Heel pain—operative results. *Foot Ankle* 1984; **5**: 16–25.

149. Stickler DE, Morley KN, Massey EW. Sural neuropathy: etiologies and predisposing factors. *Muscle Nerve* 2006; **34**: 482–4.

150. Celebrezze JPJ, Pidala MJ, Porter JA, Slezak FA. Femoral neuropathy: an infrequently reported postoperative complication. *Dis Colon Rectum* 2000; **43**: 419–22.

151. Gombar KK, Gombar S, Singh B, Sangwan SS, Siwach RC. Femoral neuropathy: a complication of the lithotomy position. *Reg Anesth* 1992; **17**: 306–8.

152. Oldenburg M, Müller RT. The frequency, prognosis and significance of nerve injuries in total hip arthroplasty. *Int Orthop* 1997; **21**: 1–3.

153. Van Veer H, Coosemans W, Pirenne J, Monbaliu D. Acute femoral neuropathy: a rare complication after renal transplantation. *Transplant Proc* 2010; **42**: 4384–8.

154. Albrecht E, Niederhauser J, Gronchi F, et al. Transient femoral neuropathy after knee ligament reconstruction and nerve stimulator-guided continuous femoral nerve block: a case series. *Anaesthesia* 2011; **66**: 850–1.

155. Kent KC, Moscucci M, Gallagher SG, iMattia ST, Skillman JJ. Neuropathy after cardiac catheterisation: incidence, clinical patterns, and long-term outcome. *J Vasc Surg* 1994; **19**: 1008–13.

156. Geiger D, Mpinga E, Steves MA, Sugarbaker PH. Femoral neuropathy: unusual presentation for recurrent large-bowel cancer. *Dis Colon Rectum* 1998; **41**: 910–13.

157. Coppack SW, Watkins PJ. The natural history of diabetic femoral neuropathy. *Q J Med* 1991; **79**: 307–13.

158. Miller EH, Benedict FE. Stretch of the femoral nerve in a dancer. A case report. *J Bone Joint Surg Am* 1985; **67**: 315–17.

159. Sammarco GJ, Stephens MM. Neurapraxia of the femoral nerve in a modern dancer. *Am J Sports Med* 1991; **19**: 413–14.

160. Yang P-C, Chang S-F. Bilateral femoral neuropathy with 'hanging leg' syndrome: report of a case. *Acta Neurol Taiwan* 2003; **12**: 136–8.

161. Pendergrass TL, Moore JH. Saphenous neuropathy following medial knee trauma. *J Orthop Sports Phys Ther* 2004; **34**: 328–34.

162. Lavee J, Schneiderman J, Yorav S, Shewach-Millet M, Adar R. Complications of saphenous vein harvesting following coronary artery bypass surgery. *J Cardiovasc Surg (Torino)* 1989; **30**: 989–91.

163. Urayama H, Misaki T, Watanabe Y, Bunko H. Saphenous neuralgia and limb edema after femoropopliteal artery by-pass. *J Cardiovasc Surg (Torino)* 1993; **34**: 389–93.

164. Mochida H, Kikuchi S. Injury to infrapatelar branch of saphenous nerve in athroscopic knee surgery. *Clin Orthop Relat Res* 1995; **320**: 88–94.

165. Fabian RH, Norcross KA, Hancock MB. Surfer's neuropathy. *N Engl J Med* 1987; **316**: 555.

166. Barrick EF. Entrapment of the obturator nerve associated with a fracture of the pelvic ring. A case report. *J Bone Joint Surg Am* 1982; **80A**: 258–61.

167. Bischoff C, Schonle PW. Obturator nerve injuries during intra-abdominal surgery. *Clin Neurol Neurosurg* 1991; **93**: 73–6.

168. Melamed NB, Satya-Murti S. Obturator neuropathy after total hip replacement. *Ann Neurol* 1983; **13**: 578–9.

169. Schmalzried TP, Amstutz HC, Dorey FJ. Nerve palsy associated with total hip replacement: risk factors and prognosis. *J Bone Joint Surg Am* 1991; **73A**: 1074–80.

170. Sorenson E, Chen JJ, Daube JR. Obturator neuropathy: causes and outcome. *Muscle Nerve* 2002; **25**: 605–7.

171. Williams PH, Trzil KP. Management of meralgia paresthetica. *J Neurosurg* 1991; **74**: 76–80.

172. Suber DA, Massey EW. Pelvic mass presenting as meralgia paresthetica. *Obstet Gynecol* 1979; **53**: 257–8.

173. Mondelli M, Rossi S, Romano C. Body mass index in meralgia paresthetica: a case-control study. *Acta Neurol Scand* 2007; **116**: 118–23.

174. Fargo MV, Konitzer LN. Meralgia paresthetica due to body armor wear in U.S. soldiers serving in Iraq: a case report and review of the literature. *Mil Med* 2007; **172**: 663–5.

175. Park JW, Kim DH, Hwang M, Bun HR. Meralgia paresthetica caused by hip-huggers in a patient with aberrant course of the lateral femoral cutaneous nerve. *Muscle Nerve* 2007; **35**: 678–80.

176. Korkmaz N, Özçakar L. Meralgia paresthetica in a policeman: the belt or the gun. *Plast Reconstr Surg* 2004; **114**: 1012–13.

177. Nahabedian MY, Dellon AL. Meralgia paresthetica: etiology, diagnosis, and outcome of surgical decompression. *Ann Plast Surg.* 1995; **35**: 590–4.

178. Mirovsky Y, Neuwirth M. Injuries to the lateral femoral cutaneous nerve during spine surgery. *Spine (Phila Pa 1976)* 2000; **25**: 1266–9.

179. Gilliatt RW, Taylor JC. Electrical changes following section of the facial nerve. *Proc R Soc Med* 1959; **52**: 1080–3.

180. Chaudry V, Cornblath DR. Wallerian degeneration in human nerves: serial electrophysiological studies. *Muscle Nerve* 1992; **15**: 687–93.

181. Denys EH. AAEM minimonograph #14: the influence of temperature in clinical neurophysiology. *Muscle Nerve* 1991; **14**: 795–811.

182. McCluskey L, Feinberg D, Cantor C, Bird S. 'Pseudo-conduction block' in vasculitic neuropathy. *Muscle Nerve* 1999; **22**: 1361–6.

183. Yoon JS, Walker FO, Cartwright MS. Ultrasonographic swelling ratio in the diagnosis of ulnar neuropathy at the elbow. *Muscle Nerve* 2008; **38**: 1231–5.

184. Boom J, Visser LH. Quantitative assessment of nerve echogenicity: comparison of methods for evaluating nerve

echogenicity in ulnar neuropathy at the elbow. *Clin Neurophysiol* 2012; **123**: 1446–53.

185. Joy V, Therimadasamy AK, Chan YC, Wilder-Smith EP. Combined doppler and B-mode sonography in carpal tunnel syndrome. *J Neurol Sci* 2011; **308**: 16–20.

186. Walker FO, Cartwright MS, Wiesler ER, Caress J. Ultrasound of nerve and muscle. *Clin Neurophys* 2004; **115**: 495–507.

187. Fischer AQ, Carpenter DW, Hartlage PL, Carroll JE, Stephens S. Muscle imaging in neuromuscular disease using computerised real-time sonography. *Muscle Nerve* 1998; **11**: 270–5.

188. Walker FO, Harpold JG, Donofrio PD, Ferrell WG. Sonographic imaging of muscle contraction and fasciculations: a comparison with electromyography. *Muscle Nerve* 1990; **13**: 33–9.

189. Vucic S, Cordato DJ, Yiannikas C, Schwartz RS, Shnier RC. Utility of magnetic resonance imaging in diagnosing ulnar neuropathy at the elbow. *Clin Neurophysiol* 2006; **117**: 590–5.

190. Jablecki CK, Andary MT, So YT, Wilkins DE, Williams FH. Literature review of the usefulness of nerve conduction studies and electromyography for the evaluation of patients with carpal tunnel syndrome. AAEM Quality Assurance Committee. *Muscle Nerve* 1993; **16**: 1392–414.

191. Uncini A, Lange DJ, Solomon M, Soliven B, Meer J, Lovelace RE. Ring finger testing in carpal tunnel syndrome: a comparative study of diagnostic utility. *Muscle Nerve* 1989; **12**: 735–41.

192. Johnson EW, Sipski M, Lammertse T. Median and radial sensory latencies to digit I: normal values and usefulness in carpal tunnel syndrome. *Arch Phys Med Rehabil* 1987; **68**: 140–1.

193. Mills KR. Orthodromic sensory action potentials from palmar stimulation in the diagnosis of carpal tunnel syndrome. *J Neurol Neurosurg Psychiatry* 1985; **48**: 250–5.

194. Tachmann W, Kaeser HE, Magun HG. Comparison of orthodromic and antidromic sensory nerve conduction velocity measurements in the carpal tunnel syndrome. *J Neurol Neurosurg Psychiatry* 1981; **224**: 257–66.

195. Preston DC, Logigian EL. Lumbrical and interossei recording in carpal tunnel syndrome. *Muscle Nerve* 1992; **15**: 1253–7.

196. Kimura J. The carpal tunnel syndrome. Localization of conduction abnormalities within the distal segment of the median nerve. *Brain* 1979; **102**: 619–35.

197. Repaci M, Torrieri F, Di Blasio F, Uncini A. Exclusive electrophysiological motor involvement in carpal tunnel syndrome. *Clin Neurophysiol* 1999; **110**: 1471–4.

198. Bhala RP. Electrodiagnosis of ulnar nerve lesions at the elbow. *Arch Phys Med Rehabil* 1976; **57**: 206–12.

199. Visser LH, Beekman R, Franssen H. Short-segment nerve conduction studies in ulnar neuropathy at the elbow. *Muscle Nerve* 2005; **31**: 331–8.

200. Todnem K, Michler RP, Wader TE, Engstrom M, Sand T. The impact of extended electrodiagnostic studies in ulnar neuropathy at the elbow. *BMC Neurol* 2009; **9**: 52.

201. Uchida Y, Sugioka Y. The value of electrophysiological examination of the flexor carpi ulnaris muscle in the diagnosis of cubital tunnel syndrome. *Electromyogr Clin Neurophysiol* 1993; **33**: 369–73.

202. Seror P. Medial antebrachial cutaneous nerve conduction study, a new tool to demonstrate mild lower brachial plexus lesions. A report of 16 cases. *Clin Neurophysiol* 2004; **115**: 2316–22.

203. Stern BJ, Krumholz A, Johns C, Scott P, Nissim J. Sarcoidosis and its neurological manifestations. *Arch Neurol* 1985; **42**: 909–17.

204. England J. The variations of neuralgic amyotrophy. *Muscle Nerve* 1999; **22**: 435–6.

205. Fraser M, Campbell IW, Ewing DJ, Clarke BF. Mononeuropathy in diabetes mellitus. *Diabetes* 1979; **28**: 96–101.

206. Albers JW, Brown MB, Sima AA, Greene DA. Frequency of median mononeuropathy in patients with mild diabetic neuropathy in the eraly diabetes intervention trial (EDIT). *Muscle Nerve* 1996; **19**: 140–6.

207. Spinner RJ, Atkinson JL, Scheithauer BW, et al. Peroneal intraneural ganglia: the importance of the articular branch. Clinical series. *J Neurosurg* 2003; **99**: 319–29.

208. Spinner RJ, Atkinson JL, Tiel RL. Peroneal intraneural ganglia: the importance of the articular branch. A unifying theory. *J Neurosurg* 2003; **99**: 330–43.

209. Young NP, Sorenson EJ, Spinner RJ, Daube JR. Clinical and electrodiagnostic correlates of peroneal intraneural ganglia. *Neurology* 2009; **72**: 447–52.

210. Grisariu S, Avni B, Batchelor TT, et al. Neurolymphomatosis: an International Primary CNS Lymphoma Collaborative Group report. *Blood* 2010; **115**: 5005–11.

211. Baehring JM, Damek D, Martin EC, Betensky RA, Hochberg FH. Neurolymphomatosis. *Neuro Oncol* 2003; **5**: 104–15.

212. Serrano P, Hernandez N, Arroyo J, de Llobet J. Bilateral bell palsy and acute HIV Type 1 infection: report of 2 cases and review. *Clin Infect Dis* 2007; **44**: e57–e61.

213. Said G, Lacroix C, Chemouilli P, et al. Cytomegalovirus neuropathy in acquired immunodeficiency syndrome: a clinical and pathological study. *Ann Neurol* 1991; **29**: 139–46.

214. Hukada H, van Rij AM, Packer SGK, McMorran PD. Pathology of acute and chronic ischaemic neuropathy in atherosclerotic peripheral vascular disease. *Brain* 1996; **119**: 1449–60.

215. Wilbourn AJ, Furlan AJ, Hulley W, Ruschhaupt W. Ischemic monomelic neuropathy. *Neurology* 1983; **33**: 447–51.

216. Stork ACJ, van der Meulen MFG, van der Pol WL, Vrancken AFJE, Franssen H, Notermans NC. Wartenberg's migrant sensory neuritis: a prospective follow-up study. *J Neurol* 2010; **257**: 1344–8.

217. Asbury AK, Picard EH, Baringer JR. Sensory perineuritis. *Arch Neurol* 1972; **26**: 302–12.

218. Simmons Z, Albers JW, Sima AAF. Case-of-the-month: perineuritis presenting as mononeuritis multiplex. *Muscle Nerve* 1992; **15**: 630–5.

219. Gruen JP, Mitchell W, Kline DG. Resection and graft repair for localized hypertrophic neuropathy. *Neurosurgery* 1998; **43**: 78–83.

220. Eisen A, Danon J. The mild cubital tunnel syndrome. *Neurology* 1974; **24**: 608–13.

221. Svernlöv B, Larsson M, Rehn K, Adolfsson l. Conservative treatment of the cubital tunnel syndrome. *J Hand Surg (Eur)* 2009; **34**: 201–7.

222. Skie M, Zeiss J, Ebraheim NA, Jackson WT. Carpal tunnel changes and median nerve compression during wrist flexion and extension seen by magnetic resonance imaging. *J Hand Surg (Am)* 1990; **15**: 934–9.

223. Szabo RM, Chidgey LK. Stress carpal tunnel pressures in patients with CTS and normal patients. *J Hand Surg (Am)* 1989; **14**: 624–7.

224. Burke DT, Burke MM, Stewart GW, Cambre A. Splinting for carpal tunnel syndrome: in search of the optimal angle. *Arch Phys Med Rehabil* 1994; **75**: 1241–4.

225. Promoselli S, Sioli P, Grossi A, Cerri C. Neutral wrist splinting in carpal tunnel syndrome: a 3- and 6-months clinical and neurophysiologic follow-up evaluation of night-only splint therapy. *Eura Medicophys* 2006; **42**: 121–6.

226. Han SE, Boland RA, Krishnan AV, et al. Ischaemic sensitivity of axons in carpal tunnel syndrome. *J Peripher Nerv Syst* 2009; **14**: 190–200.

227. Krishnan AV, Park SB, Payne M, et al. Regional differences in ulnar nerve excitability may predispose to the development of entrapment neuropathy. *Clin Neurophys* 2011; **122**: 194–8.

228. Koffman BM, Greenfield LJ, Ali II, Pirzada NA. Neurologic complications after surgery for obesity. *Muscle Nerve* 2006; **33**: 166–76.

229. Karadaş O, Tok F, Ülaş UH, Odabaşi Z. The effectiveness of traimcinolone acetonide vs. procaine hydrochloride injection in the management of carpal tunnel syndrome: a double-blind randomized clinical trial. *Arch Phys Med Rehabil* 2011; **90**: 287–92.

230. Giannini F, Passero S, Cioni R, et al. Electrophysiological evaluation of local steroid injection in carpal tunnel syndrome. *Arch Phys Med Rehabil* 1991; **72**: 738–42.

231. Visser LH, Ngo Q, Groeneweg SJ, Brekelmans G. Long term effect of local corticosteroid injection for carpal tunnel syndrome: a

relation with electrodiagnostic severity. *Clin Neurophysiol* 2012; **123**: 838–41.

232. Campbell WW. Evaluation and management of peripheral nerve injury. *Clin Neurophysiol* 2008; **119**: 1951–65.

233. Spinner RJ, Kline DG. Surgery for peripheral nerve and brachial plexus injuries or other nerve lesions. *Muscle Nerve* 2000; **23**: 680–95.

234. Terzis JK, Barmpitsioti A. Axillary nerve reconstruction in 176 posttraumatic plexopathy patients. *Plast Reconstr Surg* 2010; **125**: 233–47.

235. Weinzig N, Chin G, Mead M, et al. Recovery of sensibility after digital neurorrhaphy: a clinical investigation of prognostic factors. *Ann Plast Surg* 2000; **44**: 610–17.

236. Ray WZ, Mackinnon SE. Management of nerve gaps: autografts, allografts, nerve transfers, and end-to-side neurorrhaphy. *Exp Neurol* 2010; **223**: 77–85.

237. Nagano AO, Tsuyama N, Ochiai N, Hara T, Takahashi M. Direct nerve crossing with the intercostal nerve to treat avulsion injuries of the brachial plexus. *J Hand Surg* 1989; **14A**: 980–5.

238. Allieu Y, Cenac P. Neurotization via the spinal accessory nerve in complete paralysis due to multiple avulsion injuries of the brachial plexus. *Clin Orthop* 1988; **237**: 67–74.

239. Brandt KE, Mackinnon SE. A technique for maximizing biceps recovery in brachial plexus reconstruction. *J Hand Surg* 1993; **18A**: 726–33.

240. Cage TA, Simon NG, Bourque S, et al. Dual re-innervation of biceps muscle following side-to-side anastomotic repair of an intact median nerve to a damaged musculocutaneous nerve. *J Neurosurg* 2013; **119**: 929–33.

241. Scholten RJPM, Mink van der Molen A, Uitdehaag BMJ, Bouter LM, de Vet HCW. Surgical treatment options for carpal tunnel syndrome. *Cochrane Database of Systematic Reviews* 2007; Issue **4**: Art. No. CD003905.

242. Jarvik JG, Comstock BA, Kliot M, et al. Surgery versus non-surgical therapy for carpal tunnel syndrome: a randomised parallel-group trial. *Lancet* 2009; **374**: 1074–81.

243. Verdugo RJ, Salinas RA, Castillo JL, Cea JG. Surgical versus non-surgical treatment for carpal tunnel syndrome. *Cochrane Database of Systematic Reviews* 2008; Issue **4**: Art. No. CD001552.

244. Capasso M, Manzoli C, Uncini A. Management of extreme carpal tunnel syndrome: evidence from a long-term follow-up study. *Muscle Nerve* 2009; **40**: 86–93.

CHAPTER 13

Multiple mononeuropathies

Eleanor A. Marsh and J. Gareth Llewelyn

Introduction

Multiple mononeuropathy (MM) is a descriptive term for a peripheral nervous system (PNS) syndrome dominated by progressive multiple peripheral nerve lesions, typically asymmetric at onset, and most commonly raises the possibility of an underlying vasculitic process.

Diagnosis and clinical presentation of MM

MM is the mode of presentation in up to 30% of cases of PNS vasculitis, typically with mononeuropathies (combining motor and sensory signs relevant to an individual nerve) that are usually severe and complete [1]. These can present acutely over a few days, or with slow accumulation of asymmetric multifocal neurological deficits, sometimes punctuated by acute events. Occasionally the progression of mononeuropathies can be so rapid that, at hospital presentation, the deficits may be mistaken for that of a polyneuropathy. The peroneal nerve is preferentially affected in the lower limbs and the ulnar nerve in the upper limbs [2]. PNS vasculitis may also present with an isolated mononeuropathy, distal symmetric sensorimotor axonal polyneuropathy, or a radiculoplexus neuropathy.

A careful clinical history asking 'Where did the problem start?' and 'What did you notice after that?' may elicit the typical asymmetry in the evolution. A rapid onset with pain suggests a vasculitic/ischaemic process. A painless MM with a clear trigger such as prolonged crouching would point to hereditary neuropathy with liability to pressure palsies (HNPP) as the more likely cause (see Table 13.1).

Examination requires detailed attention to muscle wasting and muscle strength in the hands and feet—again looking for asymmetry between one limb and the other. The presence of skin changes, e.g. scattered petechiae, or palpable purpura, livedo reticularis, itchy hives, or wheals or even just painful bumps, will add weight to the suspicion of an ongoing vasculitic process (see Figs 13.1–13.3).

Table 13.1 Causes of multiple mononeuropathy

1. A primary immune-mediated vasculitic process
2. A vasculitic process resulting from other types of autoimmune conditions
3. A vasculitic process resulting from other non-autoimmune conditions
4. Multifocal demyelinating neuropathies (e.g. CIDP/MMN)
5. Other asymmetric neuropathies (e.g. hereditary/entrapment/infiltrative)

CIDP, chronic inflammatory demyelinating polyradiculoneuropathy; MMN, multifocal motor neuropathy with conduction block.

Primary immune-mediated vasculitides

In a third of patients, neuropathy is the first and only manifestation of a necrotizing primary immune-mediated vasculitis which carries a 30% mortality rate [3]. It can affect any age group and either sex equally. In addition to symptoms attributable to multiorgan involvement, patients may exhibit constitutional symptoms such as night sweats and weight loss, or a more nebulous but prominent problem of malaise that may pre-date the onset of neurological symptoms by a few weeks.

There are several schemes aimed at classifying vasculitides—according to the size of the blood vessel affected [4,5], types of organ involvement, and autoantibody profiles. One useful division is to consider whether the vasculitic process is systemic or non-systemic/localized. Another concerns the underlying type of immune process—is antibody- or immune complex-driven?

Antineutrophil cytoplasmic antibody (ANCA)-associated vasculitis (AAV) typically refers to conditions such as Wegener granulomatosis (WG), Churg–Strauss syndrome (CSS), and microscopic polyangiitis (MPA). ANCAs are specific for antigens in neutrophil granules and monocyte lysosomes. There are two staining types on indirect immunofluorescence, cytoplasmic (c-ANCA) and perinuclear (p-ANCA). Enzyme linked immunosorbent assays are then performed to identify the specific antigen targeted by the ANCA. The presence of c-ANCA with anti-proteinase 3 (anti-PR3) is highly suggestive of WG (positive in 80–90% of cases), while p-ANCA with anti-myeloperoxidase (anti-MPO) is more often encountered in those with MPA (50–80%) and CSS (42%) [6]. Importantly, ANCA negativity does not exclude the diagnosis of AAV, and false positives may be seen in systemic lupus erythematosus (SLE), rheumatoid arthritis (RA), and tuberculosis.

In ANCA-negative vasculitis, or 'immune complex' (IC) diseases, serum ICs may be deposited in blood vessel walls. Examples include Henoch–Schönlein purpura (HSP) and essential cryoglobulinaemic vasculitis.

Whilst multiorgan involvement in primary immune-mediated vasculitides is seen, the AAVs have predominant renal–pulmonary involvement whereas IC types tend to have renal–dermal involvement [7]. There are also organ- or tissue-specific vasculitides, where only the PNS is involved—a non-systemic vasculitic neuropathy (NSVN)—and long term follow up studies show that this type remains localised [8], despite the occasional presence of systemic markers (raised C-reactive protein etc.) and there is no risk of multiorgan failure.

Polyarteritis nodosa (PAN) is a medium-vessel necrotic primary systemic vasculitis. It is far less common than other AAVs. A neuropathy is seen in 60–70% of cases, normally appearing within a

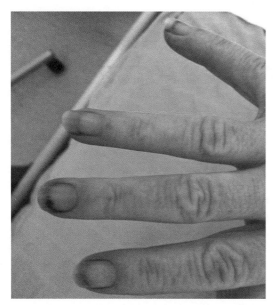

Fig. 13.1 Digital infarcts in a patient with antineutrophil cytoplasmic antibodies (ANCA)-negative vasculitis. (See also figure in colour plate section)

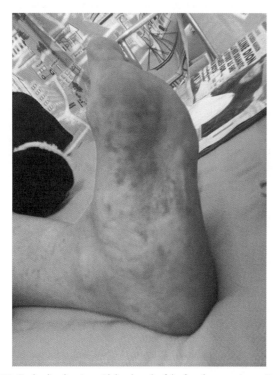

Fig. 13.2 Dusky discoloration with livedo rash of the foot (same patient as Fig. 13.1). (See also figure in colour plate section)

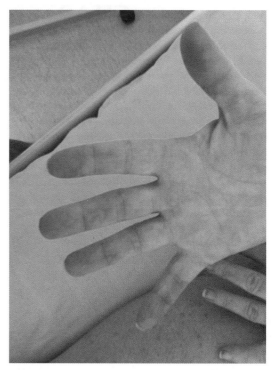

Fig. 13.3 Dusky discoloration with livedo rash of the hand (same patient as Fig. 13.1). (See also figure in colour plate section)

few months of diagnosis [9]. An association with hepatitis B is seen in a third to a half of cases [10], with the disease course in this instance being more aggressive.

WG and CSS are AAVs of small vessels. In both, the disease process starts with respiratory involvement. WG causes mucosal inflammation of nasal and paranasal structures, resulting in upper respiratory granulomas. Neurological involvement occurs in a secondary stage, usually affecting the central nervous system (CNS); however a distal symmetrical sensory neuropathy or a multiple mononeuropathy occurs in up to 10% of cases [11].

CSS normally occurs on a background of long-standing asthma or allergic rhinitis. Peripheral eosinophilia and pulmonary infiltrates are seen. More than 70% of patients with CSS have PNS involvement [12] and this tends to occur earlier and is more severe than in WG [13], with the MM pattern in 71% and a distal sensory symmetric polyneuropathy in the remaining 29% of patients [14].

MPA is an AAV that differs from WG and CSS in that lung involvement, especially that of the upper airways, is unusual. The PNS is more commonly involved (55–79%) [13] than the CNS (10–15%) [10].

HSP does not normally affect the PNS [15], but in vasculitis with cryoglobulin immune deposits PNS symptoms are an initial manifestation in 50% of cases [15]. One useful test for cryoglobulinaemia is the presence of very low levels of early complement components (especially C4) with normal or slightly low C3 levels.

A vasculitic process resulting from other autoimmune conditions

These are sometimes referred to as secondary systemic vasculitides, usually triggered by a collagen vascular disorder.

RA can be associated with a PNS vasculitis in 2–15% cases [16], normally as a late manifestation of severe seropositive disease. With the development of modern treatments, the incidence of neuropathy is declining. RA also causes a non-vasculitic entrapment neuropathy As a chronic autoimmune condition, RA may give rise to the development of cryoglobulins (in 16% of patients with RA [2]) and a consequent PNS vasculitis.

The vasculitic effects of scleroderma (systemic sclerosis) tend to manifest as plexopathy or cranial neuropathy. Up to 50% of patients with Sjögren syndrome develop a PNS vasculitis [17]. In SLE, vasculitis of the CNS is more common than in the PNS (11%) [18].

Raised concentrations of serum cryoglobulins are seen in a range of chronic infections, autoimmune disease, or haematological malignant disease, and in isolation as in essential cryoglobulinaemia. The types of cryoglobulins seen in such cases are Type 2 mixed monoclonal and polyclonal immunoglobulins. Hepatitis C is strongly associated with mixed cryoglobulinaemia, with 73–90% of patients with this condition being positive for Hepatitis C. An IC-mediated PNS vasculitis is seen in 30–70% cases of mixed cryoglobulinaemia [19]. In terms of the haematological causes, Waldenström macroglobulinaemia must be considered. This is a lymphoplasmocytic disorder characterized by proliferation of B-cell clones, which produce pathogenic immunoglobulin M (IgM). The consequent IgM can remain asymptomatic or cause immune complex-mediated systemic vasculitis.

A vasculitic process resulting from other non-autoimmune conditions

These are also referred to as secondary systemic vasculitides. In the absence of connective tissue disease, a PNS vasculitis is triggered by a known underlying condition (see Table 13.2) which induces ischaemic nerve lesions.

Diabetes mellitus is an example of such a disorder. A small proportion of diabetic patients, normally those over the age of 50 years, develop a lumbosacral radiculoplexus neuropathy. This has also been called the Bruns–Garland syndrome (historically termed diabetic amyotrophy). Patients present with acute or subacute onset pain, usually in one leg but it can be in both, and most often over the front of the thigh, but the distribution may mimic 'sciatica'.

Table 13.2 Causes of secondary systemic vasculitis

Condition inducing secondary vasculitis	Notes
Diabetes	Diabetic radiculoplexus neuropathy
Drugs	Amphetamine, propyluracil, hydralazine, interferons, non-steroidal anti-inflammatory drugs, penicillin, allopurinol, cocaine, heroin, sulphonamides, phenytoin
Viral infections	CMV, HTLV-1, hepatitis, HIV, HSV, VZV, EBV
Bacterial infections	Infective endocarditis, *Streptococcus pneumoniae*, *Haemophilus influenzae*, *Salmonella typhi*, β haemolytic streptococcus, Lyme disease, *Mycobacterium tuberculosis*, leprosy, *Treponema pallidum*
Fungal infections	*Aspergillus*, coccidioides, mucormycosis, *Histoplasma capsulatum*
Protozoal infections	*Toxoplasma gondii*, *Plasmodium falciparum*
Radiation	
Paraneoplastic	
Malignancy	
Chronic inflammatory	Sarcoidosis, inflammatory bowel disease, amyloidosis

CMV, cytomegalovirus; HTLV-1, human T lymphotrophic virus-1; HIV, human immunodeficiency virus; HSV, herpes simplex virus; VZV, varicella zoster virus; EBV, Epstein–Barr virus.

Modified from Marsh et al. [25].

Over a period of days or weeks, the pain is followed by bilateral asymmetric weakness. The natural history is that of symptoms progressing over many months with development of muscle wasting and weight loss, then some weeks of stabilization followed by some improvement in many, but not all, patients. Clinical improvement is often heralded by the regaining of body weight. This syndrome is best considered as a monophasic NSVN induced by diabetes [20].

Viral infections are interesting in that they may induce PNS vasculitis directly or as a result of mixed cryoglobulinaemia. Human immunodeficiency virus (HIV) results in PNS vasculitis in less than 1% of patients, normally in those with a CD4 count of 200–500 cells mm^{-3} [21]. HIV also predisposes to lymphoma, which may cause a PNS vasculitis in its own right. A CD4 count of less than 50 cells mm^{-3} predisposes the patient to a cytomegalovirus (CMV)-associated vasculitis [22]. However, all patients with chronic viral infections are at increased risk of primary systemic vasculitis.

Paraneoplastic causes of PNS vasculitis are important to consider, and are most commonly associated with small cell lung cancer, lymphoma, renal cell carcinoma, and other adenocarcinomas. Importantly, the well-established paraneoplastic antibodies (anti-Hu, Ri, Yo) are usually negative.

In addition to lymphoma causing a paraneoplastic PNS vasculitis, haematological lymphoproliferative malignancies are likely to induce a PNS vasculitis independently. In lymphoma, it can be very difficult to distinguish whether the associated neuropathy is due to lymphoma infiltration or vasculitic PNS involvement.

Sarcoidosis, may induce features of vasculitis. In one study, 29% of patients with sarcoidosis undergoing sural nerve biopsy showed evidence of vasculitis [23].

Multifocal demyelinating neuropathies

Chronic inflammatory demyelinating polyneuropathy (CIDP) is typically asymmetric in distribution compared with hereditary or paraproteinaemic causes of demyelinating neuropathy (see Chapter 16). Multifocal neuropathy with conduction block is very asymmetric—with weakness progressing over months in the distribution of one or two peripheral nerves but without sensory loss. Cramps and muscle twitching are common.

Other asymmetric neuropathies

Examples include focal peripheral nerve entrapment (common in diabetes mellitus, RA, amyloidosis, HNPP) or from proximal plexus infiltration or compression (common in trauma, radiotherapy, malignant infiltration, neuralgic amyotrophy, infection, hereditary neuralgic amyotrophy).

Investigation of MM

The tempo of the neuropathy often dictates the range of the initial tests. With a rapidly evolving MM, a vasculitic process is very likely and time-consuming investigations should not significantly delay the onset of treatment. Simple tests are outlined in Table 13.3.

Neurophysiology

As in other settings, neurophysiology is an adjunct to prior careful clinical evaluation, and may add important information as to whether the process is axonal or demyelinating (with implications for therapy), uniform or patchy. It also can identify a suitable sensory nerve for biopsy.

Table 13.3 Investigating multiple mononeuropathy

Looking for causes of primary immune PNS vasculitis:

- Urinalysis: proteinuria for glomerulonephritis and specific request to look for red cell casts (always pathological and strongly indicative of glomerular damage from a primary immune vasculitis in this context)
- Erythrocyte sedimentation rate
- Full blood count—eosinophilia
- Renal function
- Antinuclear antibodie/extractable nuclear antigen antibodies/ antineutrophil cytoplasmic antibodies
- Serum angiotensin-converting enzyme
- Cryoglobulins
- Glucose
- Chest X-ray—granulomatous/infiltrates

Looking for causes of secondary PNS vasculitis:

- Glucose, glucose tolerance test
- Antinuclear antibody/extractable nuclear antigen antibodies
- Blood cultures, echocardiogram
- Rhesus factor
- Chest X-ray—malignancy/sarcoidosis
- Human immunodeficiency virus
- Hepatitis B and C serology
- Lyme serology
- VDRL and TPHA
- Cryoglobulins
- Serum complement
- Serum angiotensin-converting enzyme
- Tumour markers/malignancy imaging
- Paraneoplastic antibodies

Looking for other causes of multiple mononeuropathy:

- DNA testing: *PMP22* deletion on chromosome 17 (HNPP)

PNS, peripheral nervous system; VDRL, Venereal Disease Research Laboratory [test]; TPHA, *Treponema pallidum* haemagglutination assay; HNPP, hereditary neuropathy with liability to pressure palsies

In PNS vasculitis, nerve conduction studies typically show an axonal process. Sensory nerve action potentials are reduced in amplitude or absent, with relatively normal conduction velocities and distal latencies. Compound muscle action potentials (CMAPs) may be reduced in amplitude in affected motor nerves alongside delayed or unrecordable F waves.

Occasionally conduction block may be observed. After an acute ischaemic lesion causing Wallerian degeneration, the distal stump remains capable of conducting motor impulses for a further 9 days, and in this early period the distal CMAP may be smaller than proximal ones, thus mimicking conduction block. This is a transient phenomenon and will be lost as the distal axon degenerates. The persistence of conduction block beyond this 9-day window would be more in keeping with nerve entrapment or focal demyelination as seen in inflammatory neuropathies (CIDP, MMN; see Chapter 16).

On electromyography (EMG), features of denervation in clinically weak muscles would be expected. Hence 'neurogenic-type' muscle unit potentials with reduced recruitment and spontaneous activity would be seen.

Usefulness of cerebrospinal fluid examination

This is only of value if none of the other investigations have yielded an answer, and the possibility of a malignant meningitic process has to be excluded.

Nerve and muscle biopsy

Histological evidence remains the 'gold-standard' for diagnosis of PNS vasculitis and requires the presence of both vascular inflammation (microvasculitis) and signs of vascular destruction (necrotizing change). Asymmetry in the distribution of myelinated fibres between and within fascicles is suggestive, but not by itself diagnostic, of an underlying vasculitis.

A nerve biopsy should only be considered if the possibility of a vasculitis is high and if the blood tests are uninformative. Of patients ultimately diagnosed with vasculitic neuropathy, sural nerve biopsy alone is confirmatory in 40–50% of cases, whereas combined nerve–muscle biopsy gives a positive result in 60–70% of cases [24]. In view of the fact that cellular infiltrates predominate in epineurium and have a perivascular distribution, a total, rather than fascicular nerve, biopsy is recommended, and should be processed in a laboratory used to dealing with nerve biopsies. Importantly, a negative biopsy does not exclude the diagnosis of a vasculitis.

Treatment of MM*

The treatment of vasculitis depends on its cause. The use of cyclophosphamide (CYC) and other immunosuppressive agents has transformed the prognosis of the primary immune-mediated vasculitides. There are two main phases in the treatment of PNS vasculitis [26]:

♦ Remission–induction therapy: an initial treatment that results in resolution of the manifestations of active vasculitis.

♦ Remission–maintenance therapy: a continuation of treatment for a prolonged period with the aim of maintaining control and reducing the likelihood of clinical relapses.

Remission–induction therapy

Glucocorticoids and CYC form the basis of initial treatment. Oral prednisolone is prescribed at 1 mg kg^{-1} day^{-1} (to a maximum of 80 mg day^{-1} [27]). When a rapid effect needed intravenous methylprednisolone, 1 g day–1 for 3 days, can be given before starting oral prednisolone [28].

The CYCLOPS trial showed that a single pulse of intravenous CYC (15 mg kg^{-1}; maximum dose 1.2 g—also adjusted according to age and renal function) repeated every 2 weeks for the first three pulses, then at 3-weekly intervals for another 18 weeks was equal to oral CYC at its normal dosing regime (2 mg kg^{-1} day^{-1} for 3 months and then 1.5 mg kg^{-1} day^{-1} for another 3 months, with dose adjustment for age) in providing remission–induction, but with fewer side effects [26].

It has been recommended that patients with severe or life-threatening vasculitis and significant renal failure (creatinine > 500 μmol L^{-1}) should be treated with plasma exchange in addition to the standard treatment regimes (oral prednisolone and intravenous CYC) [29].

Oral methotrexate has been shown to have similar success rates to CYC for remission–induction for early non-life-threatening

---

*This section is adapted from Marsh et al. [25].

disease without significant renal disease. However, it appears to result in more relapses at 18 months and an increased risk of progression to more widespread disease than with CYC [30].

Remission–maintenance therapy

This second phase of treatment is achieved with a combination of oral prednisolone and a steroid-sparing agent. Azathioprine at 2 mg kg^{-1} day^{-1} has been shown to be as effective as oral CYC (1.5 mg kg^{-1} day^{-1}) in preventing relapse at 18 months, but with a lower risk of serious adverse effects (10% versus 18). Oral prednisolone should be gradually tapered—the dose should not go below 15 mg day^{-1} for the first 3 months [27]. Oral methotrexate at 20–25 mg week^{-1} as an alternative to azathioprine can be used if it had been started in the remission–induction phase [31].

The treatment of vasculitis secondary to other non-autoimmune causes is focused on the underlying condition. For Hepatitis B-associated PAN, a course of oral prednisolone, followed by an antiviral agent such as interferon-alfa-2b or Lamivudine, alongside plasma exchange, may be effective [32]. In Hepatitis C-associated mixed cryoglobulinaemia a course of interferon with Ribavirin is used [33].

References

1. Zivkovic SA, Ascgerman D, Lacomis D. Vasculitic neuropathy—electrodiagnostic findings and association with malignancies. *Acta Neurol Scand* 2007; **115**: 432–6.
2. Said G, Lacroix C. Primary and secondary vasculitic neuropathy. *J Neurol* 2005; **252**: 633–41.
3. Rossi CM, Comite GD. The clinical spectrum of the neurological involvement in vasculitides. *J Neurol Sci* 2009; **285**: 13–21.
4. Hunder GG, Arend WP, Bloch DA, et al. The American College of Rheumatology 1990 criteria for the classification of vasculitis. *Arthritis Rheum* 1990; **33**: 1065–7.
5. Jeanette JC, Faulk RJ, Andrassy K, et al. Nomenclature of systemic vasculitides. Proposal of an international consensus conference. *Arthritis Rheum* 1994; **37**: 187–192.
6. Suresh E. Diagnostic approach to patients with suspected vasculitis. *Postgrad Med J* 2008; **82**: 483–8.
7. Jeanette JC, Faulk RJ. Small-vessel vasculitis. *N Engl J Med* 1997; **337**: 1512–23.
8. Dyck PJ, Benstead TJ, Conn DL, et al. Nonsystemic vasculitic neuropathy. *Brain* 1987; **110**: 843–53.
9. Guillevin L, Du LTH, Godeau P, Jais P, Wechsler B. Clinical findings and prognosis of polyarteritis nodosa and Churg–Strauss angiitis: a study in 165 patients. *Br J Rheum* 1988; **27**: 258–64.
10. Schaublin GA, Michet CJ, Dyck PJB, Burns TM. An update on the classification and treatment of vasculitic neuropathy. *Lancet Neurol* 2005; **4**: 853–65.
11. Stone JH. Limited versus severe Wegener's granulomatosis: baseline data on patients in the Wegener's granulomatosis etanercept trial. *Arthritis Rheum* 2003; **48**: 2299–309.
12. Collins MP, Kissel JT. Neuropathies with systemic vasculitis. In: Dyck PJ, Thomas PK (ed) *Peripheral Neuropathy*, 4th edn, Vol. 2, pp. 2335–404. Philadelphia, PA: Elsevier Saunders, 2004.
13. Cattaneo L, Chierici E, Pavone L, et al. Peripheral neuropathy in Wegener's granulomatosis, Churg–Stauss syndrome and microscopic polyangiitis. *J Neurol Neurosurg Psychiatry* 2007; **78**: 1119–23.
14. Seghal M, Swanson JW, DeRemee RA, Colby TV. Neurologic manifestations of Churg–Strauss syndrome. *Mayo Clinic Proc* 1995; **70**: 337–41.
15. Rossi CM, Comite GD. The clinical spectrum of the neurological involvement in vasculitides. *J Neurol Sci* 2009; **285**: 13–21.
16. Moore PM. Vasculitic neuropathies. *J Neurol Neurosurg Psychiatry* 2000; **68**: 271–6.
17. Terrier B, Lacroix C, Guillevin L, et al. Diagnostic and prognostic relevance of neuromuscular biopsy in Sjögren's syndrome-related neuropathy. *Arthritis Rheum* 2007; **57**: 1520–9.
18. Ramos-Casals M, Solans R, Roasa J, et al. Vasculitis in systemic lupus erythematosus: prevalence and clinical characteristics in 670 patients. *Medicine* 2008; **87**: 210–19.
19. Zaltron S, Puoti M, Liberini P, et al. High prevalence of peripheral neuropathy in hepatitis C virus infected patients with symptomatic and asymptomatic cryogobulinaemia. *Ital J Gastroenterol Hepatol* 1998; **30**: 391–5.
20. Llewelyn JG, Thomas PK, King RHM. Epineurial microvasculitis in proximal diabetic neuropathy. *J Neurol* 1998; **245**: 159–65.
21. Johnson RM, Barbarini G, Barbaro G. Kawasaki-like syndromes and other vasculitic syndromes in HIV-infected patients. *AIDS* 2003; **17**: S77–S82.
22. Brew BJ. The peripheral nerve complications of human immunodeficiency virus (HIV) infection. *Muscle Nerve* 2003; **28**: 542–52.
23. Vital A, Lagueny A, Ferrer X, et al. Sarcoid neuropathy: clinic-pathological study of 4 new cases and review of the literature. *Clin Neuropathol* 2008; **27**: 96–105.
24. Collins MP, Mendell JR, Periquet MI, et al. Superficial peroneal nerve/peroneus brevis muscle biopsy in vasculitic neuropathy. *Neurology* 2000; **55**: 636–43.
25. Marsh EA, Davies LM, Llewelyn JG. How to recognise and treat peripheral nervous system vasculitis. *Pract Neurol* 2013; 10 May [Epub ahead of print] doi:10.1136/practneurol-2012-000464.
26. De Groot K, Harper L, Jayne DR, et al. and EUVAS (European Vasculitis Study Group). CYCLOPS trial. Pulse versus daily oral cyclophosphamide for induction of remission in antineutrophil cyctoplasmic antibody-associated vasculitis: a randomised trial. *Ann Intern Med* 2009; **150**: 670–80.
27. De Groot K et al and EUVAS (European Vasculitis Study Group). *CYCLOPS Trial Protocol*, 2006. <http://www.vasculitis.nl/media/documents/cyclops>.
28. Hamour S, Salama AD, Pusey CD. Management of ANCA-associated vasculitis: current trends and future prospects. *Therapeut Clin Risk Manage* 2010; **6**: 253–64.
29. Lapraik C, Watts R, Bacon P, et al. BSR and BHPR guidelines for the management of adults with ANCA associated vasculitis. *Rheumatology* 2007; **46**: 1–11.
30. De Groot K, Rasmussen N, Bacon P, et al. Randomisation trial of cyclophosphamide versus methotrexate for induction of remission in early systemic antineutrophil cytoplasmic antibody associated vasculitis. *Arthritis Rheum* 2005; **52**: 2462–8.
31. Reinhold-Keller E, Fink CO, Herlyn K, et al. High rate of renal relapse in 71 patients with Wegener's granulomatosis under maintenance of remission with low-dose methotrexate. *Arthritis Rheum* 2002; **47**: 326–32.
32. Guillevin L, Francois L, Cohen P, et al. Polyarteritis nodosa related to hepatitis B virus: a prospective study with long-term observation of 41 patients. *Medicine (Baltimore)* 1995; **74**: 238–53.
33. Mazzaro C, Zorat F, Comar C, et al. Interferon plus ribavirin in patients with hepatitis C virus positive mixed cryoglobulinaemia resistant to interferon. *J Rheumatol* 2003; **30**: 1775–81.

CHAPTER 14

Plexopathy

David L. H. Bennett and Mohamed Mahdi-Rogers

Anatomy

To interpret the clinical presentation of plexus lesions, an understanding of anatomy is essential. In the brachial plexus, multiple nerve roots and their branches join and then diverge to form the terminal nerves of the upper limbs. The lumbosacral plexus is less complex than the brachial plexus and has fewer components

Brachial plexus

The brachial plexus originates from the anterior primary rami of C5, C6, C7, C8, and T1 nerve roots and extends from the upper neck to the axilla. In about 5% of people there is contribution of the C4 or T2 nerve root to the plexus. The plexus is conventionally divided into five roots (C5–T1), three trunks, (upper, middle, and lower), six divisions (three anterior, three posterior), three cords (lateral, posterior, and medial), and multiple terminal nerves (Fig. 14.1).

The anterior primary rami of the roots exit through their corresponding spinal segments, then unite to form three trunks in the supraclavicular fossa. The long thoracic and dorsal scapular nerves come directly off the roots. Clinical assessment of these nerves is useful in localizing the proximal extent of a lesion. The upper trunk is formed by the C5 and C6 roots; the middle trunk is essentially a continuation of the C7 root; and the lower trunk is formed by the C8 and T1 roots. The trunks are located superficially in the antero-inferior aspect of posterior triangle in the neck which predisposes them to traction and penetrating injuries. The suprascapular nerve which innervates the supraspinatus and infraspinatus is the only major nerve that comes off at the trunk level and branches directly from the upper trunk. Each trunk then divides into an anterior and a posterior division, giving rise to six divisions. No major nerve comes from the divisions but they serve as a useful clinical landmark in classifying plexopathies. Lesions proximal to the divisions are referred to as supraclavicular and lesions distal to the divisions as infraclavicular. Most conditions can affect any part of the plexus but supraclavicular plexopathies are more common and generally show less efficient recovery.

The divisions unite to form cords at the level of the clavicle. The posterior cord is formed by union of the three posterior divisions, the lateral cord from anterior divisions of the upper and middle trunks, and the medial cord is a direct continuation of the anterior division of the lower trunk. The cords are bound to the second portion of the axillary artery and their names derive from their anatomical relationship to the artery. The cords are the longest portion of the plexus, and each cord ends in one or more terminal nerves. The lateral pectoral, musculocutaneous, and median (lateral head) nerves (C5–C7) arise from the lateral cord; the thoracodorsal, axillary, and radial nerves

(C5–C8) originate from the posterior cord; and the medial cutaneous and antebrachial cutaneous, ulnar, and medial head of the median (C8, T1) nerves from the medial cord. Apart from the median nerve, which is derived from lateral and medial cords, all the terminal nerves originate from a single cord (Table 14.1).

Lumbosacral plexus

The lumbosacral plexus is considered a single entity but is made of two adjacent plexuses, the lumbar plexus and the sacral plexus. These two plexuses unite through the lumbosacral trunk which comprise part of the L4 nerve root anterior rami, and all L5 anterior rami.

The lumbar plexus (Fig. 14.2) comes from the anterior rami of the L1 through to L4 nerve roots, but also often receives contribution from the T12 nerve root anterior rami. These rami travel downwards and lateral to the psoas muscle where they ultimately form the plexus. The anterior rami of the L1 to L4 nerve roots divide into anterior and posterior branches within the psoas. The posterior branches of L2 to L4 anterior rami combine to form the femoral nerve. The main muscles innervated by the femoral nerve are the iliopsoas and quadriceps. The femoral nerve also gives cutaneous branches to the anteromedial thigh and continues distally as the saphenous nerve, which subserves sensation to the anteromedial lower leg and medial foot. The anterior branches of L2 to L4 become the obturator nerve, which mainly innervates the adductors of the lower limb. The lumbar plexus also gives off the lateral femoral cutaneous nerve of the thigh, the iliohypogastric, ilioinguinal, and genitofemoral nerves.

The sacral plexus originates from the lower branch of the L4 anterior rami and the anterior rami of L5 through to S4 roots (Fig. 14.3). It is situated in the pelvis and lies on the anterior surface of the piriformis muscle. Each of these anterior rami divides into an anterior and posterior division. The anterior divisions combine to form the tibial portion of the sciatic nerve and the upper four posterior divisions fuse to become the common peroneal portion. The sciatic nerve leaves the pelvis via the greater sciatic foramen, inferior to the piriformis muscle, travels down the back of the thigh to about its lower third, where it splits into the tibial and common peroneal nerves. This split can occur at any point between the sacral plexus and the lower third of the thigh. The sciatic nerve, the largest nerve in the body, innervates the hamstring muscles and all of the muscles of the lower leg and foot via its two branches, the tibial and common fibular nerves. The superior gluteal nerve, inferior gluteal nerve, and the posterior femoral cutaneous nerve are the other major nerves that come from the sacral plexus. Both the superior gluteal nerve (L4, L5, and S1), which innervates the tensor fascia lata and gluteus medius, and the inferior gluteal nerve (L5, S1, and S2), which

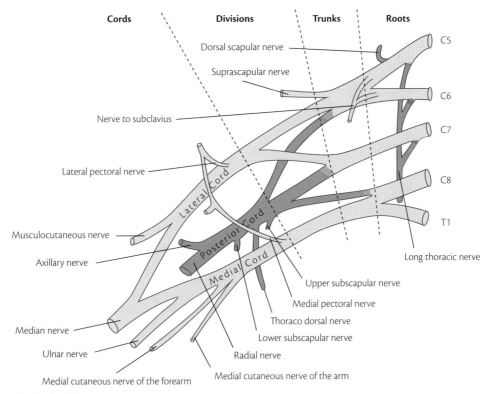

Fig. 14.1 The anatomy of the brachial plexus.

Table 14.1 The branches of the brachial plexus

Branches	Terminal nerves
Roots	
C5	Dorsal scapular
C5, C6, C7	Long thoracic
Trunks	
Upper	Suprascapular
Divisions	
Cords	
Lateral	Lateral pectoral
	Musculocutaneous
	Median
Medial	Medial pectoral
	Medial brachial
	Medial antebrachial
	Median
	Ulnar
Posterior	Subscapular
	Thoracodorsal
	Axillary
	Radial

innervates the gluteus maximus, come from the anterior divisions. The posterior femoral cutaneous nerve comes from the anterior and posterior divisions (S1 and S2 posterior divisions; S1 to S3 anterior divisions) and provides sensory innervation to the skin of the perineum and posterior surface of the lower buttock, thigh, and leg. The pudendal nerve, which innervates the external anal sphincter, also receives contribution from the sacral plexus (S2 to S4).

Clinical presentation and investigations

Clinical suspicion of a plexus lesion is raised when the distribution of weakness, reflex, or sensory loss is not confined to individual nerve or nerve roots. This differentiation can be difficult to make and some disease processes will simultaneously involve roots, plexus, and nerves (e.g. diabetes). Multiple radicular lesions may be very difficult to clinically separate from a plexus lesion. There may, however, be some clinical pointers:

• A lumbosacral plexus lesion (but not lumbar radiculopathy) may give rise to a warm, red, dry foot due to involvement of the retroperitoneal lumbar sympathetic nerves anterolateral to the vertebral bodies [1].

• Careful documentation of the pattern of weakness is very helpful in differentiating a plexus from a nerve. For instance, in the context of weakness in the sciatic distribution, additional weakness of the gluteal muscles suggests a lumbosacral plexus lesion as the superior and inferior gluteal nerves arise directly from the plexus.

• Clinical presentation may also give some clues to aetiology, e.g. when differentiating radiation plexopathy from neoplastic

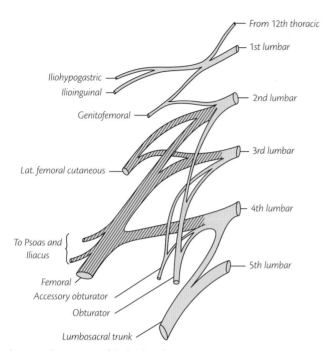

From 12th thoracic
1st lumbar
Iliohypogastric
Ilioinguinal
Genitofemoral
2nd lumbar
3rd lumbar
Lat. femoral cutaneous
4th lumbar
To Psoas and
Iliacus
5th lumbar
Femoral
Accessory obturator
Obturator
Lumbosacral trunk

Fig. 14.2 The anatomy of the lumbar plexus.

infiltration the former is associated with myokymia whilst the latter has a higher incidence of neuropathic pain.

Imaging has greatly advanced in respect to visualization of the brachial and lumbosacral plexus, despite the challenges of air/tissue interfaces and the complexity of these structures. The imaging modality of choice is usually magnetic resonance imaging (MRI) although this choice needs to be tailored to the circumstance, e.g. computed tomography (CT) myelography may be used in preference to MRI in order to detect nerve root avulsion [2]. Usually sagittal and coronal MR images are acquired including T_1- and T_2-weighted sequences with fat suppression (T_2-STIR) [3]. If there is any possibility of malignant infiltration contrast should be given. Ultrasound can also be informative if dynamic images of nerve roots and vasculature are required, e.g. in the diagnosis of thoracic outlet syndrome.

Neurophysiology provides information regarding localization of the lesion, severity, and, in traumatic plexopathies, potentially also prognosis. Reduced motor nerve amplitudes suggest motor axon loss. Most plexopathies are associated with axonal pathology. The presence of demyelination is associated with slowed motor conduction and prolonged F-waves, and conduction block may be due to inflammatory neuropathies or incomplete traumatic injury. Sensory

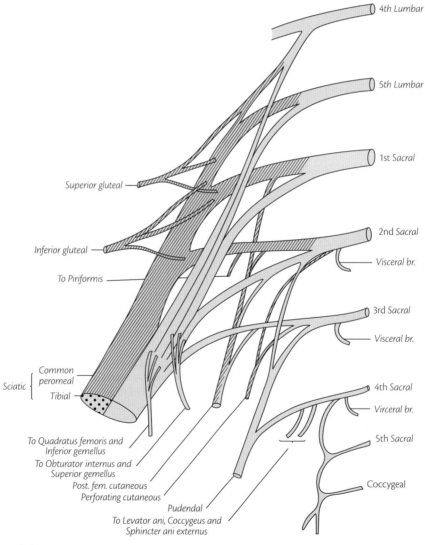

4th Lumbar
5th Lumbar
1st Sacral
Superior gluteal
2nd Sacral
Visceral br.
Inferior gluteal
To Piriformis
3rd Sacral
Visceral br.
Sciatic { Common peromeal
Tibial
4th Sacral
Virceral br.
5th Sacral
To Quadratus femoris and Inferior gemellus
To Obturator internus and Superior gemellus
Post. fem. cutaneous
Perforating cutaneous
Pudendal
To Levator ani, Coccygeus and Sphincter ani externus
Coccygeal

Fig. 14.3 The anatomy of the sacral plexus.

conduction is helpful in differentiating pre- and post-ganglionic root lesions. Following traumatic brachial plexus injury resulting in root avulsion from the spinal cord (i.e. a pre-ganglionic lesion) connectivity between distal sensory axons and their cell bodies in the dorsal root ganglion is maintained, such that sensory action potentials remain intact despite sensory loss. Evidence of denervation on electromyography (EMG) provides the most reliable indicator of motor axon loss, and through sampling multiple muscles provides information on the localization of pathology within the plexus. Some neurophysiological phenomena may be informative regarding aetiology. Myokymic discharges are recurrent bursts of repetitive firing (up to 150 Hz) of motor units in doublets, triplets, or multiplets and although such discharges are not exclusive to radiation plexopathy they are observed in up to 60% of cases (see Fig. 14.4). Lumbar puncture can be helpful in situations where there may be malignant infiltration involving the nerve roots as well as the plexus (in which cytology may reveal malignant cells) and in inflammatory neuropathies (resulting in raised cerebrospinal fluid protein).

Traumatic plexopathy

The brachial and lumbosacral plexuses can be compressed, stretched, or lacerated following trauma. The resulting injury to the plexus after such trauma can range from conduction block to complete severing of the various components of the plexus.

Brachial plexus

The most common cause of brachial plexopathy is trauma, most often seen in young males.

Mechanism of injury

Closed traction injury and open injuries are the two main types of traumatic brachial plexus injuries, with closed traction being more common. Closed traction injuries typically occur after high-velocity motor vehicle accidents, but other causes include falls from a height, objects falling on a shoulder, and sports or occupational injuries. Most closed-traction injuries result in supraclavicular plexopathies, usually upper plexopathies. These injuries occur when the upper plexus is elongated by forceful separation of the head and neck from the ipsilateral shoulder leading to stretch and sometimes rupture of the C5, C6, and C7 nerve roots [4]. Root avulsion, where the nerve root is torn from the spinal cord by high-energy traction, occurs in about 75% of traumatic supraclavicular plexopathies.

Traumatic injuries to the infraclavicular plexus are less common and mostly occur when this portion of the plexus is stretched over the humeral head in cases of shoulder dislocation and humeral fracture. Infraclavicular plexus injuries are often vascular injuries with rupture of the axillary artery occurring in up to 50% patients with severe infraclavicular plexus injuries [5].

Open traumatic brachial plexus injuries are less frequent than closed traction injuries and usually result from gunshot wounds or lacerations from knives or other sharp objects. The key difference between open and closed traction injuries is the common occurrence of damage to nearby structures such as blood vessels and lungs in open injuries. The plexus is also susceptible to secondary injury from expanding hematomas, pseudoaneurysms, and arteriovenous fistulas.

Clinical presentation

Brachial plexus injury should be suspected in patients with severe shoulder girdle injuries, particularly from motor vehicle accidents. A detailed history of the patient's symptoms and mechanism of injury should be obtained. Many patients, particularly those with multiple root avulsions, report severe pain especially in the neck, shoulder, and upper extremity. Other common complaints include sensory impairment and weakness of the affected limb. Root avulsion usually presents with marked weakness and sensory loss affecting the entire arm. All patients should undergo thorough clinical

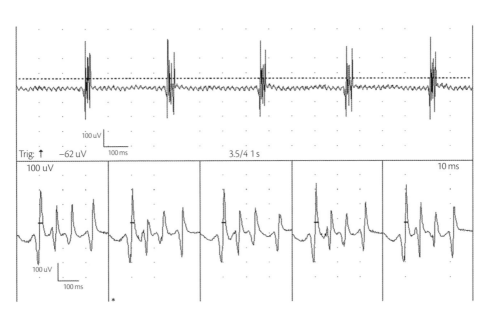

Fig. 14.4 Electromyograph demonstrating myokymic discharges associated with radiation plexopathy. This trace shows multiplets of motor unit discharges occurring in repetitive bursts. The clinical correlate is wave-like movement of the relevant myotome. Image courtesy of Dr Veronica Tan, Department of Neurophysiology, Guy's and St Thomas' NHS Trust.

examination to assess strength in muscle groups innervated by the brachial plexus. Sensory testing looking for evidence of impaired sensation in all the dermatomes helps localize the lesion. Palpation of the radial and ulnar pulses is important to determine whether there is a coexisting vascular injury. Careful examination of the cervical spine, clavicle, scapula, humerus, and their related joints should be performed to look for evidence of fractures or dislocation. Injury to the cervical sympathetic chain causing Horner syndrome can also occur in cases of root avulsion, and evidence of this such as ptosis should be noted. Examination for potential spinal cord injury is necessary, as there is a 2–5% incidence of spinal cord injury with brachial plexus injuries.

Electrodiagnostic studies are useful in traumatic brachial plexopathy to help localize the lesion, assess its severity, and determine prognosis. Nerve conduction studies may locate the level of the lesion just after injury, but the optimal timing for EMG is 4–6 weeks after the injury to ascertain whether there has been spontaneous recovery. Serial EMG in conjunction with clinical examinations is used to assess progression of recovery and make decisions about the need for surgery [6].

All patients with brachial plexus injuries should have X-ray of their cervical spine, chest, and the affected limb to determine whether there is accompanying fracture to the clavicle or ribs, or to show a raised hemidiaphragm, an indication of phrenic nerve damage. MRI plays an important role in the evaluation of patients who may require surgery for traumatic plexus injury. MRI can show the exact location of the injury, demonstrate the morphology of the injured plexus, and determine the severity of injury. Such neuroimaging helps to determine whether surgery is indicated and, if so, to plan the surgical approach.

The surgical management of nerve root avulsion (pre-ganglionic lesion) is different from that of post-ganglionic brachial plexus injuries. Imaging studies are crucial in the preoperative evaluation of patients who are to undergo surgery in order to determine whether there is evidence of root avulsion. CT myelography is the imaging modality of choice for the evaluation of root-level injuries, in particular to look for pseudomeningocoeles which are highly suggestive of root avulsion [7–9], but MRI can show both pseudomeningocoele and peripheral post-ganglionic lesions, so there is an overall advantage in its use.

Diffusion-weighted neurography and Bezier surface re-formation are newer imaging techniques for the investigation of patients with brachial plexus injury. Diffusion-weighted neurography is better than conventional MRI in distinguishing the plexus from surrounding structures; it clearly shows discontinuity in injured nerves and provides good images of the post-ganglionic brachial plexus [10]. Bezier surface re-formation is a technique that reformats CT myelographic imaging to show all the intradural nerve roots on a single image [11].

Management

The treatment of traumatic brachial plexus injuries is either conservative or surgical depending on the time from injury, the nature of the injury, its location, and its severity. Conservative management includes intensive physiotherapy, with daily passive range of movement, to ensure upper limb joint mobility and preservation of muscle strength. Early surgical exploration and repair is recommended when there is significant functional impairment, particularly following high-energy injuries because of evidence

that delaying surgery leads to poorer recovery in this situation [12]. Open injuries from a sharp object require emergency surgical exploration and direct end-to-end nerve repair if possible. If the injury is from a blunt trauma, repair may be delayed for about 3–4 weeks after initial debridement to allow the injured nerve end to become better defined.

Various types of surgical techniques are used to repair an injured brachial plexus. Nerve grafting can be beneficial in post-ganglionic ruptures but significant recovery can take up to 18 months. Nerve transfers, where a portion of a functional nerve is transferred to a denervated nerve, can be performed to restore function in pre-ganglionic injuries. In nerve root avulsion, reimplantation of nerve roots directly (or using nerve grafts) into the spinal cord can help reinstate normal function [13]. Nerve transfer is also an option in post-ganglionic injuries when surgery is late or axonal loss extensive. The effectiveness of nerve transfers in restoring strength decreases significantly with patient age and therefore reserved for younger patients.

Specific traumatic syndromes
Burner syndrome
Burner syndrome, also called Stinger syndrome, is caused by transient stretch injury to the plexus that occurs after a sudden, forceful trauma to the shoulder, usually during contact sports such as American football or rugby. The upper trunk is most commonly affected as it is stretched by traction from the downward pull of the shoulder. The characteristic symptoms are sudden, intense pain and paraesthesia in the affected upper limb. The pain is usually transient, lasting for a few minutes, and can be associated with mild weakness which is often short-lasting. Clinical examination should include assessment for accompanying spinal cord injury, and imaging of the cervical spine may be necessary in some cases. Investigations or treatment are not usually required because symptoms generally last minutes to hours. EMG is only indicated when symptoms persist for more than 3 weeks. When performed, EMG can be normal or show varying degrees of denervation, depending on the extent of weakness.

Rucksack palsy
This is a brachial plexopathy caused by stretch or traction of the upper portion of the plexus after carrying a rucksack or other device over the shoulder. This injury is most common in military personnel but can also occur in people who carry backpacks, child-carrying harnesses, or similar devices over their shoulder. This injury typically presents with unilateral weakness followed by atrophy and paraesthesiae, but pain is uncommon. The upper trunk is most commonly involved. In most patients the lesion is caused by focal conduction block and consequently recovery usually occurs within a few months of the injury. Axonal degeneration is predominant in few cases and recovery is slow and occasionally incomplete.

Lumbosacral plexus

The lumbosacral plexus is less prone to injury because of its location deep within the pelvis and the protection it has from surrounding muscles and bone. As a result, nearly all traumatic lumbosacral plexopathies are caused by penetrating trauma such as gunshot or significant high-velocity injuries such as that sustained in a motor vehicle accident. In most cases, these injuries are associated with pelvis or hip fractures or dislocation of the sacroiliac joint. Localization of lumbosacral plexus injury and evaluating the extent of injury can be difficult because accompanying skeletal injuries limit neurological examination and confound its findings. Electrodiagnosis may be useful in such situations.

Neurogenic thoracic outlet syndrome

The thoracic outlet extends from the cervical spine and mediastinum to the lower border of the pectoralis minor muscle. The outlet comprises three compartments, namely the interscalene triangle, costoclavicular space, and subcoracoid space. Thoracic outlet syndrome (TOS) is caused by compression of the brachial plexus (neurogenic TOS) and the subclavian artery or vein (vascular TOS) in any of the three compartments of the thoracic outlet.

Neurogenic TOS is a unilateral lesion that predominantly affects young to middle aged women. It is rare and has an incidence of about one per million. In neurogenic TOS, the C8–T1 fibres in the lower trunk are compressed as they cross the thoracic outlet by a taut fibrous band that extends from a cervical rib or elongated C7 transverse process to the first rib. Patients presents with pain, paraesthesia, numbness, and weakness in the medial arm and hand. The sensory symptoms, which are usually mild, can be present for a number of years before the patient seeks advice usually prompted by development of muscle weakness and wasting. The lower trunk is immediately above the band and within it the T1 fibres, below the C8 fibres, are more susceptible to compression and this leads to more prominent atrophy and weakness in the thenar muscles than other C8-innervated muscles.

In addition to the standard neurological examination, an important aspect in the clinical assessment of TOS is to determine the effects of provocative thoracic outlet compression manoeuvres in reproducing the patient's symptoms. None of these tests have a high sensitivity or specificity in making the diagnosis of neurogenic TOS but EAST (the Elevated Arm Stress Test) is considered one of the more reliable provocative tests. To perform EAST, the patient stands with their arms out and elbow bent at 90 degrees (the 'I surrender' position) and then opens and closes their hands slowly for 3 min. This manoeuvre is said to cause maximum compression of the brachial plexus and subclavian vessels by narrowing the costoclavicalar space.

Plain cervical spine X-ray may identify congenital bony anomalies such as a rudimentary cervical rib or an elongated C7 transverse process but does not reveal the radiolucent band. Electrodiagnostic studies in neurogenic TOS show reduced median and ulnar compound muscle action potential (CMAP) and low medial antebrachial cutaneous or ulnar sensory nerve action potential (SNAP). The median SNAP is normal. The medial antebrachial cutaneous sensory and median motor responses are usually more affected than that of the ulnar because the T1 fibres are more compressed than the C8 fibres. Surgical resection of the abnormal band or excision of the cervical rib usually leads to improvement or resolution of the pain and paraesthesiae and prevents further deterioration in muscle weakness and wasting.

Postmedian sternotomy plexopathy

This is similar condition to neurogenic TOS which occurs after cardiothoracic surgery requiring median sternotomy, most commonly coronary artery bypass surgery [14]. Retraction of the chest wall leading to fracture or dislocation of the first rib during surgery causes traction injury to the lower trunk of the plexus, predominantly the C8 anterior primary ramus. The C8 ramus contains motor fibres that contribute to the median, radial, and ulnar nerves, but its sensory fibres only go on to become part of the ulnar nerve. Consequently, patients present with sensory symptoms resembling those of ulnar neuropathy. Clinical examination showing weakness of muscles supplied by C8-derived median nerves such as flexor pollicis longus and C8-derived radial nerve fibres such as extensor pollicis brevis helps to differentiate this entity from an ulnar neuropathy. On nerve conduction studies, the ulnar motor and sensory responses are often more reduced in comparison to the median motor or medial antebrachial sensory responses. Management is usually conservative because the lesion is predominantly secondary to conduction block and most patients recover fully unless there is significant axonal loss.

Plexopathy related to obstetric complications

Brachial plexus

The incidence of fetal obstetric brachial plexopathy ranges from 0.4–2.0 per 1000 full-term live births [15]. Obstetric brachial plexopathy most often occur in cases of shoulder dystocia when the upper shoulder of the fetus becomes impacted against the mother's pubic symphysis requiring application of excessive lateral traction to the head and neck to free the shoulder and allow vaginal delivery. The main predisposing factor to shoulder dystocia is macrosomia (birth weight greater than 4 kg) [16,17]. Obstetric plexopathy can happen after deliveries by Caesarean section, indicating that there are other causes of obstetric plexopathy than injury from traction [18]. The majority of lesions are unilateral with a similar prevalence in both sexes. The right side is more often affected than the left.

About half of obstetric brachial plexus injuries only involve the C5 and C6 roots, a condition often referred to as Erb–Duchenne palsy [19]. In another third of cases the C7 root is affected in addition to C5 and C6 roots, and these infants present with their shoulder adducted and internally rotated, elbow extended, and wrist and fingers flexed, the so-called 'waiter's tip' posture. Other common types of injuries are paralysis of the whole arm, C5–T1 with sparing of finger flexion, C5–T1 with flail arm, and Horner syndrome. Injuries to C8–T1 which result in isolated paralysis of the hand and Horner syndrome (Klumpke palsy) is very rare and is typically caused by avulsion of the C8 and T1 roots [20]. Examination of infants with suspected obstetric plexopathy is challenging. Observation is crucial and examination should include assessment of active and passive ranges of movement. The MRC scale can be used to measure strength, but differentiating grades is difficult in these patients.

The prognosis of obstetric plexopathy is much better than in adults and many reviews have reported spontaneous recovery in 90% of cases. Two studies of the natural history of obstetric plexopathy, where surgery was not performed, found a less favourable outcome, with 22–25% of infants having significant impairment when they were older [16,21]. Infants with brachial plexus injuries should have a X-ray of the cervical spine, ipsilateral shoulder, and clavicle. Imaging with MRI or CT myelogram can detect a pseudomeningocoele in cases of nerve root avulsions. Electrodiagnosis is difficult because the child has to be sedated and special smaller electrodes are needed. Despite these problems, electrodiagnosis might be useful for prognosis and can be particularly valuable in the diagnosis of avulsion injuries. In order not to give a misleading prognosis, the electrophysiologist and referring clinician have to be aware that, in contrast to adults, EMG in children may show no evidence of denervation with preservation of motor unit potentials even in those with a completely paralysed arm [22]. It is also important to know that denervation activity can be seen within a week after delivery indicating that the injury might have occurred before delivery [23], a fact that has medicolegal implications.

Most cases of obstetric plexopathy do not require surgery but the prognosis is poor in about a quarter. When there is neurotmesis or root avulsion, spontaneous recovery is impossible and such patients require surgery but neither clinical examination nor investigations can reliably identify these types of injuries. Surgical exploration is usually advised when there is no recovery in biceps function after 3 months, in C5–T1 roots injury with flail arm presenting after a month, and when there is an upper plexopathy after breech delivery because these are typically occur after root avulsion [19]. The consensus is that performing surgery within the first year gives a better prognosis [24]. The observation period before surgery ranges from 3–9 months, and during this time physiotherapy may be beneficial.

Lumbosacral plexus

Lumbosacral plexus injury can occur in pregnant women and during delivery when the lumbosacral trunk is compressed between the mother's pelvic rim and the fetal head. This is more common in mothers with small stature or when labour is prolonged. Pain is usually the first symptom, and this radiates from the buttock down to the L5 distribution. The pain is initially intermittent but becomes constant as its severity increases. Focal weakness, usually in the form of a foot drop, may follow the pain. The underlying pathophysiology is predominantly conduction block but this can be accompanied by a degree of axon loss. The pain often subsides at or soon after delivery, but weakness may last longer. The weakness, which is mainly due to conduction block, usually resolves within 3 months of delivery.

Lumbosacral radiculoplexus neuropathy

Lumbosacral radiculoplexus neuropathy is not a pure plexopathy but a multifocal process involving the roots, plexus, and nerves. It is commonly seen in people with diabetes but a similar form can occur in non-diabetics. Diabetic radiculoplexus neuropathy (DRPN) has several other names such as diabetic amyotrophy, Bruns–Garland syndrome, diabetic motor neuropathy, or proximal diabetic neuropathy (see Chapter 17). The clinical presentation of non-diabetic lumbosacral radiculoplexus neuropathy (LRPN) has a lot in common with DRPN and only the presence of diabetes in the latter differentiate the two categories of patients. Patients with both conditions are limited by pain, weakness, sensory loss, and autonomic dysfunction. In a detailed study of 57 patients with LRPN and 33 patients with DRPN, the investigators concluded that the age of onset, disease course, nature, and distribution of symptoms and signs, laboratory findings, and outcomes are similar [25,26].

The cerebrospinal fluid protein is usually high but pleocytois is rare. The abnormalities on electrodiagnosis are usually more extensive than the clinical findings and suggest axonal degeneration rather than demyelination. Nerve conduction studies may show reduction or absence of tibial and peroneal CMAPs and sural SNAP. Asymmetry in the CMAPS and SNAPS between the two limbs is typical. EMG demonstrates fibrillation potentials, decreased recruitment, and high-amplitude motor unit potentials in lower limb and paraspinal muscles. Histopathological findings on nerve biopsy include multifocal fibre loss, perineurial thickening, neovascularization, inflammation around epineurial blood vessels, segmental demyelination, and axonal degeneration, indicating that the underlying cause of both disorders is ischaemic nerve injury secondary to microvasculitis [25,27,28].

Case series have reported benefit from corticosteroids and intravenous immunoglobulin [29]. The only randomized, double-blind, controlled trial was in DLRPN, which compared intravenous methylprednisolone, 1 g three times weekly, with decreasing dosage and frequency over 12 weeks to placebo. There was no significant difference in neurological deficit after 2 years, but neuropathic symptoms, particularly pain, improved significantly in those treated with intravenous methylprednisolone [30]. Despite the lack of clear evidence, patients who present early may be treated with immunomodulatory therapy especially intravenous methylprednisolone. Pain control is an important part of the management of patients as it common and can be disabling. Drugs such as gabapentin, duloxetine, pregabalin, amitriptyline, nortriptyline, or venlafaxine are useful in the long-term treatment of pain.

Neuralgic amyotrophy

The terminology relating to neuralgic amyotrophy can be confusing, and this condition is also known as brachial neuritis or Parsonage–Turner syndrome. Characteristic clinical features include severe pain at onset, multifocal weakness and atrophy of upper limb muscles followed by slow recovery. There may be a preceding event such as an immunization or infection. The condition is usually unilateral but there may be bilateral (often asymmetric) involvement, and recurrent forms are described. Neuralgic amyotrophy (NA) most commonly affects the upper trunk of the brachial plexus but may also involve any part of the brachial plexus, the phrenic nerve or the lumbosacral plexus. Estimations of incidence vary from between 2–20 per 100 000 per year [31,32].The simplest classification is to divide NA into idiopathic (INA) and hereditary (HNA) forms [33] accounting for approximately 90% and 10% of cases, respectively. The clinical characteristics of these two subtypes are very similar, although HNA has a younger age of onset and a greater frequency of attacks.

Clinical presentation

Severe, constant, and incapacitating pain is almost a universal feature at presentation. This usually lasts several weeks and then shows some improvement; it may be followed by pain with a more musculoskeletal rather than neuropathic quality. Weakness and muscle wasting follow the onset of pain. In the most typical presentation with involvement of the upper brachial plexus paresis affects the shoulder girdle and if the long thoracic nerve is also affected will be accompanied by winging of the scapula. There may be some patchy sensory disturbance producing numbness and paraesthesia. Involvement of the lower trunk will produce weakness of the forearm and intrinsic hand muscles, and damage to sympathetic nerves in the first thoracic root can result in vasomotor changes of the hand and a Horner syndrome.

There may be unilateral or even bilateral phrenic nerve involvement, which may be associated with minimal weakness around the shoulder girdle [34,35]. Phrenic nerve palsy results in orthopnoea (due to increased pressure from abdominal contents) and dyspnoea. This may cause sleep disturbance necessitating non-invasive respiratory support. There is often a degree of recovery in phrenic nerve function, although this may be slow [36]. NA may cause an isolated lumbosacral plexopathy; however, this is more commonly associated with diabetes (see Chapter 17). A severe or 'extended' form of NA [37] affects the brachial plexus and, in addition, nerves outside this territory such as the lumbosacral plexus, phrenic nerve, intercostal nerves, or cranial nerves such as the phrenic and accessory nerves. There may be subsequent episodes of NA which can affect different territories and recurrent attacks are more likely in the hereditary form.

The clinical course of the condition with pain at onset, a monophasic course followed by a degree of recovery is characteristic, and progression after 3 months would be unusual, which is helpful diagnostically. There is no simple diagnostic test and investigations are often carried out to exclude alternative diagnoses. MRI often shows T_2 weighted hyperintensity within the brachial plexus [38,39]. Nodularity and avid enhancement should raise concern regarding malignant infiltration. MRI imaging of the cervical spine is often performed to determine if there is multilevel cervical radiculopathy. EMG shows denervation which may have some regional variation (e.g. principally upper versus lower trunk) and there may be some patchy sensory abnormalities. It used to be thought that recovery from this condition was very good but it is now becoming clear with long-term follow-up of patients that more than 50% have significant persistent weakness, fatigue, and pain impacting on quality of life [31,38]. In appropriate cases genetic testing can be performed.

Pathophysiology

An important advance in understanding the pathophysiology of HNA is the finding that this condition can be caused by dominant mutations in the *SEPT9* gene. Mutations can take the form of missense mutations or intragenic or gene duplications [40–43]. One 645 base pair exon contains the known missense mutations and is also common to the intragenic duplications emphasizing its importance in pathogenesis. Certain mutations [c.262C>T (p.Arg88Trp)] in *SEPT9* may be associated with dysmorphic features such as epicanthic folds, dysmorphic ears, hypotelorism, and short stature [44,45]. SEPT9 is one of a family of cytoskeletal GTP-binding proteins. Recent analysis of mice lacking SEPT9 demonstrated the crucial role of this molecule, as global deletion results in embryonic lethality. Conditional deletion in fibroblasts results in abnormal cellular morphology, abnormal nuclei, and impaired cell migration [46]. Duplications of the whole gene can cause HNA [40], suggesting that there may be a dosage effect and an aberrant transcript/protein product is not essential for pathogenesis. The exact mechanism by which mutations in *SEPT9* cause HNA is unclear. Overexpression can promote filament formation and certain mutations can alter interactions with other septins and block the disassembly of filaments, suggesting that filament disassembly may have a role in pathogenesis [47,48]. In almost 50% of cases of HNA a mutation in *SEPT9* is not found, suggesting the role of other genetic factors. Hereditary neuropathy with liability to pressure palsy (HNPP) is a condition associated with patchy demyelination and the development of palsies at sites of nerve entrapment, usually secondary to haplo-insufficiency of the gene *PMP22*. This can cause a plexopathy; however, this is both genetically and clinically distinct from HNA [49]. The plexopathy associated with HNPP is usually painless, and on electrophysiological testing there is virtually always evidence of a patchy background neuropathy with conduction slowing, particularly at entrapment points.

Although genetic factors may determine the underlying risk of developing NA, there is evidence that an immune event may trigger an attack. A number of antecedent events have been associated with the development of NA, many of which involve alterations within the immune system [31], e.g. vaccination, infection, surgery, pregnancy/childbirth, and immunomodulation. Evidence for immune involvement includes the presence of lymphocytes surrounding and within the walls of epineural blood vessels in biopsy samples derived from affected nerves [50,51]. Blood lymphocytes derived from patients with NA have also been shown to have a mitogenic response to brachial plexus extract. In occasional patients antiganglioside antibodies have been found, though only in a minority of patients and at low titre [52]. Pathogenicity has not been proven, and they may simply reflect axonal damage. An interesting issue is why an autoimmune process may target one specific region of the peripheral nervous system, most commonly the brachial plexus. An interesting theory is that because the shoulder is very mobile physical factors (and up to 10% of cases are preceded by physical activity) impact on the brachial plexus and disturb the blood–nerve barrier [33].

Treatment

There is a lack of a clear evidence in the treatment of NA as noted by a Cochrane review from 2009 [53] which did not identify any randomized controlled trials. The role of the immune system in the aetiology of the condition provides a rationale for the use of corticosteroids. One open label study reported faster recovery and a reduction in pain in patients given oral prednisolone within the first month of the disease [54]. The practice in our institution would be to give a course of oral prednisolone over 2 weeks rapidly tapering to stop in the acute phase of an attack. In many cases the diagnosis may not be made in this time frame. Pain can be very debilitating, and the severe pain at onset may require opiates and agents with efficacy in the treatment of neuropathic pain such as the gabapentinoids and tricyclic antidepressants. In the long term, multidisciplinary limb rehabilitation including physiotherapy and occupational therapy may be needed.

Neoplastic and radiation-induced plexopathies

Neoplastic brachial plexopathies may be divided into primary (arising from the plexus itself) or secondary (originating from outside the plexus). The proximity of the brachial plexus to the lung, breast, and adjacent lymphatic system predispose it to external compression, infiltration, or metastatic deposits from tumours originating from these structures. In a series of 100 patients with neoplastic brachial plexopathy, lung, breast, and lymphoma accounted for about 75% of tumours affecting the plexus [55]. Soft tissue tumours such as sarcomas can also infiltrate the plexus. The lower trunk and medial cord are the most commonly involved sites in metastatic plexopathy because they are more prone to infiltration from tumour deposits in axillary lymph nodes. The majority of patients with secondary neoplastic plexopathy present with severe and constant shoulder and upper limb pain followed by progressive weakness, sensory loss, and eventually muscle atrophy.

Carcinoma at the lung apex called Pancoast tumour may cause a particular form of neoplastic plexopathy when it extends upwards to compress or infiltrate the lower trunk of the plexus. The main clinical manifestations of this condition are pain and numbness in the medial arm and progressive hand weakness. A useful localizing sign is an accompanying Horner syndrome indicating involvement of the T1 root or cervical sympathetic ganglion.

The most common cause of neoplastic lumbosacral plexopathy is infiltration or compression by a pelvic tumour. In a case series of 85 patients, over 75% of neoplastic lumbosacral plexopathies were caused by invasion or direct extension from tumours arising from the colorectal system, urogenital system (especially the cervix in women), prostate, lymphoma, and retroperitoneal or pelvic sarcomas [56]. Metastases from breast or lung account for the remainder. Bilateral lumbosacral plexopathies are most often caused by metastases from breast cancer [56].

About 70% of patients with neoplastic lumbosacral plexopathy present with gradual onset of pain [56]. When the lumbar plexus is predominantly affected the pain is typically in the lower back, hip, and anterior thigh, and when the sacral plexus is the main site of involvement pain is usually in the posterolateral thigh, leg, and foot [56]. The pain gets progressively worse and is often followed by numbness, paraesthesiae, and weakness within weeks to months. Autonomic symptoms are rare, but patients can complain of 'a hot and dry foot' as a result of involvement of the sympathetic component of the plexus [1]. The main finding on clinical examination is muscle weakness, but sensory impairment and asymmetric reflexes are also common. Sacral or sciatic notch tenderness, positive straight leg raising sign, and lower limb oedema can be seen in patients with neoplastic lumbosacral plexopathy. A rectal or pelvic mass can be palpable in up to a third of patients with neoplastic sacral plexopathy [56].

Primary neoplasms of the plexuses are less common and mostly benign. Nerve sheath tumours in the form of schwannomas or neurofibromas are the predominant primary tumours that occur in the brachial and lumbosacral plexuses. Schwannomas are slow-growing encapsulated tumours with predilection for the sensory roots. Patients with schwannomas usually present with a painless mass and paraesthesiae, which can be exacerbated by movement or touch [57]. Weakness may occur if they compress the anterior nerve root. Solitary neurofibromas are benign, unencapsulated tumours. The typical presentation of neurofibromas in the brachial plexus is pain, weakness, and numbness. Neurofibromas are usually multiple or plexiform when they occur in patients with neurofibromatosis type 1 (NF-1). Malignant peripheral nerve sheath tumours make up 14% of the primary neoplasms of the brachial plexus and are predominantly seen in patients with NF-1 or a history of radiotherapy to the plexus [58,59]. In up to 40% of cases patients with NF-1 may have solitary and plexiform neurofibromas in the abdomen and pelvic regions, and the lumbosacral plexus may be affected when these tumours occur in the retroperitoneal cavity [60].

Neurolymphomatosis is a rare condition characterized by insidious infiltration of peripheral nerves, including the plexus, by lymphoma. It can occur with our without associated pain. Fluorodeoxyglucose (FDG) positron emission tomography (PET)

is particularly sensitive to what may be a diagnostically very challenging condition [61]. Prognosis is currently similar to primary CNS lymphoma [62].

The differentiation of neoplastic infiltration of the plexus versus radiation-induced plexopathy may be very challenging. Post-radiation plexopathy is thought to arise due to radiation-induced vasculopathy and fibrosis, resulting in ischaemia of the plexus and reduced cellular proliferation. These pathologies ultimately result in axonal degeneration and, in addition, ischaemia may induce demyelination resulting in conduction block. The incidence of this complication is related to total dose [63], the dose per fraction, and whether adjuvant chemotherapy is given [64]. The onset can be anything from 1 month to decades after radiotherapy [65]. Clinically, pain is more prominent in the context of neoplastic infiltration and myokymia is more commonly observed in post-radiation plexopathy. These observations are not absolute, however, and further investigation is often essential in making this differential diagnosis.

Electrodiagnostic tests help localize the lesion to the plexus and consequently guide imaging studies. Evidence of active and chronic denervation is present in over 90% of patients and affected segments typically show reduced CMAPs with normal or borderline motor conduction velocities. EMG can often distinguish neoplastic from radiation plexopathy, as myokymia is detected in about 60% of patients with radiation plexopathy but rarely in neopastic plexopathy [66] (see Fig. 14.4).

The diagnosis of neoplastic plexopathy is aided by MRI or CT. MRI provides better anatomical detail and is more sensitive than CT [67–69]. Differentiating neoplastic from radiation plexopathy is a common clinical problem, and distinguishing the two entities can be a radiological challenge. The presence of a mass within the plexus or a patchy, asymmetric nodular enhancement of the nerve trunks is highly suggestive of a neoplastic plexopathy. Radiation-induced plexopathy is associated with diffuse fibrotic changes within the plexus. PET can also be used to evaluate patients with suspected neoplastic brachial plexopathy. In a study of 19 patients with neoplastic plexopathy from breast cancer, there was FDG avidity within the involved plexus in 14, but the specificity and sensitivity of PET for neoplastic plexopathy is not established [70]. FDG PET has also been shown to be helpful in the diagnosis of malignant peripheral nerve sheath tumours in the context of NF-1 [71].

Management of secondary neoplastic plexopathy is for the most part palliative. Adequate pain control is the predominant aim in the treatment of these patients but achieving this can be difficult. In cases where the underlying tumour is responsive to radiotherapy or specific chemotherapy, improvement in pain may occur after these treatments. Radiotherapy to the plexus has been reported to relieve pain in 46% of patients with neoplastic brachial plexopathy [55] and 15% with neoplastic lumbosacral plexopathy [56]. Neuropathic pain and dysaesthesia may be severe and refractory to treatment, but tricyclic antidepressants such as amitriptyline and desipramine, anticonvulsants such as pregabalin, gabapentin, or carbamazepine, transcutaneous electrical nerve stimulation, or regional nerve or sympathetic ganglion blocks may be of some benefit. Opiate analgesics including epidural and intrathecal morphine infusion may also be used. There are also reports of benefit from subanaesthetic doses of ketamine, an N-methyl-D-aspartate (NMDA) antagonist, in patients with intractable neuropathic pain [72]. Surgical procedures such as neurolysis, sympathectomies, stellate ganglionectomies, amputation, cordotomies, and dorsal root entry zone ablations may have an additional role in the management of pain in these patients.

For primary plexus tumours such as schwannomas and neurofibromas, surgery is indicated for pain, increase in tumour bulk, concern about malignancy, and occasionally for cosmetic reasons. Total resections of these tumours by experienced surgeons preserve function and improve pain in 90% of schwannomas, 80% of solitary neurofibromas, and 66% of neurofibromas in patients with NF-1 [73]. Plexiform neurofibromas are more difficult to excise because multiple nerve fibres are involved.

There is no treatment for radiation-induced plexopathy. However, if there is extensive fibrosis, surgical release is attempted in some cases.

Miscellaneous non-traumatic causes of plexopathy

Focal forms of chronic inflammatory demyelinating polyneuropathy (CIDP) may present as a plexopathy, and particularly the variant multifocal acquired demyelinating sensory and motor neuropathy (MADSAM; also termed Lewis–Sumner syndrome) [74]. This is usually clinically distinct from NA, being associated with less pain and having a more insidious onset. A helpful clinical sign indicating conduction block is the presence of muscle weakness in the absence of wasting. Imaging may show marked thickening and sometimes enhancement of the nerve roots and plexus (see Fig. 14.5). Neurophysiology is very helpful in confirming evidence of demyelination (see Chapter 16).

Peripheral nervous system vasculitis usually presents as a mononeuropathy multiplex but can present as plexopathy. This is, however, rare, being described in less than 6% of pathologically confirmed

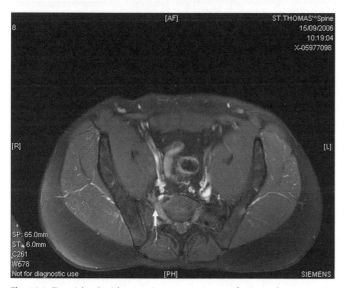

Fig. 14.5 T_1-weighted axial magnetic resonance image of spine and pelvis post-contrast. This was performed in a patient presenting with signs consistent with a right lumbosacral plexopathy and demyelinating changes on neurophysiology. Imaging showed thickened sacral nerve roots (see white arrow) merging into the sacral plexus with mild enhancement. Ultimately changes consistent with chronic inflammatory demyelinating polyneuropathy were confirmed on nerve root biopsy and the patient responded to immunosuppression.

vasculitis patients in one recent survey [75]. Infective agents should also be a consideration in the aetiology of plexopathies. This may be due to local factors such as a psoas abscess causing a lumbosacral plexopathy. Herpes zoster represents reactivation of the varicella zoster virus within dorsal root ganglia, and rarely may also cause a motor paresis and present as a plexopathy, as can HIV.

Retroperitoneal haemorrhage can lead to compartment syndromes affecting the lumbar and sacral plexuses. Anticoagulation is a major predisposing factor for retroperitoneal haemorrhage, but can also occur in patients with coagulation disorders such as haemophilia and disseminated intravascular coagulation, or from a leaking aortic aneurysm. An extensive bleed within the psoas muscle may cause psoas compartment syndrome resulting in lumbosacral plexopathy. Patients typically present with acute or subacute unilateral pain in the lower abdomen or groin radiating to the anterior thigh and medial leg. Motor deficit and sensory impairment, usually in the distribution of the obturator and femoral nerves, follow the pain. A smaller haematoma within the iliacus muscle may compress the intrapelvic portion of the femoral nerve resulting in a femoral neuropathy. Imaging with MRI or CT usually identifies the haematoma and electrodiagnosis typically shows significant axon loss in the distribution of the femoral nerve, lumbar plexus, or the lumbosacral plexus.

Retroperitoneal abscesses may also compress the lumbosacral plexus. These abscesses are usually caused by local spread from gastrointestinal, urinary, or spinal sepsis Tuberculosis is a rare cause. The collection can be demonstrated by MRI or CT, and management is by image-guided drainage.

Lumbosacral plexopathies are a complication of aneurysms of the distal aorta, iliac arteries and their branch vessels, or the surgical repair of such aneurysms. The lumbosacral plexus is injured by direct compression by aneurysms or by ischaemia from thrombotic or embolic occlusion of their vascular supply. Pain, sensory impairment, and motor deficit are often limited to one limb. The pain resembles that of sciatica and straight leg raising sign can be present, mimicking a prolapsed intervertebral disc.

References

1. Dalmau J, Graus F, Marco M. 'Hot and dry foot' as initial manifestation of neoplastic lumbosacral plexopathy. *Neurology* 1989; **39**: 871–2.
2. O'Shea K, Feinberg JH, Wolfe SW. Imaging and electrodiagnostic work-up of acute adult brachial plexus injuries. *J Hand Surg Eur* 2011; **36**: 747–59.
3. van Es HW, Bollen TL, van Heesewijk HP. MRI of the brachial plexus: a pictorial review. *Eur J Radiol* 2010; **74**: 391–402.
4. Songcharoen P, Shin AY. Brachial plexus injury: acute diagnosis and treatment. In: Berger RA, Weis APC (ed) *Hand Surgery*, pp. 1005–25. Philadelphia, PA: Lippincott, Williams & Wilkins, 2004.
5. Coene LN. Mechanisms of brachial plexus lesions. *Clin Neurol Neurosurg* 1993; **95** (Suppl): S24–S29.
6. Jones SJ, Parry CB, Landi A. Diagnosis of brachial plexus traction lesions by sensory nerve action potentials and somatosensory evoked potentials. *Injury* 1981; **12**: 376–82.
7. Carvalho GA, Nikkhah G, Matthies C, Penkert G, Samii M. Diagnosis of root avulsions in traumatic brachial plexus injuries: value of computerized tomography myelography and magnetic resonance imaging. *J Neurosurg* 1997; **86**: 69–76.
8. Walker AT, Chaloupka JC, de Lotbiniere AC, Wolfe SW, Goldman R, Kier EL. Detection of nerve rootlet avulsion on CT myelography in patients with birth palsy and brachial plexus injury after trauma. *Am J Roentgenol* 1996; **167**: 1283–7.

9. Doi K, Otsuka K, Okamoto Y, Fujii H, Hattori Y, Baliarsing AS. Cervical nerve root avulsion in brachial plexus injuries: magnetic resonance imaging classification and comparison with myelography and computerized tomography myelography. *J Neurosurg* 2002; **96** (3 Suppl): 277–84.

10. Takahara T, Hendrikse J, Yamashita T, et al. Diffusion-weighted MR neurography of the brachial plexus: feasibility study. *Radiology* 2008; **249**: 653–60.

11. Yoshioka N, Hayashi N, Akahane M, Yoshikawa T, Takeshita K, Ohtomo K. Bezier surface reformation: an original visualization technique of cervical nerve roots on myelographic CT. *Radiat Med* 2006; **24**: 600–4.

12. Kato N, Htut M, Taggart M, Carlstedt T, Birch R. The effects of operative delay on the relief of neuropathic pain after injury to the brachial plexus: a review of 148 cases. *J Bone Joint Surg Br* 2006; **88**: 756–9.

13. Carlstedt T. Nerve root replantation. *Neurosurg Clin N Am* 2009; **20**: 39–50, vi.

14. Levin KH, Wilbourn AJ, Maggiano HJ. Cervical rib and median sternotomy-related brachial plexopathies: a reassessment. *Neurology* 1998; **50**: 1407–13.

15. Kay SP. Obstetrical brachial palsy. *Br J Plast Surg* 1998; **51**: 43–50.

16. Bager B. Perinatally acquired brachial plexus palsy—a persisting challenge. *Acta Paediatr* 1997; **86**: 1214–19.

17. Levine MG, Holroyde J, Woods JR, Jr, Siddiqi TA, Scott M, Miodovnik M. Birth trauma: incidence and predisposing factors. *Obstet Gynecol* 1984; **63**: 792–5.

18. Jennett RJ, Tarby TJ. Brachial plexus palsy: an old problem revisited again. II. Cases in point. *Am J Obstet Gynecol* 1997; **176**: 1354–6.

19. Boome RS, Kaye JC. Obstetric traction injuries of the brachial plexus. Natural history, indications for surgical repair and results. *J Bone Joint Surg Br* 1988; **70**: 571–6.

20. al-Qattan MM, Clarke HM, Curtis CG. Klumpke's birth palsy. Does it really exist? *J Hand Surg Br* 1995; **20**: 19–23.

21. Sjoberg I, Erichs K, Bjerre I. Cause and effect of obstetric (neonatal) brachial plexus palsy. *Acta Paediatr Scand* 1988; **77**: 357–64.

22. van Dijk JG, Malessy MJ, Stegeman DF. Why is the electromyogram in obstetric brachial plexus lesions overly optimistic? *Muscle Nerve* 1998; **21**: 260–1.

23. Dunn DW, Engle WA. Brachial plexus palsy: intrauterine onset. *Pediatr Neurol* 1985; **1**: 367–9.

24. Grossman JA. Early operative intervention for birth injuries to the brachial plexus. *Semin Pediatr Neurol* 2000; **7**: 36–43.

25. Dyck PJ, Norell JE, Dyck PJ. Microvasculitis and ischemia in diabetic lumbosacral radiculoplexus neuropathy. *Neurology* 1999; **53**: 2113–21.

26. Dyck PJ, Norell JE, Dyck PJ. Non-diabetic lumbosacral radiculoplexus neuropathy: natural history, outcome and comparison with the diabetic variety. *Brain* 2001; **124**: 1197–207.

27. Llewelyn JG, Thomas PK, King RH. Epineurial microvasculitis in proximal diabetic neuropathy. *J Neurol* 1998; **245**: 159–65.

28. Said G, Lacroix C, Lozeron P, Ropert A, Plante V, Adams D. Inflammatory vasculopathy in multifocal diabetic neuropathy. *Brain* 2003; **126**: 376–85.

29. Thaisetthawatkul P, Dyck PJ. Treatment of diabetic and nondiabetic lumbosacral radiculoplexus neuropathy. *Curr Treat Options Neurol* 2010; **12**: 95–9.

30. Dyck PJB, O'Brien P, Bosch P. The multi-center double-blind controlled trial of IV methylprednisolone in diabetic lumbosacral radiculoplexus neuropathy. *Neurology* 2006; **66** (Suppl 2): A191.

31. van Alfen N, van Engelen BG. The clinical spectrum of neuralgic amyotrophy in 246 cases. *Brain* 2006; **129**: 438–50.

32. Beghi E, Kurland LT, Mulder DW, Nicolosi A. Brachial plexus neuropathy in the population of Rochester, Minnesota, 1970–1981. *Ann Neurol* 1985; **18**: 320–3.

33. van Alfen N. Clinical and pathophysiological concepts of neuralgic amyotrophy. *Nat Rev Neurol* 2011; **7**: 315–22.

34. Lahrmann H, Grisold W, Authier FJ, Zifko UA. Neuralgic amyotrophy with phrenic nerve involvement. *Muscle Nerve* 1999; **22**: 437–42.

35. Tsao BE, Ostrovskiy DA, Wilbourn AJ, Shields RW, Jr. Phrenic neuropathy due to neuralgic amyotrophy. *Neurology* 2006; **66**: 1582–4.

36. Hughes PD, Polkey MI, Moxham J, Green M. Long-term recovery of diaphragm strength in neuralgic amyotrophy. *Eur Respir J* 1999; **13**: 379–84.

37. Byrne E. Extended neuralgic amyotrophy syndrome. *Aust NZ J Med* 1987; **17**: 34–8.

38. van Alfen N, van der Werf SP, van Engelen BG. Long-term pain, fatigue, and impairment in neuralgic amyotrophy. *Arch Phys Med Rehabil* 2009; **90**: 435–9.

39. Gaskin CM, Helms CA. Parsonage–Turner syndrome: MR imaging findings and clinical information of 27 patients. *Radiology* 2006; **240**: 501–7.

40. Collie AM, Landsverk ML, Ruzzo E, et al. Non-recurrent *SEPT9* duplications cause hereditary neuralgic amyotrophy. *J Med Genet* 2010; **47**: 601–7.

41. Kuhlenbaumer G, Hannibal MC, Nelis E, Schirmacher A, Verpoorten N, Meuleman J, et al. Mutations in *SEPT9* cause hereditary neuralgic amyotrophy. *Nat Genet* 2005; **37**: 1044–6.

42. Landsverk ML, Ruzzo EK, Mefford HC, et al. Duplication within the *SEPT9* gene associated with a founder effect in North American families with hereditary neuralgic amyotrophy. *Hum Mol Genet* 2009; **18**: 1200–8.

43. Hannibal MC, Ruzzo EK, Miller LR, et al. *SEPT9* gene sequencing analysis reveals recurrent mutations in hereditary neuralgic amyotrophy. *Neurology* 2009; **72**: 1755–9.

44. Laccone F, Hannibal MC, Neesen J, Grisold W, Chance PF, Rehder H. Dysmorphic syndrome of hereditary neuralgic amyotrophy associated with a *SEPT9* gene mutation—a family study. *Clin Genet* 2008; **74**: 279–83.

45. Ueda M, Kawamura N, Tateishi T, et al. Phenotypic spectrum of hereditary neuralgic amyotrophy caused by the *SEPT9* R88W mutation. *J Neurol Neurosurg Psychiatry* 2010; **81**: 94–6.

46. Fuchtbauer A, Lassen LB, Jensen AB, et al. Septin9 is involved in septin filament formation and cellular stability. *Biol Chem* 2011; **392**: 769–77.

47. Nagata K, Kawajiri A, Matsui S, et al. Filament formation of MSF-A, a mammalian septin, in human mammary epithelial cells depends on interactions with microtubules. *J Biol Chem* 2003; **278**: 18538–43.

48. Sudo K, Ito H, Iwamoto I, Morishita R, Asano T, Nagata K. SEPT9 sequence alterations causing hereditary neuralgic amyotrophy are associated with altered interactions with SEPT4/SEPT11 and resistance to Rho/Rhotekin-signaling. *Hum Mutat* 2007; **28**: 1005–13.

49. Chance PF, Lensch MW, Lipe H, Brown RH, Sr, Brown RH, Jr, Bird TD. Hereditary neuralgic amyotrophy and hereditary neuropathy with liability to pressure palsies: two distinct genetic disorders. *Neurology* 1994; **44**: 2253–7.

50. Klein CJ, Dyck PJ, Friedenberg SM, Burns TM, Windebank AJ, Dyck PJ. Inflammation and neuropathic attacks in hereditary brachial plexus neuropathy. *J Neurol Neurosurg Psychiatry* 2002; **73**: 45–50.

51. Suarez GA, Giannini C, Bosch EP, et al. Immune brachial plexus neuropathy: suggestive evidence for an inflammatory-immune pathogenesis. *Neurology* 1996; **46**: 559–61.

52. van Eijk JJ, van Alfen N, Tio-Gillen AP, et al. Screening for antecedent Campylobacter jejuni infections and anti-ganglioside antibodies in idiopathic neuralgic amyotrophy. *J Peripher Nerv Syst* 2011; **16**: 153–6.

53. van Alfen N, van Engelen BG, Hughes RA. Treatment for idiopathic and hereditary neuralgic amyotrophy (brachial neuritis). *Cochrane Database Syst Rev* 2009; **3**: CD006976.

54. van Eijk JJ, van Alfen N, Berrevoets M, van der Wilt GJ, Pillen S, van Engelen BG. Evaluation of prednisolone treatment in the acute phase of neuralgic amyotrophy: an observational study. *J Neurol Neurosurg Psychiatry* 2009; **80**: 1120–4.

55. Kori SH, Foley KM, Posner JB. Brachial plexus lesions in patients with cancer: 100 cases. *Neurology* 1981; **31**: 45–50.

56. Jaeckle KA, Young DF, Foley KM. The natural history of lumbosacral plexopathy in cancer. *Neurology* 1985; **35**: 8–15.

57. Knight DM, Birch R, Pringle J. Benign solitary schwannomas: a review of 234 cases. *J Bone Joint Surg Br* 2007; **89**: 382–7.

58. Lusk MD, Kline DG, Garcia CA. Tumors of the brachial plexus. *Neurosurgery* 1987; **21**: 439–53.

59. Dart LH, Jr, MacCarty CS, Love JG, Dockerty MB. Neoplasms of the brachial plexus. *Minn Med* 1970; **53**: 959–64.

60. Tonsgard JH, Kwak SM, Short MP, Dachman AH. CT imaging in adults with neurofibromatosis-1: frequent asymptomatic plexiform lesions. *Neurology* 1998; **50**: 1755–60.

61. Rosso SM, de Bruin HG, Wu KL, van den Bent MJ. Diagnosis of neurolymphomatosis with FDG PET. *Neurology* 2006; **67**: 722–3.

62. Baehring JM, Damek D, Martin EC, Betensky RA, Hochberg FH. Neurolymphomatosis. *Neuro Oncol* 2003; **5**: 104–15.

63. Amini A, Yang J, Williamson R, et al. Dose constraints to prevent radiation-induced brachial plexopathy in patients treated for lung cancer. *Int J Radiat Oncol Biol Phys* 2012; **82**: e391–e398.

64. Pierce SM, Recht A, Lingos TI, et al. Long-term radiation complications following conservative surgery (CS) and radiation therapy (RT) in patients with early stage breast cancer. *Int J Radiat Oncol Biol Phys* 1992; **23**: 915–23.

65. Bowen J, Gregory R, Squier M, Donaghy M. The post-irradiation lower motor neuron syndrome neuronopathy or radiculopathy? *Brain* 1996; **119**: 1429–39.

66. Roth G, Magistris MR, Le FD, Desjacques P, Della SD. [Post-radiation branchial plexopathy. Persistent conduction block. Myokymic discharges and cramps]. *Rev Neurol (Paris)* 1988; **144**: 173–80.

67. Qayyum A, MacVicar AD, Padhani AR, Revell P, Husband JE. Symptomatic brachial plexopathy following treatment for breast cancer: utility of MR imaging with surface-coil techniques. *Radiology* 2000; **214**: 837–42.

68. Taylor BV, Kimmel DW, Krecke KN, Cascino TL. Magnetic resonance imaging in cancer-related lumbosacral plexopathy. *Mayo Clin Proc* 1997; **72**: 823–9.

69. Thyagarajan D, Cascino T, Harms G. Magnetic resonance imaging in brachial plexopathy of cancer. *Neurology* 1995; **45**: 421–7.

70. Ahmad A, Barrington S, Maisey M, Rubens RD. Use of positron emission tomography in evaluation of brachial plexopathy in breast cancer patients. *Br J Cancer* 1999; **79**: 478–82.

71. Ferner RE, Golding JF, Smith M, et al. [18F]2-fluoro-2-deoxy-D-glucose positron emission tomography (FDG PET) as a diagnostic tool for neurofibromatosis 1 (NF1) associated malignant peripheral nerve sheath tumours (MPNSTs): a long-term clinical study. *Ann Oncol* 2008; **19**: 390–4.

72. Hoffmann V, Coppejans H, Vercauteren M, Adriaensen H. Successful treatment of postherpetic neuralgia with oral ketamine. *Clin J Pain* 1994; **10**: 240–2.

73. Spinner RJ, Kline DG. Surgery for peripheral nerve and brachial plexus injuries or other nerve lesions. *Muscle Nerve* 2000; **23**: 680–95.

74. Lewis RA, Sumner AJ, Brown MJ, Asbury AK. Multifocal demyelinating neuropathy with persistent conduction block. *Neurology* 1982; **32**: 958–64.

75. Bennett DL, Groves M, Blake J, et al. The use of nerve and muscle biopsy in the diagnosis of vasculitis: a 5 year retrospective study. *J Neurol Neurosurg Psychiatry* 2008; **79**: 1376–81.

CHAPTER 15

Polyneuropathies: axonal

Camiel Verhamme and Ivo N. van Schaik

General introduction

Polyneuropathy may be defined as a diffuse, generally symmetrical, length-dependent disease of two or more nerves. The onset and duration of symptoms determine whether the polyneuropathy is categorized as (sub)acute or chronic [1]. Furthermore, polyneuropathies can be categorized as pure motor, pure sensory, or sensorimotor, and finally the clinical pattern and distribution of abnormalities should be taken into account to determine whether it is uniform, and thus symmetrical, or multifocal. The majority of axonal polyneuropathies are of the chronic, uniform, symmetrical type. The estimated prevalence of chronic, uniform, symmetrical symptomatic polyneuropathy ranges between 0.09% [95% confidence interval (CI) 0.08–0.10%] in population-based studies and 1.3% (95% CI 0.5–3.2%) in case–control studies [2]. The multifocal axonal neuropathies, also known as multiple mononeuropathies (or mononeuritis multiplex), have a much lower incidence and are discussed in Chapter 13.

Although the axonal polyneuropathies are a group of diseases with a wide and heterogeneous range of aetiologies, the presenting signs and symptoms are often quite similar. To arrive at the correct diagnosis and therapy in a patient with an axonal polyneuropathy is therefore a clinical challenge. For more extensive descriptions we refer to textbooks devoted to peripheral neuropathies [3–5].

Clinical picture, symptoms, and signs

The clinical picture of the most prevalent, chronic, uniform symmetrical sensorimotor axonal polyneuropathy is characterized by symmetric, sensory more than motor involvement of peripheral nerves in a length-dependent way. Onset is insidious and initial manifestations progress gradually. Due to the length-dependent character, signs and symptoms start in the lower extremities. Typical initial complaints are toe-tip tingling, loss of feeling in a stocking–glove distribution, and walking problems due to instability. Pain, often lancinating sharp or burning, can be a first symptom. When the disease progresses, normally over years, sensory loss will spread and eventually the lower legs and hands may become involved. Development of manifest muscle weakness is rare, but the patient may complain of muscle cramps and twitching. If motor impairment develops, it remains confined to the feet, lower legs, and intrinsic hand muscles.

Neurological examination may reveal loss of function of small and large sensory nerve fibres: diminished pain, temperature, vibration, touch, and joint-position sensation, and mild allodynia in the feet. Ankle reflexes are absent or diminished with relative preservation of the knee and arm deep tendon reflexes. There may be gait disturbances. In general, abnormalities found with neurological examination are mild.

Although most chronic axonal polyneuropathies are sensorimotor, pure motor and pure sensory forms do exist. Asymmetries may point to a multifocal character, and thus to a multiple mononeuropathy. Severe pains, asymmetry, predominant motor impairment, pure sensory, fast progression, and autonomic involvement are all characteristics not normally found in a chronic axonal polyneuropathy and should be a reason to consider other neuropathies (e.g. predominant motor involvement may point in the direction of demyelinating neuropathy). These red flags should also prompt for a search into specific aetiologies (Table 15.1).

The clinical picture of isolated small-fibre neuropathy is characterized by usually painful paraesthesiae (burning sensation, tingling) and spontaneous shooting, or stabbing pains [6]. Allodynia or hyperalgesia may be present. Autonomic complaints include altered sweating, facial flushing, dry eyes or mouth, erectile dysfunction, orthostatic hypotension, and gastrointestinal disturbances. Neurological examination may indicate small-fibre dysfunction with disturbed temperature and pain sensation, or may be normal.

Patients with a sensory neuronopathy complain at onset of pain and paraesthesiae with asymmetric distribution. The arms are more and earlier involved than the legs. At a later stage numbness, limb ataxia, and pseudoathetotic movements of the hands are prominent features, while the pain decreases. The neurological examination shows reduced or absent deep tendon reflexes and involvement of all modalities of sensation.

Electrophysiology (Table 15.2)

In patients with uniform axonal polyneuropathies the hallmarks in nerve conduction studies are low compound muscle action potential (CMAP) and sensory nerve action potential (SNAP) amplitudes in a distal–proximal gradient, but normal or only slightly slowed nerve conduction velocities, not in the range of the slow nerve conduction velocities as found in demyelinating neuropathies [7]. Electromyography (EMG) may show signs of denervation (fibrillations and positive sharp waves) and reinnervation (long-duration motor unit potentials, which may be polyphasic) with poor recruitment. More subtle signs may be prolonged latencies of the soleus H reflex and prolonged minimal F wave latencies or absent F waves.

In patients with multiple mononeuropathies, there are asymmetries in motor or sensory involvement. In severe cases, the widespread abnormalities may mimic a diffuse axonal polyneuropathy.

In patients with small-fibre neuropathies nerve conduction studies and EMG are normal, but other investigations like temperature discrimination and skin biopsy for assessment of small-fibre density are abnormal.

Table 15.1 Specific aetiologies in relation to red flags

Symptoms	Diagnosis	Ancillary investigations
Severe pains	Vasculitis	CBC, ESR, CRP, ANA, ANCA, anti-SSA, anti-SSB, rheumatoid factor, Hepatitis B and C serologies, cryoglobulins
	Intoxication (alcohol, arsenic exposure, thallium, thalidomide)	Specific screen for intoxication, liver enzymes
	Diabetes mellitus	Fasting blood glucose, HbA1c
	Diabetic amyotrophy (proximal diabetic neuropathy)	Fasting blood glucose, HbA1c
	HIV	HIV
	Sarcoidosis	Di-hydroxy vitamin D, ACE, CSF, FDG-PET/CT-thorax
	Neuroborreliosis	Lyme serology and CSF
	Sjögren syndrome	ESR, ANA, rheumatoid factor, anti-SSA, anti-SSB, lip biopsy
	Acute intermittent porphyria	PBG, D-Ala (urine) or Ala-dehydratase (serum)
	Amyloidosis	Serum protein electrophoresis and immunofixation, TTR, amyloid mass spectrometry, abdominal wall fat biopsy
	Hereditary: HSN/HSAN, Fabry disease	HS(A)N-specific genes (see Chapter 9), alpha-galactosidase A (enzyme and gene) (Fabry disease)
Asymmetry	Vasculitis	CBC, ESR, CRP, ANA, ANCA, anti-SSA, anti-SSB, rheumatoid factor, hepatitis B and C serologies, cryoglobulins
	Sensory neuronopathy	Paraneoplastic antibodies, CT-chest
	Syphilis	*Treponema pallidum*, lues serology
	Sarcoidosis	Di-hydroxy vitamin D, ACE, CSF, FDG-PET/CT-thorax
	Amyloidosis	Serum protein electrophoresis and immunofixation, TTR, amyloid mass spectrometry, abdominal wall fat biopsy
Predominant motor	AMAN	Anti-GM1 antibodies, CSF
	Thyrotoxicosis	TSH, T4
	Hyperparathyroidism	Calcium, phosphate
	Toxic (lead, dapsone, nitrofurantoin)	Specific screen for intoxication, liver enzymes
	Acute intermittent porphyria	PBG, D-Ala (urine) or Ala-dehydratase (serum)
	Neuroborreliosis	Lyme serology and CSF
Pure sensory	Chemotherapy (cisplatinum, pyridoxin, thalidomide, vincristine)	
	Paraproteinaemia (IgM-MGUS)	Anti-MAG antibodies
	Sjögren syndrome	ESR, ANA, rheumatoid factor, anti-SSA, anti-SSB, labial salivary gland biopsy
	HIV	HIV
	Paraneoplastic neuro(no)pathy	Paraneoplastic antibodies, CT-chest
	Vitamin E deficiency	Vitamin E
	Idiopathic sensory neuropathy	
	Hereditary: HSN/HSAN, Friedreich ataxia	HS(A)N-specific genes (see Chapter 9) HS(A)N1: *SPTCL1* gene, frataxin gene
	Isolated small-fibre neuropathy	See Table 15.6
Fast progression	Vasculitis	CBC, ESR, CRP, ANA, ANCA, anti-SSA, anti-SSB, rheumatoid factor, hepatitis B and C serologies, cryoglobulins
	Paraneoplastic neuro(no)pathy	Paraneoplastic antibodies, CT-chest
	Malignant transformation of MGUS	IgG/IgM/IgA
	Neuroborreliosis	Lyme serology and CSF

(continued)

Table 15.1 Continued

Symptoms	Diagnosis	Ancillary investigations
	Acute intermittent porphyria	PBG, D-Ala (urine) or Ala-dehydratase (serum)
	Intoxication (thallium, organophosphates, arsenic exposure)	Intoxication screen, liver enzymes
Autonomic disturbances	Diabetes mellitus	Fasting blood glucose, HbA1c
	Alcohol	Liver enzymes
	Amyloidosis	Serum protein electrophoresis and immunofixation, TTR, amyloid mass spectrometry, abdominal wall fat biopsy
	Paraneoplastic	Paraneoplastic antibodies, CT-chest
	Sjögren syndrome	ESR, ANA, rheumatoid factor, anti-SSA, anti-SSB, labial salivary gland biopsy
	Vasculitis	CBC, ESR, CRP, ANA, ANCA, anti-SSA, anti-SSB, rheumatoid factor, hepatitis B and C serologies, cryoglobulins
	Acute intermittent porphyria	PBG, D-Ala (in urine) or Ala-dehydratase (serum)
	Infection (HIV, leprae)	HIV serology, skin biopsy (leprae)
	Intoxication (arsenic exposure, mercury, acrylamide)	Specific screen for intoxication, liver enzymes
	Hereditary: HSN/HSAN	HS(A)N-specific genes (see Chapter 9) HS(A)N1: *SPTCL1* gene
	Idiopathic sensory neuronopathy	

ACE, angiotensin-converting enzyme; Ala, alanine; AMAN, acute motor axonal neuropathy; ANA, antinuclear antibody; ANCA, antineutrophil cytoplasmic antibody; CBC, complete blood cell count; CRP, C-reactive protein; CSF, cerebrospinal fluid; CT, computed tomography; D-Ala, D-alanine; ESR, erythrocyte sedimentation rate; FDG, fluorodeoxyglucose; GM1, monosialotetrahexosylganglioside; Hb, haemoglobin; HIV, human immunodeficiency virus; HSAN, hereditary sensory and autonomic neuropathy; HSN, hereditary sensory neuropathy; IgM, immunoglobulin M; MAG, myelin-associated glycoprotein; MGUS, monoclonal gammopathy of unknown significance; PBG, porphobilinogen; PET, positron emission tomography; SSA, Sjögren syndrome A; SSB, Sjögren syndrome B; T4, thyroxine; TTR, transthyretin; TSH, thyroid-stimulating hormone.

In patients with sensory neuronopathies the hallmarks in nerve conduction studies are low or absent SNAP amplitudes with spared CMAPs.

Diagnostic algorithm

History and neurological examination combined with the results of electrophysiological testing will guide the further search for an aetiology. Onset and duration determine whether the neuropathy is categorized as (sub)acute or chronic. In clinical practice an arbitrary cut off of 6 weeks is useful. Next the polyneuropathy should be categorized as pure motor, pure sensory, or sensorimotor, and finally the clinical pattern and distribution of abnormalities should be taken into account: focal, multifocal, or uniform symmetrical. The electrodiagnostic testing will distinguish axonal and

Table 15.2 Summary of electrodiagnostic abnormalities

	Axonal polyneuropathy	Small-fibre neuropathy	Sensory neuronopathy	Demyelinating polyneuropathy
Motor conduction studies				
Distal CMAP amplitude	↓ or absent	Normal	Normal	Normal or ↓
Conduction velocity	Normal or slightly↓	Normal	Normal	↓↓↓
Conduction block	None	None	None	May be present
Sensory conduction studies				
Distal SNAP amplitude	↓ or absent	Normal	↓ or absent	Normal or ↓
Conduction velocity	Normal or slightly ↓	Normal	Normal or slightly ↓	↓↓↓
Needle EMG				
Spontaneous muscle fibre activity	May be present	None	None	May be present
MUP	May be long-duration and polyphasic	Normal	Normal	Normal or long-duration and polyphasic
Distribution of abnormalities	Uniform or multifocal. Most often distal; legs >> arms	Uniform. Most often distal; legs >> arms	Uniform	Uniform or multifocal. May be proximal

CMAP, compound muscle action potential; SNAP, sensory nerve action potential; EMG, electromyography; MUP, motor unit potential [7].

demyelinating neuropathies. The differential diagnosis of a demyelinating neuropathy is discussed in Chapter 16.

This leads to the algorithms for axonal neuropathies shown in Figs 15.1 and 15.2.

Ancillary investigations

Many causes are rare and ancillary investigations should only be performed if diagnostic clues are present. A thoroughly taken history should reveal the use of medication, alcohol, or other toxic agents. A patient already known to have diabetes or chronic renal insufficiency will eliminate the necessity for further diagnostic work-up only if symptoms and signs fit the typical clinical picture. A family history and a search for foot deformity may be helpful in diagnosing Charcot–Marie–Tooth Type 2. The minimal set of laboratory tests should encompass complete blood cell count (CBC), fasting blood sugar, renal function, liver enzymes, serum protein electrophoresis and immunofixation, vitamin B_1 and B_{12}, thyroid screening test, and haemoglobin. In Table 15.3 the causes listed in Figs 15.1 and 15.2 are ordered alphabetically with suggestions for specific ancillary investigations.

The diagnosis of chronic idiopathic axonal neuropathy should only be made in a patient over the age of 45 years with a chronic sensorimotor axonal polyneuropathy without any cause after diagnostic work-up. In a patient younger than 45 the search should be extended and longer follow-up is necessary before concluding to an idiopathic neuropathy.

In patients with symptoms and signs consistent with small-fibre involvement and normal electrophysiological studies, a diagnosis of an isolated small-fibre neuropathy should be considered.

Specific causes

In this section short descriptions of the most prevalent axonal polyneuropathies, multiple mononeuropathies, sensory neuronopathies, and small-fibre neuropathies due to specific causes are given. For some causes we refer to other chapters, e.g. the chapters on inherited peripheral nerve diseases (Charcot–Marie–Tooth, Chapter 8; hereditary sensory and motor neuropathies, Chapter 9; familial amyloid, Chapter 10; inherited metabolic, Chapter 11;

Table 15.3 Diseases mentioned in Figures 15.1 and 15.2 (in alphabetical order) with suggested ancillary investigations

Autoimmune hepatitis	ASAT, ALAT, total IgG, ANA, SMA, anti-LKM-1, or anti-LC1, liver biopsy
Acute intermittent porphyria	PBG, D-Ala (urine) or Ala-dehydratase (serum)
Acute motor axonal neuropathy	Anti-GM1 antibodies, CSF
Amyloidosis	Serum protein electrophoresis and immunofixation, TTR, amyloid mass spectrometry, abdominal wall fat biopsy
Axonal CMT (type 2)	Specific genes (see Chapter 8)
Arsenic exposure	Arsenic
Chronic idiopathic axonal polyneuropathy	Per exclusion
Cryoglobulinaemia	Cryoglobulins, Hepatitis C serology
Critical illness polyneuropathy	
Diabetes mellitus, including diabetic amyotrophy	Fasting blood glucose, HbA1c
Diabetic amyotrophy	Fasting blood glucose, HbA1c
Friedreich ataxia	Frataxin gene
Hereditary sensory autonomic neuropathy	Specific genes (see Chapter 9)
HIV	HIV
Hyperparathyroidism	Calcium, phosphate
Hypoglycaemia/hyperinsulinaemia	Fasting blood glucose
Hypothyroidism	TSH, FT4
Idiopathic sensory neuropathy	
Inherited disorders of fat absorption leading to vitamin E deficiency	Specific genes (see Chapter 11)
Intoxications (alcohol, glue, arsenic exposure)	Specific screen for intoxication, liver enzymes
Lead neuropathy	Lead
Leprae	Serology, skin biopsy
Medication (platinum based, antibiotic)	
Mitochondrial neuropathies	
Neuroborreliosis	Lyme serology and CSF

(continued)

Table 15.3 Continued

Nitrofurantoin	
Paraneoplastic neuro(no)pathy	Paraneoplastic antibodies, CT-chest
Paraproteinaemia (monoclonal gammopathy of undetermined significance)	Serum protein electrophoresis and immunofixation, IgM, anti-MAG antibodies
Polycythaemia vera	Hb, MCV
Primary biliary cirrhosis	Bilirubin, ammonia
Radiation-induced neuropathy	
Rheumatoid arthritis	CBC, ESR, CRP, rheumatoid factor, anti-cyclic citrullinated peptide antibodies
Spinocerebellar ataxia with neuropathy	Specific genes
Sarcoidosis	Di-hydroxy vitamin D, ACE, CSF, FDG-PET/CT-thorax
Sjögren syndrome	ESR, ANA, rheumatoid factor, anti-SSA, anti-SSB, labial salivary gland biopsy
Systemic lupus erythematosus	CBC, ESR, CRP, ANA, anti-Sm, anti-dsDNA
Syphilis	*Treponema pallidum*, lues serology
Thyrotoxicosis	TSH, FT4
Vasculitis	CBC, ESR, CRP, ANA, ANCA, anti-SSA, anti-SSB, rheumatoid factor, hepatitis B and C serologies, cryoglobulins
Vitamins	Serum vitamin levels

ACE, angiotensin-converting enzyme; Ala, alanine; ALAT, alanine aminotransferase; ANA, antinuclear antibody; ANCA, antineutrophil cytoplasmic antibody; anti-LC1, anti-liver cytosol antibody Type 1; ASAT, aspartate aminotransferase; CBC, complete blood cell count; CMT, Charcot–Marie–Tooth; CRP, C-reactive protein; CSF, cerebrospinal fluid; CT, computed tomography; D-Ala, D-alanine; dsDNA, double-stranded DNA; ESR, erythrocyte sedimentation rate; FDG, fluorodeoxyglucose; GM1, monosialotetrahexosylganglioside; Hb, haemoglobin; HIV, human immunodeficiency virus; IgG, immunoglobulin G; LKM-1, liver kidney microsome-1; MAG, myelin-associated glycoproteins; MCV, mean corpuscular volume; PBG, porphobilinogen; PET, positron emission tomography; SMA, smooth muscle antibody; SSA, Sjögren syndrome A; SSB, Sjögren syndrome B; T4, thyroxine; TTR, transthyretin; TSH, thyroid-stimulating hormone.

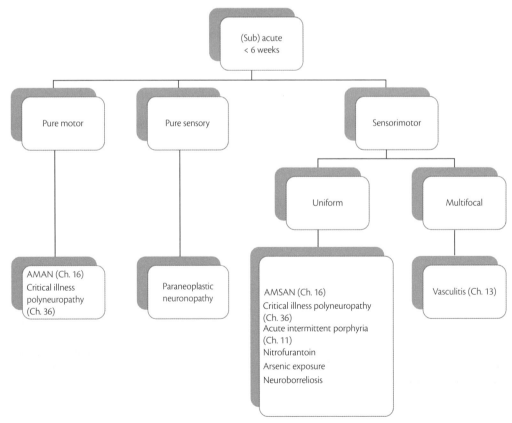

Fig. 15.1 Acute/subacute axonal neuropathies. AMAN, acute motor axonal neuropathy; AMSAN, acute motor and sensory axonal neuropathy. The chapter in which the specific neuropathy is discussed is indicated.

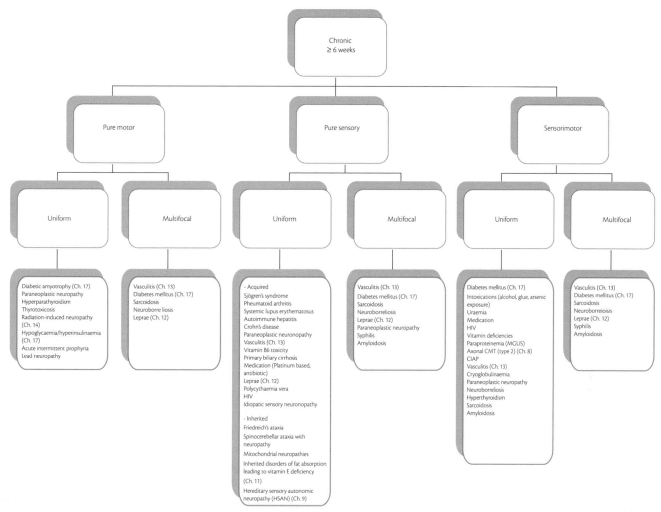

Fig. 15.2 Chronic axonal neuropathies. CIAP, chronic idiopathic axonal polyneuropathy; CMT, Charcot–Marie–Tooth disease; HIV, human immunodeficiency virus; HSAN, hereditary sensory and autonomic neuropathy; MGUS, monoclonal gammopathy of unknown significance. The chapter in which the specific neuropathy is discussed is indicated.

multiple mononeuropathies, Chapter 13), diabetes mellitus (Chapter 17), and ICU acquired weakness (Chapter 36).

Uremic polyneuropathy

Uremic polyneuropathy is a common complication of end-stage renal disease [8]. It generally only develops with glomerular filtration rates below about 12 ml min^{-1} and creatinine levels greater than 400–500 µmol L^{-1} [9]. The clinical picture is that of a typical chronic axonal sensorimotor polyneuropathy [8]. Secondary restless legs is often an important complaint [10]. Renal transplantation is effective in the prevention and (partial) reversal of uremic polyneuropathy [11,12]. Haemodialysis and peritoneal dialysis tend to retard its progression [8].

Thyroid-related neuropathies

Hypothyroidism may lead to a chronic axonal sensorimotor polyneuropathy in which sensory symptoms dominate in the majority of patients [13,14]. Coexistent myopathy may explain proximal weakness. Muscle tendon reflexes are depressed in the arms and are often absent in the legs. If reflexes are present there may be prolonged relaxation ('hung-up'). Most patients experience considerable improvement with thyroid hormone replacement therapy [13]. It is of note that carpal tunnel syndrome is more prevalent in patients with untreated hypothyroidism [13,14].

There is some uncertainty regarding polyneuropathy as a complication of hyperthyroidism. In patients with newly diagnosed hyperthyroidism a substantial portion had predominantly sensory signs compatible with a sensorimotor axonal neuropathy early in the cause of the disease. These signs resolved rapidly and completely following treatment [13].

Infection-related neuropathies

Human immunodeficiency virus (HIV)-associated peripheral neuropathies

Peripheral neuropathy is common in individuals infected with HIV (Table 15.4). The distal symmetric sensorimotor neuropathy is the most common type. Despite the introduction of highly active antiretroviral therapy (HAART), this form remains prevalent, causing substantial disability [15,16]. The other types are rare. The aetiology is diverse and only partially caused by the HIV infection itself. Opportunistic infections, neurotoxicity of medication, dietary and vitamin deficiencies, and other diseases associated with HIV, like diabetes mellitus, may cause a polyneuropathy. Acute and chronic inflammatory demyelinating polyneuropathies (AIDP and CIDP) do occur in patients with HIV infection, although it is unclear

Table 15.4 Human immunodeficiency virus (HIV)-associated peripheral nervous system disorders

Disorder	Disease stage	Clinical features	Course	Ancillary investigations
Distal sensorimotor polyneuropathy		Distal sensory loss and neuropathic pain; depressed or absent ankle reflexes		EMG
HIV associated	Late		Subacute or chronic	
Antiretroviral toxic	Any stage		Subacute; rarely acute with lactic acidosis	
Multiple mononeuropathy	Early or late	Multifocal cranial/peripheral nerve weakness/sensory loss; painful	Subacute or chronic	EMG, CMV
Small-fibre neuropathy	Any stage	Distal neuropathic pain, autonomic symptoms	Subacute or chronic	EMG, skin biopsy, quantitative sensory testing
Sensory neuronopathy	Any stage	Pain and paraesthesiae in asymmetric distribution; numbness in arms and legs, ataxia	Subacute	EMG
Seroconversion neuropathy	Early	Generalized systemic illness, mononeuropathies	Acute	EMG, HIV
Acute/chronic inflammatory demyelinating polyradiculoneuropathy	Early	Quadriparesis; acral paraesthesia	Acute/subacute or chronic	EMG, CSF
Progressive polyradiculopathy	Late	Bladder dysfunction, paraesthesiae; lumbosacral pain, saddle anaesthesia; rapidly progressive flaccid paraparesis, leg hyporeflexia	Acute	EMG; CSF; CMV; VZV
Diffuse infiltrative lymphocytosis syndrome	Late	Sicca syndrome; symmetric > asymmetric sensorimotor, sensory loss, mild weakness, burning pain	Acute/subacute	EMG; serum CD8 hyperlymphocytosis; nerve biopsy CD8+ T-cell infiltrates
Motor neuron disease	Early > late	Motor dysfunction, muscle wasting with upper motor neuron signs; bulbar dysfunction; hyperreflexia	Subacute	EMG

EMG, electromyography; CMV, cytomegalovirus; VZV, varicella zoster virus.

Adapted from [17].

whether the frequency is higher than in the general population and they do not behave differently in patients with HIV infection.

Lyme neuroborreliosis

Lyme disease or Lyme borreliosis is caused by several genospecies of *Borrelia burgdorferi*, a spirochaete transmitted by ticks [18]. It is the most common vector-borne bacterial infection in temperate regions of the Northern Hemisphere. The hallmark of the early localized phase is erythema migrans [19]. In 10–15% of untreated patients the disease disseminates and neurological symptoms usually occur 1–12 weeks after the tick bite [20]. It is of importance that patients may present with these symptoms without a history of prior signs or symptoms suggestive of earlier Lyme disease. Lymphocytic meningitis is the most common central nervous system manifestation. Cranial neuropathies are the most common peripheral nervous system manifestation, the facial nerve being most often affected, in a substantial proportion of patients bilaterally. The other common peripheral nervous system manifestations are often painful, mono- or polyradicolopathy (Garin–Bujadoux–Bannwarth syndrome), multiple mononeuropathy, and brachial/lumbosacral plexopathy. In patients who have more longstanding

disease a relatively mild, slowly evolving, symmetric polyneuropathy is fairly common, but detailed studies suggest that this is in fact a confluent multiple mononeuropathy [21]. Several guidelines on diagnosis and management have been developed [20,22].

Nutritional neuropathies

Thiamin (vitamin B₁)

Thiamine is an important cofactor for enzymes involved in amino acid and carbohydrate metabolism. The most common causes for a vitamin B_1 deficiency are chronic alcoholism and recurrent vomiting (i.e. hyperemesis gravidarum). Other causes are chronic renal dialysis, prolonged parenteral feeding, ulcerative colitis, gastric resection surgery, and jejuno-ileal bypass surgery. Deficiencies due to insufficient intake are rare in developed countries. Continuous supplementation is necessary as body stores are relatively low and can be depleted from the healthy body in 18 days [23]. The first symptoms of a vitamin B_1 deficiency are fatigue, irritability, and muscle cramps, and usually develop in days to weeks. However, subclinical deficiencies may lead to acute symptomatology after heavy physical exercise and infections. Symptoms of a polyneuropathy start after a longer period and consist of sensory loss and burning sensations in the feet and toes. If the deficiency prolongs, sensory loss increases and symptoms progress proximally in the legs; some loss of strength in the feet and lower legs may become apparent and may involve the hands. Many of the described causes actually should be on standard supplementation. Improvement after supplementation takes several months.

Pyridoxine (vitamin B$_6$)

Pyridoxine (vitamin B$_6$) deficiency is very rare and is associated with the use of isoniazid and hydralazine [24,25], pregnancy, chronic peritoneal dialysis, and alcoholism. Due to adequate standard supplementation, deficiencies in the first three groups are rare. However, pyridoxine excess with high daily doses (200 mg to 10 g), most often in feeding supplements, may lead to distal sensory polyneuropathy or neuronopathy in a dose-dependent manner [26]. Pyridoxine excess neuropathy is reversible after stopping excess supplementation. Symptoms may increase 2–3 weeks afterwards (coasting) [27]. The majority of symptoms may disappear within 6 months, but complete recovery may take 2–3 years.

Cobalamin (vitamin B$_{12}$)

Cobalamin, or vitamin B$_{12}$, is an essential vitamin that cannot be synthesized by humans. Causes of vitamin B$_{12}$ deficiency are: inadequate gastric production of intrinsic factor (pernicious anaemia, atrophic gastritis, gastrectomy) or from disorders of the terminal ileum (resection or inflammatory bowel disease), large bacterial or parasitic infections that divert cobalamin from the host, proton pump inhibitors, and exposure to nitrous oxide. Dietary deficiency is rare but may result from a strictly vegetarian diet. Besides the possible presence of a megablastic anaemia, the most important neurological manifestations are subacute combined degeneration of the dorsal (posterior) and lateral spinal columns, polyneuropathy, cognitive impairments, and, less often, optic neuropathy [28]. Patients may only have symptoms of polyneuropathy. Onset is typically with distal paraesthesiae, usually in the legs, but the hands may be affected first. An unsteady gait is common. Large-fibre sensory modalities (vibration and proprioception) are affected with sparing of small-fibre modalities. Differentiating peripheral nerve from spinal cord manifestations can be difficult. Loss of ankle jerks is the best clinical evidence of peripheral nerve involvement. The combined spinal cord manifestations may lead to hyperreflexia of the other muscle stretch reflexes and extensor plantar responses. First the cobalamin is measured in the serum. If low (<200 pg ml^{-1}; <148 pmol L^{-1}), this is consistent with cobalamin deficiency. If the results are in the normal range (>300 pg ml^{-1}; >221 pmol L^{-1}) cobalamin deficiency is unlikely. If the results are borderline (200–300 pg ml^{-1}; 148–221 pmol L^{-1}), cobalamin deficiency is possible. Then, additionally, specific metabolic intermediates (methylmalonic acid and homocysteine), which accumulate if cobalamin-dependent reactions are blocked, should be investigated [29].

Toxic neuropathies

Toxic neuropathies include those caused by pharmaceutical agents, industrial toxins, heavy metals, drugs, and alcohol [30]. Medication use should be considered in every patient with the clinical picture of a polyneuropathy, and firmly addressed during history-taking. It is of importance to also specifically ask for over-the-counter medication such as vitamin supplements (vitamin B$_6$). Besides medication, there should be enough attention during history-taking given to other toxic agents which may cause a polyneuropathy like recreational drugs (glue-sniffing, nitrous oxide), the use of metals during hobbies, and alcohol. Physical examination should include skin, nails, and hair to search for suggestions of a systemic intoxication. Most of these polyneuropathies are progressive as long as the exposure continues and lead to a symmetrical, distal, sensory or sensorimotor polyneuropathy.

Medication

A selected list of medications associated with polyneuropathies is given in Table 15.5. Many chemotherapeutic drugs have significant neuropathic side effects. These neurotoxic side effects substantially affect the quality of life of patients with cancer, and may require a dose reduction, delay, or even premature termination of potentially successful treatment [30].

Most medication-associated polyneuropathies lead to an axonal polyneuropathy in which sensory fibres are more affected than motor fibres. An exception is cisplatinum which leads to a sensory neuronopathy [30]. Severe sensory ataxia with the Lhermitte phenomenon as a consequence of centripetal degeneration of spinal cord posterior columns may lead to significant loss of function. Other exceptions are amiodarone, perhexiline, and gold which may show a predominantly demyelinating polyneuropathy with more prominent muscle weakness.

Metals

The most important metals for toxic neuropathy are lead, arsenic, and thallium. The neuropathy usually occurs in the context of a systemic illness involving the gastrointestinal system, the hematopoietic system, and the central nervous system [31]. Lead poisoning in adults has the typical clinical triad of abdominal pain and constipation, anaemia, and neuropathy. Lead poisoning in adults leads to a painless, progressive motor neuropathy in which the upper limbs are more affected than the lower limbs with localized weakness that may be asymmetrical [31]. The neuropathy associated with arsenic and thallium ingestion often is preceded for several days by an acute gastrointestinal illness. A sensorimotor polyneuropathy appears between several days and weeks following a single dose and may progress for weeks [32]. In chronic or repeated intoxications, progression will occur over a longer interval [31]. Both thallium and arsenic intoxication may show typical Mees lines in the fingernails and toenails, but alopecia is only found several weeks after thallium exposure.

Ethanol (alcohol)

In the past alcohol-related polyneuropathy appeared in patients with nutritional (thiamin) deficiencies. This hampered a proper distinction between the thiamin deficiency and the direct toxic effect of the alcohol in the development of the axonal sensorimotor polyneuropathy. The evidence on both sides was recently reviewed again and the authors concluded that alcohol-related polyneuropathy should be regarded as a toxic rather than nutritional neuropathy [33]. There are no strict criteria about how much alcohol needs to be consumed over a specific duration to lead to a polyneuropathy, but a cumulative lifetime dose effect is suggested [33].

Table 15.5 Selected medications associated with neuropathy

Chemotherapeutic drugs	Cardiovascular drugs	Antibiotics/antivirals	CNS agents	Miscellaneous agents
Bortezomib	**Amiodarone**	**Dapsone**	**Nitrous oxide**	**Colchicine**
Ixabepilone	**Perhexiline**	**Isoniazid**	Chlorprothixene	**Dichloroacetate**
Platinum compounds (cisplatin, carboplatin, and oxaliplatin)		**Linezolid**	Glutethimide	**Etanercept**
Suramin		**Metronidazole**	Phenelzine	**Infliximab**
Taxanes		**Nucleoside reverse transcriptase inhibitors (NRTIs) ddI, ddC, d4T**	Phenytoin	**Pyridoxine (vitamin B$_6$) excess**
Thalidomide (R analogue lenalidomide)		Chloroquine		Allopurinol
Vinca alkaloids		Chloramphenicol		Interferons: alpha 2a, -2b
5-Azacitidine		Fluroquinolones		Leflunomide
5-Fluorouracil		Griseofulvin		Sulphasalazine
Clioquinol		Nitrofurantoin		Triazole antifungals
Cytarabine		Podophyllin resin		Cimetidine Disulfiram
Etoposide				Penicillamine
Gemcitabine				
Ifosfamide				
Misonidazole				
Teniposide				

Bold text indicates the more common or better established causes of neuropathy.

Adapted from [30].

The clinical picture is that of a typical chronic axonal sensorimotor polyneuropathy, but prominent pain in both feet may be the presenting symptom.

Paraneoplastic neuropathies

The paraneoplastic neurological syndrome represents the remote effects of cancer on the nervous system. The paraneoplastic neuropathies are one of its major constituents. Depending on the form of the neuropathy, it may be classified as classical or non-classical [34]. The classical paraneoplastic neuropathies are subacute sensory neuronopathy, Lambert–Eaton myasthenic syndrome, and chronic intestinal pseudo-obstruction. The non-classical are motor neuron disease-like, Guillain–Barré syndrome, brachial neuritis, subacute/chronic sensorimotor neuropathy, neuropathy with vasculitis, autonomic neuropathy, and neuromyotonia. They may occur in parallel and with extensive variation. Depending on the grade of certainty, this may lead to the diagnosis of a definite or possible paraneoplastic disorder [34]. The sensory neuronopathies, with or without motor involvement, are by far the most prevalent type [35]. The onset of sensory neuronopathy is usually subacute and rapidly progressive, but may be acute, subacute, or chronic progressive. Numbness and paraesthesiae may begin in the limbs or face and spread to other regions, including the trunk, or may begin more diffusely. Marked asymmetries may occur. In about 50% of patients the upper limbs are affected first. Sensory disturbances typically begin distally, but the distribution is often asymmetric and multifocal in a non-length-dependent manner. Ataxia and gait difficulty are usually early and prominent complaints, aside from shooting or aching limb pains, burning and dysaesthesiae. About half of the patients with features of a sensory neuronopathy also have distal motor involvement, resulting in a sensorimotor neuronopathy. It is

unknown whether additional motor involvement in some patients could be 'motor neuronopathy' affecting the anterior horn cells or distal axonal neuropathy [35]. Dysautonomia may present as an isolated syndrome, but more commonly concomitantly with sensory neuronopathies, limbic, or brainstem encephalitis [35]. Autoimmune neuropathies (chronic inflammatory demyelinating polyradiculoneuropathy and Guillain–Barré syndrome) have been described as paraneoplastic syndromes, but recently were found in such a low percentage in a large study that the authors suggest that an association by chance is likely [35]. End-plate disorders like Lambert–Eaton myasthenic syndrome are discussed in Chapter 21.

In a subgroup of patients onconeural antibodies can be detected which are directed against neural antigens expressed by the tumour, suggesting an underlying autoimmune process. Among various autoantibodies associated with paraneoplastic syndrome, anti-Hu and anti-CV2/CRMP-5 antibodies are frequently associated with paraneoplastic neuropathy.

Although paraneoplastic neuropathy frequently precedes the detection of malignancy by months or years, it should also be considered in patients who are already undergoing or have completed treatment for malignancies. When paraneoplastic neurological syndromes are suspected and no cancer is found by conventional investigations, a whole-body fluorodeoxyglucose (FDG)-positron emission tomography (PET) or FDG-PET/computed tomography scan may be indicated. Recommendations for screening for tumours in paraneoplastic syndromes have recently been proposed [36].

Chronic idiopathic axonal polyneuropathy

Even after extensive investigations and long-term follow-up, a cause of chronic axonal polyneuropathy cannot be found in approximately 20% of patients [37] and in these cases the disorder is termed chronic idiopathic axonal polyneuropathy (CIAP) [38], also known in the literature as cryptogenic (sensory) polyneuropathy. Typically, onset is slow, often in the sixth decade, with gradual progression over years [39]. There is a predominance of distal sensory or sensorimotor impairments in the legs (more than in the hands), and some patients experience neuropathic pain [40]. Electrodiagnostic studies are compatible with an axonal polyneuropathy [37,39,41]. Patients remain ambulatory with generally minimal disability [39–42]. In several studies a lower age limit of 45 years was introduced, as the majority of inherited polyneuropathies presents at a younger age [38,39]. However, the lower age limit of 45 years is a safe guideline in clinical practice as well. This means that in a patient younger than 45 the search should be extended, and longer follow-up is necessary before concluding to an idiopathic neuropathy.

Isolated small-fibre neuropathies

In isolated small-fibre neuropathy thinly myelinated (A-delta) and unmyelinated (C) fibres are affected, leading to disturbances in pain and temperature sensation and/or autonomic functions. The clinical picture is characterized by usually painful paraesthesiae (burning sensation, tingling) and spontaneous shooting or stabbing pains [6]. Allodynia or hyperalgesia may be present. Autonomic complaints include changed sweating, facial flushing, dry eyes or mouth, erectile dysfunction, orthostatic hypotension, and gastrointestinal disturbances. Onset is in adulthood. Neurological examination may show indications for small-fibre dysfunction with disturbed temperature and pain sensation, or may be normal. Sensory modalities subserved by the large myelinated fibres (touch-pressure, vibration sense, joint position) are spared. Strength and tendon reflexes are preserved. Electrodiagnostic studies are normal, and the diagnosis is confirmed by demonstration of reduced intra-epidermal nerve fibre density or abnormal quantitative sensory testing. Known underlying causes are listed in Table 15.6, of which diabetes mellitus is most prevalent. A relatively large group remains idiopathic. Recently, in this idiopathic group a gain of function mutations in sodium channels $Na_V1.7$ and $Na_V1.8$ were found [43, 44]. Isolated small-fibre neuropathy may evolve to include large fibres, and one may search for aetiology in this pattern. In the differential diagnosis of a small-fibre neuropathy are tarsal tunnel syndrome, erythromelalgia, Morton neuroma, bilateral L5/S1 radiculopathy, plantar fasciitis, tendonitis, arthritis, and bursitis.

Sjögren syndrome

Sjögren syndrome disease is a chronic inflammatory disorder associated with reduced tear production (keratoconjuctivitis sicca) and dry mouth (xerostomia), the so-called sicca syndrome [45]. Signs of a sensory neuronopathy, or ganglionopathy, are numbness and paraesthesiae that may begin in the limbs or face and spread to other regions, including the trunk. Ataxia and forthcoming gait difficulties are often a clue to arrive at the diagnosis. An association between sensory ganglionopathy and inflammatory or immune-mediated disorders was first found in Sjögren syndrome but has since been discovered in other autoimmune diseases, such as rheumatoid arthritis, systemic lupus erythematosus, and autoimmune hepatitis [46].

Table 15.6 Causes of an isolated small-fibre neuropathy with suggested ancillary investigations

Causes	Investigations
Idiopathic	
Diabetes mellitus and abnormal oral glucose tolerance	Fasting blood glucose, HbA1c, oral glucose tolerance test
Alcohol misuse	
Paraproteinaemia (monoclonal gammopathy of undetermined significance, amyloidosis)	Serum protein electrophoresis and immunofixation, TTR, amyloid mass spectrometry, abdominal wall fat biopsy
HIV	HIV
Medication (antiretroviral, chemotherapeutics, vitamin B₆) and intoxications	
Paraneoplastic	Paraneoplastic antibodies, CT-chest
Sjögren syndrome	ESR, ANA, rheumatoid factor, anti-SSA, anti-SSB, labial salivary gland biopsy
Vasculitis (Wegener granulomatosis, SLE)	CBC, ESR, CRP, ANA, ANCA, anti-SSA, anti-SSB, rheumatoid factor, hepatitis B and C serologies, cryoglobulins
Sarcoidosis	Di-hydroxy vitamin D, ACE, CSF, FDG-PET/CT-thorax
Guillain–Barré syndrome	CSF
Post-infectious (e.g. EBV, influenza)	
Hyperlipidaemia	Lipid profile
Coeliac disease	IgA anti-endomysial antibodies, antitransglutaminase antibodies
Leprae	Serology, skin biopsy
Fabry disease	Alpha-galactosidase A
Tangier disease	Cholesterol, HDL
Hereditary sensory (autonomic) neuropathy, Charcot–Marie–Tooth Type 2B	HS(A)N-specific genes (see Chapter 9)HS(A)N1: SPTCL1 gene; CMT2B, RAB7 gene
Erythromelalgia/erythromelalgia, burning feet syndrome	Sodium channel $Na_V1.7$ mutations

ACE, angiotensin-converting enzyme; ANA, antinuclear antibody; ANCA, antineutrophil cytoplasmic antibody; CBC, complete blood cell count; CRP, C-reactive protein; CSF, cerebrospinal fluid; CT, computed tomography; EBV, Epstein–Barr virus; ESR, erythrocyte sedimentation rate; FDG, fluorodeoxyglucose; Hb, haemoglobin; HIV, human immunodeficiency virus; HS(A)N, hereditary sensory (and autonomic) neuropathy; IgA, immunoglobulin A; PET, positron emission tomography; SSA, Sjögren syndrome A; SSB, Sjögren syndrome B; TTR, transthyretin.

References

1. Hughes RA. Peripheral neuropathy. *Br Med J* 2002; **324**: 466–9.
2. Biegstraaten M, Mengel E, Marodi L, et al. Peripheral neuropathy in adult type 1 Gaucher disease: a 2-year prospective observational study. *Brain* 2010; **133**: 2909–19.
3. Mendell JR, Kissel JT, Cornblath DR. *Diagnosis and Management of Peripheral Nerve Disorders*. New York: Oxford University Press, 2001.

4. Herskovitz S, Scelsa SN, Schaumburg HH. *Peripheral Neuropathies in Clinical Practice*. New York: Oxford University Press, 2010.

5. Dyck PJ, Thomas PK. *Peripheral Neuropathy*, 4th edn. Philadelphia, PA: Elsevier Saunders, 2005.

6. Holland NR, Crawford TO, Hauer P, Cornblath DR, Griffin JW, McArthur JC. Small-fiber sensory neuropathies: clinical course and neuropathology of idiopathic cases. *Ann Neurol* 1998; **44**: 47–59.

7. Preston DC, Shapiro BE. *Electromyography and Neuromuscular Disorders: Clinical-Electrophysiologic Correlations*, 2nd edn. Boston, MA: Butterworth-Heinemann, 2005.

8. Krishnan AV, Kiernan MC. Uremic neuropathy: clinical features and new pathophysiological insights. *Muscle Nerve* 2007; **35**: 273–90.

9. Savazzi GM, Migone L, Cambi V. The influence of glomerular filtration rate on uremic polyneuropathy. *Clin Nephrol* 1980; **13**: 64–72.

10. Gigli GL, Adorati M, Dolso P, et al. Restless legs syndrome in end-stage renal disease. *Sleep Med* 2004; **5**: 309–15.

11. Said G, Boudier L, Selva J, Zingraff J, Drueke T. Different patterns of uremic polyneuropathy: clinicopathologic study. *Neurology* 1983; **33**: 567–74.

12. Fraser CL, Arieff AI. Nervous system complications in uremia. *Ann Intern Med* 1988; **109**: 143–53.

13. Duyff RF, Van den Bosch J, Laman DM, van Loon BJ, Linssen WH. Neuromuscular findings in thyroid dysfunction: a prospective clinical and electrodiagnostic study. *J Neurol Neurosurg Psychiatry* 2000; **68**: 750–5.

14. Eslamian F, Bahrami A, Aghamohammadzadeh N, Niafar M, Salekzamani Y, Behkamrad K. Electrophysiologic changes in patients with untreated primary hypothyroidism. *J Clin Neurophysiol* 2011; **28**: 323–8.

15. Ellis RJ, Rosario D, Clifford DB, et al. Continued high prevalence and adverse clinical impact of human immunodeficiency virus-associated sensory neuropathy in the era of combination antiretroviral therapy: the CHARTER Study. *Arch Neurol* 2010; **67**: 552–8.

16. Maschke M, Kastrup O, Esser S, Ross B, Hengge U, Hufnagel A. Incidence and prevalence of neurological disorders associated with HIV since the introduction of highly active antiretroviral therapy (HAART). *J Neurol Neurosurg Psychiatry* 2000; **69**: 376–80.

17. Simpson DM. Selected peripheral neuropathies associated with human immunodeficiency virus infection and antiretroviral therapy. *J Neurovirol* 2002; **8** (Suppl 2): 33–41.

18. O'Connell S. Lyme borreliosis: current issues in diagnosis and management. *Curr Opin Infect Dis* 2010; **23**: 231–5.

19. Dandache P, Nadelman RB. Erythema migrans. *Infect Dis Clin North Am* 2008; **22**: 235–60, vi.

20. Mygland A, Ljostad U, Fingerle V, Rupprecht T, Schmutzhard E, Steiner I. EFNS guidelines on the diagnosis and management of European Lyme neuroborreliosis. *Eur J Neurol* 2010; **17**: 8–16.

21. Halperin JJ. Nervous system Lyme disease. *Infect Dis Clin North Am* 2008; **22**: 261–74, vi.

22. Halperin JJ, Shapiro ED, Logigian E, et al. Practice parameter: treatment of nervous system Lyme disease (an evidence-based review): report of the Quality Standards Subcommittee of the American Academy of Neurology. *Neurology* 2007; **69**: 91–102.

23. Koffman BM, Greenfield LJ, Ali II, Pirzada NA. Neurologic complications after surgery for obesity. *Muscle Nerve* 2006; **33**: 166–76.

24. Carlson HB, Anthony EM, Russel WF, Jr, Middlebrook G. Prophylaxis of isoniazid neuropathy with pyridoxine. *N Engl J Med* 1956; **255**: 119–22.

25. Snider DE, Jr. Pyridoxine supplementation during isoniazid therapy. *Tubercle* 1980; **61**: 191–6.

26. Schaumburg H, Kaplan J, Windebank A, et al. Sensory neuropathy from pyridoxine abuse. A new megavitamin syndrome. *N Engl J Med* 1983; **309**: 445–8.

27. Berger AR, Schaumburg HH, Schroeder C, Apfel S, Reynolds R. Dose response, coasting, and differential fiber vulnerability in human toxic neuropathy: a prospective study of pyridoxine neurotoxicity. *Neurology* 1992; **42**: 1367–70.

28. Hemmer B, Glocker FX, Schumacher M, Deuschl G, Lucking CH. Subacute combined degeneration: clinical, electrophysiological, and magnetic resonance imaging findings. *J Neurol Neurosurg Psychiatry* 1998; **65**: 822–7.

29. Pruthi RK, Tefferi A. Pernicious anemia revisited. *Mayo Clin Proc* 1994; **69**: 144–50.

30. Manji H. Toxic neuropathy. *Curr Opin Neurol* 2011; **24**: 484–90.

31. Windebank AJ. Metal neuropathy. In: Dyck PJ, Thomas PK (ed) *Peripheral Neuropathy*, 4th edn, pp. 2527–51. Philadelphia, PA: Elsevier Saunders, 2005.

32. Le Quesne PM, McLeod JG. Peripheral neuropathy following a single exposure to arsenic. Clinical course in four patients with electrophysiological and histological studies. *J Neurol Sci* 1977; **32**: 437–51.

33. Mellion M, Gilchrist JM, de la Monte S. Alcohol-related peripheral neuropathy: nutritional, toxic, or both? *Muscle Nerve* 2011; **43**: 309–16.

34. Antoine JC, Camdessanche JP. Peripheral nervous system involvement in patients with cancer. *Lancet Neurol* 2007; **6**: 75–86.

35. Giometto B, Grisold W, Vitaliani R, Graus F, Honnorat J, Bertolini G. Paraneoplastic neurologic syndrome in the PNS Euronetwork database: a European study from 20 centers. *Arch Neurol* 2010; **67**: 330–5.

36. Titulaer MJ, Soffietti R, Dalmau J, et al. Screening for tumours in paraneoplastic syndromes: report of an EFNS task force. *Eur J Neurol* 2011; **18**: 19-e3.

37. McLeod JG, Tuck RR, Pollard JD, Cameron J, Walsh JC. Chronic polyneuropathy of undetermined cause. *J Neurol Neurosurg Psychiatry* 1984; **47**: 530–5.

38. Notermans NC, Wokke JH, Franssen H, et al. Chronic idiopathic polyneuropathy presenting in middle or old age: a clinical and electrophysiological study of 75 patients. *J Neurol Neurosurg Psychiatry* 1993; **56**: 1066–71.

39. Notermans NC, Wokke JH, Van der GY, Franssen H, van Dijk GW, Jennekens FG. Chronic idiopathic axonal polyneuropathy: a five year follow up. *J Neurol Neurosurg Psychiatry* 1994; **57**: 1525–7.

40. Hughes RA, Umapathi T, Gray IA, et al. A controlled investigation of the cause of chronic idiopathic axonal polyneuropathy. *Brain* 2004; **127**: 1723–30.

41. Vrancken AF, Franssen H, Wokke JH, Teunissen LL, Notermans NC. Chronic idiopathic axonal polyneuropathy and successful aging of the peripheral nervous system in elderly people. *Arch Neurol* 2002; **59**: 533–40.

42. Erdmann PG, Teunissen LL, van Genderen FR, et al. Functioning of patients with chronic idiopathic axonal polyneuropathy (CIAP). *J Neurol* 2007; **254**: 1204–11.

43. Faber CG, Hoeijmakers JG, Ahn HS, et al. Gain of function Na$_v$1.7 mutations in idiopathic small fiber neuropathy. *Ann Neurol* 2012; **71**: 26–39.

44. Faber CG, Lauria G, Merkies IS, et al. Gain-of-function Na$_v$1.8 mutations in painful neuropathy. *Proc Natl Acad Sci USA* 2012; **109**: 19444–9.

45. Sheikh SI, Amato AA. The dorsal root ganglion under attack: the acquired sensory ganglionopathies. *Pract Neurol* 2010; **10**: 326–34.

46. Sghirlanzoni A, Pareyson D, Lauria G. Sensory neuron diseases. *Lancet Neurol* 2005; **4**: 349–61.

CHAPTER 16

Polyneuropathies: demyelinating

Pieter A. van Doorn and Judith Drenthen

General introduction

The most important differences between Guillain–Barré syndrome (GBS), chronic inflammatory demyelinating polyneuropathy (CIDP), multifocal motor neuropathy (MMN), and monoclonal gammopathy of undetermined significance (MGUS) polyneuropathy (MGUSP) are the speed of progression and the severity of disease. Progression of GBS is fast (within days to weeks), intermediate in CIDP (generally at least 2 months), and slow in MMN and in most patients with a paraproteinaemic neuropathy, especially in those with MGUSP. The severity of weakness differs between these disorders. Associated signs of systemic illness can sometimes be found in patients with paraproteinaemic neuropathy. Electrophysiological investigation is essential for the diagnosis, especially in CIDP and MMN, and—if indicated—to separate GBS into the demyelinating (acute inflammatory demyelinating polyneuropathy, AIDP) or axonal (acute motor axonal neuropathy, AMAN) variety. Cerebrospinal fluid (CSF) examination often reveals increased protein in GBS, CIDP, and sometimes in MMN. The courses of disease, the diagnostics including the characteristic electrophysiological findings (see Tables 16.1 and 16.2), and the differential diagnosis and treatment options are discussed.

Electrophysiology

Classically, features of 'demyelination' on electrophysiological examination are presumed to be caused by damage to the myelin sheath. However, in some neuropathies, such as MMN, the 'demyelinating' features might be caused by pathological activity of antibodies at or near the node of Ranvier. The classical features of demyelination are: increased distal motor latency (DML), decreased motor nerve conduction velocity (mNCV), excessive temporal dispersion (TD), and the presence of conduction block (CB). TD is defined as a prolonged duration of the compound muscle action potential (CMAP) on proximal stimulation versus distal stimulation. It is caused by a difference in the conduction times of the slowest and fastest axons within a nerve segment. CB is defined as a reduction in the amplitude (or area) of the CMAP obtained by proximal versus distal stimulation of motor nerves in the absence of abnormal TD. Electrophysiological studies are useful in the diagnostic workup of neuropathies. The electrophysiological studies show differences in the type and distribution of 'demyelinating' abnormalities in the various immune-mediated neuropathies [1]. When a demyelinating neuropathy is suspected, temperature is an important variable to take into account. If the skin temperature is below 32°C, the limbs should preferably be warmed prior to the electrophysiological investigation because this can influence the obtained values.

Guillain–Barré syndrome

Introduction

GBS is a rapidly progressive polyneuropathy that can result in complete paralysis with respiratory failure within 24–48 h. The disorder was first described in 1916 by the French neurologists Guillain, Barré, and Strohl in two soldiers who developed acute paralysis with areflexia and who finally recovered spontaneously [2]. They reported the combination of a raised protein with a normal cell count in the cerebrospinal fluid (CSF), or 'dissociation albuninocytologique', a feature that differentiated GBS from poliomyelitis. The incidence of GBS is 1.2–2.3 per 100 000 per year [3] with a linear increase with age. Men are about 1.5 times more frequently affected than women. There has been substantial progress in our understanding of the immunobiology of GBS over the past years [4–7]. GBS is a post-infectious polyradiculoneuropathy. In about 60% of cases GBS is preceded either by diarrhoea (due to *Campylobacter jejuni*) or by an upper respiratory tract infection 1–3 weeks before onset of weakness [8]. GBS is generally considered to be monophasic, but recurrences are reported in 2–5% of patients [9].

Diagnosis

GBS is a descriptive diagnosis for which there are no specific diagnostic tests. The combination of rapidly progressive, relatively symmetric weakness in the arms and legs with or without sensory disturbances, hypo- or areflexia, in the absence of a CSF cellular reaction, remains the hallmark for diagnosis [10]. In typical cases, among the first symptoms are pain, numbness, paraesthesia, or weakness in the limbs. Pain in GBS is under-recognized. Approximately 30% of patients already have moderate to severe pain 1 week before the onset of weakness. This pain is mainly located at the extremities and the back, and might lead to inappropriate orthopaedic referral and a delay in making the diagnosis.

By definition, the weakness in GBS reaches its maximum within 4 weeks, but most patients have already reached their nadir within 2 weeks. Patients then have a plateau phase of variable duration, ranging from days to several weeks or months. This phase is followed by a recovery phase of variable duration (Fig. 16.1). Cranial

Table 16.1 Speed of progression, severity, signs, cerebrospinal fluid (CSF) protein and electrophysiological examination in the demyelinating polyneuropathies

Disease	Speed of progression	Severity	Motor/sensory	Symmetry	CSF protein	Electrophysiology
GBS	+++	+++	M or M/S	Yes	↑	Demyelinating or axonal
CIDP	++	++	M or M/S	Yes	↑	Demyelinating
MMN	+	+	M (multifocal)	No	(↑)	Motor nerve conduction blocks
IgM anti-MAG MGUSP	+	+	S > M	Yes	–	Increased distal motor latencies
Other MGUSP	+	+	S > M or S	Yes	–	Often mild abnormalities

GBS, Guillain–Barré syndrome; CIDP, chronic inflammatory demyelinating polyneuropathy; MMN, multifocal motor neuropathy; IgM, immunoglobulin M; MGUSP, monoclonal gammopathy of undetermined significance polyneuropathy; MAG, myelin-associated glycoprotein; M, motor; S, sensory; MS, motor and sensory; ↑, increased; –, normal.

Table 16.2 Electrophysiological abnormalities in various immune-mediated neuropathies

Electrophysiological features	AIDP	AMAN/AMSAN	MFS	CIDP	MMN	IgM anti-MAG
DML	↑	N	N	↑	(↑)	↑ ↑
Motor NCV	↓	N	N	↓	(↓)	↓
Motor CB	+	N	N	+	++	(+)
Motor TD	+	N	N	+	(+)	(+)
Distal CMAP amplitude	(↓)	↓	N	(↓)	(↓)	(↓)
Sensory abnormality	+*	+†	(+)	+	N	+

AIDP, acute inflammatory demyelinating polyneuropathy; AMAN, acute motor axonal neuropathy; AMSAN, acute motor and sensory axonal neuropathy; CIDP, chronic inflammatory demyelinating polyneuropathy; MMN, multifocal motor neuropathy; MAG, myelin associated glycoprotein; DML, distal motor latency; NCV, nerve conduction velocity; CB, conduction block; TD, temporal dispersion; CMAP, compound muscle action potential; +, frequently present; N, normal; ↓, decreased; ↑, increased; ++ and ↑ ↑, key feature; symbol between brackets, feature can be present.

*Sometimes sural sparing.

†Abnormal in AMSAN, not in AMAN.

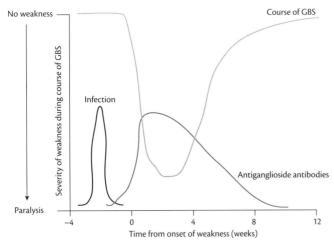

Fig. 16.1 Infections, antiganglioside antibodies and course of disease in Guillain–Barré syndrome (GBS).

nerve palsies, if present, most frequently involve facial palsies (in 25–45% of all GBS cases), 10–15% have swallowing difficulties, and oculomotor weakness occurs in about 5–10%. The diagnostic criteria for typical GBS are shown in Table 16.3. A proposal for GBS criteria especially made for vaccine safety and epidemiological purposes has recently been published [3]. Weakness usually affects all limb muscles equally; however, variants with predominantly distal or proximal weakness exist. If only the legs are involved, other lumbosacral pathology should be excluded (see the section Differential diagnosis). CSF examination is commonly performed in patients suspected of having GBS. Typically, the CSF shows an increased protein content with normal CSF white cell count. If the number of cells is increased (> 50 × 10^6 L^{-1}), other diagnoses should be suspected. Levels of protein in the CSF of GBS patients are often normal in the first week, but are increased in more than 90% of patients at the end of the second week. In Miller Fisher syndrome (MFS) it was shown that the percentage of patients with raised CSF total protein increased from 25% in the first week to 84% in the third week [11,12].

GBS can be divided into AIDP, which is by far the most frequent form in the western world, AMAN, which is much more frequent in Japan and China, acute motor and sensory axonal neuropathy (AMSAN), MFS, and other variants [5,6]. Electrophysiological examination can be helpful to confirm the diagnosis in clinically difficult cases. EMG is required for subclassifying GBS into subgroups like AMAN and AIDP.

Electrophysiological examination in GBS

In AIDP, electrophysiological features are most prominent at 2–3 weeks after onset of weakness. Electrophysiological examination can show features of demyelination (prolonged DML, decreased

Table 16.3 Diagnosis of typical Guillain–Barré syndrome

Features required for diagnosis:
• Progressive weakness in both arms and both legs
• Areflexia (or decreased tendon reflexes)

Features strongly supporting diagnosis:
• Progression of symptoms over days to 4 weeks
• Relative symmetry of symptoms
• Mild sensory symptoms or signs
• Cranial nerve involvement, especially bilateral weakness of facial muscles
• Autonomic dysfunction
• Pain (often present)
• High concentration of protein in cerebrospinal fluid (CSF)
• Typical electrodiagnostic features

Features that should raise doubt about the diagnosis:
• Severe pulmonary dysfunction with limited limb weakness at onset
• Severe sensory signs with limited weakness at onset
• Bladder or bowel dysfunction at onset
• Fever at onset
• Sharp sensory level
• Slow progression with limited weakness without respiratory involvement (consider subacute or chronic inflammatory demyelinating polyneuropathy)
• Marked persistent asymmetry of weakness
• Persistent bladder or bowel dysfunction
• Increased number of mononuclear cells in CSF (> 50 × 10^6 L^{-1})
• Polymorphonuclear cells in CSF

Table adapted from Asbury and Cornblath [10].

NCV, conduction blocks, temporal dispersion, and prolonged F-wave latency) in motor and/or sensory nerves [7]. In early AIDP, however, nerve conduction studies (NCS) may be normal (up to 13%) or non-diagnostic. Roughly 30% of patients have a sural sparing pattern in the early phase of the disease [normal sural sensory nerve action potential (SNAP) with absent or reduced median and ulnar SNAPs]. Needle electromyography (EMG) shows reduced motor unit action potential recruitment. Spontaneous activity, when present, is related to secondary axonal degeneration and is associated with less complete recovery. Over the years, multiple sets of electrophysiological criteria have been developed to identify demyelination in GBS patients [13]. However, no set is universally accepted. Furthermore, criteria for an abnormal study may not always be met, especially in the early disease course or in mildly affected patients. The characteristic electrophysiological features in AM(S)AN are reduced or absent distal CMAPs and the absence of demyelinating features. In AMAN, SNAPs and sensory nerve conductions are normal. The entity is named AMSAN when sensory abnormalities are also present. Classification into AIDP and AMAN is often difficult in the early phase of the disease, since some nerves of AM(S)AN patients can show prolonged DMLs in the early phase. These DMLs resolve rapidly in time, whereas in AIDP they progressively increase [14]. Another presumed entity of AMAN is acute motor CB neuropathy (AMCBN). Electrophysiological studies show reduction of distal CMAP amplitudes and early partial motor CB with normal sensory conductions [15,16].

Miller Fisher syndrome

MFS is a rare variant of GBS, accounting for approximately 5% of cases. Typical MFS presents with the triad of ophthalmoplegia, ataxia, and areflexia. Ataxia predominantly affects the gait and trunk, with the limbs relatively spared. The prognosis of MFS, even without specific treatment, is considered to be relatively good [17,18]. Most patients with MFS have immunoglobulin G (IgG) autoantibodies to the ganglioside GQ1b or GT1a. Some patients have incomplete MFS or initially have cranial nerve dysfunction and subsequently develop weakness in the extremities (MFS–GBS overlap syndrome). If there is severe weakness as in GBS, these patients should be treated as GBS. In typical MFS, electrophysiological examination often shows only mild abnormalities. H-reflexes are absent, and sensory abnormalities may be found. Motor nerve abnormalities, if any, are moderate and might show increased F-wave latency. In MFS–GBS overlap syndrome the motor nerve abnormalities can be more extensive, with features of demyelination and low CMAP amplitudes.

Differential diagnosis of GBS

Generally, diagnosing GBS is not difficult. However, in some cases, and especially in children and in patients presenting with a lot of pain, it can be a challenge (Table 16.4). Studies in preschool children showed that there can be a diagnostic delay because of a refusal to walk and pain in the legs, initially suggesting such as a myopathy, coxitis, or discitis [19,20].

Pain in GBS

Pain is a common and severe symptom in patients with GBS. Recognition of pain is important, especially in patients who are unable to communicate due to intubation. Pain occurs in up to 89% of all patients. Thirty-six per cent of patients experience pain in the 2 weeks preceding the onset of weakness. The pain is mainly located in the extremities and back. The severity of the pain correlates with sensory loss, the severity of the disease at its nadir, and the presence of diarrhoea [21]. In 38% of patients, pain lasts for at least a year. This is more likely in patients who suffered from a more severe form of GBS and in those who had pain in the acute phase [21]. The pathophysiology of pain in GBS is poorly understood. Hypothesized mechanisms include: nerve root swelling giving low back pain or radiating pain in the legs; inflammatory factors that generate pain via the nervi nervorum innervating the nerve trunks; demyelination of large sensory nerve fibres that may cause painful dysaesthesiae; and dysfunction of small nerve fibres, causing burning neuropathic pain. Interestingly, low intra-epidermal nerve fibre density in the acute phase of GBS appears to be associated with the presence and severity of neuropathic pain in the acute phase.

Autonomic failure

Autonomic dysfunction often occurs in GBS [22]. In a prospective study, 39% of patients had tachycardia, 9% bradycardia, 67% hypertension, 11% hypotension, 46% gastrointestinal dysfunction, and 20% bladder dysfunction (L. Ruts, Department of Neurology, Havenziekenhuis, Rotterdam, The Netherlands, personal communication). Recognition of autonomic dysfunction is important because it can result in severe complications and even death. Three to 10% of GBS patients die, presumably partly due to (sudden) autonomic failure. Currently it is not possible to predict which patients will develop serious autonomic failure.

Table 16.4 Differential diagnosis of Guillain–Barré syndrome

Intracranial/spinal cord: Brainstem encephalitis, meningitis carcinomatosis/lymphomatosis, transverse myelitis, cord compression
Anterior horn cells: Poliomyelitis, West Nile virus
Spinal nerve roots: Compression, inflammation (e.g. cytomegalovirus, Lyme borreliosis), leptomeningeal malignancy
Peripheral nerves: Chronic inflammatory demyelinating polyneuropathy, drug-induced neuropathy, porphyria, critical illness polyneuropathy, vasculitis, diphtheria, vitamin B_1 deficiency (beri-beri), heavy metal or drug intoxication, tick paralysis, metabolic disturbances (hypokalaemia, hypophosphataemia, hypermagnesia, hypoglycaemia)
Neuromuscular junction: Myasthenia gravis, botulism, organophosphate poisoning
Muscle: Critical illness polyneuromyopathy, polymyositis, dermatomyositis, acute rhabdomyolysis

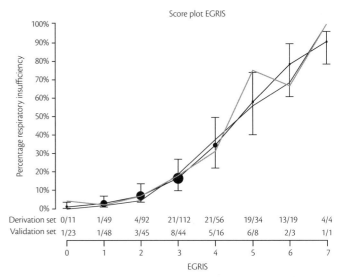

Fig. 16.2 The Erasmus GBS (Guillain–Barré syndrome) respiratory insufficiency score (EGRIS)—the predicted percentage of patients with respiratory insufficiency needing artificial ventilation. (With permission from Walgaard C et al., *Ann Neurol* 2010; **67**: 781–7).

Treatment

General care in GBS

Patients with GBS need multidisciplinary care to prevent and manage potentially fatal complications [22]. Issues that require attention are prophylaxis for deep vein thrombosis, cardiac and haemodynamic monitoring, pain management, management of possible bladder and bowel dysfunction, adequate eye care (especially in case of facial nerve palsy), psychosocial support, and rehabilitation. Since approximately 20–25% of severely involved GBS patients need artificial ventilation, regular measurements of vital capacity and respiratory frequency is required [23]. Timely transfer to an intensive care unit (ICU) should be considered if respiratory function deteriorates. The Erasmus GBS Respiratory Insufficiency Scale (EGRIS) [24] is a simple scale that can be used at hospital admission to predict the chance of needing artificial ventilation, and thus may indicate whether a patient preferentially needs to be admitted to an ICU. Prediction is based upon three simple clinical factors (Fig. 16.2).

Many patients and their relatives benefit from contacting a patients' organization such as the GBS/CIDP Foundation International (<http://www.GBS-CIDP.org>).

Immunotherapy [25]

Plasma exchange (PE) has been proven to be beneficial when applied within the first 4 weeks after onset, but the largest effect was seen when started early (within the first 2 weeks) [26,27]. The usual PE regimen consists of a total exchange of about five plasma volumes in four to six treatments during 2 weeks [28]. The first randomized controlled trial (RCT) on the use of intravenous immunoglobulin (IVIg) (0.4 g IVIg kg^{-1} bodyweight day^{-1} for five consecutive days) was published in 1992, demonstrating that IVIg is as effective as PE [29]. IVIg nowadays has replaced PE as the preferred treatment in many centres, mainly because of its greater convenience and availability. However, IVIg is expensive and may not be ubiquitously available. The Cochrane review on the use of IVIg in GBS showed that there

was no difference between IVIg and PE with respect to the improvement in disability grade after 4 weeks, the duration of mechanical ventilation, mortality, or residual disability [30]. The combination of PE followed by IVIg was not significantly better than PE or IVIg alone [31]. Oral steroids or intravenous methylprednisolone, 500 mg day^{-1} for five consecutive days, alone are not beneficial in GBS [25]. The combination of IVIg and intravenous methylprednisolone was not more effective than IVIg alone, but there might be some additional short-term effect of this combined treatment when a correction was made for known prognostic factors [32]. Although there is an effect of immunotherapy on the course of GBS, new studies aiming to improve short- and long-term outcome, especially in patients who currently still have a poor prognosis, are urgently needed.

Should mildly affected patients be treated?

'Mildly affected' can be arbitrarily defined as still being able to walk. A retrospective study demonstrated that these patients frequently have residual disabilities. RCTs evaluating the effect of IVIg in mildly affected patients are not available [33]. A French trial studied the effect of PE in patients who could walk with or without aid, but not run. Onset of motor recovery was faster in patients who received two PE sessions compared with none [34]. Based on this study there could be an indication to also treat mildly affected GBS patients with PE.

Should patients with MFS be treated?

No RCTs have been performed on the effect of PE or IVIg in patients with MFS [35]. Observational studies suggested that the final outcome in patients with MFS is generally good [36].

What to do if a patient continues to deteriorate after treatment?

A proportion of GBS patients continue to deteriorate after PE or a standard course of IVIg. In these cases, and in other patients with a poor prognosis, it is unknown whether additional treatment should be given. A small open study suggested that a repeated course of IVIg might be effective in severe unresponsive GBS patients. Whether a second course of IVIg is effective in a selected group of severely affected GBS patients is currently being investigated.

What to do if a patient deteriorates after initial improvement?

About 10% of GBS patients deteriorate after initial improvement or stabilization following IVIg treatment ('treatment-related clinical fluctuation') [37]. Although no RCT has evaluated the effect of a repeated IVIg course in this condition, it is common practice to give a second IVIg course (2 g kg^{-1} in 2–5 days) since these patients are likely to improve after reinitiating IVIg. It is considered that these patients may have a prolonged immune response that causes ongoing nerve damage needing treatment for a longer period of time. Some of these GBS patients may even have several episodes of deterioration. This often raises the question of whether these patients have GBS or CIDP with acute onset (A-CIDP) (Fig. 16.3). A-CIDP should be suspected when patients have three or more deteriorations or when they have a subsequent deterioration after 8 weeks from onset of GBS [37]. Once it is clear that the patient has A-CIDP, treatment for CIDP should be initiated.

Prognosis and chronic symptoms of GBS

About one-third of GBS patients remain able to walk independently; this condition can be considered as relatively 'mild GBS'. About 20–25% of those with 'severe GBS' require artificial ventilation despite treatment with IVIg or PE. Additionally about 20% of the 'severe GBS' patients are unable to walk unaided after 6 months. The prognosis for independent walking can be determined early in the course of disease using the modified Erasmus Guillain–Barré Outcome Score (mEGOS) (Fig. 16.4) [38,39]. Sixty to 80% of patients report severe fatigue, even years after disease onset [40]. A 12-week programme of bicycle exercise training was likely to be effective in severely fatigued but neurologically well recovered GBS and stable CIDP patients [41]. A RCT, however, is still awaited. Furthermore, 3–6 years after onset many patients still experience a great impact on their social life and ability to perform daily activities [42]. More than a third of patients have moderate to severe pain for at least 1 year after onset [21]. So far, there is no clue about how to prevent pain, and controlled studies on how to treat the different forms of pain in chronic GBS are lacking. It seems advisable to treat neuropathic pain in GBS in the same way as pain in other polyneuropathies.

Immunobiology

Studies in humans and animals have convincingly shown that GBS, at least in specific subgroups, is caused by an infection-induced aberrant immune response against peripheral nerves [4,5,7,43]. A substantial number of patients have serum antiganglioside antibodies.

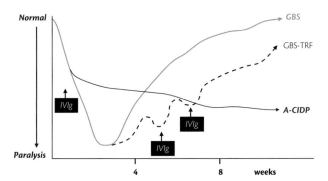

Fig. 16.3 Guillain–Barré syndrome (GBS), treatment-related fluctuations (TRF) and acute-onset chronic inflammatory demyelinating polyneuropathy (A-CIDP) (IVIg, intravenous immunoglobulin).

These antibodies are directed against lipo-oligosaccharide (LOS) structures on microorganisms such as *Campylobacter jejuni* and cross-react with peripheral nerves [5,44]. This may induce complement activation and destruction of nerves, and antibody activity against sodium channels [4,5,45]. In an animal model for GBS this cascade could be prevented when complement activation was blocked with eculizumab [46].

Immunopathological differences were found between GBS patients with AIDP and AMAN. In AIDP, the presumed mode of action is the binding of autoantibodies to myelin antigens and activation of complement on the outer surface of Schwann cells, leading to vesicular degeneration of myelin [47]. So far, no specific antibodies against single gangliosides related to the AIDP variant have been identified, but recent studies have shown that antibodies to various ganglioside complexes are probably involved.* Antiganglioside antibodies are predominantly found in GBS patients with oculomotor disturbances, in AMAN, and in MFS. In patients with AMAN, IgG anti-GM1 or GD1a autoantibodies bind to the nodal axolemma and activate complement. Subsequently this can lead to the destruction of sodium channel clusters, detachment of the paranodal myelin, and axonal degeneration, with invasion of macrophages into the periaxonal space [5,47]. In MFS patients, antibodies against the gangliosides GQ1b and GT1a are involved. The GQ1b epitope is expressed mainly in the paranodal regions of the extramedullary portion of the cranial nerves involved in ocular movement, compatible with the neurological findings in these patients. Although about one person in a thousand develops GBS after *C. jejuni* diarrhoea, real outbreaks of GBS do not occur. The specific genetic *C. jejuni* type does not fully determine whether someone gets GBS. Additionally, there is a great variability in the symptoms and severity of GBS, implying that host factors—such as single nucleotide polymorphisms (SNPs)—also play a role in the cascade of the immune response in GBS [5,43,48].*

Future directions

New treatment options for GBS are needed because the prognosis in many patients is still poor. Studies on the effect of a second IVIg course in patients with a poor prognosis based upon the mEGOS are ongoing [38,39].

Recent experiments indicate that agents that interfere with complement activation are potentially attractive candidates for testing in GBS [46]. Since it is now possible to more accurately predict a poor outcome in individual patients, new drugs or regimens could be tested especially in this restricted GBS population. New trials investigating less aggressive treatments are also needed for mildly affected patients, and possibly also for patients with MFS. More attention should be paid to pain, autonomic dysfunction, and severe fatigue, which are serious and often not well-recognized symptoms.

Chronic inflammatory demyelinating polyneuropathy

Introduction

By definition, in CIDP the symptoms of weakness and often also sensory disturbances develop over a period of at least 8 weeks

*That work has been published since this chapter was completed. See Rinaldi S, Brennan KM, Kalna G, et al. Antibodies to heteromeric glycolipid complexes in Guillain–Barré syndrome. *PloS One* 2013; **8**(12): e82337, doi: 10.1371/journal.pone.0082337.

Predicted probability to be unable to walk

at 4 weeks, 3 and 6 months according to mEGOS (n = 394)

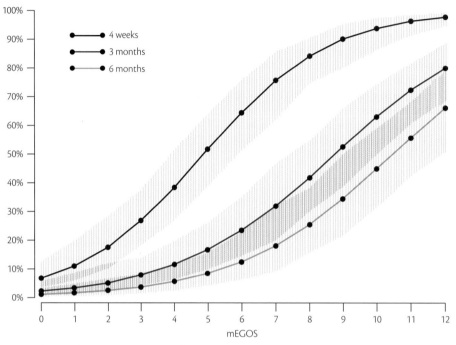

Fig. 16.4 The modified Erasmus Guillain–Barré Outcome Score (mEGOS). Predicted fraction of patients unable to walk independently at 4 weeks (black lines), 3 months (dark green lines), and 6 months (light green lines) on the basis of the mEGOS at day 7 of admission. The grey areas around the coloured lines represent 90% confidence intervals. (With permission from Walgaard C et al., *Neurology* 2011; **76**: 968–75)

[49,50]. Some patients, however, have a faster onset similar to GBS, and are diagnosed as A-CIDP [37]. CIDP may have a chronic progressive, stepwise progressive, or relapsing–remitting course. There are several sets of criteria available for the diagnosis of CIDP [49–51]. These criteria rest upon a combination of clinical, electrophysiological, and laboratory features, particularly used to exclude some other disorders that may appear as CIDP. CIDP is a treatable disorder. IVIg, steroids, and PE are effective in the majority of patients. Most patients require long-term treatment for at least 6 months to several years [52]. The precise pathophysiological cause of CIDP is not well known. There is a continuing debate about whether CIDP can be considered as the chronic form of GBS [53]. Diagnostic criteria for CIDP are provided in Tables 16.5–16.7.

Diagnosis

The diagnosis of CIDP may be challenging [50]. Typical CIDP is characterized by symmetric proximal and distal weakness and sensory dysfunction of the arms and legs and reduced or absent tendon reflexes. The symptoms have a chronically progressive, stepwise, or recurrent course, developing over at least 2 months. The typical presentation of symmetric weakness and sensory disturbances occurs in approximately 80% of cases. Pure motor CIDP occurs in fewer than 5% of cases; pure sensory CIDP is much rarer and is described in isolated case reports. About 10–15% of CIDP patients initially have a course that mimics (usually less severe) GBS [37,54]. The diagnosis of CIDP is generally based on clinical features and electrophysiological studies. CSF examination, and sometimes a nerve biopsy, or magnetic resonance (MR) examinations of the

spinal roots, brachial plexus, and lumbosacral plexus may provide supportive information, but these are not required for diagnosis. Analysis of the CSF often reveals an elevated protein content with normal cell count. Magnetic resonance imaging (MRI) might show swelling of the brachial and/or lumbar plexuses with increased signal intensity on T_2-weighted images with or without contrast enhancement. In the diagnostic workup, blood tests need to be done to detect/exclude concomitant disease. It is recommended to test for serum and urine paraproteins, fasting glucose, complete blood count, renal function, liver function, antinuclear factor, and thyroid function [50]. If clinically indicated, other tests such as *Borrelia burgdorferi* serology, HIV, lues serology, extractable nuclear antigen antibodies, angiotensin-converting enzyme, DNA (especially *PMP22* duplication and connexin 32 mutations) to detect hereditary neuropathy, or a nerve biopsy (usually not indicated) can be performed [50].

Electrophysiological examination

Electrodiagnostic examination requires features of demyelination to diagnose CIDP. Electrophysiological investigation usually shows symmetrical, multifocal features of demyelination in arm and leg nerves. These features are increased DML, decreased mNCV, TD, and CB (Fig. 16.5). Typically, both sensory and motor nerve examinations are abnormal, but pure motor forms and pure sensory forms exist. For the diagnosis of CIDP, several sets of clinical and electrophysiological criteria for demyelination are available. They are based on the presence of the various demyelinating features. In patients with longer disease duration, more demyelinating features appear

Table 16.5 Clinical diagnostic criteria for chronic inflammatory demyelinating polyneuropathy (CIDP)

Inclusion criteria:

(a) Typical CIDP

- Chronic progressive, stepwise, or recurrent symmetric proximal and distal weakness and sensory dysfunction of all extremities, generally developing over at least 2 months; cranial nerves may be affected
- Absent or reduced tendon reflexes in all extremities

(b) Atypical CIDP (still considered CIDP)

- Predominantly distal (DADS without paraprotein)
- Asymmetric (MADSAM) or Lewis-Sumner syndrome
- Pure motor or pure sensory

Exclusion criteria:

- Prominent sphincter disturbance
- *Borrelia burgdorferi*, drug or toxin exposure (e.g. amiodarone), diphtheria
- Hereditary demyelinating neuropathy (especially CMT1A)
- Multifocal motor neuropathy
- IgM anti-MAG monoclonal gammopathy
- Other causes for demyelinating neuropathy including POEMS, osteosclerotic myeloma, lumbosacral radiculoplexus neuropathy, PNS lymphoma, amyloidosis

DADS, distal acquired demyelinating symmetric polyneuropathy; MADSAM, multifocal acquired demyelinating sensory and motor neuropathy; CMT1A, Charcot–Marie–Tooth Type 1A; IgM, immunoglobulin M; MAG, myelin-associated glycoprotein; POEMS, polyneuropathy, organomegaly, endocrinopathy, monoclonal protein, and skin changes; PNS, peripheral nervous system.

Adapted from European Federation of Neurological Societies/Peripheral Nerve Society CIDP guideline [50].

on electrophysiological examination. But secondary axonal loss also occurs in later phases. In early phases, diagnosing CIDP can sometimes be difficult. More extensive electrophysiological investigation, such as excitability testing and somatosensory evoked potentials might reveal abnormalities that point to demyelination [55].

Treatment of CIDP

Three treatments have proven to be effective in CIDP: steroids [56–58], PE [59], and IVIg [60]. There is no clear preference for steroids over IVIg. PE is a much more invasive treatment and is generally

Table 16.6 Electrodiagnostic criteria for chronic inflammatory demyelinating polyneuropathy

Definite (at least one of the following):

- Prolonged distal motor latency
- Reduced motor conduction velocity
- Prolonged F-wave latency or absent F-waves
- Partial conduction block
- Abnormal temporal dispersion
- Increase in duration of distal compound muscle action potential

Probable:

- Less prominent criteria present in at least two nerves

Possible:

- Less prominent criteria in only one nerve

Adapted from European Federation of Neurological Societies/Peripheral Nerve Society CIDP guideline [50].

Table 16.7 Supportive criteria for chronic inflammatory demyelinating polyneuropathy (CIDP)

CSF protein elevated and leucocytes < 30 × 10^6 L^{-1}
MRI gadolinium enhancement and/or hypertrophy of cauda equina, nerve roots, or plexus
Abnormal sensory electrophysiology
Clinical improvement following immunomodulatory treatment
Nerve biopsy (usually not indicated) showing demyelination and/or remyelination

CSF, cerebrospinal fluid; MRI, magnetic resonance imaging.

Adapted from European Federation of Neurological Societies/Peripheral Nerve Society CIDP guideline [50].

considered as a second- or third-line option. Currently, there is no evidence that other treatments are effective in CIDP [61,62].

Steroids

The advantages of steroids are their availability and low initial cost, but side effects can be serious. Trials investigating the use of steroids in CIDP have focused on relatively short (6 weeks) or intermediate (6 months) treatment durations [57,58,63–65]. Side effects during this period were generally mild, but in some patients treatment side effects necessitated discontinuation of treatment. Recent RCTs did not prove, but seem to indicate, that patients treated with pulse dose steroids (monthly oral dexamethasone 40 mg day^{-1} for four consecutive days; or monthly intravenous methylprednisolone 500 mg day^{-1} for four consecutive days) might have a higher chance of achieving remission than with standard dose prednisolone (starting with 60 mg day^{-1}, slowly tapering over at least 6 months) or treatment with IVIg [57,58]. A follow-up study found that patients receiving pulse steroid treatment not only had a faster improvement than with standard prednisolone treatment, but also had slightly longer remissions, relative fewer relapses, and fewer adverse events [65]. Since a lot of patients require steroids for many months it is advocated to start osteoporosis prophylaxis at or shortly after start of steroids, especially in the elderly population. Note that patients with a pure motor form of CIDP may deteriorate within days after starting treatment with steroids for reasons that are still unknown.

Plasma exchange

PE is effective, but clear disadvantages are its limited availability, high cost, and the relatively invasive procedure [59]. Patients treated with PE may improve rapidly, but need regular treatment to avoid clinical deterioration. In severe cases a suggested PE regimen starts with five sessions in 2 weeks, followed by one PE session every other week. PE is generally not the first choice of treatment, but could be an effective option, e.g. in patients with severe diabetes (contraindication for steroids) or when IVIg is not available. Some patients may require a combination of treatments, e.g. steroids and PE, in order to achieve a relatively good clinical condition.

Immunoglobulins

Immunoglobulins can be administered intravenously (IVIg) or subcutaneously (SCIg). Trials in CIDP have investigated IVIg (starting with 2.0 g kg^{-1} bodyweight administered over 2–5 days), and showed that IVIg is an effective treatment [60]. The overall response rate varies between 50 and 80% [60,65–71]. About 15% of

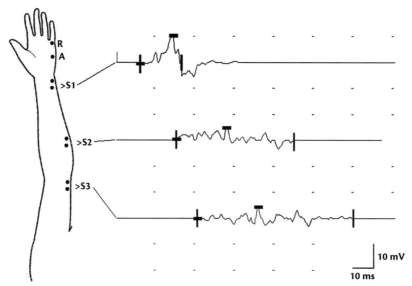

Fig. 16.5 Ulnar motor nerve conduction study in a patient with severe chronic inflammatory demyelinating polyneuropathy, showing prolonged distal motor latency, decreased motor nerve conduction velocity (mNCV) and temporal dispersion. When the ulnar nerve is stimulated at more proximal sites (S1→S2→ S3), compound muscle action potentials (CMAPs) of increasing latency are recorded. The distal motor latency is increased (12.8 ms). The mNCV is 14 m s^{-1} in the forearm and 8 m s^{-1} over the elbow. CMAP amplitudes are 1.1 mV at the wrist and 0.6 mV at the distal and proximal elbow. The duration of the CMAP is 21 ms at the wrist, 59 ms at the distal elbow, and 79 ms at the proximal elbow (temporal dispersion).

patients treated with one or two courses of IVIg remain in remission [70]. Whether this occurred spontaneously or was induced by treatment is not known. IVIg generally acts quickly (within 7–14 days), although in the ICE trial about half of patients needed at least two courses of IVIg before an effect on the modified INCAT disability score could be measured [67,72]. The vast majority of patients need intermittent IVIg treatment (with a frequency of once every 2–4 weeks) during many months or several years to maintain the improvement. Since administration of IVIg requires good vascular access, long-term IVIg treatment might cause problems in some patients. Furthermore, IVIg treatment is expensive. On the other hand, IVIg in general is well tolerated and has only a few and mostly mild infusion-related side effects [73]. Serious adverse effects are rare and can include thromboembolic events, renal failure (mainly in patients with pre-existing renal failure), anaphylaxis (especially in patients with IgA deficiency), or aseptic meningitis.

Small studies also described a positive effect of SCIg in patients with CIDP [74,75]. The effect of SCIg is now being evaluated in RCTs. The rationale is the notion that SCIg might be more convenient for patients and might induce much more stable serum IgG levels. Whether these RCTs show that SCIgG is effective in CIDP, and whether patients benefit from more stable IgG levels, is awaited.

Comparison between steroids, plasma exchange, and IVIg

IVIg, PE, and steroids are effective in CIDP. IVIg and PE are equally effective when compared in a single-blind, controlled crossover trial of CIDP patients assigned to a 6-week course of PE or IVIg (0.2–0.4 g kg^{-1} administered weekly) [76]. A randomized double-blind, crossover trial showed that IVIg (2 g kg^{-1} given over 1 or 2 days) is not significantly better than oral prednisolone during a treatment period of 6 weeks (tapered from 60 to 10 mg daily during that period) [64]. The treatment duration in this trial, however, was too short to make a judgement about differences in side effects. A RCT comparing IVIg 0.5 g kg^{-1} day^{-1} for 4 days with pulsed methylprednisolone 0.5 g for 4 days given every month for 6 months showed that IVIg was less frequently discontinued because of inefficacy, adverse events, or intolerance compared with intravenous methylprednisolone [58]. Also, IVIg acted more quickly than intravenous methylprednisolone. However, when the treatment was stopped after 6 months, significantly more patients who were on IVIg worsened and required further therapy compared with the methylprednisolone-treated patients. Therefore, if one aims to induce remission, pulsed high-dose steroid treatment may be advocated above IVIg. However, if a fast response needs to be achieved, or when side effects of steroids are seriously feared, IVIg (or PE) seems to be the preferred treatment. For pure motor CIDP, IVIg treatment should be the first choice, and if corticosteroids are used patients should be monitored closely for deterioration.

Management of IVIg treatment during long-term follow-up

In most IVIg studies, patients are initially treated with a total dose of 2 g IVIg kg^{-1} administered in fractions over 2–5 days. Based on the published studies and on our experience, it seems that clinical improvement after IVIg in general can be judged within 7–14 days after starting treatment. Some patients, however, may require a second dose of IVIg before clear improvement can be observed. When a CIDP patient improves after IVIg, there seems to be a small but significant chance (about 15%) that no further treatment will then be needed. The vast majority (about 85%) will need repeated administration of IVIg to maintain the improved condition. It is important to regularly test whether a patient on IVIg treatment still needs IVIg (at least once every 4–6 months). Mainly because of a short treatment interval, and sometimes very high IVIg dosages, it may be necessary to eventually add an immunosuppressive drug. However, is it not known which drug is (most) effective.

Potentially effective agents

Over the years smaller non-controlled studies have reported positive effects of immunosuppressive agents such as azathioprine, cyclosporine, interferon-beta, methotrexate, or mycophenolate.

A Cochrane analysis concluded that there is inadequate evidence to ascertain whether, azathioprine, or any other immunosuppressive drug, is beneficial in CIDP [61]. Therefore, there is an urgent need for trials evaluating the effect of immunosuppressive or immunomodulatory drugs in CIDP [53,77–79]. One parallel group open study of azathioprine for 9 months involving 27 participants did not show a positive effect [80]. A potential problem in evaluating a new drug can be selection bias, when only patients who are refractory to standard treatments are included in such studies.

Prognostic factors related to improvement

A better outcome is related to younger age at onset, relapsing–remitting course, and absence of axonal damage [81]. We have recently reviewed a series of over 140 CIDP patients and found that all patients with a relapsing course improved after IVIg treatment (P. A. van Doorn, Erasmus MC, Rotterdam, the Netherlands, personal communication). Most studies suggest that axonal degeneration is a poor prognostic factor for improvement after immunomodulatory treatment. It is not known whether treatment can diminish the long-term axonal degeneration that typically accompanies disease progression.

Timing of treatment

Once the diagnosis of CIDP is clear, immunomodulatory treatment should be initiated when the patient exceeds a certain level of disability. Some patients have minor symptoms. In these patients spontaneous recovery can be awaited. Besides medication, attention has to be paid to rehabilitation and managing symptoms such as foot drop, fatigue, and pain. One study indicates that a well-structured physical training programme, three times a week for 12 consecutive weeks, can help to reduce severe fatigue and improve quality of life in GBS but possibly also in patients with CIDP [41].

Lewis–Sumner syndrome

Multifocal acquired demyelinating sensory and motor neuropathy (MADSAM), also known as Lewis–Sumner syndrome (LSS), is a rare multifocal acquired immune-mediated neuropathy [82]. This disorder presents with asymmetrical weakness and sensory loss, and is worse in the arms. Besides the asymmetric and focal distribution, it is rather similar to CIDP in its symptoms and response to treatment. LSS is usually treated with corticosteroids or IVIg. Differentiation from MMN (see the section Multifocal motor neuropathy) is important because LSS often responds to corticosteroids whereas MMN may worsen [83].

Electrophysiological examination shows multifocal and asymmetrical demyelinating features in both sensory and motor nerves. The predominant feature is persistent CB. However, other signs of segmental demyelination, such as segmental conduction slowing and TD, are typically seen, even in clinically unaffected nerves [84]. To demonstrate a CB can be a challenge since some lesions may be proximal or in nerves that are difficult to stimulate. Less conventional electrophysiological techniques, such as nerve-root stimulation, magnetic stimulation, inching techniques, and use of F-wave studies, may be required to convincingly demonstrate CB.

Multifocal motor neuropathy

Introduction

MMN is a rare inflammatory neuropathy characterized by chronic slowly progressive asymmetric, predominantly distal, limb weakness without sensory loss [85–87] (Table 16.8). The age of onset may be wide (between 20 and 75 years). However, in almost 80% of patients, the first symptoms appear before the age of 50. Men are affected more commonly than women, with an approximate male:female ratio of 2.7:1. Typically there is weakness without significant wasting in early disease (in contrast to lower motor neuron-predominant amyotrophic lateral sclerosis). MMN is a treatable disorder and should be differentiated from motor neuron disorders and other immune-mediated neuropathies. The low incidence of MMN (0.6 per 100.000) makes it difficult to conduct proper clinical trials. Although the underlying pathological mechanisms of MMN are unclear, MMN is considered to be an immune-mediated neuropathy: IgM anti-GM1 antibodies are present in between 30 and 80% of MMN patients, MRI changes may demonstrate swollen nerve roots, and most patients improve after IVIg. Although in the majority of MMN patients IgM anti-GM1 antibodies are present, they are not specific for MMN [88]. Anti-GM1 antibodies have been reported to occur in other dysimmune neuropathies are well. These antibodies may cause changes in the nodal and perinodal structures leading to conduction failure.

Diagnosis

There are several sets of diagnostic criteria. In the European Federation of Neurological Societies/Peripheral Nerve Society (EFNS/PNS) guideline, the occurrence of abnormalities compatible with MMN in at least two motor nerves is required [86], though others advocate that these abnormalities only need to be present in at least one motor nerve [85]. Electrophysiological assessment is essential for diagnosing MMN. Other supportive criteria are elevated IgM antiganglioside GM1 antibodies, increased CSF protein (<1 g L^{-1}), MRI showing increased signal on T_2-weighted imaging and nerve swelling of the brachial plexus, and objective clinical improvement following IVIg treatment [85,86].

Symptoms

Weakness usually starts in the forearm or hand muscles, but the first symptoms may present in the distal leg (in up to 25% of cases).

Table 16.8 Clinical criteria for multifocal motor neuropathy

Core criteria:
- Slowly or stepwise progressive, focal, asymmetric limb weakness. Motor involvement in at least two nerves*
- No objective sensory abnormalities (minor vibration sense abnormalities in lower limbs may be present)

Supportive clinical criteria:
- Predominant upper limb involvement
- Decreased or absent tendon reflexes in affected limb
- Absence of cranial nerve involvement
- Cramps or fasciculations in affected limb
- Response to immunomodulatory treatment

Exclusion criteria:
- Upper motor neuron signs
- Marked bulbar involvement
- Sensory involvement (more than the second core criterion)
- Diffuse symmetric weakness during initial phase of disease

*It has been suggested that abnormalities need to be present in at least one nerve, if otherwise typical features [85].

Criteria adapted from the EFNS guideline [86].

Almost all patients with symptom onset in the legs eventually develop weakness in the arms. In the first years after onset, muscle atrophy is usually mild compared with weakness. However, in patients with longer disease duration muscle atrophy can be more substantial. Other motor symptoms include cramps and fasciculations, which are reported in more than half of patients. Tendon reflexes are normally low or absent in weakened muscles, although normal and brisk reflexes may be found in up to 15% of patients. Typically there is no involvement of cranial nerves [85,86].

MMN has a steadily progressive disease course with a gradual decline in muscle strength, despite the beneficial effects of treatment with IVIg [85,86]. Remission is very uncommon. Severe functional impairment of the arms is reported by 20% of patients, and severe fatigue that interferes with activities of daily living is experienced by more than half of patients. Patients do not develop weakness of the respiratory muscles and have a normal life expectancy.

Electrophysiological examination

MMN is electrophysiologically characterized by the presence of persistent, multifocal, (partial) CBs in motor nerves outside the usual sites of nerve compression [89] (Fig. 16.6). Besides CBs, other features of demyelination can also be observed, e.g. increased TD, nerve conduction slowing, and low distal CMAPs (due to distal CB). In addition, features of secondary axonal degeneration can be found (i.e. needle EMG abnormalities and decreased distal compound muscle action), but not as profusely present as in motor neuron disorders. Sensory conduction is normal, and also in segments of motor CB. Electrophysiological abnormalities are most likely to be found in long motor nerves of the arms (median and ulnar nerves) and are more often present in nerves innervating weakened muscles. Yet approximately one-third of the electrophysiological abnormalities are found in nerves innervating non-weakened muscles [90].

Treatment

Intravenous or subcutaneous immunoglobulin

IVIg is effective in most patients, and is the treatment of choice in MMN [86,91–94]. The effect of IVIg, however, may decline over years and many patients develop progressive symptoms due to axonal degeneration [95]. It is suggested that early IVIg treatment may prevent axonal degeneration to a certain extent. The treatment regime is more or less the same as in CIDP.

In one randomized, single-blinded trial and in a few open-label studies SCIg seemed to be effective [96]. These studies suggested that SCIg is feasible, safe, and therapeutically equivalent to IVIg. However, large controlled studies are currently lacking.

Steroids and PE

Steroids are ineffective, and can even worsen the symptoms of MMN (as in pure motor CIDP) [85,86]. Surprisingly, PE is not effective in patients with MMN [85,86].

Other immunosuppressive agents

Small studies have described improvement of weakness upon administration of cyclophosphamide. This treatment, however, is toxic and not appealing to use in this chronic condition. Also, larger studies are lacking [97,98]. Several other immunosuppressive therapies have been investigated in small, open-labelled studies. Uncontrolled studies have suggested beneficial effects of interferon-beta, cyclosporine, methotrexate, azathioprine, and mycophenolate in some patients with MMN. A RCT, however, did not show a positive effect of mycophenolate [99]. Treatment with a monoclonal antibody against complement C5 (eculizumab) in an open study in 13 MMN patients being treated with IVIg showed that the drug could be administered safely in conjunction with IVIg, but did not indicate that eculizumab could reduce the IVIg dosage [100]. Several small studies have tested

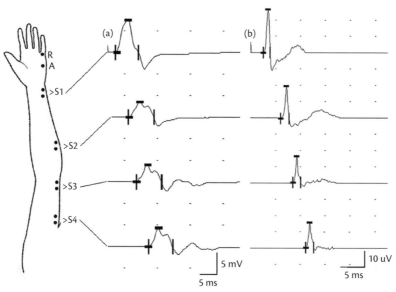

Fig. 16.6 Ulnar motor and sensory nerve conduction study in a patient with multifocal motor neuropathy. When the ulnar nerve is stimulated at more proximal sites (S1→S2→S3→S4), compound muscle action potentials (CMAPs) and sensory nerve action potentials of increasing latency are recorded. (a) Motor nerve conduction velocity is 38 m s^{-1} in the forearm; 48 m s^{-1} over the elbow and 47 m s^{-1} in the upper arm. CMAP amplitudes are 7.5 mV at the wrist, 3.6 mV at the distal elbow, 3.6 mV at the proximal elbow, and 3.7 mV at the axilla. The reduction of CMAP amplitude over the forearm is consistent with a conduction block. (b) Sensory nerve conduction study is normal, there is no conduction block over the forearm. (NB: note the different scaling.)

rituximab as a treatment for MMN, both as monotherapy and as add-on treatment. The results from these studies are inconsistent [85,86,98].

Future directions

To guide the search for new effective treatments for patients with MMN, new studies investigating the (immuno)pathology and pathophysiology are eagerly awaited. Future treatment strategies should particularly aim to prevent axon loss.

Paraproteinaemic neuropathies

Introduction

Patients with a paraproteinaemic neuropathy clinically often have a distal acquired demyelinating symmetric polyneuropathy (DADS) [101]. This heterogeneous group of neuropathies is most frequently associated with the presence of a MGUS. A monoclonal gammopathy, however, can also occur in the context of malignancy such as Waldenström macroglobulinaemia, plasmocytoma, multiple myeloma, primary amyloidosis, or in POEMS (polyneuropathy, organomegaly, endocrinopathy, monoclonal protein, and skin changes) [102]. Therefore, patients with a paraproteinaemic neuropathy should be investigated for a malignant plasma cell dyscrasia The coexistence of a polyneuropathy and a monoclonal gammopathy represents a relatively common but complex problem [103]. In older patients in particular it is often not clear whether an IgG monoclonal protein is associated with the polyneuropathy because the prevalence of these monoclonal proteins increases with age. MGUS is more likely to be causing the neuropathy if the paraprotein is IgM, especially when antibodies against myelin-associated glycoprotein (MAG) can be detected and the clinical phenotype is a chronic distal sensory or sensorimotor neuropathy.

What to do with a positive paraprotein result in the neuromuscular clinic

Patients with a chronic polyneuropathy in which a paraprotein has been detected, usually with immunoelectrophoresis or immunofixation, require further investigation. The question is whether or not the paraprotein is related pathogenically to the polyneuropathy. First, it is important to have information about both the heavy (IgM, IgG, or IgA) and light (kappa or lambda) chains. In relatively younger patients, or with an IgM paraprotein plus antibodies against MAG, and prolonged distal latencies with EMG examination, there is a much higher chance that the paraprotein is related to the polyneuropathy. All patients with a monoclonal protein should be asked for 'B-symptoms' (like weight loss, night sweating, loss of appetite). The following should be considered in patients with a paraprotein [102]:

1. Physical examination for peripheral lymphadenopathy, hepatosplenomegaly, macroglossia, and signs of POEMS syndrome (see the section POEMS).

2. Total IgG, IgA, and IgM concentrations, random urine collection for detection of Bence-Jones protein (free light chains).

3. Additional blood tests including a full blood count, renal and liver function, calcium, phosphate, erythrocyte sedimentation rate, C-reactive protein, uric acid, beta 2-microglobulin, lactate dehydrogenase, rheumatoid factor, serum cryoglobulins.

4. Radiographic skeletal survey and CT of chest, abdomen, and pelvis (to detect lymphadenopathy, hepatosplenomegaly, or malignancy).

5. Serum vascular endothelial growth factor (VEGF) levels if POEMS syndrome is suspected.

In our clinic a haematologist is consulted for all patients with a chronic polyneuropathy and a paraprotein to evaluate the presence of a malignant plasma cell dyscrasia. If a malignant plasma cell dyscrasia is suspected a more extensive workup is required, which includes bone marrow examination.

In patients with MGUS the serum level of the paraprotein and the IgG, IgM, and IgA concentrations should be checked at least yearly and even more frequently when B-symptoms, a sudden worsening of the polyneuropathy, or any other suspicion for a higher risk of malignant transformation are present [102].

Monoclonal gammopathy of undetermined significance

MGUS can only be diagnosed when there is no indication of a haematological malignancy. MGUS accounts for two-thirds of paraproteinaemic neuropathies [104].

IgG or IgA MGUS

IgG or IgA MGUS is defined by the presence of all of the following [102]:

1. serum monoclonal component ≤ 30 g L^{-1}

2. Bence-Jones proteinuria ≤ 1 g per 24 h

3. no lytic or sclerotic lesions in bone

4. no anaemia, hypercalcaemia, or chronic renal insufficiency

5. bone marrow plasma cell infiltration <10%.

Neuropathic findings in patients with an IgG or IgA MGUS are heterogeneous, but can also be similar to CIDP. In patients with a CIDP-like neuropathy, the detection of IgG or IgA MGUS does not justify a different therapeutic approach from CIDP without a paraprotein [105].

Electrophysiological examination can show abnormalities of the motor nerves, sensory nerves, or both and it can show features of demyelination, axonal loss, or both [106].

IgM MGUS

IgM MGUS is defined by the presence of both of the following [102]:

1. no lymphoplasmacytic infiltration on bone marrow biopsy, or equivocal infiltration with negative phenotypic studies

2. no signs or symptoms suggesting tumour infiltration (e.g. constitutional symptoms, hyperviscosity syndrome, organomegaly).

Patients with IgM paraproteinaemic demyelinating neuropathy usually have predominantly distal, chronic (duration over 6 months), slowly progressive, symmetric, predominantly sensory impairment with ataxia, relatively mild or no weakness, and often a tremor. Especially when there are clearly prolonged distal motor latencies it is most strongly associated with the presence of IgM anti-MAG antibodies. IgM anti-MAG neuropathy may respond to immunomodulatory therapies. A RCT suggested a response to the combination of cyclophosphamide and steroids [107]. A recent Cochrane review concluded that there is inadequate reliable evidence from trials of immunotherapies in anti-MAG neuropathy to form an evidence-based conclusion supporting any particular immunotherapy treatment [108]. The publication of a large RCT on the use of rituximab is eagerly awaited.

The electrophysiological hallmark of IgM anti-MAG polyneuropathy is generalized demyelinative slowing, mainly located in the distal segments and more marked in the lower limbs [109]. The increase in distal motor latency is disproportionate to the proximal NCV. This can be demonstrated by several standardized electrophysiological measures, including the terminal latency index. Sensory responses are often attenuated or absent.

Amyloidosis

The presence of a MGUS with a painful (mostly axonal) neuropathy, autonomic disturbances, weight loss, macroglossia, an enlarged liver or spleen, or a cardiomyopathy should point to the presence of amyloidosis (see Chapter 10). The diagnosis rests on the demonstration of amyloid in liver, nerve, or abdominal fat [102,103].

POEMS

Polyneuropathy, organomegaly, endocrinopathy, and monoclonal protein, with associated skin changes, or POEMS syndrome, usually has an underlying osteosclerotic myeloma with IgA or IgG lambda paraprotein, but may also be associated with Castleman disease (angiofollicular lymph node hyperplasia). POEMS neuropathy has clinical features similar to those of CIDP, and highlights the need for a thorough general physical as well as neurological examination. Many patients are initially thought to have CIDP or MGUS. The pathogenesis of POEMS syndrome is not well understood, but overproduction of VEGF, probably secreted by plasmacytomas, is likely to be responsible for most of the characteristic symptoms [110].

The prognosis for patients with POEMS varies considerably. The median survival has been estimated as 12–33 months, with survival up to 165 months with extensive therapy [111]. The most commonly identified causes of death were cardiorespiratory failure and infection. Survival is not affected by the number of POEMS features, although clubbing and extravascular volume overload are associated with shorter survival. The neuropathy may be unrelenting and contribute to progressive disability and eventual cardiorespiratory failure and pneumonia. Stroke and myocardial infarction, which may or may not be related to the POEMS syndrome, also are observed causes of death. The optimal treatment of POEMS syndrome involves eliminating the plasma cell clone, and this may include local therapy of a plasmacytoma with surgery or radiation therapy, using systemic chemotherapy or even autologous stem cell transplantation [111].

Electrophysiological examination shows demyelinating abnormalities in both sensory and motor nerves. The slowing of nerve conduction is more prominent in intermediate nerve segments than in distal nerve segments. The presence of CBs and TD is rare. Lower limb nerves are more severely involved than upper limb nerves, resulting in greater axonal loss in the lower extremities [112].

CANOMAD

Chronic ataxic neuropathy, ophthalmoplegia, monoclonal protein, cold agglutinins and disialosyl antibodies (CANOMAD) represents a rare syndrome that can be considered to be a chronic variant of MFS. Patients have antibodies against the gangliosides GD1b and GQ1b. Although there are only a few cases published in the literature, the CANOMAD syndrome presents a consistent clinical picture, with the main feature being chronic sensory ataxic neuropathy. Clinically, there is a loss of kinaesthesia with relative preservation of muscle strength and small-fibre sensation. Patients typically present with gait and upper limb ataxia. Paraesthesiae in the hands are also frequently present. Despite the absence of significant limb weakness in most cases, the majority of cases have cranial nerve involvement (mainly ophthalmoplegia, dysphagia, and dysarthria) at any stage of the syndrome. The clinical course of CANOMAD often extends over decades, sometimes interspersed with episodes of motor and sensory cranial nerve involvement. No treatment trials have been published. Data on responses are limited to single case descriptions. Both PE and IVIg have been used with benefit in some cases. PE may be complicated by agglutination in the extracorporeal arm of the system, and reinfusion fluid temperatures should be controlled carefully. The role of other treatments has not been evaluated systematically [113].

The most striking electrophysiological feature is an amplitude reduction or absence of SNAPs. Motor conduction abnormalities are found in approximately 50% of patients, even when clinical motor involvement is absent. Electrophysiological findings are heterogeneous. CANOMAD can present features of demyelination or of axonal damage, with variable denervation changes on needle EMG.

References

1. Franssen H. Electrophysiology in demyelinating polyneuropathies. *Expert Rev Neurother* 2008; **8**: 417–31.
2. Guillain G, Barré JA, Strohl A. Sur un syndrome de radiculo-nevrite avec hyperalbuminose du liquide cephalorachidien sans reaction cellulaire. Remarques surles caracteres cliniques et graphiques des reflexes tendineux. *Bull Soc Med Hop Paris* 1916; **28**: 1462–70.
3. Sejvar JJ, Kohl KS, Gidudu J, et al. Guillain–Barré syndrome and Fisher syndrome: case definitions and guidelines for collection, analysis, and presentation of immunization safety data. *Vaccine* 2011; **29**: 599-612.
4. Willison HJ. The immunobiology of Guillain–Barré syndromes. *J Peripher Nerv Syst* 2005; **10**: 94–112.
5. Yuki N, Hartung HP. Guillain–Barré syndrome. *N Engl J Med* 2012; **366**: 2294–304.
6. Van Doorn PA, Ruts L, Jacobs BC. Clinical features, pathogenesis, and treatment of Guillain–Barré syndrome. *Lancet Neurol* 2008; **7**: 939–50.
7. Hughes RA, Cornblath DR. Guillain–Barré syndrome. *Lancet* 2005; **366**: 1653–66.
8. Jacobs BC, Rothbarth PH, Van Der Meché FG, et al. The spectrum of antecedent infections in Guillain–Barré syndrome: a case-control study. *Neurology* 1998; **51**: 1110–15.
9. Kuitwaard K, van Koningsveld R, Ruts L, et al. Recurrent Guillain–Barré syndrome. *J Neurol Neurosurg Psychiatry* 2009; **80**: 56–9.
10. Asbury AK, Cornblath DR. Assessment of current diagnostic criteria for Guillain–Barré syndrome. *Ann Neurol* 1990; **27** (Suppl): S21–S24.
11. Van Der Meché FG, van Doorn PA. Guillain–Barré syndrome and chronic inflammatory demyelinating polyneuropathy: immune mechanisms and update on current therapies. *Ann Neurol* 1995; **37** (Suppl 1): S14–S31.
12. Fokke C, van den Berg B, Drenthen J, Walgaard C, van Doorn PA, Jacobs BC. Diagnosis of Guillain–Barré syndrome and validation of Brighton criteria. *Brain* 2013; Oct 26 (Epub ahead of print), doi: 10.1093/brain/awt285
13. Uncini A, Yuki N. Electrophysiologic and immunopathologic correlates in Guillain–Barré syndrome subtypes. *Expert Rev Neurother* 2009; **9**: 869–84.

14. Kuwabara S, Ogawara K, Misawa S, et al. Does *Campylobacter jejuni* infection elicit 'demyelinating' Guillain–Barré syndrome? *Neurology* 2004; 63: 529–33.

15. Capasso M, Caporale CM, Pomilio F, et al. Acute motor conduction block neuropathy. Another Guillain–Barré syndrome variant. *Neurology* 2003; 61: 617–22.

16. Kuwabara S, Yuki N. Axonal Guillain–Barré syndrome: concepts and controversies. *Lancet Neurol* 2013; 12: 1180–8.

17. Mori M, Kuwabara S, Yuki N. Fisher syndrome: clinical features, immunopathogenesis and management. *Expert Rev Neurother* 2012; 12: 39–51.

18. Overell JR, Hsieh ST, Odaka M, et al. Treatment for Fisher syndrome, Bickerstaff's brainstem encephalitis and related disorders. *Cochrane Database Syst Rev* 2007: CD004761.

19. Roodbol J, de Wit MC, Walgaard C, et al. Recognizing Guillain–Barré syndrome in preschool children. *Neurology* 2011; 76: 807–10.

20. Korinthenberg R, Schessl J, Kirschner J. Clinical presentation and course of childhood Guillain–Barré syndrome: a prospective multicentre study. *Neuropediatrics* 2007; 38: 10–17.

21. Ruts L, Drenthen J, Jongen JL, et al. Pain in Guillain–Barré syndrome: a long-term follow-up study. *Neurology* 2010; 75: 1439–47.

22. Hughes RA, Wijdicks EF, Benson E, et al. Supportive care for patients with Guillain–Barré syndrome. *Arch Neurol* 2005; 62: 1194–8.

23. Lawn ND, Fletcher DD, Henderson RD, et al. Anticipating mechanical ventilation in Guillain–Barré syndrome. *Arch Neurol* 2001; 58: 893–8.

24. Walgaard C, Lingsma HF, Ruts L, et al. Prediction of respiratory insufficiency in Guillain–Barré syndrome. *Ann Neurol* 2010; 67: 781–7.

25. Hughes RA, Swan AV, Raphael JC, et al. Immunotherapy for Guillain–Barré syndrome: a systematic review. *Brain* 2007; 130: 2245–57.

26. The Guillain–Barré Syndrome Study Group. Plasmapheresis and acute Guillain–Barré syndrome. *Neurology* 1985; 35: 1096–104.

27. Efficacy of plasma exchange in Guillain–Barré syndrome: role of replacement fluids. French Cooperative Group on Plasma Exchange in Guillain–Barré syndrome. *Ann Neurol* 1987; 22: 753–61.

28. Raphael JC, Chrevret S, Hughes RA, Annane D. Plasma exchange for Guillain–Barré syndrome. *Cochrane Database Syst Rev* 2012; 7: CD001798.

29. Van der Meché FG, Schmitz PI. A randomized trial comparing intravenous immune globulin and plasma exchange in Guillain–Barré syndrome. Dutch Guillain–Barré Study Group. *N Engl J Med* 1992; 326: 1123–9.

30. Hughes RA, Swan AV, van Doorn PA. Intravenous immunoglobulin for Guillain-Barré syndrome. *Cochrane Database Syst Rev* 2012; 7: CD002063.

31. Randomised trial of plasma exchange, intravenous immunoglobulin, and combined treatments in Guillain–Barré syndrome. Plasma Exchange/Sandoglobulin Guillain–Barré Syndrome Trial Group. *Lancet* 1997; 349: 225–30.

32. Van Koningsveld R, Schmitz PI, van der Meché FG, et al. Effect of methylprednisolone when added to standard treatment with intravenous immunoglobulin for Guillain–Barré syndrome: randomised trial. *Lancet* 2004; 363: 192–6.

33. van Koningsveld R, Schmitz PI, Ang CW, et al. Infections and course of disease in mild forms of Guillain–Barré syndrome. *Neurology* 2002; 58: 610–14.

34. Appropriate number of plasma exchanges in Guillain–Barré syndrome. The French Cooperative Group on Plasma Exchange in Guillain–Barré Syndrome. *Ann Neurol* 1997; 41: 298–306.

35. Overell JR, Hsieh ST, Odaka M, et al. Treatment for Fisher syndrome, Bickerstaff's brainstem encephalitis and related disorders. *Cochrane Database Syst Rev* 2007: CD004761.

36. Yuki N. Fisher syndrome and Bickerstaff brainstem encephalitis (Fisher–Bickerstaff syndrome). *J Neuroimmunol* 2009; 215: 1–9.

37. Ruts L, Drenthen J, Jacobs BC, van Doorn PA. Distinguishing acute-onset CIDP from fluctuating Guillain–Barré syndrome: a prospective study. *Neurology* 2010; 74: 1680–6.

38. Van Koningsveld R, Steyerberg EW, Hughes RA, et al. A clinical prognostic scoring system for Guillain–Barré syndrome. *Lancet Neurol* 2007; 6: 589–94.

39. Walgaard C, Lingsma HF, Ruts L, et al. Early recognition of poor prognosis in Guillain–Barré syndrome. *Neurology* 2011; 76: 968–75.

40. Merkies IS, Schmitz PI, Samijn JP, et al. Fatigue in immune-mediated polyneuropathies. European Inflammatory Neuropathy Cause and Treatment (INCAT) Group. *Neurology* 1999; 53: 1648–54.

41. Garssen MP, Bussmann JB, Schmitz PI, et al. Physical training and fatigue, fitness, and quality of life in Guillain–Barré syndrome and CIDP. *Neurology* 2004; 63: 2393–5.

42. Bernsen RA, de Jager AE, Schmitz PI, Van Der Meché FG. Residual physical outcome and daily living 3 to 6 years after Guillain–Barré syndrome. *Neurology* 1999; 53: 409–10.

43. Van Doorn PA, Ruts L, Jacobs BC. Clinical features, pathogenesis, and treatment of Guillain–Barré syndrome. *Lancet Neurol* 2008; 7: 939–50.

44. Ang CW, Jacobs BC, Laman JD. The Guillain–Barré syndrome: a true case of molecular mimicry. *Trends Immunol* 2004; 25: 61–6.

45. Susuki K, Rasband MN, Tohyama K, et al. Anti-GM1 antibodies cause complement- mediated disruption of sodium channel clusters in peripheral motor nerve fibers. *J Neurosci* 2007; 27: 3956–67.

46. Halstead SK, Zitman FM, Humphreys PD, et al. Eculizumab prevents anti-ganglioside antibody-mediated neuropathy in a murine model. *Brain* 2008; 131: 1197–208.

47. Griffin JW, Li CY, Ho TW, et al. Pathology of the motor-sensory axonal Guillain–Barré syndrome. *Ann Neurol* 1996; 39: 17–28.

48. Kuijf ML, Geleijns K, Ennaji N, et al. Susceptibility to Guillain–Barré syndrome is not associated with CD1A and CD1E gene polymorphisms. *J Neuroimmunol* 2008; 205: 110–12.

49. Research criteria for diagnosis of chronic inflammatory demyelinating polyneuropathy (CIDP). Report from an Ad Hoc Subcommittee of the American Academy of Neurology AIDS Task Force. *Neurology* 1991; 41: 617–18.

50. European Federation of Neurological Societies/Peripheral Nerve Society Guideline on management of chronic inflammatory demyelinating polyradiculoneuropathy: report of a joint task force of the European Federation of Neurological Societies and the Peripheral Nerve Society—First Revision. *J Peripher Nerv Syst* 2010; 15: 1–9.

51. Koski CL, Baumgarten M, Magder LS, et al. Derivation and validation of diagnostic criteria for chronic inflammatory demyelinating polyneuropathy. *J Neurol Sci* 2009; 277: 1–8.

52. Gorson KC, van Schaik IN, Merkies IS, et al. Chronic inflammatory demyelinating polyneuropathy disease activity status: recommendations for clinical research standards and use in clinical practice. *J Peripher Nerv Syst* 2010; 15: 326–33.

53. Koller H, Kieseier BC, Jander S, Hartung HP. Chronic inflammatory demyelinating polyneuropathy. *N Engl J Med* 2005; 352: 1343–56.

54. McCombe PA, Pollard JD, McLeod JG. Chronic inflammatory demyelinating polyradiculoneuropathy. A clinical and electrophysiological study of 92 cases. *Brain* 1987; 110: 1617–30.

55. French CIDP Study Group. Recommendations on diagnostic strategies for chronic inflammatory demyelinating polyradiculoneuropathy. *J Neurol Neurosurg Psychiatry* 2008; 79: 115–18.

56. Hughes RA, Mehndiratta MM. Corticosteroids for chronic inflammatory demyelinating polyradiculoneuropathy. *Cochrane Database Syst Rev* 2012; 8: CD002062.

57. Van Schaik IN, Eftimov F, van Doorn PA, et al. Pulsed high-dose dexamethasone versus standard prednisolone treatment for chronic inflammatory demyelinating polyradiculoneuropathy (PREDICT study): a double-blind, randomised, controlled trial. *Lancet Neurol* 2010; 9: 245–53.

58. Nobile-Orazio E, Cocito D, Jann S, et al. Intravenous immunoglobulin versus intravenous methylprednisolone for chronic inflammatory demyelinating polyradiculoneuropathy: a randomised controlled trial. *Lancet Neurol* 2012; **11**: 493–502.

59. Mehndiratta MM, Hughes RA. Plasma exchange for chronic inflammatory demyelinating polyradiculoneuropathy. *Cochrane Database Syst Rev* 2012; **9**:CD003906.

60. Eftimov F, Winer JB, Vermeulen M, et al. Intravenous immunoglobulin for chronic inflammatory demyelinating polyradiculoneuropathy. *Cochrane Database Syst Rev* 2009; CD001797.

61. Mahdi-Rogers M, Swan AV, van Doorn PA, Hughes RA. Immunomodulatory treatment other than corticosteroids, immunoglobulin and plasma exchange for chronic inflammatory demyelinating polyradiculoneuropathy. *Cochrane Database Syst Rev* 2010; CD003280.

62. Randomised controlled trial of methotrexate for chronic inflammatory demyelinating polyradiculoneuropathy (RMC trial): a pilot, multicentre study. *Lancet Neurol* 2009; **8**: 158–64.

63. Dyck PJ, O'Brien PC, Oviatt KF, et al. Prednisone improves chronic inflammatory demyelinating polyradiculoneuropathy more than no treatment. *Ann Neurol* 1982; **11**: 136–41.

64. Hughes R, Bensa S, Willison H, et al. Randomized controlled trial of intravenous immunoglobulin versus oral prednisolone in chronic inflammatory demyelinating polyradiculoneuropathy. *Ann Neurol* 2001; **50**: 195–201.

65. Eftimov F, Vermeulen M, van Doorn PA, et al. Long-term remission of CIDP after pulsed dexamethasone or short-term prednisolone treatment. *Neurology* 2012; **78**: 1079–84.

66. Hahn AF, Bolton CF, Zochodne D, Feasby TE. Intravenous immunoglobulin treatment in chronic inflammatory demyelinating polyneuropathy. A double-blind, placebo- controlled, cross-over study. *Brain* 1996; **119**: 1067–77.

67. Hughes RA, Donofrio P, Bril V, et al. Intravenous immune globulin (10% caprylate-chromatography purified) for the treatment of chronic inflammatory demyelinating polyradiculoneuropathy (ICE study): a randomised placebo-controlled trial. *Lancet Neurol* 2008; **7**: 136–44.

68. Mendell JR, Barohn RJ, Freimer ML, et al. Randomized controlled trial of IVIg in untreated chronic inflammatory demyelinating polyradiculoneuropathy. *Neurology* 2001; **56**: 445–9.

69. Van Doorn PA, Brand A, Strengers PF, et al. High-dose intravenous immunoglobulin treatment in chronic inflammatory demyelinating polyneuropathy: a double-blind, placebo-controlled, crossover study. *Neurology* 1990; **40**: 209–12.

70. Van Doorn PA, Vermeulen M, Brand A, et al. Intravenous immunoglobulin treatment in patients with chronic inflammatory demyelinating polyneuropathy. Clinical and laboratory characteristics associated with improvement. *Arch Neurol* 1991; **48**: 217–20.

71. Vermeulen M, van Doorn PA, Brand A, et al. Intravenous immunoglobulin treatment in patients with chronic inflammatory demyelinating polyneuropathy: a double blind, placebo controlled study. *J Neurol Neurosurg Psychiatry* 1993; **56**: 36–9.

72. Latov N, Deng C, Dalakas MC, et al. Timing and course of clinical response to intravenous immunoglobulin in chronic inflammatory demyelinating polyradiculoneuropathy. *Arch Neurol* 2010; **67**: 802–7.

73. Donofrio PD, Bril V, Dalakas MC, et al. Safety and tolerability of immune globulin intravenous in chronic inflammatory demyelinating polyradiculoneuropathy. *Arch Neurol* 2010; **67**: 1082–8.

74. Cocito D, Serra G, Falcone Y, Paolasso I. The efficacy of subcutaneous immunoglobulin administration in chronic inflammatory demyelinating polyneuropathy responders to intravenous immunoglobulin. *J Peripher Nerv Syst* 2011; **16**: 150–2.

75. Lee DH, Linker RA, Paulus W, et al. Subcutaneous immunoglobulin infusion: a new therapeutic option in chronic inflammatory demyelinating polyneuropathy. *Muscle Nerve* 2008; **37**: 406–9.

76. Dyck PJ, Litchy WJ, Kratz KM, et al. A plasma exchange versus immune globulin infusion trial in chronic inflammatory demyelinating polyradiculoneuropathy. *Ann Neurol* 1994; **36**: 838–45.

77. Kuitwaard K, van Doorn PA. Newer therapeutic options for chronic inflammatory demyelinating polyradiculoneuropathy. *Drugs* 2009; **69**: 987–1001.

78. Hartung HP, Lehmann HC, Willison HJ. Peripheral neuropathies: establishing common clinical research standards for CIDP. *Nat Rev Neurol* 2011; **7**: 250–1.

79. Vallat JM, Sommer C, Magy L. Chronic inflammatory demyelinating polyradiculoneuropathy: diagnostic and therapeutic challenges for a treatable condition. *Lancet Neurol* 2010; **9**: 402–12.

80. Dyck PJ, O'Brien P, Swanson C, et al. Combined azathioprine and prednisone in chronic inflammatory-demyelinating polyneuropathy. *Neurology* 1985; **35**: 1173–6.

81. Iijima M, Yamamoto M, Hirayama M, et al. Clinical and electrophysiologic correlates of IVIg responsiveness in CIDP. *Neurology* 2005; **64**: 1471–5.

82. Lewis RA, Sumner AJ, Brown MJ, Asbury AK. Multifocal demyelinating neuropathy with persistent conduction block. *Neurology* 1982; **32**: 958–64.

83. Lewis RA. Multifocal motor neuropathy and Lewis Sumner syndrome: two distinct entities. *Muscle Nerve* 1999; **22**: 1738–9.

84. Lewis RA. Neuropathies associated with conduction block. *Curr Opin Neurol* 2007; **20**: 525–30.

85. Vlam L, van der Pol WL, Cats EA, et al. Multifocal motor neuropathy: diagnosis, pathogenesis and treatment strategies. *Nat Rev Neurol* 2012; **8**: 48–58.

86. European Federation of Neurological Societies/Peripheral Nerve Society guideline on management of multifocal motor neuropathy. Report of a joint task force of the European Federation of Neurological Societies and the Peripheral Nerve Society—first revision. *J Peripher Nerv Syst* 2010; **15**: 295–301.

87. Muley SA, Parry GJ. Multifocal motor neuropathy. *J Clin Neurosci* 2012; **19**: 1201–9.

88. Kuijf ML, van Doorn PA, Tio-Gillen AP, et al. Diagnostic value of anti-GM1 ganglioside serology and validation of the INCAT-ELISA. *J Neurol Sci* 2005; **239**: 37–44.

89. Nobile-Orazio E. Multifocal motor neuropathy. *J Neuroimmunol* 2001; **115**: 4–18.

90. Van Asseldonk JT, Van den Berg LH, Van den Berg-Vos RM, et al. Demyelination and axonal loss in multifocal motor neuropathy: distribution and relation to weakness. *Brain* 2003; **126**: 186–98.

91. Azulay JP, Blin O, Pouget J, et al. Intravenous immunoglobulin treatment in patients with motor neuron syndromes associated with anti-GM1 antibodies: a double-blind, placebo-controlled study. *Neurology* 1994; **44**: 429–32.

92. Van den Berg LH, Kerkhoff H, Oey PL, et al. Treatment of multifocal motor neuropathy with high dose intravenous immunoglobulins: a double blind, placebo controlled study. *J Neurol Neurosurg Psychiatry* 1995; **59**: 248–52.

93. Federico P, Zochodne DW, Hahn AF, et al. Multifocal motor neuropathy improved by IVIg: randomized, double-blind, placebo-controlled study. *Neurology* 2000; **55**: 1256–62.

94. Leger JM, Chassande B, Musset L, et al. Intravenous immunoglobulin therapy in multifocal motor neuropathy: a double-blind, placebo-controlled study. *Brain* 2001; **124**: 145–53.

95. Cats EA, van der Pol WL, Piepers S, et al. Correlates of outcome and response to IVIg in 88 patients with multifocal motor neuropathy. *Neurology* 2010; **75**: 818–25.

96. Harbo T, Andersen H, Hess A, et al. Subcutaneous versus intravenous immunoglobulin in multifocal motor neuropathy: a randomized, single-blinded cross-over trial. *Eur J Neurol* 2009; **16**: 631–8.

97. Pestronk A, Cornblath DR, Ilyas AA, et al. A treatable multifocal motor neuropathy with antibodies to GM1 ganglioside. *Ann Neurol* 1988; **24**: 73–8.

98. Umapathi T, Hughes RA, Nobile-Orazio E, Leger JM. Immunosuppressant and immunomodulatory treatments for multifocal motor neuropathy. *Cochrane Database Syst Rev* 2012; **4**: CD003217.

99. Piepers S, Van dB-V, van der Pol WL, et al. Mycophenolate mofetil as adjunctive therapy for MMN patients: a randomized, controlled trial. *Brain* 2007; **130**: 2004–10.

100. Fitzpatrick AM, Mann CA, Barry S, et al. An open label clinical trial of complement inhibition in multifocal motor neuropathy. *J Peripher Nerv Syst* 2011; **16**: 84–91.

101. Katz JS, Saperstein DS, Gronseth G, et al. Distal acquired demyelinating symmetric neuropathy. *Neurology* 2000; **54**: 615–20.

102. European Federation of Neurological Societies/Peripheral Nerve Society Guideline on management of paraproteinemic demyelinating neuropathies. Report of a Joint Task Force of the European Federation of Neurological Societies and the Peripheral Nerve Society--first revision. *J Peripher Nerv Syst* 2010; **15**: 185–95.

103. Rajabally YA. Neuropathy and paraproteins: review of a complex association. *Eur J Neurol* 2011; **18**: 1291–8.

104. Kyle R, Dyck P. Neuropathy associated with the monoclonal gammopathies. In: Dyck PJ, Thomas PC (ed) *Peripheral Neuropathy*, 4th edn, vol. 2, pp. 2255–76. Philadelphia, PA: Elsevier Saunders, 2005.

105. Allen D, Lunn MP, Niermeijer J, Nobile-Orazio E. Treatment for IgG and IgA paraproteinaemic neuropathy. *Cochrane Database Syst Rev* 2007; CD005376.

106. Ramchandren S, Lewis RA. An update on monoclonal gammopathy and neuropathy. *Curr Neurol Neurosci Rep* 2012; **12**: 102–10.

107. Niermeijer JM, Eurelings M, van der Linden MW, et al. Intermittent cyclophosphamide with prednisone versus placebo for polyneuropathy with IgM monoclonal gammopathy. *Neurology* 2007; **69**: 50–9.

108. Lunn MP, Nobile-Orazio E. Immunotherapy for IgM anti-myelin-associated glycoprotein paraprotein-associated peripheral neuropathies. *Cochrane Database Syst Rev* 2012; **5**: CD002827.

109. Kaku DA, England JD, Sumner AJ. Distal accentuation of conduction slowing in polyneuropathy associated with antibodies to myelin-associated glycoprotein and sulphated glucuronyl paragloboside. *Brain* 1994; **117**: 941–7.

110. Kuwabara S, Dispenzieri A, Arimura K, et al. Treatment for POEMS (polyneuropathy, organomegaly, endocrinopathy, M-protein, and skin changes) syndrome. *Cochrane Database Syst Rev* 2012 ; **6**: CD006828.

111. Dispenzieri A, Kyle RA, Lacy MQ, et al. POEMS syndrome: definitions and long-term outcome. *Blood* 2003; **101**: 2496–506.

112. Sung JY, Kuwabara S, Ogawara K, et al. Patterns of nerve conduction abnormalities in POEMS syndrome. *Muscle Nerve* 2002; **26**: 189–93.

113. Willison HJ, O'Leary CP, Veitch J, et al. The clinical and laboratory features of chronic sensory ataxic neuropathy with anti-disialosyl IgM antibodies. *Brain* 2001; **124**: 1968–77.

CHAPTER 17

Diabetic neuropathy

Stephen A. Goutman, Andrea L. Smith,
Stacey A. Sakowski, and Eva L. Feldman

Introduction

Diabetes is a metabolic disorder characterized by hyperglycaemia. The two major forms of diabetes are Type 1, resulting from a deficiency of insulin, and Type 2, resulting from a resistance to insulin [1]. The prevalence of diabetes in the United States is 8.3% of the population and in Europe 8.5% of the population, with an estimated annual treatment cost of $174 billion in the United States and $106 billion in Europe [2,3]. Diabetes is the most common cause of neuropathy in the United States. The peripheral nervous system is affected in up to 60–70% of patients with all types of diabetes [2,4], with the majority of cases representing a distal symmetric sensorimotor polyneuropathy that is estimated to occur in 10.7–59% of patients with diabetes during the course of the disease [4–6]. This range reflects the varying criteria used to diagnose the polyneuropathy, including whether clinical evaluations alone, electrodiagnostic studies alone, or a combination of the two are required to satisfy the diagnosis [5,7]. Given that changes in reflexes and sensation are a component of normal aging [5], using a standard clinical evaluation for diagnosing a polyneuropathy may overestimate the number of people affected.

Classification of diabetic neuropathies

Diabetes is implicated in a range of peripheral nervous system abnormalities. These abnormalities can be classified broadly into a generalized typical polyneuropathy (distal symmetric neuropathy), generalized atypical polyneuropathy (small-fibre neuropathy, autonomic neuropathy), and focal neuropathies (including ischaemic mononeuropathies, compression mononeuropathies, and regional or multifocal neuropathic syndromes) (Table 17.1) [8–10]. These classifications present in a variety of patterns (Fig. 17.1) and are described in detail in the rest of this section.

Distal symmetric sensorimotor polyneuropathy

The distal symmetric sensorimotor polyneuropathy typical in diabetics is an insidious onset of symmetrical numbness, paraesthesiae, and pain, mostly in the distal lower limbs without subjective complaints of peripheral nerve dysfunction such as weakness [11]. Objective examination findings include loss of ankle jerks, glove and stocking sensory loss to pinprick and light touch, and impaired vibration and proprioception in the toes. Weakness is uncommon, but if present is localized to the distal lower extremity, involving the intrinsic foot muscles or ankle dorsiflexors [11–13]. Alternative presentations, such as those with a wider distribution of weakness, should raise the suspicion of an alternative diagnosis. A formal definition of the typical diabetic sensorimotor polyneuropathy (DSPN) was established by the Toronto Diabetic Neuropathy Expert Group in 2009, which defined it as a 'symmetrical, length-dependent sensorimotor polyneuropathy attributable to metabolic and microvessel alterations as a result of chronic hyperglycemia exposure (diabetes) and cardiovascular risk covariates' [10]. The expert group noted that DSPN can be first diagnosed via nerve conduction studies (NCS), and the coexistence of retinopathy and nephropathy (Kimmelstiel–Wilson syndrome) would support diabetes as the underlying cause of DSPN, as both of these factors infer an increased risk of developing DSPN [4,11,14].

Although axon loss is the classic pathophysiological process of DSPN, the earliest electrodiagnostic findings in DSPN are slowing of the conduction velocities (CVs) [15]. Moreover, while the degree of CV slowing does not meet formal criteria for demyelination, it does correlate with the degree of axon loss in the DSPN. Importantly, the degree of CV slowing in DSPN is out of proportion to that in amyotrophic lateral sclerosis which is also characterized by axon loss [16–18]. There may be different electrophysiological patterns when comparing the upper and lower limbs, with the lower limbs predisposed to an axon loss pattern with reduced amplitudes and the upper limbs predisposed to demyelination characterized by reduced CVs, albeit not meeting formal criteria for acquired demyelination [19].

At the time of diagnosis of diabetes, symptomatic DSPN occurs in 1.5% of patients, although the prevalence of DSPN using a combination of electrodiagnostic and clinical criteria ranges from 7.6 to

Table 17.1 Classification of diabetic neuropathy

Generalized typical polyneuropathy
Distal symmetric sensorimotor polyneuropathy
Generalized atypical polyneuropathy
Small-fibre neuropathy
Autonomic neuropathy
Focal neuropathies
Ischaemic mononeuropathies
Compression mononeuropathies
Regional or multifocal neuropathic syndromes

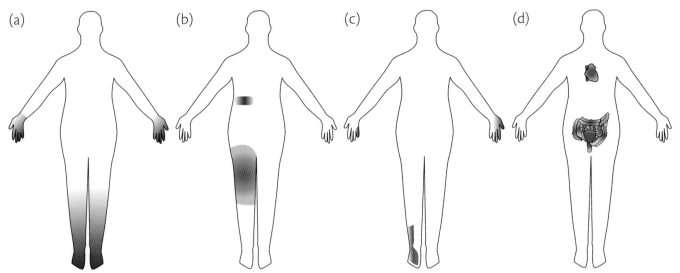

Fig. 17.1 Patterns of nerve injury in diabetic neuropathy. Clinicians should be aware of all potential patterns of nerve injury because they have implications for the assessment and treatment of patients with diabetes. For example, patients with diabetes can have radiculopathy without a disc herniation or degenerative changes in the spine. This knowledge could prevent unnecessary spine surgery in cases where imaging results are equivocal. Furthermore, patients with diabetes can have more than one pattern of nerve injury, and the clinician needs to ask patients about specific symptoms such as autonomic involvement, which is often overlooked.

The following patterns of nerve injury are shown in the figure: distal symmetrical polyneuropathy (DSP), small fibre predominant neuropathy, and treatment-induced neuropathy (a); radiculoplexopathy and radiculopathy (b); mononeuropathy and mononeuritis multiplex (c); and autonomic neuropathy and treatment-induced neuropathy (d). Small fibre predominant neuropathy has the same pattern as DSP but neurological examination and electrodiagnostic studies give quite different results, which can help the clinician to distinguish between these types of neuropathy. Diabetic radiculoplexopathy can be responsive to immunotherapy and, in contrast to most nerve injury in patients with diabetes, usually improves with time. Treatment-induced neuropathy is an under-recognized disorder. Unlike the other peripheral manifestations of diabetes, this disorder is caused by overaggressive control of glucose levels.

Reprinted from: *The Lancet Neurology*, Volume 11 (issue 6), Callaghan et al, Diabetic neuropathy: clinical manifestations and current treatments, pp. 521–34, Copyright (2012), with permission from Elsevier.

15.2% of patients [20] and increases to 41.9% at 10 years [5]. The prevalence range for DSPN at the time of diagnosis of diabetes is dependent on how many NCS abnormalities are required to meet the diagnosis of DSPN [20]. The American Diabetes Association (ADA) recommends four criteria for the diagnosis of diabetes:

1. haemoglobin A1c ≥ 6.5%,

2. fasting plasma glucose ≥ 126 mg dl^{-1} (7.0 mmol L^{-1}),

3. 2-h plasma glucose ≥ 200 mg dl^{-1} (11.1 mmol L^{-1}) during an oral glucose tolerance test using a glucose load of 75 g anhydrous glucose, or

4. random plasma glucose ≥ 200 mg dl^{-1} (11.1 mmol L^{-1}) in a patient with symptoms of hyperglycaemia [21].

Importantly, impaired glucose tolerance (IGT) is also associated with abnormalities of large nerve function [22]. Moreover, glucose tolerance testing may be better at detecting diabetes or IGT when compared with studies of fasting glucose or haemoglobin A1c in patients with symptoms of polyneuropathy [23,24]. Those with painful symptoms may have an increased likelihood of an impairment of glucose tolerance [25] and may actually have preferential involvement of the small fibres (see section on Small-fibre neuropathy) [26]. Therefore, it is recommended to routinely obtain 2-h glucose tolerance tests in all patients presenting with symptoms of DSPN.

When evaluating a patient with DSPN with confirmed diabetes or glucose intolerance, it is also important to consider other factors that cause neuropathy, such as toxins, medications, vitamin deficiencies, or paraproteinaemias [27,28]. In addition, it is important to assess for other conditions where the patient's examination findings are not consistent with DSPN. For example, if there is proximal or distal upper limb weakness, proximal lower limb weakness, or a wider distribution of lower limb weakness, electrodiagnostic testing is useful to screen for alternative diagnoses. Specifically, chronic inflammatory demyelinating polyneuropathy (CIDP) may occur in patients with diabetes, although it is debated whether the incidence of CIDP is higher in diabetic patients [29,30]. Helpful examination findings to suggest CIDP in diabetic patients include motor symptoms greater than sensory symptoms, weakness beyond what is expected for DSPN, and imbalance [31]. Findings on NCS will show evidence of acquired demyelination. Importantly, these patients may respond to intravenous immunoglobulin [32,33].

Sural nerve biopsies in patients with diabetes can show a variety of findings. Patients with untreated diabetes and without symptoms of DSPN show segmental demyelination and remyelination. Patients with untreated diabetes and symptoms of DSPN show both axonal degeneration and segmental demyelination and remyelination. Patients with treated diabetes and longstanding DSPN show axonal degeneration [34].

Mononeuropathies

Median mononeuropathy at the wrist, or carpal tunnel syndrome (CTS), is the most common type of mononeuropathy seen in diabetic patients [4]. In a group of patients with only mild diabetic neuropathy, 23% have been shown to have electrodiagnostic evidence of this entity [35]. In patients with bilateral median mononeuropathy at the wrist, there is a higher prevalence of diabetes [36], although whether DM is a risk factor for CTS is less certain [37]. There may be a role for surgical release in diabetic patients with CTS; however, not all studies report an improved clinical outcome [38,39]. The incidence of cranial neuropathies is higher in patients with diabetes compared with those patients without [40]. Involved cranial nerves include VII, III, and VI. When cranial nerve III is affected a typical symptom is ophthalmoparesis as the conditions tends to spare the pupil function, although it can be involved [41]. Other mononeuropathies frequent in diabetic patients include ulnar neuropathy [42,43], common fibular neuropathy [44], and lateral femoral cutaneous neuropathy [45]. A femoral neuropathy has been described in patients with diabetes [46], although this more likely represents the diabetic lumbosacral radiculoplexus neuropathy (see section Diabetic radiculoplexus neuropathies).

Diabetic radiculoplexus neuropathies

Diabetic radiculoplexus neuropathies (DRPNs) are a group of disorders with an acute-to-subacute clinical presentation characterized by pain and weakness. As a group, they have been variably described in the medical literature, and whether they represent a spectrum of a single disease mechanism or individual entities is not yet determined. In general, the different presentations can be divided into those affecting the cervical roots and brachial plexus, the thoracic roots, and the lumbosacral roots and plexus. Although diabetic cachexia (see section Diabetic cachexia) may be a combination of a thoracic radiculopathy and lumbosacral radiculoplexus neuropathy, due to its dramatic clinical presentation this entity is described separately.

Diabetic lumbosacral radiculoplexus neuropathy (DLRPN) has been referred to as diabetic myelopathy [47], diabetic amyotrophy [48], and subacute proximal diabetic neuropathy [49]. Patients typically do not have a long history of diabetes and the presenting symptom is progressive, asymmetric pain (which is non-specific and may be sharp, aching, or burning) in the proximal lower limb or thigh, along with weakness and atrophy of the pelvifemoral muscles over a period of weeks to months [47,50–52]. Autonomic symptoms in the limb are also noted. There is a tendency to involve the thigh. Recovery is spontaneous. The motor symptoms are more pronounced than the sensory symptoms and, if present, the sensory abnormalities are typically distal and symmetric. However, others have suggested the presentation is acute in onset and affects patients with a long history of diabetes, and therefore there may be a spectrum of abnormalities lumped under the same term [53]. The cause may be an ischaemic microscopic vasculitis with secondary segmental demyelination [50].

Diabetic cervical radiculoplexus neuropathy is the upper extremity correlate to the lumbosacral form. It presents with pain followed by weakness and is either unilateral or asymmetric [54,55]. Patients may have symptoms localized to the cervical segments or a concurrent or prior history of radiculoplexus neuropathies affecting the thoracic or lumbosacral segments. Symptoms gradually resolve. There is equal involvement of the upper, middle, and lower brachial plexus, distinct from non-diabetic inflammatory brachial plexopathies, which tend to involve the upper plexus.

Diabetic proximal neuropathy

A subacute diabetic proximal neuropathy has been described [56]. These patients present with bilateral proximal lower extremity weakness that may not be symmetric, and a reduction of reflexes in the legs. Patients may have pain and weight loss with evidence of autonomic dysfunction. Electrodiagnostic evaluation shows evidence of axon loss, but signs of demyelination such as conduction block, temporal dispersion, and prolonged distal latencies can be seen as well. The needle examination supports a polyradiculopathy. Suggested diagnostic criteria include:

- subacute progression of weakness over 1–3 month period,
- bilateral involvement or unilateral involvement that becomes bilateral within 2 months,
- reduced or absent patellar reflex,
- increased cerebrospinal fluid protein concentration,
- progression of symptoms for 2 months,
- electrodiagnostic evidence of a polyradiculoneuropathy [56].

This clinical entity has similarities to other diagnostic labels including DLRPN, diabetic amyotrophy, or femoral neuropathy, with the major distinction of a bilateral versus unilateral process. The electrodiagnostic testing does not usually meet the criteria for CIDP. The symptoms of subacute diabetic proximal neuropathy are not as widespread compared with CIDP, and the autonomic involvement is more severe.

The presence of diabetes does not exclude other neuropathies from occurring. Therefore it is important that studies evaluate for conditions such as CIDP, keeping in mind that NCS with diabetes can show findings characteristic of CIDP with the exception of increased evidence of axon loss such as reduced sural sensory and ulnar motor amplitude [57].

Diabetic truncal neuropathy

Diabetic truncal neuropathy typically presents with pain, paraesthesiae, and dysaesthesiae in the anterior and/or posterior thorax, but can also lead to weakness of the abdominal muscles [58]. The symptoms are usually unilateral, can worsen at night, and may mimic symptoms of acute coronary syndrome, cholecystitis, or appendicitis [59]. Affected patients typically have a history of diabetes; however, this can be the initial presentation of the disease [60]. EMG of the paraspinal and, when normal, the intracostal and/or abdominal, muscles can identify abnormal spontaneous activity [60].

Diabetic cachexia

Diabetic neuropathic cachexia is an acute-to-subacute painful process associated with weight loss, anorexia, autonomic dysfunction, and peripheral neuropathy [61,62]. Pain is characteristically in the lower extremities and worse at night. Weight loss can be profound (up to 50%). Patients typically have a history of mild diabetes without the sequelae of chronic diabetes such as retinopathy or nephropathy, although their examination may show evidence of an underlying DSPN. Spontaneous resolution is typical. Occasionally, there is an association with an improvement in glucose control, such as after initiating an insulin regimen.

Diabetic autonomic neuropathy

Diabetes may affect the sympathetic and parasympathetic autonomic nervous systems leading to functional abnormalities in the cardiovascular, gastrointestinal, and genitourinary systems, in addition to defects in sudomotor and pupillary responses (Table 17.2)

Table 17.2 Autonomic dysfunction in diabetes

Cardiovascular

Orthostatic hypotension

Reduced ejection fraction

Systolic dysfunction

Decreased diastolic filling

Prolonged or dispersed QT interval

Increased resting heart rate

Poor heart rate response to exercise

Painless myocardial infarction

Gastrointestinal

Oesophageal dysmotility: dysphagia, retrosternal discomfort, gastro-oesophageal reflux

Gastroparesis: nausea/vomiting, bloating, abdominal pain, early satiety

Constipation (most common) or diarrhoea (may alternate with constipation or may be explosive)

Impaired gallbladder motility: diarrhoea, abdominal pain

Decreased anal sphincter tone: leakage of stool

Urogenital

Erectile dysfunction

Impaired testicular pain sensation

Retrograde ejaculation

Loss of sensation of bladder filling

Reduced urinary flow

Sudomotor

Anhidrosis/hyperhydrosis

Respiratory

Reduced airway tone: increased risk of obstructive sleep apnoea

Impaired ventilatory response to hypoxia/hypercapnia

Impairment of bronchoconstriction

Pupillary function

Small unreactive pupils

Reproduced from: *Practical Neurology*, Little et al., **7**, 82–92, 2007 with permission from BMJ Publishing Group Ltd.

[63]. Symptoms include orthostatic hypotension, diarrhoea, vomiting, gustatory sweating, bladder distension, and impotence [64,65]. The prevalence of autonomic neuropathy ranges from 54 to 66% of patients with Type 1 diabetes, and from 59 to 73% of those with Type 2 diabetes [65]. Even patients with IGT show abnormalities of sudomotor functioning based on quantitative sudomotor axon reflex testing (QSART) [66]. The pathological changes in patients with diabetic autonomic neuropathy include larger nerve cells in the sympathetic ganglion with granules or vacuoles, inflammatory cellular infiltrations in autonomic nerve bundles and ganglia, neuromata in the pancreas, reduction of cells in the intermediolateral columns of the spinal cord, eosinophilic bodies in the smooth muscles, and loss of myelinated fibres in the vagus nerve [64].

Standard tests exist to evaluate the autonomic nervous system, and careful attention must be paid to medication, concurrent illness, or other confounding factors upon performing these evaluations [67]. Testing of sympathetic function includes the response of blood pressure to head-up tilt and QSART, and testing of parasympathetic function includes the response of heart rate to deep breathing. Complete testing of the autonomic nervous system in diabetic neuropathy is outside the scope of this chapter (reviewed in [67]).

Cardiac autonomic neuropathy (CAN) is a disorder resulting from denervation of autonomic fibres that innervate the heart and blood vessels, resulting in the symptoms of orthostatic hypotension, exercise intolerance, intra-operative cardiovascular lability, silent myocardial ischaemia, and resting tachycardia [68,69]. In patients with insulin-dependent diabetes, risk factors for the development of CAN include increased haemoglobin A1c, hypertension, DSPN, and retinopathy [70]. In addition, in insulin-dependent diabetes, the presence of autonomic neuropathy may be associated with left ventricular hypertrophy and diastolic dysfunction [71]. It is important to recognize this entity in diabetic patients as it can result in cardiac arrhythmias, sudden death, and increased mortality [68,69,72–75]. It is possible, however, that the increased mortality is due to the complications associated with nephropathy and hypertension [74]. The earliest abnormality in CAN is vagus nerve dysfunction, as this is the longest nerve of the autonomic nervous system; this results in unopposed sympathetic activity on the heart that can be detected by a reduced heart rate variability (HRV) [72]. Abnormalities of HRV may be seen within 2 years of the diagnosis of diabetes [76]. Various instruments exist to evaluate autonomic symptoms including the Survey of Autonomic Symptoms [77] and the Autonomic Symptom Profile [78].

While a full review of autonomic symptoms as a result of diabetic autonomic neuropathy is outside the scope of this chapter, certain troubling symptoms should be noted. Pupillary symptoms can result in impaired dark adaptation [79] leading to difficulties with vision and driving at night. The mechanism is thought to be secondary to either decreased sympathetic activity or increased parasympathetic activity, and abnormalities of the pupil may proceed CAN [80,81]. Furthermore, patients with early pupillary abnormalities may be at a higher risk of microvascular complications, such as retinopathy and microalbuminuria, in the future [80]. Diabetic gastroparesis as a result of delayed gastric emptying causes symptoms of abdominal bloating and fullness and may lead to significant difficulties with disease control, including impaired absorption of oral medications and blood glucose concentrations [63,82,83]. Treatment focuses on glucose control, frequent small meals, avoidance of foods that delay gastric emptying, and certain prokinetic medications [84]. Another problematic disorder is diabetic diarrhoea which leads to frequent watery stools that may cause incontinence due to poor sphincter tone [63,84]. Finally, the impact of diabetes on the genitourinary system may impair sexual and urinary function. In men this results in erectile dysfunction and retrograde ejaculation, and in women in painful intercourse and impaired vaginal lubrication [63,85]. Bladder dysfunction in men causes weak detrusor contractility resulting in straining, weak stream, and post-void dribbling, and in women causes incontinence. There is also an increased risk of urinary tract infections [63,85].

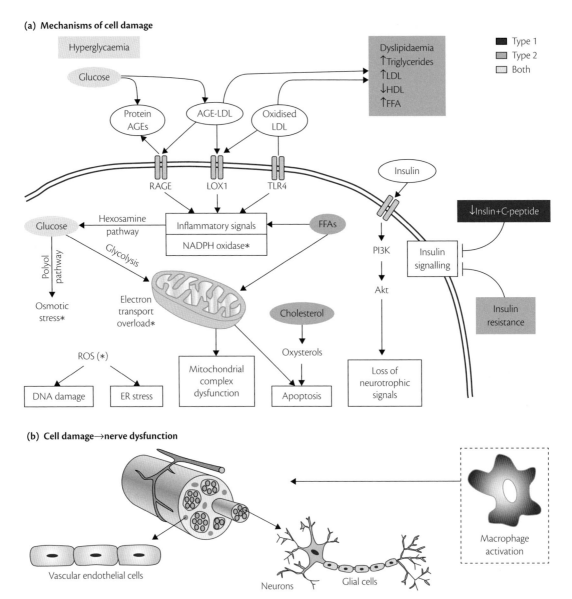

Fig. 17.2 Mechanisms of diabetic neuropathy. Factors linked to Type 1 diabetes, Type 2 diabetes, and both cause DNA damage, endoplasmic reticulum stress, mitochondrial complex dysfunction, apoptosis, and loss of neurotrophic signalling (a). This cell damage can occur in neurons, glial cells, and vascular endothelial cells, as well as triggering macrophage activation, all of which can lead to nerve dysfunction and neuropathy (b). The relative importance of the pathways in this network will vary with cell type, disease profile, and time. AGE, advanced glycation end products; LDL, low-density lipoprotein; HDL, high-density lipoprotein; FFA, free fatty acids; ROS, reactive oxygen species (red star); ER, endoplasmic reticulum; PI3K, phosphatidylinositol-3-kinase; LOX1, oxidized LDL receptor 1; RAGE, receptor for advanced glycation end products; TLR4, toll-like receptor 4.

Reprinted from: *The Lancet Neurology*, Volume 11 (issue 6), Callaghan et al, Diabetic neuropathy: clinical manifestations and current treatments, pp. 521–534, Copyright (2012), with permission from Elsevier.

Small-fibre neuropathy

As opposed to abnormalities of the large nerve fibres that lead to weakness, areflexia, and impaired proprioception, small fibre neuropathies (SFNs) preferentially affect the small-diameter myelinated and unmyelinated fibres, leading to neuropathic pain with subsequent diminished pain and temperature sensation [86]. The particular presentation of 'burning feet' is a characteristic complaint [87]. A shallow skin biopsy, usually of 3 mm in diameter at a proximal and distal location in the leg, can be used to determine the intra-epidermal nerve fibre (IENF) density, which is a reliable test to assess for a SFN [88]. A reduced distal IENF can be present

in diabetic patients with no symptoms of neuropathy, and in those patients with an underlying large fibre neuropathy the reduction of IENF is expected to be greater than in those patients without a large fibre neuropathy.

Treatment-induced diabetic neuropathy

A syndrome characterized by acute onset of pain and autonomic dysfunction has been described [89]. These cases share a correction of glucose control in what is typically a patient with previously poor glycaemic control. The pain is often severe and is not responsive to monotherapy or even polytherapy. Autonomic symptoms include orthostatic intolerance. In some female patients with Type 1 diabetes, intentional withholding of insulin for the purpose of weight loss (diabetic anorexia) precedes the treatment-induced diabetic neuropathy. Although there is an improvement in pain and autonomic function, patients can have worsening retinopathy.

Pathogenesis of diabetic neuropathy

Various mechanisms are implicated in the pathogenesis of diabetic neuropathy and are broadly divided among metabolic, ischaemic, and autoimmune classifications (Fig. 17.2). These mechanisms are only briefly discussed here and the interested reader is directed to more detailed reviews [90–92]. Pathways implicated in the metabolic pathogenesis of diabetic neuropathy include the polyol pathway, the hexosamine pathway, the protein kinase C (PKC) pathway, the advanced glycation endproducts (AGEs) pathway, the poly(ADP-ribose) polymerase (PARP) pathway, and oxidative stress and apoptosis [90]. In combination, abnormalities of these pathways lead to the formation of reactive oxygen species (ROS) due to an imbalance of the mitochondrial redox state of the cell.

Aldose reductase (AR) reduces toxic aldehydes to inactive alcohol; however, in the hyperglycaemic state, AR, consuming the cofactor NADPH, reduces glucose to sorbitol [91,92]. As a consequence of the consumed NADPH, this cofactor cannot aid in the regeneration of reduced glutathione which helps mediate the effects of intracellular oxidative stress. Sorbitol is then oxidized to fructose via sorbitol dehydrogenase with the reduction of NAD+ to NADH [93]. Increased fructose leads to glycation and further depletion of NADPH. Finally, this pathway leads to the formation of diacylglycerol (DAG) with activates the PKC pathway [94,95]. This activation leads to an increase in a series of factors that lead to further remodelling of blood vessels, leading the to microvascular complications of diabetes [90,91,96]. There is also upregulation of the hexosamine pathway [90–92]. This pathway ultimately results in the increased production of transforming growth factor beta and plasminogen activator inhibitor-1 which causes capillary and vascular occlusion [97,98]. This pathway is upregulated by the increased concentration of fructose-6-phosphate from the increased glycolysis as a result of increased intracellular glucose. Intracellular hyperglycaemia results in the formation of AGEs which can modify axons, Schwann cells, endothelial cells, basement vessels, and the extracellular matrix [99]. Similarly, the PARP pathway is activated by oxidative–nitrosative stress. The overall result of this pathway is that glycolytic intermediates lead to activation of PKC and formation of AGEs [90].

These processes in combination lead to oxidative stress and apoptosis via ROS production or a reduction in glutathione. As a result, cellular function, including mitochondrial function, is impaired, which can cause cell apoptosis [90]. Inflammation also plays a role in the pathogenesis of diabetic neuropathy via the production of tumour necrosis factor (TNF)-α, TNF-β, and NF-κB. Furthermore, the upregulation of cyclooxygenase-2 (COX-2) and inducible nitric oxide synthase (iNOS) promotes ongoing inflammation and thus ongoing damage to nerves [90]. It is also possible that abnormalities in growth factor activity, including nerve growth factor (NGF), insulin-like growth-factor-1 (IGF-1), and neurotrophin 3 (NT3), play a role in the pathogenesis of diabetic neuropathy.

Treatment

The hallmark of treatment is glucose control. A large study of 1441 patients with insulin-dependent diabetes showed that more intensive therapy either decreased the incidence of neuropathy (defined by clinical and electrodiagnostic or autonomic abnormalities) or slowed the onset of symptoms [100], and this was associated with reduced abnormalities on NCS [101]. Moreover, the effect of early intensive glucose control reduced the incidence of DSPN and CAN even after a decade of the therapy [102]. Patients should also be instructed on appropriate foot care to avoid diabetic ulcerations as a source of local or systemic infection [103].

Whether DLRPN, and other forms of DRPN, require treatment is still a topic of debate, as spontaneous improvement is the rule. In a retrospective review of 44 patients with subacute diabetic proximal neuropathy, Pascoe et al. identified 12 patients who received treatment consisting of prednisone, plasma exchange, or intravenous immunoglobulin (IVIg) [56]. Nine of the 12 improved, two were unchanged, and one was worse. There was no statistically significant improvement comparing the treatment group with the non-treatment group. In another study, 15 patients were treated with either plasma exchange, IVIg, or prednisone, and although there was no placebo group the authors felt the symptoms improved more rapidly due to the treatment [104]. Krendel et al. treated 15 patients with prednisone or IVIg and added azathioprine or cyclophosphamide in others, and felt that patients improved; however, they only selected patients who were 'disabled by progressive weakness' [105]. Reports also exist detailing patients who did not improve following immunomodulation therapy [106]. Ongoing studies are needed to determine the role of these therapies in patients with DLRPN [107].

Several treatments can be used to treat pain related to DSPN or a small-fibre neuropathy; however, these must be individualized to the patient based on medication preferences and comorbidities. Guidelines do exist for the treatment of this pain, and have been reviewed elsewhere [10,108]. First-line therapies include tricyclic antidepressants, serotonin–norepinephrine reuptake inhibitors, and voltage-gated calcium channel alpha-2-delta ligands. Opioids are an acceptable second-line therapy; however, the side effects of especially long-term use should be considered. Topical agents may also play a role in treatment, especially for focal pain. These options include capsaicin and lidocaine creams, among others.

Symptom scales

Criteria exist to characterize the severity of DSPN. The Neuropathy Symptom Profile (NSP) is a questionnaire to evaluate patient-reported symptoms of neuropathy [109]. Its proposed usefulness includes screening an at-risk population for neuropathy, evaluating patients longitudinally, comparing various forms of neuropathy, and for use during research. The Neuropathy Impairment Score (NIS) is a scoring system for a group of muscles, reflexes, and sensation [110]. This scale can be performed on the lower limbs only (NIS-LL) if desired. The Neuropathy Disability Score (NDS) is a comprehensive neurological examination that allows for a systemic assessment of the presence and severity of neuropathy [34]. The Michigan Neuropathy Screening Instrument (MNSI) was devised as a brief screening tool to evaluate outpatients with a history of diabetes for DSPN [7]. This tool consists of two parts: (1) 15 'yes or no' questions pertaining to foot symptoms, and (2) a foot examination including reporting foot deformities, dry skin, callus, infection, or ulceration, vibration assessment, and ankle reflexes. The clinical portion of the MNSI is a good screening tool for diabetes, with a sensitivity of 80% and specificity of 95%. The Michigan Diabetic Neuropathy Scale (MDNS) provides a way to confirm the diagnosis of DSPN and consists of a clinical neurological examination and NCS. Examination includes an evaluation of sensation (including the modalities of vibratory threshold perception, pain, and light touch), deep tendon reflexes, and muscle strength [7]. Finally, the Utah Early Neuropathy Scale (UENS) is a scale to assess sensory and small fibre abnormalities and may be useful to detect and study the early manifestations of neuropathy [111]. This scale grades according to toe extensor strength, pin sensation, presence of allodynia or hyperaesthesia, vibration and proprioception sense, and deep tendon reflexes.

Conclusion/summary

Diabetes is implicated in a wide array of abnormalities of peripheral nervous system function. Recognition of these entities is essential for primary and secondary prevention, appropriate management of symptoms, targeting evaluations, and avoiding unnecessary tests in uncommon presentations of diabetic neuropathies.

References

1. Powers AC. Diabetes mellitus. In: Longo D, Fauci A, Kasper DL, Hauser SL, Jameson JL, Loscalzo J (ed) *Harrison's Principles of Internal Medicine*, 18th edn, pp. 2968–3002. New York: McGraw-Hill, 2012.

2. Centers for Disease Control and Prevention. *National Diabetes Fact Sheet: National Estimates and General Information on Diabetes and Prediabetes in the United States, 2011*. Atlanta, GA: US Department of Health and Human Services, Centers for Disease Control and Prevention, 2011. Available from: <http://www.cdc.gov/diabetes/pubs/factsheet11.htm?loc=diabetes-statistics#citation>.

3. International Diabetes Federation. *IDF Diabetes Atlas*, 5th edn, 2009 [update]. Available from: <http://www.idf.org/diabetesatlas/europe>.

4. Dyck PJ, Kratz KM, Karnes JL, et al. The prevalence by staged severity of various types of diabetic neuropathy, retinopathy, and nephropathy in a population-based cohort: the Rochester Diabetic Neuropathy Study. *Neurology*, 1993; **43**: 817–24.

5. Partanen J, Niskanen L, Lehtinen J, et al. Natural history of peripheral neuropathy in patients with non-insulin-dependent diabetes mellitus. *N Engl J Med* 1995; **333**: 89–94.

6. Boulton AJ, Knight G, Drurym J, Ward JD. The prevalence of symptomatic, diabetic neuropathy in an insulin-treated population. *Diabetes Care* 1985; **8**: 125–8.

7. Feldman EL, Stevens MJ, Thomas PK, Brown MB, Canal N, Greene DA. A practical two-step quantitative clinical and electrophysiological assessment for the diagnosis and staging of diabetic neuropathy. *Diabetes Care* 1994; **17**: 1281–9.

8. Podwall D, Gooch C. Diabetic neuropathy: clinical features, etiology, and therapy. *Curr Neurol Neurosci Rep* 2004; **4**: 55–61.

9. Dyck PJ, Albers JW, Andersen H, et al. Diabetic polyneuropathies: update on research definition, diagnostic criteria and estimation of severity. *Diabetes Metab Res Rev* 2011; **27**: 620–8.

10. Tesfaye S, Boulton AJ, Dyck PJ, et al. Diabetic neuropathies: update on definitions, diagnostic criteria, estimation of severity, and treatments. *Diabetes Care* 2010; **33**: 2285–93.

11. Martin MM. Diabetic neuropathy; a clinical study of 150 cases. *Brain* 1953; **76**: 594–624.

12. Dyck PJ, Karnes JL, O'Brien PC, Litchy WJ, Low PA, Melton LJ, 3rd. The Rochester Diabetic Neuropathy Study: reassessment of tests and criteria for diagnosis and staged severity. *Neurology* 1992; **42**: 1164–70.

13. England JD, Gronseth GS, Franklin G, et al. Distal symmetric polyneuropathy: a definition for clinical research: report of the American Academy of Neurology, the American Association of Electrodiagnostic Medicine, and the American Academy of Physical Medicine and Rehabilitation. *Neurology* 2005; **64**: 199–207.

14. Cohen JA, Jeffers BW, Faldut D, Marcoux M, Schrier RW. Risks for sensorimotor peripheral neuropathy and autonomic neuropathy in non-insulin-dependent diabetes mellitus (NIDDM). *Muscle Nerve* 1998; **21**: 72–80.

15. Mulder DW, Lambert EH, Bastron JA, Sprague RG. The neuropathies associated with diabetes mellitus. A clinical and electromyographic study of 103 unselected diabetic patients. *Neurology* 1961; **11**: 275–84.

16. Wilson JR, Stittsworth JD, Jr, Kadir A, Fisher MA, et al. Conduction velocity versus amplitude analysis: evidence for demyelination in diabetic neuropathy. *Muscle Nerve* 1998; **21**: 1228–30.

17. Herrmann DN, Ferguson ML, Logigian EL. Conduction slowing in diabetic distal polyneuropathy. *Muscle Nerve* 2002; **26**: 232–7.

18. Abu-Shakra SR, Cornblath DR, Avila OL, et al. Conduction block in diabetic neuropathy. *Muscle Nerve* 1991; **14**: 858–62.

19. Bagai K, Wilson JR, Khanna M, Song Y, Wang L, Fisher MA. Electrophysiological patterns of diabetic polyneuropathy. *Electromyogr Clin Neurophysiol* 2008; **48**: 139–45.

20. Lehtinen JM, Uusitupa M, Siitonen O, Pyörälä K. Prevalence of neuropathy in newly diagnosed NIDDM and nondiabetic control subjects. *Diabetes* 1989; **38**: 1307–13.

21. Standards of medical care in diabetes—2012. *Diabetes Care*, 2012; **35** (Suppl 1): S11–S63.

22. de Neeling JN, Beks PJ, Bertelsmann FW, Heine RJ, Bouter LM. Peripheral somatic nerve function in relation to glucose tolerance in an elderly Caucasian population: the Hoorn study. *Diabet Med* 1996; **13**: 960–6.

23. Singleton JR, Smith AG, Bromberg MB. Painful sensory polyneuropathy associated with impaired glucose tolerance. *Muscle Nerve* 2001; **24**: 1225–8.

24. Hoffman-Snyder C, Smith BE, Ross MA, Hernandez J, Bosch EP. Value of the oral glucose tolerance test in the evaluation of chronic idiopathic axonal polyneuropathy. *Arch Neurol* 2006; **63**: 1075–9.

25. Novella SP, Inzucchi SE, Goldstein JM. The frequency of undiagnosed diabetes and impaired glucose tolerance in patients with idiopathic sensory neuropathy. *Muscle Nerve* 2001; **24**: 1229–31.

26. Sumner CJ, Sheth S, Griffin JW, Cornblath DR, Polydefkis M. The spectrum of neuropathy in diabetes and impaired glucose tolerance. *Neurology* 2003; **60**: 108–11.

27. Smith AG, Singleton JR. The diagnostic yield of a standardized approach to idiopathic sensory-predominant neuropathy. *Arch Intern Med* 2004; **164**: 1021–5.

28. Gorson KC, Ropper AH. Additional causes for distal sensory polyneuropathy in diabetic patients. *J Neurol Neurosurg Psychiatry* 2006; **77**: 354–8.

29. Sharma KR, Cross J, Farronay O, Ayyar DR, Shebert RT, Bradley WG. Demyelinating neuropathy in diabetes mellitus. *Arch Neurol* 2002; **59**: 758–65.

30. Laughlin RS, Dyck PJ, Melton LJ, III, Leibson C, Ransom J, Dyck PJ. Incidence and prevalence of CIDP and the association of diabetes mellitus. *Neurology* 2009; **73**: 39–45.

31. Haq RU, Pendlebury WW, Fries TJ, Tandan R. Chronic inflammatory demyelinating polyradiculoneuropathy in diabetic patients. *Muscle Nerve* 2003; **27**: 465–70.

32. Sharma KR, Cross J, Ayyar DR, Martinez-Arizala A, Bradley WG. Diabetic demyelinating polyneuropathy responsive to intravenous immunoglobulin therapy. *Arch Neurol* 2002; **59**: 751–7.

33. Stewart JD, McKelvey R, Durcan L, Carpenter S, Karpati G. Chronic inflammatory demyelinating polyneuropathy (CIDP) in diabetics. *J Neurol Sci* 1996; **142**: 59–64.

34. Dyck PJ, Sherman WR, Hallcher LM, et al. Human diabetic endoneurial sorbitol, fructose, and myo-inositol related to sural nerve morphometry. *Ann Neurol* 1980; **8**: 590–6.

35. Albers JW, Brown MB, Sima AA, Greene DA. Frequency of median mononeuropathy in patients with mild diabetic neuropathy in the early diabetes intervention trial (EDIT). Tolrestat Study Group For Edit (Early Diabetes Intervention Trial). *Muscle Nerve* 1996; **19**: 140–6.

36. Zambelis T, Tsivgoulis G, Karandreas N. Carpal tunnel syndrome: associations between risk factors and laterality. *Eur Neurol* 2010; **63**: 43–7.

37. Becker J, Nora DB, Gomes I, et al. An evaluation of gender, obesity, age and diabetes mellitus as risk factors for carpal tunnel syndrome. *Clin Neurophysiol* 2002; **113**: 1429–34.

38. Thomsen NO, Cederlund R, Rósen I, Björk J, Dahlin LB. Clinical outcomes of surgical release among diabetic patients with carpal tunnel syndrome: prospective follow-up with matched controls. *J Hand Surg Am* 2009; **34**: 1177–87.

39. Mondelli M, Padua L, Reale F, Signorini AM, Romano C. Outcome of surgical release among diabetics with carpal tunnel syndrome. *Arch Phys Med Rehabil* 2004; **85**: 7–13.

40. Watanabe K, Hagura R, Akanuma Y, et al. Characteristics of cranial nerve palsies in diabetic patients. *Diabetes Res Clin Pract* 1990; **10**: 19–27.

41. Greco D, Gambina F, Maggio F. Ophthalmoplegia in diabetes mellitus: a retrospective study. *Acta Diabetol* 2009; **46**: 23–6.

42. Schady W, Abuaisha B, Boulton AJ. Observations on severe ulnar neuropathy in diabetes. *J Diabetes Complications* 1998; **12**: 128–32.

43. Acosta JA, Hoffman SN, Raynor EM, Nardin RA, Rutkove SB. Ulnar neuropathy in the forearm: A possible complication of diabetes mellitus. *Muscle Nerve* 2003; **28**: 40–5.

44. Katirji MB, Wilbourn AJ. Common peroneal mononeuropathy: a clinical and electrophysiologic study of 116 lesions. *Neurology* 1988; **38**: 1723–8.

45. Parisi TJ, Mandrekar J, Dyck PJ, Klein CJ. Meralgia paresthetica: relation to obesity, advanced age, and diabetes mellitus. *Neurology* 2011; **77**: 1538–42.

46. Calverley JR, Mulder DW. Femoral neuropathy. *Neurology* 1960; **10**: 963–7.

47. Garland H, Taverner D. Diabetic myelopathy. *Br Med J* 1953; **1**(4825): 1405–8.

48. Garland H. Diabetic amyotrophy. *Br Med J* 1955; **2**(4951): 1287–90.

49. Williams IR, Mayer RF. Subacute proximal diabetic neuropathy. *Neurology* 1976; **26**: 108–16.

50. Dyck PJ, Norell JE. Microvasculitis and ischemia in diabetic lumbosacral radiculoplexus neuropathy. *Neurology* 1999; **53**: 2113–21.

51. Garland H. Diabetic amyotrophy. *Br J Clin Pract* 1961; **15**: 9–13.

52. Chokroverty S, Reyes MG, Rubino FA. Bruns–Garland syndrome of diabetic amyotrophy. *Trans Am Neurol Assoc* 1977; **102**: 173–7.

53. Asbury AK. Proximal diabetic neuropathy. *Ann Neurol* 1977; **2**: 179–80.

54. Katz JS, Saperstein DS, Wolfe G, et al. Cervicobrachial involvement in diabetic radiculoplexopathy. *Muscle Nerve* 2001; **24**: 794–8.

55. Massie R, Mauermann ML, Dyck PJB. Diabetic cervical radiculoplexus neuropathy. In: *135th Meeting of the American Neurological Association.* San Francisco, CA, 2010.

56. Pascoe MK, Low PA, Windebank AJ, Litchy WJ. Subacute diabetic proximal neuropathy. *Mayo Clin Proc* 1997; **72**: 1123–32.

57. Gorson KC, Ropper AH, Adelman LS, Weinberg DH. Influence of diabetes mellitus on chronic inflammatory demyelinating polyneuropathy. *Muscle Nerve* 2000; **23**: 37–43.

58. Stewart JD. Diabetic truncal neuropathy: topography of the sensory deficit. *Ann Neurol* 1989; **25**: 233–8.

59. Ellenberg M. Diabetic truncal mononeuropathy—a new clinical syndrome. *Diabetes Care* 1978; **1**: 10–13.

60. Kikta DG, Breuer AC, Wilbourn AJ. Thoracic root pain in diabetes: the spectrum of clinical and electromyographic findings. *Ann Neurol* 1982; **11**: 80–5.

61. Godil A., Berriman D, Knapik S, Norman M, Godil F, Firek AF. Diabetic neuropathic cachexia. *West J Med* 1996; 165: 382–5.

62. Ellenberg M. Diabetic neuropathic cachexia. *Diabetes* 1974; **23**: 418–23.

63. Vinik AI, Maser RE, Mitchell BD, Freeman R. Diabetic autonomic neuropathy. *Diabetes Care* 2003; **26**: 1553–79.

64. Duchen LW, Anjorin A, Watkins PJ, Mackay JD. Pathology of autonomic neuropathy in diabetes mellitus. *Ann Intern Med* 1980; **92**: 301–3.

65. Low PA, Benrud-Larson LM, Sletten DM, et al. Autonomic symptoms and diabetic neuropathy: a population-based study. *Diabetes Care* 2004; **27**: 2942–7.

66. Grandinetti A, Chow DC, Sletten DM, et al. Impaired glucose tolerance is associated with postganglionic sudomotor impairment. *Clin Auton Res* 2007; **17**: 231–3.

67. Kahn R. Proceedings of a consensus development conference on standardized measures in diabetic neuropathy. Autonomic nervous system testing. *Diabetes Care* 1992; **15**: 1095–103.

68. Ewing DJ, Campbell IW, Clarke BF. Assessment of cardiovascular effects in diabetic autonomic neuropathy and prognostic implications. *Ann Intern Med* 1980; **92**: 308–11.

69. Maser RE, Mitchell BD, Vinik AI, Freeman R. The association between cardiovascular autonomic neuropathy and mortality in individuals with diabetes: a meta-analysis. *Diabetes Care* 2003; **26**: 1895–901.

70. Witte DR, Tesfaye S, Chaturvedi N, Eaton SE, Kempler P, Fuller JH. Risk factors for cardiac autonomic neuropathy in type 1 diabetes mellitus. *Diabetologia* 2005; **48**: 164–71.

71. Taskiran M, Rasmussen V, Rasmussen B, et al. Left ventricular dysfunction in normotensive Type 1 diabetic patients: the impact of autonomic neuropathy. *Diabet Med* 2004; **21**: 524–30.

72. Pop-Busui R. Cardiac autonomic neuropathy in diabetes: a clinical perspective. *Diabetes Care* 2010; **33**: 434–41.

73. Soedamah-Muthu SS, Chaturvedi N, Witte DR, et al. Relationship between risk factors and mortality in type 1 diabetic patients in Europe: the EURODIAB Prospective Complications Study (PCS). *Diabetes Care* 2008; **31**: 1360–6.

74. Orchard TJ, Lloyd CE, Maser RE, Kuller LH. Why does diabetic autonomic neuropathy predict IDDM mortality? An analysis from the Pittsburgh Epidemiology of Diabetes Complications Study. *Diabetes Res Clin Pract* 1996; **34** (Suppl): S165–S171.

75. O'Brien IA, McFadden JP, Corrall RJ. The influence of autonomic neuropathy on mortality in insulin-dependent diabetes. *Q J Med* 1991; **79**: 495–502.

76. Pfeifer MA, Weinberg CR, Cook DL, et al. Autonomic neural dysfunction in recently diagnosed diabetic subjects. *Diabetes Care* 1984; **7**: 447–53.

77. Zilliox L, Peltier AC, Wren PA, et al. Assessing autonomic dysfunction in early diabetic neuropathy: the Survey of Autonomic Symptoms. *Neurology* 2011; **76**: 1099–105.

78. Suarez GA, Opfer-Gehrking TL, Offord KP, Atkinson EJ, O'Brien PC, Low PA. The Autonomic Symptom Profile: a new instrument to assess autonomic symptoms. *Neurology* 1999; **52**: 523–8.

79. Karavanaki K, Baum JD. Coexistence of impaired indices of autonomic neuropathy and diabetic nephropathy in a cohort of children with type 1 diabetes mellitus. *J Pediatr Endocrinol Metab* 2003; **16**: 79–90.

80. Maguire AM, Craig ME, Craighead A, et al. Autonomic nerve testing predicts the development of complications: a 12-year follow-up study. *Diabetes Care* 2007; **30**: 77–82.

81. Cahill M, Eustace P, de Jesus V. Pupillary autonomic denervation with increasing duration of diabetes mellitus. *Br J Ophthalmol* 2001; **85**: 1225–30.

82. Jones KL, Russo A, Stevens JE, Wishart JM, Berry MK, Horowitz M. Predictors of delayed gastric emptying in diabetes. *Diabetes Care* 2001; **24**: 1264–9.

83. Horowitz M, Fraser R. Disordered gastric motor function in diabetes mellitus. *Diabetologia* 1994; **37**: 543–51.

84. Sellin JH, Chang EB. Therapy insight: gastrointestinal complications of diabetes--pathophysiology and management. *Nat Clin Pract Gastroenterol Hepatol* 2008; **5**: 162–71.

85. Fedele D. Therapy insight: sexual and bladder dysfunction associated with diabetes mellitus. *Nat Clin Pract Urol* 2005; **2**: 282–90 [quiz 309].

86. Holland NR, Crawford TO, Hauer P, Cornblath DR, Griffin JW, McArthur JC. Small-fiber sensory neuropathies: clinical course and neuropathology of idiopathic cases. *Ann Neurol* 1998; **44**: 47–59.

87. Periquet MI, Novak V, Collins MP, et al. Painful sensory neuropathy: prospective evaluation using skin biopsy. *Neurology* 1999; **53**: 1641–7.

88. European Federation of Neurological Societies/Peripheral Nerve Society Guideline on the use of skin biopsy in the diagnosis of small fiber neuropathy. Report of a joint task force of the European Federation of Neurological Societies and the Peripheral Nerve Society. *J Peripher Nerv Syst* 2010; **15**: 79–92.

89. Gibbons CH, Freeman R. Treatment-induced diabetic neuropathy: a reversible painful autonomic neuropathy. *Ann Neurol* 2010; **67**: 534–41.

90. Edwards JL, Vincent AM, Cheng HT, Feldman EL. Diabetic neuropathy: mechanisms to management. *Pharmacol Ther* 2008; **120**: 1–34.

91. Brownlee M. Biochemistry and molecular cell biology of diabetic complications. *Nature* 2001; **414**: 813–20.

92. Brownlee M. The pathobiology of diabetic complications: a unifying mechanism. *Diabetes* 2005; **54**: 1615–25.

93. Feldman, E.L., M.J. Stevens, and D.A. Greene, *Pathogenesis of diabetic neuropathy. Clin Neurosci*, 1997. 4(6): p. 365–70.

94. Yamagishi S. Uehara K, Otsuki S, Yagihashi S. Differential influence of increased polyol pathway on protein kinase C expressions between endoneurial and epineurial tissues in diabetic mice. *J Neurochem* 2003; **87**: 497–507.

95. Uehara K, Yamagishi S, Otsuki S, Chin S, Yagihashi S. Effects of polyol pathway hyperactivity on protein kinase C activity, nociceptive peptide expression, and neuronal structure in dorsal root ganglia in diabetic mice. *Diabetes* 2004; **53**: 3239–47.

96. Das Evcimen N, King GL. The role of protein kinase C activation and the vascular complications of diabetes. *Pharmacol Res* 2007; **55**: 498–510.

97. Kolm-Litty V, Sauer U, Nerlich A, Lehmann R, Schleicher ED. High glucose-induced transforming growth factor beta1 production is mediated by the hexosamine pathway in porcine glomerular mesangial cells. *J Clin Invest* 1998; **101**: 160–9.

98. Du XL, Edelstein D, Rossetti L, et al. Hyperglycemia-induced mitochondrial superoxide overproduction activates the hexosamine pathway and induces plasminogen activator inhibitor-1 expression by increasing Sp1 glycosylation. *Proc Natl Acad Sci USA* 2000; **97**: 12222–6.

99. Wada R, Yagihashi S. Role of advanced glycation end products and their receptors in development of diabetic neuropathy. Ann NY *Acad Sci* 2005; **1043**: 598–604.

100. The effect of intensive treatment of diabetes on the development and progression of long-term complications in insulin-dependent diabetes mellitus. The Diabetes Control and Complications Trial Research Group. *N Engl J Med* 1993; **329**: 977–86.

101. Effect of intensive diabetes treatment on nerve conduction in the Diabetes Control and Complications Trial. *Ann Neurol* 1995; **38**: 869–80.

102. Pop-Busui R, Herman WH, Feldman EL, et al. DCCT and EDIC studies in type 1 diabetes: lessons for diabetic neuropathy regarding metabolic memory and natural history. *Curr Diab Rep* 2010; **10**: 276–82.

103. Little AA, Edwards JL, Feldman EL. Diabetic neuropathies. *Pract Neurol* 2007; **7**: 82–92.

104. Jaradeh SS, Prieto TE, Lobeck LJ. Progressive polyradiculoneuropathy in diabetes: correlation of variables and clinical outcome after immunotherapy. *J Neurol Neurosurg Psychiatry* 1999; **67**: 607–12.

105. Krendel DA, Costigan DA, Hopkins LC. Successful treatment of neuropathies in patients with diabetes mellitus. *Arch Neurol* 1995; **52**: 1053–61.

106. Zochodne DW, Isaac D, Jones C. Failure of immunotherapy to prevent, arrest or reverse diabetic lumbosacral plexopathy. *Acta Neurol Scand* 2003; **107**: 299–301.

107. Dyck PJ, Windebank AJ. Diabetic and nondiabetic lumbosacral radiculoplexus neuropathies: new insights into pathophysiology and treatment. *Muscle Nerve* 2002; **25**: 477–91.

108. Callaghan BC, Cheng HT, Stables CL, Smith AL, Feldman EL. Diabetic neuropathy: clinical manifestations and current treatments. *Lancet Neurol* 2012; **11**: 521–34.

109. Dyck PJ, Karnes J, O'Brien PC, Swanson CJ. Neuropathy Symptom Profile in health, motor neuron disease, diabetic neuropathy, and amyloidosis. *Neurology* 1986; **36**: 1300–8.

110. Dyck PJ, Davies JL, Litchy WJ, O'Brien PC. Longitudinal assessment of diabetic polyneuropathy using a composite score in the Rochester Diabetic Neuropathy Study cohort. *Neurology* 1997; **49**: 229–39.

111. Singleton JR, Bixby B, Russell JW, et al. The Utah Early Neuropathy Scale: a sensitive clinical scale for early sensory predominant neuropathy. *J Peripher Nerv Syst* 2008; **13**: 218–27.

CHAPTER 18

Peripheral nerve hyperexcitability disorders

David Hilton-Jones

Introduction

The peripheral nerve hyperexcitability disorders (PNHDs) are defined by variable combinations of symptoms and signs reflecting the consequences of hyperexcitability of motor, sensory, and autonomic nerves. Whilst many specific inherited and acquired causes are recognized (Table 18.1), most cases of PNHD are idiopathic. Autoimmunity is the basis of some idiopathic cases, and may also be relevant in some cases associated with a specific acquired peripheral nerve disorder.

The terminology surrounding PNHD, with respect to the clinical phenomenology and neurophysiological accompaniments of motor nerve hyperexcitability, is complex, confused, and overall rather unilluminating. Terms that have been used to describe the clinical features include twitches, cramps, fasciculations, benign fasciculation, myokymia, undulating myokymia, syndrome of continuous muscle fibre activity, Isaacs syndrome, Isaacs–Mertens syndrome, carpopedal spasm, tetany, the Chvostek sign, the Trousseau sign, cramp-fasciculation syndrome, neuromyotonia, and rippling muscle. Electromyographic (EMG) findings include fasciculation potentials, doublet, triplet, and multiplet discharges (with high intraburst frequency), continuous motor unit discharges, myokymic discharges, and after-discharges (Fig. 18.1). To add to the confusion, some words (e.g. fasciculation, myokymia) are use to describe both clinical and electromyographic features, but not necessarily always the same phenomenon! A lumper's gross simplification is that the patient with PNHD may complain of a wide range of muscle symptoms, which are associated with EMG features indicating that the muscle is simply responding to peripheral nerve discharges. But the spectrum is enormous, and ranges from fasciculation alone, or localized cramping that might otherwise be considered 'physiological', to a profoundly disabling disorder of widespread muscle stiffness and delayed relaxation ('neuromyotonia') which may be accompanied by encephalopathy (Morvan syndrome). Symptoms may be generalized, or restricted to the area of distribution of a single peripheral nerve.

Although motor nerve features dominate, there is evidence in some cases of sensory and autonomic nerve hyperactivity. Sensory symptoms include paraesthesia and pain. Excessive sweating may be due either to heat generated by excessive activity or autonomic nerve involvement, and the latter is also suggested by rare cases with evidence of smooth muscle involvement (e.g. the oesophagus, causing dysphagia [1], or bronchial smooth muscle, causing bronchospasm [2]).

Acquired disorders

'Simple' cramps

There are few people who have not experienced cramp, typically affecting the calf muscles. There is no clear distinction between such simple cramps, sometimes called physiological cramps, and the mildest forms of PNHD, but features of the latter include great frequency, more widespread distribution (e.g. hands, trunk muscles), and the detection of additional features such as fasciculation. All forms of cramping, even if not caused by, may be exacerbated by a wide range of physiological and metabolic variables which must be considered in every case [3].

Metabolic disorders

As noted, metabolic changes, including those brought on by exercise, may precipitate or exacerbate cramping. Commonly cited causes include dehydration (e.g. with diarrhoea, vomiting, diuretics, exercise), uraemia, haemodialysis, pregnancy, and hypothyroidism. Rather more specifically, peripheral nerve hyperexcitability (PNH) can be a pronounced feature of hypocalcaemia (and hypomagnesaemia). Because other clinical features of these disorders may be absent, serum calcium and magnesium and renal and thyroid function should be assessed in all patients presenting with PNHD.

Drugs and toxins

Any neurotoxic drug may cause features of PNHD, typically fasciculation and cramping, as well as dysaesthesia and sensory loss. PNH has been particularly associated with the organoplatinum compounds, such as oxaliplatin [4].

Neurotoxins associated with PNHS include animal venoms (e.g. snake, spider, and jellyfish venom; latrodectism is the term given to the clinical syndrome induced by venom from various spiders including the black widow and Australian redback). The release of acetylcholine by peripheral nerves leads to severe muscle cramping/spasm. Neurotoxins act directly on the nerves, but another mechanism leading to PNH is when a toxin induces a secondary immune response leading to production of antivoltage-gated potassium channel (anti-VGKC) antibodies, as in a dramatic case of neuromyotonia induced by a wasp sting [5].

Pyridostigmine is used for symptomatic treatment of myasthenia gravis and related conditions. It blocks cholinesterase activity at neuromuscular junctions, and therefore prolongs the action of acetylcholine. Whilst that helps muscle weakness due to myasthenia,

Table 18.1 Causes of peripheral nerve hyperexcitability

Acquired:
Metabolic disorders
Drugs and toxins
Neuropathies
• Acute inflammatory demyelinating polyneuropathy (Guillain–Barré syndrome) • Chronic inflammatory demyelinating polyneuropathy • Brachial plexus neuropathy (neuralgic amyotrophy) • Radiation-induced neuropathy/plexopathy • Focal/compressive • Axonal neuropathy
Anterior horn cell: preceding anterior horn cell disease (amyotrophic lateral sclerosis/motor neuron disease)
Autoimmune: tumour-associated (thymoma, small cell lung cancer)
Idiopathic
Inherited:
Neurogenic disorders

• Peripheral neuropathies (e.g. Charcot–Marie–Tooth disease)
• Spinal muscular atrophies
    Proximal (e.g. *SMN*-related)
    Distal
   Kennedy syndrome
• Episodic ataxia type 1 (*KCNA1* mutations)
• *KCNQ2* mutations

it causes overstimulation of muscles that are less affected by the disease, and common symptoms include cramping, particularly of the hands, and lower eyelid 'myokymia'. It is important to have an appreciation of this, because in patients with autoimmune myasthenia there is an increased incidence of PNHD due to acquisition of anti-VGKC antibodies (see section on Autoimmune disorders) and the phenomenology may be similar.

Neuropathies

PNHD may be seen in association with acquired, immune-mediated neuropathies (acute inflammatory demyelinating polyneuropathy/Guillain–Barré syndrome, chronic inflammatory demyelinating polyneuropathy (CIDP), multifocal motor neuropathy with conduction block, brachial and lumbar plexus neuropathy/neuralgic amyotrophy), neuropathies caused by physical damage (compression- or radiation-induced neuropathy/plexopathy) and with apparently idiopathic axonal neuropathy. There is potential confusion with respect to the latter, as there is some evidence that anti-VGKC-related PNH may lead to secondary axonal damage [6], and therefore a potential 'chicken and egg' situation. Focal neuropathies (e.g. compression, trauma, radiation) of course show symptoms and signs of focal PNH.

When associated with structural damage (e.g. compression or radiation), the PNH is a direct consequence (although potentially via several complex mechanisms) of local nerve damage [7]. Hemifacial spasm due to compression, e.g. by a vascular loop, is a well-known, albeit restricted, example. When PNH is associated with one of the immune-mediated neuropathies there are two possible underlying mechanisms. Firstly, the consequences of nerve damage, and secondly the development of immune-mediated PNH

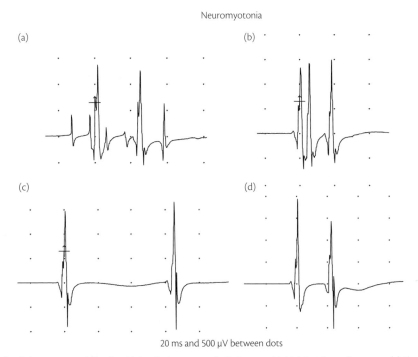

Neuromyotonia

(a)   (b)

(c)   (d)

20 ms and 500 μV between dots

Fig. 18.1 The characteristic finding in 'neuromyotonia' is of multiplet single motor unit discharges with high intraburst frequency. (a) Short burst of neuromyotonic discharge with an intraburst frequency of about 50–100 Hz. (b) Triplet motor unit repeat discharge—the intraburst frequency of the first two is about 200 Hz. (c) Doublet motor unit discharge—intraburst frequency about 15 Hz. (d) Doublet motor unit discharge—intraburst frequency about 45 Hz. (Figure courtesy of Dr Robin Kennett.)

either with anti-VGKC antibodies (see section on Autoimmune disorders) or other, as yet unidentified, antibodies. Guillain–Barré syndrome and CIDP have been reported with anti-VGKC antibodies in association with Isaacs syndrome [8,9].

Anterior horn cell disorders

Fasciculation and cramp are common, and often presenting, symptoms/signs of amyotrophic lateral sclerosis/motor neuron disease (ALS/MND). A practical difficulty may be differentiating between those patients having a benign 'cramp/fasciculation' syndrome, who can be reassured accordingly, and those having early features of ALS/MND. The presence of wasting, weakness, and reflex changes clearly supports the latter. Several studies have looked at predictive features, including patterns of distribution of fasciculation, neurophysiological findings, etc., but the final conclusion has to be that surveillance for several years is the only certain way of excluding progression [10–12].

Autoimmune disorders

The observation that PNH was sometimes seen in association with other autoimmune disorders, particularly myasthenia gravis, and as a paraneoplastic phenomenon (thymoma and lung cancer), suggested autoimmunity as a cause and led to the subsequent identification of anti-VGKC antibodies [13–15]. More recent studies have shown that these antibodies are in fact mainly directed at proteins complexing with the potassium channel, rather than the channel itself, and are thus now known as VGKC-complex antibodies—they include LGI-1 and CASPR2, but undoubtedly others remain to be identified. Clinical phenotypes show marked overlap with the antibody specificities, but broadly speaking limbic encephalitis is more frequently associated with LGI-1 than CASPR2, and vice versa for PNH [16], whereas in Morvan syndrome there are high titres to CASPR2 [17].

The clinical syndrome that led to the discovery of this pathway comprises acquired onset, at any age, of varying combinations and severities of muscle stiffness, cramps, twitching, myokymia, slow muscle relaxation after contraction, muscle hypertrophy, and increased sweating. Serum creatine kinase is often modestly elevated. An early description was by Isaacs, who used the term 'continuous muscle fibre activity', hence the earlier eponymous labelling of this condition as Isaacs syndrome [18,19]. Mertens showed that the muscle was responding to PNH and coined the term 'neuromyotonia' [20], and Isaacs–Mertens syndrome became another eponymous descriptor. Morvan syndrome describes neuromyotonia in association with central nervous system (CNS) involvement (insomnia, delirium, hallucinations), with the CNS features being due to central action of the VGKC-complex antibodies. Subsequently patients were identified with CNS involvement without PNH and presenting with features of limbic encephalitis, spawning a whole new area of autoimmune encephalitides [21,22].

Not all patients presenting with 'neuromyotonia' have anti-VGKC-complex antibodies, but have clear evidence of an autoimmune basis to their disorder in terms of responsiveness to immunotherapies. As noted, it is likely that antibodies against other components of the VGKC-complex, or indeed against unrelated proteins, remain to be identified. In clinical practice, many patients are seen with varying combinations of muscle twitching and cramps some of which may be *formes frustes* of 'neuromyotonia' as already described, but a majority do not have anti-VGKC-complex antibodies and have no obvious association with other autoimmune disorders. Many respond well to symptomatic treatments (see section on Treatment) and so are not exposed to immunomodulatory approaches, such as plasma exchange, intravenous immunoglobulin, or immunosuppression—so it remains uncertain whether they have an immune disorder. Despite the observation of associations with other autoimmune disorders and neoplasia, the majority of cases, whether with anti-VGKC-complex antibodies or not, appear to be idiopathic in origin.

Inherited disorders

A number of inherited disorders affecting the motor nerves, from the anterior horn cell to terminal branches, may be associated with PNH (see Table 18.1). The most common features of PNH are muscle twitching and cramping. In most cases there are additional neuromuscular features to aid differential diagnosis.

Peripheral neuropathies

Cramping is common in the hereditary motor and sensory neuropathies (HMSN). In one paediatric study, a third of patients with HMSN Type 1A were troubled by calf cramps [23]. It is also seen in axonal neuropathies, in some rare forms of which neuromyotonia has been a prominent feature [24,25].

Spinal muscular atrophies

Cramping is relatively common in the various forms of proximal spinal muscular atrophy associated with homozygous *SMN* mutations. Polyminimyoclonus (trembling of the fingers) may be seen, and twitching ('fibrillation') of the tongue, a finer movement than tongue fasciculation in ALS/MND. Such features are usually accompanied by obvious proximal muscle weakness and wasting, but rarely cramping may precede such developments [26].

Distal spinal muscular atrophy is much less common than the proximal variety, and relatively few specific genetic causes have been identified. Scattered case reports, not surprisingly, describe patients with cramps and muscle twitching.

Kennedy syndrome (X-linked spinal and bulbar muscular atrophy) is due to an unstable CAG trinucleotide repeat expansion in the androgen receptor gene. Symptoms and signs of PNH are common, with tremor, muscle twitching, especially in the perioral/mental region, and cramping, typically preceding any significant weakness [27,28].

Episodic ataxia Type 1

Mutations in the neuronal voltage-gated potassium channel gene, *KCNA1*, are most commonly associated with episodic ataxia and myokymia. However, there is considerable phenotypic variability and patients have been reported with marked features of PNH (variously described as myokymia and neuromyotonia) without ataxia [29,30]. *KCNA1* mutations should be excluded when there is a family history of apparent PNH, even in the absence of ataxia. Other genes may be involved, and families with apparent autosomal dominant inheritance of neuromyotonia have been reported without an identified mutation in *KCNA1* or several related genes [31]. Mutations in the potassium channel gene *KCNQ2* cause a form of benign familial neonatal epilepsy; a unique mutation in one family was also associated with later onset of myokymia [32].

Differential diagnosis

Similar symptoms and signs to those already described may be seen in both CNS and myopathic disorders, although the EMG features usually allow easy differentiation from PNHD.

CNS disorders may cause muscle spasms, stiffness, and delayed relaxation, but not localized twitching/fasciculation/myokymia or an abnormal reaction to muscle percussion (myotonia). In stiff person syndrome there is centrally driven continuous motor unit activity, with the latter showing normal morphology.

Myotonia (with stiffness, delayed relaxation, percussion myotonia) is seen in myotonic dystrophies Types 1 and 2, myotonia congenita (chloride channelopathy), and paramyotonia congenita (sodium channelopathy, with associated hyperkalaemic periodic paralysis).

The phenomenon of 'rippling muscle' may be due to PNH when electromyography shows motor unit activity, but two other forms are recognized which arise from muscle. Mutations in the caveolin (CAV3) gene may cause rippling muscle, muscle mounding on percussion, and 'percussion-induced rapid contractures' (PIRCS), which are electrically silent, and are also associated with limb-girdle muscular dystrophy Type 1C and asymptomatic hyperCKaemia [33,34]. Rarely, electrically silent rippling (as opposed to rippling due to PNH and anti-VGKC antibodies, discussed in the section Autoimmune disorders) has been reported in patients with myasthenia gravis, and is presumed to have an autoimmune basis [35,36].

In the extremely rare condition Schwartz–Jampel syndrome, due to mutations affecting the basement membrane protein perlecan, there is abnormal muscle activity resembling myotonia, with blepharophimosis and an unusual facial appearance due to abnormal muscle activity [37]. Electromyography shows activity akin to myotonia/complex repetitive discharges but differing somewhat from both.

In metabolic myopathies, particularly glycogenolytic disorders (e.g. McArdle disease), localized exercise-induced muscle cramps/spasms are electrically silent.

Treatment

It is a *sine qua non* that if a specific treatable cause of PNH is identified then it should be treated in its own right, or that if PNH is induced by a drug or toxin that agent should be removed. However, in many instances either no specific cause is identified or the cause has no specific treatment, and the only option is symptomatic treatment.

Muscle 'twitching', which includes fasciculation, often causes patients great anxiety but does not in itself usually merit drug therapy. Furthermore, the symptomatic treatment options listed in this section often have no discernible effect on such twitching. Treatments are required when cramping and pain are major features, or when they are associated with CNS involvement. Some patients appear to have significant discomfort without necessarily very obvious cramping, and may merit treatment.

The main treatment options include the use of 'membrane-stabilizing drugs' and, in those cases with an immune basis, immunomodulatory or immunosuppressive therapies. Quinine is a time-honoured treatment for cramp. In mild cases it may prove to be effective and safe, but is very dangerous in excess. The 'membrane-stabilizing/anticonvulsant' drugs lamotrigine, carbamazepine, valproate, phenytoin, gabapentin, pregabalin, oxcarbazepine, and probably others of similar ilk may all be effective [38]. The principle of low initial dosage and gradual titration, as in treating epilepsy, applies. Other agents reported to be helpful in treating simple cramps include vitamin B, naftidrofuryl, and calcium-channel blockers [39].

If the PNH has an immune basis, e.g. with anti-VGKC antibodies, then immunotherapies are effective. In some cases of uncertain aetiology, when no specific antibodies have been identified, it is a successful response to such treatment that may prove the immune basis of the condition. In the short term, plasma exchange and intravenous immunoglobulin therapy are effective [5,40]. For long-term treatment, immunosuppression with prednisolone and azathioprine or alternative second-line immunosuppressant drugs is effective, although formal trials are lacking [38].

References

1. Braune S, Hentschel M, Glocker FX, Lücking CH. Involvement of the esophagus in the cramp-fasciculation syndrome. *Muscle Nerve* 1998; **21**: 802–4.
2. De Entrambasaguas M, Ortega-Albás JJ, Martínez-Lozano MD, Díaz JR. Bronchial involvement in the cramp-fasciculation syndrome. *Eur Neurol* 2006; **56**: 124–6.
3. Miller TM, Layzer RB. Muscle cramps. *Muscle Nerve* 2005; **32**: 431–42.
4. Lucchetta M, Lonardi S, Bergamo F, et al. Incidence of atypical acute nerve hyperexcitability symptoms in oxaliplatin-treated patients with colorectal cancer. *Cancer Chemother Pharmacol* 2012; **70**: 899–902.
5. Turner MR, Madkhana A, Ebers GC, et al. Wasp sting induced autoimmune neuromyotonia. *J Neurol Neurosurg Psychiatry* 2006; **77**: 704–5.
6. Rubio-Agusti I, Perez-Miralles F, Sevilla T, et al. Peripheral nerve hyperexcitability: a clinical and immunologic study of 38 patients. *Neurology* 2011; **76**: 172–8.
7. Delanian S, Lefaix JL, Pradat PF. Radiation-induced neuropathy in cancer survivors. *Radiother Oncol* 2012; **105**: 273–82.
8. Myers KA, Baker SK. Late-onset seropositive Isaacs' syndrome after Guillain–Barré syndrome. *Neuromuscul Disord* 2009; **19**: 288–90.
9. Odabasi Z, Joy JL, Claussen GC, Herrera GA, Oh SJ. Isaacs' syndrome associated with chronic inflammatory demyelinating polyneuropathy. *Muscle Nerve* 1996; **19**: 210–15.
10. De Carvalho M, Swash M. Fasciculation-cramp syndrome preceding anterior horn cell disease: an intermediate syndrome? *J Neurol Neurosurg Psychiatry* 2011; **82**: 459–61.
11. Simon NG, Kiernan MC. Fasciculation anxiety syndrome in clinicians. *J Neurol* 2013; **260**: 1743–7.
12. Singh V, Gibson J, McLean B, Boggild M, Silver N, White R. Fasciculations and cramps: How benign? Report of four cases progressing to ALS. *J Neurol* 2011; **258**: 573–8.
13. Vernino S, Lennon VA. Ion channel and striational antibodies define a continuum of autoimmune neuromuscular hyperexcitability. *Muscle Nerve* 2002; **26**: 702–7.
14. Hart IK, Maddison P, Newsom-Davis J, Vincent A, Mills KR. Phenotypic variants of autoimmune peripheral nerve hyperexcitability. *Brain* 2002; **125**: 1887–95.
15. Newsom-Davis J, Buckley C, Clover L, et al. Autoimmune disorders of neuronal potassium channels. *Ann NY Acad Sci* 2003; **998**: 202–10.
16. Klein CJ, Lennon VA, Aston PA, et al. Insights from LGI1 and CASPR2 potassium channel complex autoantibody subtyping. *J Am Med Assoc Neurology* 2013; **70**: 229–34.
17. Irani SR, Pettingill P, Kleopa KA, et al. Morvan syndrome: clinical and serological observations in 29 cases. *Ann Neurol* 2012; **72**: 241–55.
18. Isaacs H, Frere G. Syndrome of continuous muscle fibre activity. Histochemical, nerve terminal and end plate study of two cases. *S Afr Med J* 1974; **48**: 1601–7.

19. Isaacs H, Heffron JJA. The syndrome of 'continuous muscle fibre activity' cured: further studies. *J Neurol Neurosurg Psychiatry* 1974; **37**: 1231–5.

20. Mertens HG, Ricker K. Übererregbarkeit der γ-Motoneurone beim 'Stiff-man'-Syndrom. *Klin Wochenschr* 1968; **46**: 33–42.

21. Buckley C. Autoimmune neurological diseases. *Medicine (UK).* 2012; **40**: 553–7.

22. Vincent A, Bien CG, Irani SR, Waters P. Autoantibodies associated with diseases of the CNS: new developments and future challenges. *Lancet Neurol* 2011; **10**: 759–72.

23. Blyton F, Ryan MM, Ouvrier RA, Burns J. Muscle cramp in pediatric Charcot–Marie–Tooth disease type 1A: prevalence and predictors. *Neurology* 2011; **77**: 2115–18.

24. Maurelli M, Candeloro E, Egitto MT, Alfonsi E. Hereditary motor and sensory neuropathy type II (HMSN-II) and neurogenic muscle hypertrophy: a case report and literature review. *Neurol Sci* 1998; **19**: 184–8.

25. Zimoń M, Baets J, Almeida-Souza L, et al. Loss-of-function mutations in HINT1 cause axonal neuropathy with neuromyotonia. *Nat Genet* 2012; **44**: 1080–3.

26. Bussaglia E, Tizzano EF, Illa I, Cervera C, Baiget M. Cramps and minimal EMG abnormalities as preclinical manifestations of spinal muscular atrophy patients with homozygous deletions of the SMN gene. *Neurology* 1997; **48**: 1443–5.

27. Finsterer J. Perspectives of Kennedy's disease. *J Neurol Sci* 2010; **298**: 1–10.

28. Lee JH, Shin JH, Park KP, et al. Phenotypic variability in Kennedy's disease: implication of the early diagnostic features. *Acta Neurol Scand* 2005; **112**: 57–63.

29. Kinali M, Jungbluth H, Eunson LH, et al. Expanding the phenotype of potassium channelopathy: severe neuromyotonia and skeletal deformities without prominent episodic ataxia. *Neuromuscul Disord* 2004; **14**: 689–93.

30. Poujois A, Antoine JC, Combes A, Touraine RL. Chronic neuromyotonia as a phenotypic variation associated with a new mutation in the KCNA1 gene. *J Neurol* 2006; **253**: 957–9.

31. Falace A, Striano P, Manganelli F, et al. Inherited neuromyotonia: a clinical and genetic study of a family. *Neuromuscul Disord* 2007; **17**: 23–7.

32. Dedek K, Kunath B, Kananura C, Reuner U, Jentsch TJ, Steinlein OK. Myokymia and neonatal epilepsy caused by a mutation in the voltage sensor of the KCNQ2 K+ channel. *Proc Natl Acad Sci USA* 2001; **98**: 12272–7.

33. Vann Den Bergh PYK, Gérard JM, Elosegi JA, Manto MU, Kubisch C, Schoser BGH. Novel missense mutation in the caveolin-3 gene in a Belgian family with rippling muscle disease. *J Neurol Neurosurg Psychiatry* 2004; **75**: 1349–51.

34. Vorgerd M, Bolz H, Patzold T, Kubisch C, Malin JP, Mortier W. Phenotypic variability in rippling muscle disease. *Neurology* 1999; **52**: 1453–9.

35. Zelinka L, McCann S, Budde J, et al. Characterization of the in vitro expressed autoimmune rippling muscle disease immunogenic domain of human titin encoded by TTN exons 248–249. *Biochem Biophys Res Commun* 2011; **411**: 501–5.

36. Schoser B, Jacob S, Hilton-Jones D, et al. Immune-mediated rippling muscle disease with myasthenia gravis: a report of seven patients with long-term follow-up in two. *Neuromuscul Disord* 2009; **19**: 223–8.

37. Arikawa-Hirasawa E, Le AH, Nishino I, et al. Structural and functional mutations of the perlecan gene cause Schwartz–Jampel syndrome, with myotonic myopathy and chondrodysplasia. *Am J Hum Genet* 2002; **70**: 1368–75.

38. Skeie GO, Apostolski S, Evoli A, et al. Guidelines for treatment of autoimmune neuromuscular transmission disorders. *Eur J Neurol* 2010; **17**: 893–902.

39. Katzberg HD, Khan AH, So YT. Assessment: symptomatic treatment for muscle cramps (an evidence-based review): report of the Therapeutics and Technology Assessment Subcommittee of the American Academy of Neurology. *Neurology* 2010; **74**: 691–6.

40. Jaben EA, Winters JL. Plasma exchange as a therapeutic option in patients with neurologic symptoms due to antibodies to voltage-gated potassium channels: a report of five cases and review of the literature. *J Clin Apheresis* 2012; **27**: 267–73.

Neuromuscular Junction: Inherited and Acquired

CHAPTER 19

Inherited myasthenic syndromes

Jacqueline Palace and Sarah Finlayson

Introduction

Congenital myasthenic syndromes (CMS) are a heterogeneous group of inherited disorders of neuromuscular junction (NMJ) transmission. In contrast to transient neonatal myasthenia (TNM), these syndromes are caused by mutations in genes that encode proteins of the NMJ, and have no immunological basis. The advent of molecular genetic techniques in the late twentieth century allowed significant advances in our understanding of the underlying mechanisms of NMJ pathophysiology to be made, including clear identification of genetic subtypes. No fewer than 17 genes have so far been identified (Table 19.1) as causing CMS, many of which involve private mutations. Accurate prevalence data are difficult to ascertain. An analysis of genetically confirmed cases found an overall UK prevalence of 3.8 per million. However, this varied considerably between regions, ranging from 1.6 to 6.7 per million in different UK strategic health authorities (SHAs) or devolved nations. Furthermore, within SHAs there is clustering, with some areas demonstrating prevalence as high as 13 per million [1] (and authors' unpublished observations). Although this variability may be partially explained by differences in the racial composition of populations and familial clustering it is likely that many patients are undiagnosed.

Fatigable muscle weakness presenting early in life is the hallmark of this group of disorders as a whole, but each genetic subtype of CMS has typical phenotypic characteristics which will be discussed in detail in this chapter. Eye signs can often be of considerable help in directing genetic testing (Table 19.2). Importantly there are a number of effective treatments in routine use for CMS and the genetic subtype determines the treatment choice (Table 19.3).

Congenital myasthenia has a variable impact on patients' lives, with the spectrum of those harbouring pathogenic mutations ranging from asymptomatic to having severe physical disabilities. Multidisciplinary care with emphasis on pragmatic solutions in areas of day to day life such as schooling, work, or personal care is essential. With the exception of the autosomal dominant slow channel syndrome, CMS is inherited in an autosomal recessive pattern. Thus genetic counselling plays an important role, particularly where there is a family history of consanguinity.

The neuromuscular junction

Normal neuromuscular transmission is a robust process that elicits muscle contraction in response to a nerve terminal action potential. The electrical nerve impulse is transduced into chemical energy in the form of synaptic neurotransmitter acetylcholine (ACh) and then back to electrical energy, generating an action potential within the muscle.

The synapse acts as a switch with rapid and precise control over movement. Although each nerve action potential yields a muscle contraction in a 1:1 ratio the amount of neurotransmitter released by the nerve is estimated to be three to five times over the threshold for generating a muscle action potential [2]. This overcompensation is termed the 'safety factor' and means that transmission does not fail under normal conditions.

The safety factor is reliant on both structural and functional integrity at the synapse. While presynaptic neurotransmitter release can be modulated almost immediately in response to shifting requirements, the structure of the postsynaptic region cannot [2]. However, the architecture of the postsynaptic region exhibits specific features that allow an economical and effective response to neurotransmitter release, thereby conserving the safety factor.

The neurotransmitter ACh is packaged in synaptic vesicles within the nerve terminal (Fig. 19.1). The vesicles cluster in areas termed 'active zones'. Vesicle exocytosis is stimulated by calcium influx triggered by the nerve action potential, releasing ACh into the synaptic cleft. The postsynaptic membrane has deep folds, the openings of which are situated opposite the active zones. Acetylcholine receptors (AChR) are concentrated at high density on the crests of these folds.

Adult AChR are pentameric structures comprising alpha (α), beta (β), delta (δ), and epsilon (ϵ) subunits in a ratio of 2:1:1:1 (Fig. 19.2). A separate gene encodes each subunit. The fetal form of AChR contains a gamma (γ) subunit in place of the ϵ subunit, and is thought to play a role in organogenesis of the nerve–muscle junction [3]. AChR are ligand gated ion channels. Channel opening is triggered by ACh binding which allows a flow of cations through the central pore, thereby depolarizing the postsynaptic muscle membrane and generating an endplate potential (EPP). If the EPP reaches threshold an action potential and ultimately contraction of the muscle occur.

The narrow morphology of the interfold spaces and clusters of voltage-gated sodium channels at the depths of the folds both serve to amplify the neurotransmitter effect, thereby making efficient use of the available ACh. The basal lamina within the cleft is a single-layer extracellular matrix rich in proteins and glycoproteins not found at non-synaptic regions. These include laminin, agrin, and acetylcholinesterase (AChE) which terminates NMJ transmission by enzymatically cleaving ACh into acetate and choline. The

Table 19.1 Congenital myasthenic syndromes (CMS)

Syndrome	Gene	Protein
Presynaptic:		
Choline acetyltransferase (ChAT)	CHAT	Choline acetyltransferase
Synaptic:		
Acetylcholinesterase deficiency (COLQ)	COLQ	Collagen-like subunit tail of acetylcholinesterase
LAMB2	LAMB2	Laminin beta2 subunit
Postsynaptic:		
Acetylcholine receptor (AChR) deficiency	CHRNE*	AChR epsilon subunit
	CHRNA	AChR alpha subunit
	CHRNB	AChR beta subunit
	CHRND	AChR delta subunit
Kinetic abnormalities (fast and slow channel syndrome)	CHRNE	
	CHRNA	
	CHRNB	
	CHRND	
Rapsyn	RAPSN	Receptor associated protein of the synapse
DOK7	DOK7	Downstream of kinase 7
MuSK	MUSK	Muscle-specific tyrosine kinase
GFPT1	GFPT1	Glutamine-fructose-6-phosphate transaminase 1
DPAGT1	DPAGT1	Dolichyl-phosphate (UDP-N-acetylglucosamine) N-acetylglucosamine phosphotransferase 1
ALG2	ALG2	An alpha-1,3-mannosyltransferase
ALG14	ALG14	Interacts with other proteins to form a multiglycosyltransferase complex
Agrin	AGRN	Agrin
Sodium channel	SCN4A	Skeletal muscle sodium channel ($Na_v1.4$)
Escobar syndrome†	CHRNG	AChR gamma subunit

*Predominantly CHRNE affected.

†Consequences of muscle weakness during early gestation causes phenotype. Neuromuscular transmission is thought to be normal postnatally.

resulting choline is transported back to the nerve terminal, where it is recycled by choline acetyltransferase (ChAT).

Several genes involved in different aspects of the formation and maintenance of this specialized synapse have now been identified. Mutations in these genes can disrupt structure and/or function by various methods, but ultimately result in loss of the safety factor and failure of NMJ transmission. While some genes, such as *RAPSN* or *DOK7*, are associated with individual syndromes the genes encoding AChR subunits are associated with more than one subtype of CMS and may be implicated in fast or slow channel syndrome or AChR deficiency syndrome. Figure 19.3 shows the percentage distribution of CMS subtypes occurring in the UK and Republic of Ireland.

Individual syndromes

Presynaptic

Choline acetyltransferase (ChAT) deficiency

The enzyme ChAT is active in the presynaptic nerve terminal where it functions in the resynthesis of ACh molecules. This condition is typically associated with sudden episodes of respiratory distress with apnoea and bulbar weakness, and patients may be relatively strong in between such crises. Symptoms may be apparent from birth and continue episodically following initial improvement. However, affected children may be normal at birth and develop episodic apnoeas later during infancy or in childhood. The respiratory weakness may be prolonged, requiring days to weeks of artificial ventilation [4], and infection is a common precipitant of these crises, which tend to reduce with age. There may be a background of other myasthenic symptoms. The condition is rare, but the published literature would suggest that while ptosis is a feature the extraocular muscles are spared [5]. Decrement on repetitive nerve stimulation (RNS), and increased jitter on single-fibre electromyography (SFEMG), may not be apparent in affected patients, particularly if they are tested between episodes. To demonstrate abnormal NMJ transmission it has been recommended that the tested muscle should be fatigued, either with exercise or with 10 Hz stimulation for up to 5 min [6]. This is challenging in the young. AChE inhibitors are helpful in providing symptomatic relief, as may be 3,4-diaminopyridine (3,4-DAP), which stimulates presynaptic ACh release. There is a theoretical concern that 3,4-DAP might further diminish the limited presynaptic ACh stores, but this does not appear to be a problem in practice. Prophylactic AChE treatment is advocated by some sources [6,7] as a means to reduce life-threatening apnoeas. The older

Table 19.2 Typical ocular signs of congenital myasthenic syndromes

Subtype	Ophthalmoplegia	Ptosis	Other
AChR deficiency	Severe to complete	Moderate to severe	
Fast channel syndrome	Severe to complete	Moderate to severe	
Slow channel syndrome	Mild to moderate > absent	Mild to moderate > absent	
Rapsyn	Absent	Mild to moderate	Strabismus frequent, often mild
DOK7	Absent	Moderate to severe	
ChAT*	Absent	Present	
COLQ	Present or absent	Present or absent	Slow pupillary response to light

*Rare. The published literature would suggest ophthalmoplegia is absent.

Table 19.3 Treatment options for congenital myasthenic syndromes

Subtype	Treatment options
ChAT	AChE inhibitors, 3,4-DAP (see text)
AChR deficiency	AChE inhibitors, 3,4-DAP
Rapsyn	AChE inhibitors, 3,4-DAP
Fast channel syndrome	AChE inhibitors, 3,4-DAP
Slow channel syndrome	Fluoxetine, quinidine
Acetylcholinesterase deficiency (COLQ)	Ephedrine, salbutamol
DOK7	Ephedrine, salbutamol, 3,4-DAP*

AChE, acetylcholinesterase; 3,4-DAP, 3,4-diaminopyridine.

*May also worsen symptoms.

classifications of 'familial myasthenic syndrome' and 'CMS with episodic apnoea' were attributed to a presynaptic abnormality. It is now appreciated that episodic apnoeas are also typical features in rapsyn and fast channel CMS.

Synaptic

Acetylcholinesterase (AChE) deficiency (COLQ CMS)

Mutations in the AChE collagen-like tail subunit gene (*COLQ*) account for approximately 6% of genetically diagnosed CMS. At the normal NMJ this subunit tail anchors the enzyme to the basal lamina where it terminates neuromuscular transmission by hydrolysing ACh. *COLQ* mutation causes loss of this enzyme, resulting in prolonged ACh lifetime in the synapse with consequent desensitization of the AChR, prolonged EPPs and depolarization blockade. In addition these prolonged endplate currents cause the muscle endplate to be bombarded with cations, leading to a secondary excitotoxic myopathy. As a result the postsynaptic architecture is disrupted with loss of junctional folding. Typically the condition causes severe and progressive weakness from birth or early infancy. However, later onset and milder phenotypes are also recognized. Weakness often affects the respiratory muscles, with both respiratory crises and chronic hypoventilation occurring. Prevalence of eye

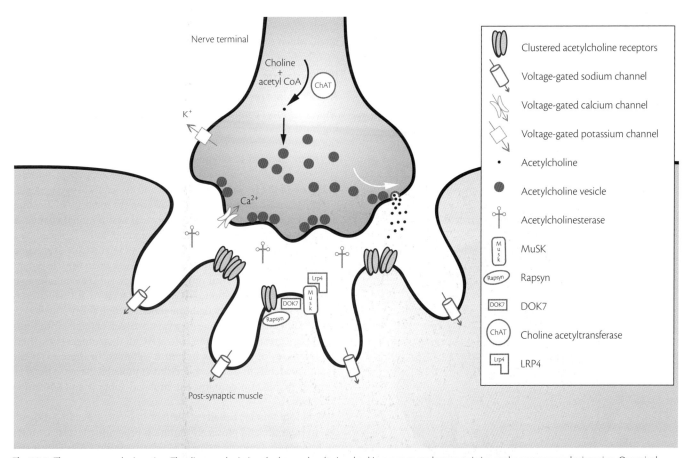

Fig. 19.1 The neuromuscular junction. The diagram depicting the key molecules involved in neuromuscular transmission at the neuromuscular junction. On arrival of the nerve action potential at the presynaptic terminal, calcium ions influx through the voltage-gated calcium channel, causing fusion of synaptic vesicles containing acetylcholine (ACh) with the presynaptic membrane. The ACh is released by exocytosis. Sodium ions move in through cation channels causing endplate potentials. Subsequent opening of the voltage-gated sodium ion channels trigger muscle action potentials leading to actin–myosin coupling and muscle contraction. See text for further details. LRP4, low-density lipoprotein receptor-related protein 4.

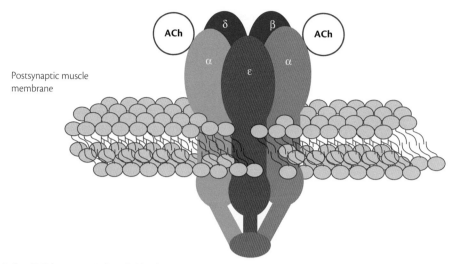

Fig. 19.2 The adult acetylcholine (ACh) receptor. Di-liganded binding of ACh to the α subunits triggers opening of the central ion channel.

signs is variable in COLQ CMS. While ptosis and ophthalmoplegia are common they were both absent in just over 18% of patients in the largest published case series [8]. A slow pupillary response to light has classically been described, but was only demonstrated in 25% of patients within the same case series. Neurophysiological tests may show a repetitive compound muscle action potential (CMAP) response to single stimuli. This can also be seen in conditions other than COLQ CMS, including the slow channel syndrome, or in cholinergic toxicity secondary to excess pyridostigmine or 3,4-DAP or organophosphate poisoning. Patients may improve with ephedrine [9] or oral salbutamol, both of which are adrenergic agonists. Their mechanism of action is incompletely understood, but both drugs are thought to improve the secondary myopathy by stabilizing the postsynaptic muscle membrane. The main side effects to consider with these agents are insomnia and cardiac effects such as tachycardia

and hypertension [10]. We routinely perform initial and follow-up blood pressure and electrocardiography. Importantly, patients with COLQ CMS and some other subtypes can experience significant clinical deterioration with AChE inhibitor or 3,4-DAP medication (Table 19.4). Paradoxically there may be initial short-term improvement, which can mislead.

Postsynaptic

Acetylcholine receptor deficiency

This is the most common of the CMS subtypes with genetic screening most often revealing two different mutations in the ε subunit (i.e. compound heterozygotes). A common mutation, 1267delG, has been reported to be present on at least one allele in 20% of a large cohort of patients [11]. This arises from an ancient founder mutation in the Indian subcontinent and is usually associated with a relatively mild phenotype [12]. However, the majority of kinships have private mutations. Although normal maturational change in receptor conformation causes fetal γ subunits to be replaced by ε subunits during late gestation, low levels of fetal AChR expression continue into adulthood and can be increased when muscle is denervated. Thus the survival of patients with ε subunit mutations is probably due to utilization of background fetal AChR which may function more effectively than the mutated adult form. The degree of this compensatory change may vary between patients, with some retaining a greater proportion of fetal AChR than others [11]. There are few cases of mutations in non-ε subunits. In these cases the phenotype tends to be severe and this is probably because the fetal form of AChR also contains the mutated subunit and so cannot compensate.

Symptom onset is usually at birth or in infancy. Feeding difficulties in early life and ptosis are common presenting features. Motor milestones are typically delayed. Unlike in rapsyn CMS, which also results in a functional deficiency of AChR, arthrogryposis is not a typical feature. While early 'worsenings' do occur in AChR deficiency they are not as dramatic as the crises seen in rapsyn or ChAT CMS. Ophthalmoplegia is striking in this type of CMS, where it is invariably a feature and virtually complete. Generalized weakness is

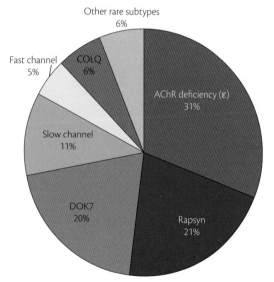

Fig. 19.3 Occurrence of congenital myasthenic syndrome subtypes within the UK and Republic of Ireland. AChR deficiency (ε), acetylcholine receptor deficiency due to ε subunit mutation.

Table 19.4 Patient subtypes and clinical deterioration with acetylcholinesterase (AChE) inhibitor or 3,4-diaminopyridine (3,4-DAP) medication

Subtype	Typically worsen with	
	AChE inhibitors	3,4-DAP
Slow channel syndrome	+	+
Acetylcholinesterase deficiency (COLQ)	+	+
DOK7	+	+/−

typically present. Mild bulbar weakness is not uncommon, and respiratory weakness may be a feature. The severity of this condition is highly variable, but most patients have a stable lifetime course. However, as with other types of CMS, exacerbation can occur with infection. Patients tend to have a good sustained response to cholinesterase inhibitors. 3,4-DAP is often used as a second-line agent in combination with cholinesterase inhibitors. Anecdotally, 3,4-DAP appears to have a better effect at reducing ptosis than pyridostigmine. Despite the other beneficial effects of these medications they tend to have no or little effect on the ophthalmoplegia seen in AChR deficiency and other subtypes.

Kinetic abnormalities

Some mutations in either α, β, δ, or ε subunits lead to a change in the kinetic properties of the channel. Those that cause abnormally brief channel openings result in fast channel syndrome [13,14], and conversely slow channel syndrome results from abnormally prolonged AChR channel opening. Despite the contrasting pathophysiology, both ultimately lead to loss of safety factor and failure of neuromuscular transmission.

Fast channel syndrome

Here channel openings are brief as a result of either abnormally rapid closure of the channel or reduced probability of channel opening, or a combination of both mechanisms [15]. Typically, genetic analysis reveals one fast channel mutation combined with a low expresser or null mutation on the second allele. Thus far mutations in the α, δ, and ε subunits have been reported. A common fast channel mutation, εP121L, was identifiable in at least one allele in 90% of a UK series [16].

Patients with fast channel syndrome tend to be symptomatic from birth or early infancy. In the same UK case series, where early history was available, all patients presented at birth with bulbar symptoms [16]. Other symptoms at onset included ptosis, hypotonia, weak cry, and respiratory symptoms, which were common—with some infants requiring respiratory support at birth. Congenital stridor was reported in two patients, one of whom had bilateral vocal cord paralysis documented following microlaryngobronchoscopy. Arthrogryposis was reported in three. Notably this has not been reported thus far in AChR deficiency syndrome. The major concern in fast channel syndrome is of sudden life-threatening apnoeas often leading to repeated admissions to intensive care. These deteriorations may occur outwith episodes of infection and can be dramatic. In contrast to rapsyn and ChAT CMS, patients commonly remain weak in between crises. Involvement of a respiratory specialist is usually necessary and parents and carers should be trained

in cardiopulmonary resuscitation. Respiratory function may be normal between crises. In the UK series apnoeic attacks ceased in those who had survived childhood. Ophthalmoplegia is generally complete, although often not initially recognized, and is typically accompanied by ptosis. Patients usually respond to pyridostigmine, although the effect may diminish over time and the addition of 3,4-DAP may be needed.

Slow channel syndrome

This is the only dominantly inherited CMS. Here the mutation results in abnormally prolonged AChR channel opening with consequent prolonged EPPs. Like AChE deficiency it is associated with a depolarization blockade and nerve conduction studies can show repetitive CMAP to single stimuli. This overstimulation of muscle and the prolonged EPPs lead to a secondary excitotoxic myopathy. Mutations occur in any of the adult receptor subunits, although about 70% of UK cases are affected by the α subunit point mutation αG153S [17]. Different mechanisms underlie the altered channel kinetics and depend upon the site of the mutation. Mutations in the extracellular N2 domain tend to cause increased affinity of the receptor for ACh molecules, whereas mutations in the pore-lining M2 domain usually result in stabilization and hence prolongation of the open state. The age of onset of symptoms is widely variable but tends to be later than in the majority of other CMS subtypes. Most patients present in childhood with neck flexion weakness or difficulty running. Some patients are affected from birth, but the typical early problems of feeding difficulties and apnoea seen frequently in other subtypes are not common. Onset is recognized in the third and even fourth decade. Overall this condition tends to be milder than the other subtypes and asymptomatic relatives are occasionally identified. A pattern of selective weakness of cervical and upper limb muscles, particularly affecting the distal arm and hand, has been identified [18,19]. Within the hand, thumb abduction weakness is striking [17]. While ophthalmoplegia is common it does not tend to be as severe as in AChR deficiency or fast channel syndrome, and down gaze and adduction are relatively spared. Treatment for slow channel syndrome relies on medications which block the AChR when in its open state. Thus the channel opening times and resulting cationic overload of the muscle endplate are reduced. Both quinidine and fluoxetine are in routine use. Evidence that one is superior to the other is lacking. However, fluoxetine is the drug of choice as quinidine requires therapeutic drug monitoring and carries the risk of QT interval prolongation. The adverse effect of AChE inhibitors or 3,4-DAP is the same as that described for AChE deficiency.

Rapsyn

Rapsyn (receptor associated protein of the synapse) is a key protein in the initiation and maintenance of synaptic structures and specifically in clustering of AChR at the muscle endplate. Clustering assays using muscle cells expressing rapsyn mutations show a reduced number of ACh receptors [20]. However, rapsyn CMS presents a distinctly different phenotype compared with AChR deficiency syndromes due to AChR subunit mutations.

The N88K missense mutation is a common cause of rapsyn CMS in Europeans [21]. Genotypic analysis has shown that this mutation arises from a common ancient Indo-European ancestor. Over 90% of rapsyn CMS patients harbour the N88K mutation on at least one allele, making genetic screening for rapsyn mutations relatively straightforward [11].

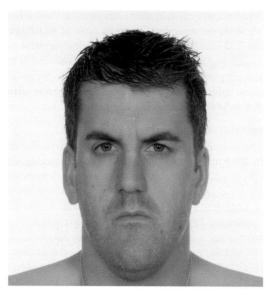

Fig. 19.4 Facial dysmorphism in a patient with rapsyn congenital myasthenic syndrome.

Two phenotypes of this recessive CMS have been described, early and late onset [22]. The typical early onset pattern is of presentation at birth or early infancy with respiratory failure, feeding difficulties, or generalized hypotonia. Fetal akinesia *in utero* gives rise to characteristic dysmorphic facies (Fig. 19.4) and usually mild arthrogryposis which tends to resolve with physiotherapy. Patients commonly have a high arched palate, a feature that is not usually seen in other forms of CMS. Weakness is typically generalized and includes facial muscles. Ophthalmoplegia is not a feature, but ptosis may be present. Strabismus, usually divergent, is very common in rapsyn CMS and is a useful distinguishing feature. However, the main caveat to this is the high frequency of strabismus, convergent more than divergent, in the general population.

Exacerbations are frequent in the first few years of life and usually, but not always, occur in the context of intercurrent infection. Similar to ChAT CMS these episodic exacerbations can be associated with respiratory failure and apnoea and little weakness in between attacks. Although the frequency and severity of these life-threatening crises diminish during childhood and usually resolve around 6 years of age [22], the good response to AChE inhibitors, with or without 3,4-DAP, justifies early treatment to reduce early morbidity and mortality.

Less frequently patients present later in life, in adolescence or adulthood. Presentation in the fifth decade has been described [22]. Their symptoms are milder than those with a typical early onset pattern and it is possible that early involvement has been overlooked. Homozygous N88K mutations are detected in both early and late-onset phenotypes. Late-onset rapsyn CMS may mimic autoimmune myasthenia gravis (AIMG). However, a useful differentiating sign when present is ankle dorsiflexion weakness which is unusual in acquired myasthenia gravis but not uncommon in CMS. Rapsyn CMS has a good long-term prognosis; it often improves during childhood and many adults are able to substantially reduce or even stop treatment.

DOK7

DOK7 (downstream of kinase 7) is a cytoplasmic protein that is essential for normal synaptogenesis. It interacts with MuSK (muscle-specific kinase) signalling pathways responsible for post-synaptic differentiation including AChR clustering. Mutations in DOK7 result in a synaptopathy with abnormally simplified NMJs bearing postsynaptic endplate regions with reduced junctional folding. It is postulated that such postsynaptic changes alter retrograde signalling giving rise to the small presynaptic regions that have also been described [23]. Individual receptor subunits and AChE are normal in structure and function. Most patients harbour at least one truncating frameshift mutation in exon 7 [11,24].

Although it has only recently been identified, DOK7 is the third most common CMS in the UK and may rise in position. Infants are often asymptomatic with normal early motor milestones and onset is usually in early childhood, presenting with difficulties in walking. However, some patients have earlier symptoms such as ptosis, and more severe cases may present with neonatal stridor or feeding difficulties from birth [25]. Weakness in DOK7 CMS is usually generalized and most often proximal predominant in the limbs giving rise to a limb-girdle phenotype. Features that help to distinguish this from other subtypes are tongue wasting (Fig. 19.5) and sparing of the extraocular muscles. Ptosis is often moderate to severe. Bulbar and respiratory weakness are common and can present later in the course of the disease. In addition to fatigable weakness, worse towards the end of the day, DOK7 patients can report variation in their symptoms over longer time periods, i.e. weeks to months. Sudden dramatic fluctuations are not typical of DOK7 CMS. The protein encoded by *DOK7* is expressed in cardiac muscle [24], but the condition does not appear to be associated with cardiomyopathy and electrocardiograms are typically normal. Patients often have a slowly progressive clinical course. Muscle biopsy tends to show mild myopathic change and the associated myopathic features may be the cause of the progressive weakness and the worsening commonly seen with AChE inhibitors (although a temporary initial response may be noted). 3,4-DAP may also

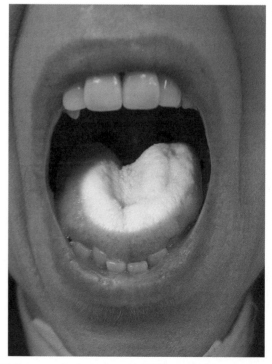

Fig. 19.5 Tongue wasting in a patient with DOK7 congenital myasthenic syndrome.

worsen symptoms but can sometimes reduce DOK7 CMS weakness. Ephedrine [26] or oral salbutamol are the mainstay of treatment; improvement tends to develop slowly, over many months, but may eventually be dramatic.

Other rarer subtypes

To date at least eight further genes encoding a protein present at the NMJ have been associated with a CMS. All are extremely rare.

CMS caused by mutation in *SCN4A*, the gene encoding the Na$_V$1.4 sodium channel of skeletal muscle, has been reported in one patient. This patient had generalized fatigable weakness and recurrent episodes of respiratory and bulbar muscle weakness from birth. The mode of inheritance is unclear [27].

Mutations in *GFPT1* (glutamine-fructose-6-phosphate transaminase 1) have been identified as causing a recessive form of CMS with limb-girdle weakness in a similar pattern to DOK7 CMS. The condition differs from DOK7 in that the facial muscles are spared and tubular aggregates are seen on muscle biopsy. Additionally there is a good response to AChE inhibitors. GFPT1 is a rate-limiting cytoplasmic enzyme at the beginning of the hexosamine biosynthesis pathway, the obligatory source of essential amino sugars involved in protein and lipid glycosylation [28].

A major product of the hexosamine biosynthesis pathway, uridine diphosphate *N*-acetylglucosamine, acts as an essential substrate for N-linked protein glycosylation, a ubiquitous post-translational modification which can affect protein folding and stability. Most recently, mutations in three genes which encode early components of the N-linked glycosylation pathway, *DPAGT1* [29,30], *ALG2*, and *ALG14* [31], have been associated with congenital myasthenic syndromes similar in phenotype to GFPT1 CMS. Thus far, minimal craniobulbar features with a normal range of eye movements have been reported in these conditions. Tubular aggregates have been reported in muscle biopsy in both the DPAGT1 and ALG2 subtypes, but were not seen in the one patient with *ALG14* mutations who had undergone muscle biopsy. Similar to CMS caused by *GFPT1* mutations, a good response to AChE inhibitors is reported in patients with DPAGT1 CMS and in the individual patients with ALG2 and ALG14 subtypes where this medication had been tried.

Mutations in *AGRN* [32] and *MUSK*, both of which code for key proteins involved in postsynaptic differentiation, have been shown to cause congenital myasthenia. Neural agrin, the product of *AGRN*, is released by the nerve terminal and activates MuSK. Muscle biopsy of a patient with mutant MuSK demonstrated abnormal postsynaptic AChR clustering and presynaptic nerve terminal sprouting [33].

One case of a synaptic CMS due to mutation in *LAMB2*, the gene encoding the basal lamina glycoprotein subunit laminin beta2, has been reported [34]. The patient had congenital nephrosis and ocular malformations in addition to myasthenia.

Escobar syndrome

Mutations in the γ subunit cause defective fetal AChR, leading to fetal akinesia and subsequent dysmorphism. Characteristically severe arthrogryposis multiplex congenita (AMC) and multiple pterygium are seen. Other features can include scoliosis, pulmonary hypoplasia, neonatal respiratory distress, craniofacial dysmorphism, low-set ears, arachnodactyly, and cryptorchism in males. Reduced intrauterine movement is normally reported and there is often a history of recurrent spontaneous abortion [3].

The condition is recessive, and mutations lead to an impaired, truncated, or absent γ subunit. The fetal form of AChR is considered to be important in NMJ organogenesis in addition to NMJ transmission. In humans the transgression from fetal to adult AChR occurs gradually in the late perinatal and early neonatal period. Thus affected children show no signs of myasthenia after birth and EMG did not show evidence of myasthenia in any of the five children tested in a published case series [3].

Transient neonatal myasthenia (TNM)

This is due to placental transfer of maternal AChR antibodies to the fetus. It is not genetically inherited, though like many of the CMS subtypes presents at birth. Reported incidence is variable but probably affects between 10 and 20% of the offspring of mothers with AIMG [35–37]. While it is reportedly more frequent in mothers with active disease than those in remission there are no predictive maternal risk factors [35]. There are contrasting reports of the relationship between maternal antibody levels and whether a child is affected or not. Furthermore, infants with AChR antibodies in their serum may be asymptomatic [35]. Affected children may exhibit poor feeding, a weak cry, reduced movements, or respiratory weakness, although symptoms usually resolve within weeks. Treatment is with AChE inhibitors and, if severe, plasma exchange [7]. Recent evidence suggests that the composition of total maternal antibody can affect outcome. A high fetal:adult AChR antibody ratio can lead to AMC and was described in three siblings with persistent weakness following TNM [38]. The risk of TNM in infants of mothers with MuSK MG is unclear [37].

When no genetic diagnosis is found

It is evident that there are undiscovered candidate genes, with an estimated 10–20% of CMS patients having no genetically determined abnormality. CMS can share clinical features with primary muscle, mitochondrial, and neurogenic disorders. In the absence of an identified genetic abnormality affecting a component of the NMJ, muscle biopsy and neurophysiological techniques, particularly repetitive nerve stimulation and SFEMG, play key roles in establishing the diagnosis of a CMS.

A common clinical dilemma is that of trying to distinguish between congenital myasthenia and seronegative myasthenia gravis. The standard anti-AChR radioimmunoprecipitation assay detects AChR antibodies in approximately 80% of patients with generalized myasthenia gravis. The remaining 20%, excluding the variable proportion that have antibodies to MuSK, are termed seronegative. The recent development of a cell-based assay, using rapsyn to cluster AChRs to the cell surface has allowed detection of low-affinity AChR antibodies in 66% of a group of 38 'seronegative' patients [39]. Despite such advances, there will still be patients with a suspected NMJ disorder in whom neither antibodies nor a genetic mutation can be identified. Clinical features that point more towards an autoimmune rather than an inherited process are: (1) asymmetry of clinical findings (ptosis being an exception in that it may be asymmetrical in CMS also), (2) later onset of disease, (3) acute onset from normality to ongoing non-resolving weakness (i.e. not a typical crisis), and (4) spontaneous resolution, which appears common in childhood acquired myasthenia gravis. Symptom onset at birth or early infancy is strongly suggestive of congenital myasthenia. A trial of immunomodulatory therapy

Table 19.5 Key features directing genetic testing

• Marked restriction of extraocular muscles directs initial testing towards the ε AChR subunit
• In the UK, CMS with normal eye movements should be initially tested for *RAPSN* and *DOK7* mutations and rapsyn is a strong suspect where strabismus or joint contractures have been a feature
• Worsening with AChE inhibitors, progression, later onset, and myopathic features are attributes of slow channel syndrome, COLQ, and DOK7 CMS
• Acute respiratory crises are characteristic of rapsyn, fast channel, and ChAT CMS, although can occur as a fluctuation in other types

AChR, Acetylcholine receptor; CMS, congenital myasthenic syndromes; AChE, acetylcholinesterase; ChAT, choline acetyltransferase.

(e.g. plasma exchange or intravenous immunoglobulin), or immunosuppression (e.g. steroids) may be appropriate, to which most patients with immune myasthenia respond but none with CMS do.

Summary

◆ Inherited myasthenias are rare but increasingly recognized.

◆ Characteristic phenotypes for each subtype are described but the spectrum is widening.

◆ It is worthwhile pursuing a definite genetic diagnosis as this guides prognosis, genetic counselling, and, most importantly, treatment choice.

◆ Considering the relative frequency of the different CMS mutations in the UK an algorithm of screening the AChR ε subunit when ophthalmoparesis is present, and *RAPSN* and *DOK7* when it is not, will identify about 75% of mutation-positive CMS.

Key features directing genetic testing are listed in Table 19.5.

References

1. Lashley D, Burke G, Palace J, Beeson D, Goldsworthy C, Newsom-Davis J. Prevalence and geographical distribution of UK congenital myasthenic syndrome patients referred to the Oxford National Specialist Commissioning Advisory Group service. ABN Abstracts. *J Neurol Neurosurg Psychiatry* 2007; **78**: 1014–38.

2. Wood SJ, Slater CR. Safety factor at the neuromuscular junction. *Prog Neurobiol* 2001; **64**: 393–429.

3. Hoffmann K, Müller JS, Stricker S, et al. Escobar syndrome is a prenatal myasthenia caused by disruption of the acetylcholine receptor fetal γ subunit. *Am J Hum Genet* 2006; **79**: 303–12.

4. Beeson D, Hantaï D, Lochmüller H, Engel AG. 126th International Workshop: Congenital Myasthenic Syndromes, 24–26 September 2004, Naarden, The Netherlands. *Neuromuscul Disord* 2005; **15**: 498–512.

5. Kraner S, Laufenberg I, Strassburg HM, Sieb JP, Steinlein OK. Congenital myasthenic syndrome with episodic apnea in patients homozygous for a CHAT missense mutation. *Arch Neurol* 2003; **60**: 761–3.

6. Kaminski HJ. *Myasthenia Gravis and Related Disorders.* Berlin: Springer, 2008.

7. Parr JR, Jayawant S. Childhood myasthenia: clinical subtypes and practical management. *Dev Med Child Neurol* 2007; **49**: 629–35.

8. Mihaylova V, Müller JS, Vilchez JJ, et al. Clinical and molecular genetic findings in COLQ-mutant congenital myasthenic syndromes. *Brain* 2008; **131**: 747–59.

9. Bestue-Cardiel M, de Cabezón-Alvarez AS, Capablo-Liesa JL, et al. Congenital endplate acetylcholinesterase deficiency responsive to ephedrine. *Neurology* 2005; **65**: 144–6.

10. *British National Formulary*, 61st edn. London: British Medical Association and Royal Pharmaceutical Society, 2011.

11. Palace J, Beeson D. The congenital myasthenic syndromes. *J Neuroimmunol* 2008; **201–202**: 2–5.

12. Morar B, Gresham D, Angelicheva D, et al. Mutation history of the Roma/Gypsies. *Am J Hum Genet* 2004; **75**: 596–609.

13. Ohno K, Wang HL, Milone M, et al. Congenital myasthenic syndrome caused by decreased agonist binding affinity due to a mutation in the acetylcholine receptor epsilon subunit. *Neuron* 1996; **17**: 157–70.

14. Wang HL, Milone M, Ohno K, et al. Acetylcholine receptor M3 domain: stereochemical and volume contributions to channel gating. *Nat Neurosci* 1999; **2**: 226–33.

15. Engel AG, Sine SM. Current understanding of congenital myasthenic syndromes. *Curr Opin Pharmacol* 2005; **5**: 308–21.

16. Palace J, Lashley D, Bailey S, et al. Clinical features in a series of fast channel congenital myasthenia syndrome. *Neuromuscul Disord* 2012; **22**: 112–17.

17. Finlayson S, Beeson D, Palace J. Congenital myasthenic syndromes: an update. *Pract Neurol* 2013; **13**: 80–91.

18. Engel AG, Lambert EH, Mulder DM, et al. A newly recognized congenital myasthenic syndrome attributed to a prolonged open time of the acetylcholine-induced ion channel. *Ann Neurol* 1982; **11**: 553–69.

19. Oosterhuis HJ, Newsom-Davis J, Wokke JH, et al. The slow channel syndrome. Two new cases. *Brain* 1987; **110**: 1061–79.

20. Burke G, Cossins J, Maxwell S, et al. Rapsyn mutations in hereditary myasthenia. *Neurology* 2003; **61**: 826–8.

21. Müller JS, Mildner G, Müller-Felber W, et al. Rapsyn N88K is a frequent cause of congenital myasthenic syndromes in European patients. *Neurology* 2003; **60**: 1805–10.

22. Burke G, Cossins J, Maxwell S, et al. Distinct phenotypes of congenital acetylcholine receptor deficiency. *Neuromuscul Disord* 2004; **14**: 356–64.

23. Palace J, Lashley D, Newsom-Davis J, et al. Clinical features of the DOK7 neuromuscular junction synaptopathy. *Brain* 2007; **130**: 1507–15.

24. Okada K, Inoue A, Okada M, et al. The muscle protein Dok-7 is essential for neuromuscular synaptogenesis. *Science* 2006; **312**: 1802–5.

25. Jephson CG, Mills NA, Pitt MC, et al. Congenital stridor with feeding difficulty as a presenting symptom of Dok7 congenital myasthenic syndrome. *Int J Pediatr Otorhinolaryngol* 2010; **74**: 991–4.

26. Lashley D, Palace J, Jayawant S, Robb S, Beeson D. Ephedrine treatment in congenital myasthenic syndrome due to mutations in DOK7. *Neurology* 2010; **74**: 1517–23.

27. Tsujino A, Maertens C, Ohno K, et al. Myasthenic syndrome caused by mutation of the SCN4A sodium channel. *Proc Natl Acad Sci USA* 2003; **100**: 7377–82.

28. Senderek J, Müller JS, Dusl M, et al. Hexosamine biosynthetic pathway mutations cause neuromuscular transmission defect. *Am J Hum Genet* 2011; **88**: 162–72.

29. Belaya K, Finlayson S, Slater CR, et al. Mutations in DPAGT1 cause a limb-girdle congenital myasthenic syndrome with tubular aggregates. *Am J Hum Genet* 2012; **91**: 193–201.

30. Finlayson S, Palace J, Belaya K, et al. Clinical features of congenital myasthenic syndrome due to mutations in DPAGT1. *J Neurol Neurosurg Psychiatry* 2013; **84**: 1119–25.

31. Cossins J, Belaya K, Hicks D, et al. Congenital myasthenic syndromes due to mutations in ALG2 and ALG14. *Brain* 2013; **136**: 944–56.

32. Huzé C, Bauché S, Richard P, et al. Identification of an agrin mutation that causes congenital myasthenia and affects synapse function. *Am J Hum Genet* 2009; **85**: 155–67.

33. Chevessier F, Faraut B, Ravel-Chapuis A, et al. MUSK, a new target for mutations causing congenital myasthenic syndrome. *Hum Mol Genet* 2004; **13**: 3229–40.

34. Maselli RA, Ng JJ, Anderson JA, et al. Mutations in LAMB2 causing a severe form of synaptic congenital myasthenic syndrome. *J Med Genet* 2009; **46**: 203–8.

35. Papazian O. Topical review article: transient neonatal myasthenia gravis. *J Child Neurol* 1992; **7**: 135–41.

36. Oosterhuis HJ. The natural course of myasthenia gravis: a long term follow up study. *J Neurol Neurosurg Psychiatry* 1989; **52**: 1121–7.

37. Evoli A. Acquired myasthenia gravis in childhood. *Curr Opin Neurol* 2010; **23**: 536–40.

38. Oskoui M, Jacobson L, Chung WK, et al. Fetal acetylcholine receptor inactivation syndrome and maternal myasthenia gravis. *Neurology* 2008; **71**: 2010–12.

39. Leite MI, Jacob S, Viegas S, et al. IgG1 antibodies to acetylcholine receptors in 'seronegative' myasthenia gravis. *Brain* 2008; **131**: 1940–52.

CHAPTER 20

Myasthenia gravis

Saiju Jacob, Stuart Viegas, and David Hilton-Jones

Introduction

Myasthenia gravis (MG) is the most common of the disorders of neurotransmission. MG is an autoimmune disorder, with antibodies directed against postsynaptic targets. The first to be recognized, and the most common, are antibodies against the nicotinic acetylcholine receptor (AChR). More recently antibodies against muscle-specific kinase (MuSK) and low-density lipoprotein receptor-related protein 4 (LRP4) have been recognized. A proportion of cases do not have a clear easily demonstrable antibody and are described as being 'seronegative', but there are several lines of evidence which indicate that an immune mechanism is likely to be responsible, with antibodies directed against other, as yet unidentified, postsynaptic proteins. Clinical and experimental findings have confirmed that both the commonly identified antibodies are pathogenic, and MG remains the prototypical autoimmune channelopathy. It is heterogeneous with respect to age of onset, severity, involvement of specific muscle groups, and thymic changes.

The hallmark of the condition is fatigable muscle weakness. A clinical diagnosis is supported by the detection of serum autoantibodies, together with neurophysiological evidence of impaired neurotransmission, although in a proportion of cases one or the other may be absent. The majority of cases respond to acetylcholinesterase inhibitors and immunosuppressive drugs, but good evidence for the use of the latter drugs is often lacking and more randomized control studies are required. Thymectomy may also be useful in younger patients. Newer biological agents are now being studied in refractory MG.

MG should be distinguished from some rarer disorders of neurotransmission in which other autoimmune, genetic, or toxic aetiologies are responsible. An overview of the differential diagnosis will be discussed later, with congenital myasthenia outlined in detail in Chapter 19 and the Lambert–Eaton myasthenic syndrome in Chapter 21.

Epidemiology of MG

The annual incidence of MG is reported to be 2.5–20 per million [1] with a recent meta-analysis of 55 studies calculating a pooled incidence rate of 5.3 per million person-years (confidence interval, CI, 4.4–6.1) [2]. There appears to be a bimodal distribution, with female predominance in early onset MG cases (onset < 40 years) and a male predominance amongst late-onset (> 40 years) cases [3]. The incidence amongst the early onset group appears to be static, whilst that of the late-onset group is increasing, with older-onset cases often being under-recognized [4]. A recent meta-analysis calculated a pooled prevalence rate of 77.7 per million (CI, 64–93 per million) [2].

With the exception of the association with thymoma (found in 10% of MG cases) no specific cause can be identified in the remaining patients. It is likely that the most important predisposing factor is an individual's immunogenetic make-up, with unknown environmental factors then being required to trigger the development of the condition. An intriguing example of this interaction is seen in those patients who develop MG after treatment with D-penicillamine, with these individuals often possessing the HLA-DR1 haplotype.

The most compelling evidence for genetic susceptibility comes from the different human leucocyte antigen (HLA) associations that exist for MG associated with AChR antibodies in both the early and late forms [5], and MuSK antibodies [6,7]. Other important evidence is the finding of increased concordance amongst monozygotic (35.5%) and dizygotic (4–5%) twins [8]. Finally, patients with MG, in common with other organ-specific autoimmune conditions, often demonstrate an increased frequency of other autoimmune disorders amongst first-degree relatives.

Physiology of neuromuscular transmission

The neuromuscular junction (NMJ) is a chemical synapse, approximately 100 nm thick, formed between the end of the motor nerve terminal and the voluntary muscle (see Fig. 19.1). The presynaptic nerve terminal contains synaptic vesicles, each containing up to 10 000 molecules of acetylcholine (ACh). In response to a nerve action potential, the voltage-gated calcium channels (VGCCs) in the presynaptic terminal open, leading to influx of calcium ions into the nerve terminal. This triggers fusion of the vesicles to the presynaptic membrane, by a process which requires the coordinated assembly of SNARE (soluble NSF attachment protein receptor) proteins. SNARE proteins like syntaxin 1, SNAP25, and synaptobrevin help form a tight fusion complex of the vesicles to the presynaptic membrane. (It is worth noting that different botulinum toxins work by binding to one or other of these SNARE proteins, thus decreasing the release of ACh, causing impaired neuromuscular transmission.)

Once the ACh molecules are released by exocytosis from the fused synaptic vesicles, they bind to the nicotinic AChRs present in the postsynaptic muscle membrane. This causes transient opening of the intrinsic cation channels and muscle membrane depolarization, leading to miniature endplate potentials (MEPPs). When multiple vesicles are released simultaneously, depending on the strength of the nerve impulse, a critical threshold is reached causing an endplate potential (EPP). The number of vesicles released per nerve impulse is approximately 50 to 300, and is called the quantal content. In response to the EPPs, the postsynaptic voltage-gated sodium channels (VGSCs) open, triggering an action potential. The muscle action potential leads to calcium ions being released from the sarcoplasmic reticulum, which then bind to troponin C and cause actin–myosin-mediated muscle contraction.

Rapid and effective neuromuscular transmission depends on the tight clustering of AChRs at the postsynaptic membrane, which is mediated by rapsyn and also by other closely associated proteins including MuSK and DOK7. Once the action potential is propagated, the presynaptic voltage-gated potassium channels (VGKCs) open, causing repolarization of the nerve membrane back to its resting level. The excess ACh in the synaptic cleft is broken down by acetylcholinesterase, anchored in the synaptic space by collagen-Q (ColQ), thus terminating the signal.

The amplitude of EPPs usually exceeds the depolarization threshold for VGSC activation and is defined as the 'safety factor'. The safety factor of neuromuscular transmission is reduced by insufficient presynaptic ACh release (e.g. Lambert–Eaton myasthenic syndrome), antibodies to postsynaptic membrane proteins (autoimmune myasthenia), or mutations in the NMJ proteins (congenital myasthenia). This means that the EPPs are not sufficient to cause membrane depolarization, leading to muscle weakness.

AChR is a transmembrane glycoprotein, which is arranged as a pentamer formed of four subunits. Fetal AChRs are formed of two α and one each of β, δ, and γ subunits. The γ subunit is replaced in adult receptors by the ε subunit. The ACh-binding site is formed between the α subunit and the δ or γ/ε subunits. Most AChR antibodies are directed against the extracellular N-terminal region of the α-subunit, called the main immunogenic region—which is close to, but distinct from, the ACh-binding sites.

Pathophysiology

The majority of patients with MG have antibodies directed against the nicotinic AChR with a variable proportion of the remaining cases having antibodies directed against MuSK. Both antibodies bind to the extracellular domains of the native molecule.

Both AChR and MuSK antibodies are directly pathogenic and not just markers of the disease. They satisfy the strict criteria for causation in antibody-mediated diseases:

1. Both antibodies are specific to MG, with autoantigens on postsynaptic muscle membrane that are involved in neurotransmission.

2. Passive transfer of immunoglobulin G (IgG) from MG patients to mice produces weakness and evidence of impaired neurotransmission [9,10]. Similarly, transient maternal–fetal transfer of disease has been reported in both serological forms of MG [11,12].

3. Active immunization in animals with the respective autoantigen is capable of replicating the human disease with similar clinical and electrophysiological features [13,14].

4. The observation that lowering antibody levels with immunosuppressive therapy, or more directly with plasma exchange [15,16], leads to clinical improvement is further evidence as to the pathogenic nature of these antibodies.

AChR antibodies induce loss of functional numbers of AChR by three mechanisms. Firstly, the antibodies can induce complement-mediated destruction of the postsynaptic architecture [17]. These antibodies are predominantly of the complement-fixing IgG1 and IgG3 subclass [18]. Secondly, the antibodies can act in a divalent fashion by cross-linking surface AChRs, leading to an accelerated rate of internalization and subsequent degradation [19]. Finally, the antibodies can directly inhibit AChR function, which may be due either to impaired ACh-binding or prevention of its normal function as an ion channel. The relevant contribution of each of these factors is unknown, but the latter is thought to be the least prominent effector mechanism [20].

The precise mechanism by which MuSK antibodies cause disease remains uncertain. The antibodies are typically of the non-complement-fixing IgG4 subclass [21], which act in a monovalent fashion and so are unable to cross-link antigen [22]. This suggests that effector mechanisms may be different from those of AChR antibodies. To date, limited human pathological studies have demonstrated morphologically normal NMJs, with normal numbers of AChRs and virtually no complement deposition [23]. However, *in vitro* studies have demonstrated complement-fixing IgG1 antibodies to MuSK, albeit at a lower level than the IgG4 antibodies [24]. In contrast, both active immunization [14] and passive transfer [10] models have demonstrated loss of postsynaptic AChRs in clinically weak animals. There is also growing evidence that the antibodies may have an additional presynaptic effect [10,25] leading to failure of apposition between the pre- and postsynaptic structures. MuSK is critical not only to the development of the NMJ [26] but also for maintenance of the adult NMJ. RNA interference to impair the synthesis of MuSK resulted in disassembly of the NMJ, although the maximum effects took 6 weeks [27]. It may well be that a reduction in neurotransmission in MuSK MG results from changes in AChR distribution or function as a consequence of alterations in MuSK activity.

Recently, antibodies directed against LRP4 have been identified in a proportion of previously 'seronegative' MG patients [28,29]. An active immunization model has since been described, with potential pathogenic mechanisms involving a reduction in agrin-induced MuSK activation and AChR clustering [30]. The LRP4 antibodies are found to be highly specific for myasthenia and are predominantly IgG1, capable of activating the complement pathway.

The thymus gland is responsible for the generation of T cells, with self-tolerance mechanisms necessary for the deletion of autoreactive T cells. The thymus has a critical role in the development of AChR MG. Within the thymus, AChR expression is normally observed on muscle-like myoid cells within the medullary epithelium. In early onset MG, the thymus is typically enlarged, containing germinal centres with specific B- and T-cell regions. These thymic B cells are able to spontaneously synthesize AChR antibodies [31]. Similar histological changes are also seen in 'seronegative' MG cases, but not in MuSK MG [32]. In late-onset MG, the thymus is usually atrophic, without these germinal centres. Tumours of the thymus are found in 10% of MG cases. These are typically epithelial in origin, and have a tendency to spread locally even if the histology is benign.

Clinical features

Myasthenia typically manifests as fatigable muscle weakness, i.e. the weakness worsens with activity and is relieved by rest. Symptoms are typically worse later in the day. It is thought that the earliest description of myasthenia is that by Thomas Willis, an

Oxford-born physician who in 1672 gave a report of a woman who had long-standing paralysis [33]:

> ...in the mornings, they are able to walk firmly...or to take up any heavy thing. Before noon, the stock of the spirits being spent, which had flowed into the muscles, they are scarce able to move hand or foot...A prudent and honest woman has this spurious palsie since many years, not only in her members (limbs) but also in her tongue. Some time she can speak freely,...but, after she has spoke long, hastily or eagerly, she becomes as mute as a fish; nor can she recover the use of her voice under an hour or two....

Although medical historians argue whether this was indeed a description of MG, it typically describes fatigable muscle weakness which is relieved by rest.

The characteristic fatigability and fluctuating nature of the disease was described almost two centuries later by Wilhelm Heinrich Erb [34,35] and Samuel Goldflam [36]; the disease was thereby referred to as Erb–Goldflam disease. Sir William Gowers described features of a typical patient in his manual around this time [37]. In 1895, the disease was renamed as 'myasthenia gravis pseudopara-lytica' by Friedrich Jolly [38]. One of the earliest English-language case series of 60 patients was published soon afterwards [39].

Myasthenia may be clinically classified as affecting only the extraocular muscles (ocular MG), or affecting peripheral and bulbar muscles as well (generalized MG). Patients with generalized MG may have antibodies against AChR or MuSK. Arbitrarily, AChR MG patients may be subdivided into early or late-onset MG, according to age of onset (Table 20.1).

Ocular myasthenia

Muscle weakness in myasthenia typically begins around the eye, i.e. droopy eyelids (ptosis) and double vision (diplopia) due to ophthalmoplegia. Other causes of ptosis and ophthalmoplegia include mitochondrial disorders (chronic progressive external ophthalmoplegia), oculopharyngeal muscular dystrophy, and thyroid ophthalmopathy (although proptosis is more common). However, the majority of these patients will develop symptoms elsewhere over a period of time. Ocular myasthenia (OMG) is defined as occurring in those patients who have myasthenic symptoms and signs restricted to the extraocular muscles (EOM) for at least 2 years.

This is based on the observation that the majority (up to 90%) of OMG patients who develop generalized symptoms will do so within the first year [40,41], with almost 60% generalizing in the initial 6 months [42]. Twenty per cent of all MG patients may have OMG [43,44]. However, there is considerable racial variation, with up to 50% of Chinese MG patients reported as having purely ocular symptoms in cohort studies [45,46].

OMG can occur at any age with no clear HLA association [47,48]. Even though the symptoms and signs are restricted to the EOM, some patients show subclinical evidence of systemic disease by the presence of abnormal neurophysiology in the peripheral muscles [49,50]. AChR antibody is present in only about 50%, compared with about 85% with generalized disease [51,52]. In addition, the thymus is more likely to be normal (mild hyperplasia is seen in about 30%), without clear evidence of benefit from thymectomy [48].

Clinically, ptosis may be unilateral or bilateral, is usually asymmetric, and patients usually complain of concomitant diplopia, although ptosis can occur in isolation for long periods of time [53]. OMG typically has wide variation in its severity, and patients may also complain of dizziness, unsteady gait, blurred vision, or visual 'confusion' [54]. On examination, the less affected lid may be hyper-retracted in concordance with the Hering law of equal innervation. One of the commonly observed signs, which is considered relatively specific for OMG, is the drooping of the contralateral lid with passive elevation of a ptotic lid. When the patient looks down for 15 seconds and then rapidly looks up, the ptotic eyelid overshoots and then slowly droops to the previous ptotic position. This sign, named the Cogan lid twitch sign, is due to transient improvement of lid strength after resting of the levator palpebrae superioris muscle.

Generalized MG

In approximately 85% of patients, the weakness spreads from the EOM to elsewhere in the body, usually within the first 2 years of onset. Commonly facial muscles are affected causing difficulty in smiling (vertical smile— 'myasthenic snarl'), inability to puff the cheeks out, and difficulty in closing the eyelids tight. Proximal weakness in the limbs more frequently affects the shoulder girdle

Table 20.1 Clinical and immunological subtypes of myasthenia gravis (MG)

Clinical subgroup	Immunological subgroup	Proportion of all MG (%)	Age of onset (years)	M:F	Clinical features	AChR antibodies	MuSK antibodies	Thymus
Ocular MG		15–25	4–90	3:2	Ptosis, ophthalmoplegia	Approx. 50%	Very rare	Mild hyperplasia (30%)
Generalized MG	Early onset AChR MG	20–25	10–40	1:3	Ptosis, ophthalmoplegia, generalized weakness	Approx. 85%	Absent	Hyperplasia (>80%)
	Late-onset AChR MG	30–40	>40	3:2	Ptosis, ophthalmoplegia, generalized weakness	Approx. 60%	Absent	Atrophy
	MuSK MG	5–8	2–70	1:3	Predominant ocular, facial and bulbar weakness	Absent	100%	Normal or atrophied
	Clustered AChR MG	3–6	10–70	1:2	Ptosis, ophthalmoplegia, generalized weakness	Clustered AChR antibodies using CBA	Absent	Mild hyperplasia
	Seronegative MG	2–5	10–70	1:2	Ptosis, ophthalmoplegia, generalized weakness	Not detectable by RIA or CBA	Absent	Mild hyperplasia

AChR, acetylcholine receptor; MuSK, muscle-specific kinase; CBA, cell-based immunofluorescence assay; RIA, radioimmunoassay.

than the hip girdle. Other causes of limb girdle weakness include limb girdle muscular dystrophies, inflammatory myopathies, toxic and endocrine myopathies, mitochondrial disorders, congenital myasthenic syndromes, and late-onset congenital myopathies.

Weakness of the long finger extensors and small hand muscles is not uncommon, but distal weakness in the lower limbs is rare. Neck flexor weakness is almost invariably present. Neck extensor weakness is much less common and is more often seen in older men when it can present as 'dropped head syndrome'. Other causes of dropped head syndrome include motor neuron disease, inflammatory myopathies, metabolic myopathies (e.g. carnitine deficiency), myotonic dystrophy, inflammatory neuropathies (i.e. Guillain–Barré syndrome, chronic inflammatory demyelinating polyneuropathy), and isolated neck extensor myopathy. Patients tend to complain more of pain and stiffness in the neck than weakness per se, although some will say they have to hold their head up by supporting their chin. Bulbar muscle involvement leads to difficulty in chewing, swallowing, and speech, with these activities fatiguing with continuing effort.

Clinical scoring systems have been defined to describe the severity of myasthenia, including that by Ossermann [55] and more recently by the Myasthenia Gravis Foundation of America (MGFA) [56]. The MGFA scoring ranges from I (ocular) to V (ventilator dependent), with II, III, and IV representing mild, moderate, or severe generalized weakness. Grades II, III, and IV are also subdivided into (a) or (b), based on the absence or presence of bulbar muscle involvement, respectively.

Myasthenic crisis

Myasthenic crisis occurs when neuromuscular weakness leads to respiratory failure requiring airway protection or ventilatory support. It affects up to 12–16% of myasthenia patients usually within 2–3 years after diagnosis (median interval 8 months) [57,58]. Potential triggers include recent respiratory infections, bulbar dysfunction and risk of aspiration pneumonia, recent thymectomy or significant surgery, and non-compliance or withdrawal of required medication. Drugs that can potentially worsen myasthenia include certain antibiotics, anaesthetic agents, antiarrhythmics, and antihypertensives (Table 20.2). Myasthenic crisis is potentially fatal and must be managed in an intensive care unit. Although early and rigorous treatments have improved the general prognosis of patients with myasthenia, there is still a small group of patients who develop this life-threatening complication [59].

Myasthenic crisis may manifest in two types of patients: either in those with a pre-existing diagnosis of myasthenia or in those who present for the first time in crisis. All patients with myasthenia presenting with worsening bulbar symptoms should be evaluated for impending myasthenic crisis. However, when dealing with respiratory weakness in a patient known to have myasthenia it has also to be borne in mind that: (1) drugs used to treat myasthenia itself can cause symptoms similar to myasthenic crisis (Table 20.2), (2) patients with myasthenia can present with other conditions causing respiratory muscle weakness (Table 20.3), and, rarely, (3) the initial diagnosis itself could have been wrong (especially in 'seronegative' patients).

Patients may or may not have a history of increasing muscle weakness prior to their current presentation. Bulbar muscle weakness may be triggered by a variety of factors (Table 20.2). Increasing double vision and swallowing difficulties are seen in some patients preceding the onset of respiratory symptoms. Tachypnoea,

Table 20.2 Factor worsening myasthenia gravis and potentially precipitating myasthenic crisis

PHARMACOLOGICAL TRIGGERS
Medications related to myasthenia
• Withdrawal of cholinesterase inhibitors (especially when symptoms not fully controlled)
• Sudden increase or initiation of steroids
Other medications (most are rare, but particular care should be taken with the ones in bold text)
• Antibiotics
• Aminoglycosides—**gentamicin**, amikacin, streptomycin, **telithromycin**, etc.
• Quinolones—ciprofloxacin, levofloxacin
• Tetracyclines
• Anaesthetic agents
• **Succinylcholine**
• Antiarrhythmics
• Quinidine
• Procainamide
• Antihypertensives
• Beta-blockers
• Calcium channel blockers—verapamil
• Antimalarials
• **Chloroquine**
• Antirheumatic drugs
• **Penicillamine**
• Chemotherapy
• Cisplatin
• Miscellaneous
• Magnesium salts,
• Epsom salts
• **Botulinum toxin**
• Iodinated contrast agents
PATHOLOGICAL TRIGGERS
Infections
• Viral and bacterial respiratory tract infections
• Aspiration pneumonia
• Other severe systemic infections
Physical stress
• Trauma
• Postoperative—thymectomy
Electrolyte imbalance
• Hypokalaemia
• Hypophosphataemia
Anaemia
PHYSIOLOGICAL TRIGGERS
• Pregnancy and menstruation (rare)

intercostal indrawing, and nasal flaring may be early signs, although not necessarily in all patients. Subsequently there is reduced chest expansion and quieter breath sounds on auscultation, tachycardia, and a rise in arterial blood pressure. It should be borne in mind that

Table 20.3 Differential diagnosis of myasthenia gravis and myasthenic crisis

Diagnosis	Principal signs	Investigations
Guillain–Barré syndrome	Initial proximal weakness, some distal sensory symptoms, absent reflexes	Lumbar puncture, NCS
Other myopathies (e.g. acid maltase)	Proximal weakness, no sensory changes	Raised CK, EMG, muscle biopsy
Cervical myelopathy (structural or inflammatory)	Usually subacute onset, sensory level, urinary retention	MRI, LP
Motor neuron disease	Usually with clear preceding history, muscle fasciculation and wasting, brisk reflexes	EMG
Brainstem stroke/inflammation	Other cranial nerve signs, altered consciousness, brisk reflexes, sensory signs	MRI, LP
Botulism	History of intravenous drug abuse, weakness spreading caudally, autonomic disturbances (sluggish pupillary responses, dry eyes)	EMG
Lambert–Eaton myasthenic syndrome	Rare; subacute proximal leg weakness, autonomic symptoms	EMG, VGCC antibodies
Organophosphate poisoning	History of pesticide use, chemical warfare, symptoms similar to cholinergic crisis	RBC acetylcholinesterase levels
Cholinergic crisis	Salivation, lachrymation, diarrhoea, urinary incontinence, bradycardia, miosis, bronchospasm (in addition to muscle weakness and respiratory failure)	Drug history and clinical signs

NCS, nerve conduction studies; CK, creatine kinase; EMG, electromyogram; MRI, magnetic resonance imaging; LP, lumbar puncture; VGCC, voltage-gated calcium channel; RBC, red blood cell.

in patients with myasthenia, the ventilation and perfusion capacity of the lungs is usually intact and hence the oxygen saturation and arterial blood gases (ABG) will be normal until quite late in the crisis and are therefore inappropriate measures. Close monitoring of the forced vital capacity (FVC) is essential. A FVC of <15 ml kg^{-1} indicates the immediate need for admission to intensive care, but a steady worsening of previously observed values in forced expiratory volume (FEV) or FVC should prompt intensive care treatment and/or intubation even above this threshold.

Diagnosis of myasthenia

Myasthenia gravis is clinically suspected with an appropriate history of fatigable muscle weakness in the absence of sensory symptoms. To elicit fatigability, patients are often tested before and after a brief amount of muscle exertion—a sustained up-gaze for a few seconds to elicit weakness of the eyelids, repeated abduction/adduction at the shoulder for testing limb strength (often useful to exercise one shoulder and compare with the non-fatigued side), or neck flexion against sustained resistance, if the weakness is not apparent otherwise. Deep tendon reflexes and sensory examination are normal.

Bed-side tests for diagnosis include the ice-pack test (application of crushed ice in a latex glove over the ptotic eyelid, leading to eyelid opening) and the edrophonium (Tensilon®) test (transient improvement in objective muscle weakness after intravenous injection of the acetylcholinesterase inhibitor). However, both tests give false positive and false negative results, particularly in inexperienced hands, and edrophonium has the potential to cause serious bradycardias (hence atropine, a cardiac monitor, and resuscitation equipment should be readily available). Neither test should be needed in the vast majority of patients.

Neurophysiological examination is most informative when performed by an experienced clinician. False negative results are common, especially in OMG, and over-interpretation of minor decrement leads to false positive results. Repetitive nerve stimulation (RNS) at 3–10 Hz may produce a decrement of more than 10% in over 50% of patients with generalized MG [60]. RNS has particularly low sensitivity in OMG.

Single-fibre EMG (Fig. 20.1), demonstrating an increase in jitter (i.e. the time interval between the two action potentials from two adjacent muscle fibres, after voluntary activation) or failure of excitation ('blockade') of the second action potential, is more than 90% sensitive, even in OMG, when appropriate muscles are sampled. But it should be noted that denervation also increases jitter. It has to be noted that in MuSK MG, limb muscle neurophysiology is often normal, this being a predominantly oculobulbar disease.

Up to 85% of patients with generalized MG and 50% of OMG patients have antibodies against AChR as measured by standard radioimmunoprecipitation (using ^{125}I-labelled bungarotoxin) or enzyme-linked immunosorbent assay (ELISA) techniques. Approximately 5% of patients have antibodies against rapsyn-clustered AChR when they are measured using a cell-based immunofluorescence assay, thereby detecting AChR antibodies with lower affinity [24]. AChR antibodies are predominantly IgG1 or IgG3 and are hence capable of activating complement [24], which could be contributing to the pathogenesis and hence might be amenable to specific anticomplement therapy.

A further 5–8% of patients with generalized MG have antibodies against a different muscle membrane protein, MuSK—also analysed by radioimmunoassay, using ^{125}I-labelled MuSK. Unlike AChR antibodies, MuSK antibodies are predominantly of the IgG4 subclass and do not usually activate complement (although in vitro studies show some complement-fixing IgG1 antibodies as well [24]).

LRP4 is a newly identified receptor for agrin and is needed for the formation of NMJs [61]. Recently, antibodies against LRP4 have been described in a variable number of patients with MG without antibodies to AChR or MuSK (i.e. the 'double seronegatives') [28,29,62]. They can be seen in 2–45% of patients who are negative for AChR and MuSK antibodies, but the true incidence is unknown because of limited studies.

All patients with a diagnosis of myasthenia should undergo a chest scan (usually a computed tomography scan) to look for thymus enlargement. Thymic abnormalities are seen in over a third of myasthenic patients with thymic hyperplasia being common in patients with early onset AChR MG (Table 20.1). Thymic

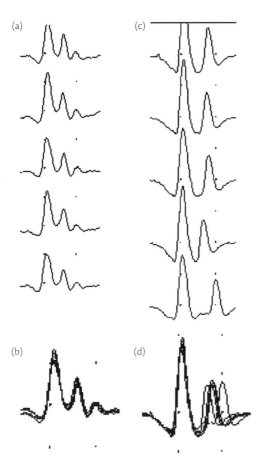

Fig. 20.1 Single-fibre electromyogram recording from the orbicularis oculi muscle. Five consecutive discharges (a, c) were recorded and superimposed (b, d) to measure the variability of interdischarge intervals. (a), (b) Traces showing normal jitter of 24 μs. (c), (d) Traces showing increased jitter of 90 μs in a patient with myasthenia. (The illustration shows only five consecutive discharges, but practically at least 20 discharges are taken before jitter is calculated.)

hyperplasia causes expansion of the perivascular spaces containing germinal centres, which are considered to be the autosensitization sites producing AChR antibodies. Thymoma, a neoplasm of the cortical epithelium is seen in 10% of people with MG, and conversely 30% of patients with thymoma develop MG [63]. Thymomas may not produce AChR antibodies, but help in the pathogenesis of MG by exporting mature CD4+ T cells and inhibiting the production of T_{Reg} cells [64]. Patients with thymoma may have other autoantibodies [skeletal muscle antibodies and ryanodine receptor (RyR) antibodies], but their exact pathogenic role in MG is unknown and they are not useful in routine clinical practice.

Treatment of MG

In a mildly affected individual, symptomatic treatment with an anticholinesterase drug alone may give adequate symptom control. However, that is the exception and most will require some form of immunosuppression, with the aim of inducing pharmacological remission of the disease.

Symptomatic treatment involves the use of an acetylcholinesterase inhibitor, which increases the amount of available acetylcholine, thereby enhancing neurotransmission. The most commonly employed drug is pyridostigmine, whilst neostigmine is an

alternative option in some countries. The typical maximum dose is 360 mg daily (divided into four or five separate doses). Above that level, side effects (diarrhoea, abdominal cramps, bowel and urinary urgency) tend to increase rapidly without additional benefit. Much higher doses can precipitate a cholinergic crisis. Propatheline, or another antimuscarinic drug, is useful for counteracting troublesome gastrointestinal symptoms.

Corticosteroids such as prednisolone are central to the immunosuppressive treatment strategy employed in MG. The evidence base for this remains limited, but many years of experience have led to an overwhelming consensus amongst MG experts. The introduction of a corticosteroid can be associated with a transient worsening of MG, and it should therefore be introduced slowly, especially in cases with significant weakness and bulbar involvement. A more rapid escalation should only be undertaken in a hospital setting. The target dose is 1.5 mg kg^{-1} on alternate days (maximum 100 mg) in generalized MG and 0.75 mg kg^{-1} on alternate days in OMG (maximum 60 mg). Once remission is achieved, the dose should be reduced slowly, aiming for the lowest maintenance dose necessary. Common adverse effects are mood disturbance, altered sleep, weight gain, gastric irritation, diabetes mellitus, hypertension, cataracts, osteoporosis, and susceptibility to infections. In our experience steroid myopathy is extremely rare with an alternate-day prednisolone regime. If it does occur, it can cause considerable difficulties—we have seen patients given higher and higher doses of steroids for presumed myasthenic weakness. The appropriate prophylaxis and management of osteoporosis in patients on steroids remains controversial and current best-practice guidelines should be followed.

Steroid-sparing agents, including azathioprine, mycophenolate mofetil, ciclosporin, tacrolimus, methotrexate, and cyclophosphamide, are widely used but the evidence base in terms of preferred drug and the timing of introduction is weak. Many patients with OMG can be managed on a relatively low dose of prednisolone and don't need such additional treatment. But many patients with generalized MG need unacceptably high doses of prednisolone and require a steroid-sparing agent. On the basis of limited studies [65] and extensive personal experience we use azathioprine as the first agent, as do many others. Some introduce azathioprine at the same time as initiating prednisolone for generalized MG, on the grounds that many will need a steroid-sparing drug and that, as it is slow to achieve maximum benefit, it is best introduced early. On the other hand, some patients may eventually manage on an acceptably small dose of prednisolone and the azathioprine will be unnecessary. About 10% of patients are intolerant of azathioprine. For these reasons there is an argument in favour of delaying its introduction until it is clear that it is necessary.

The largest (but still relatively small) trial of azathioprine [65] demonstrated its steroid-sparing effect in MG and also showed that it takes 12–18 months to achieve maximal effect. The drug is metabolized to 6-metacaptopurine, which inhibits DNA and RNA synthesis, thereby interfering with T-cell function. The target dose is 2.5 mg kg^{-1}. Common adverse effects are nausea, vomiting, liver dysfunction, and bone marrow suppression. Regular blood monitoring is therefore required and care should be exercised in those individuals known to have low levels of thiopurine methyltransferase (TPMT). It is believed to be safe in pregnancy, which is an important issue for young female MG patients. Whether there is an increased risk of malignancy with long-term use in

MG remains controversial, but this should be discussed with the patient.

Mycophenolate mofetil is a drug that suppresses the cell-mediated immune response and antibody production. Early retrospective studies showed some promise, with the drug being well tolerated and remission being achieved earlier than with azathioprine [66]. However, more recent randomized controlled studies failed to demonstrate a significant steroid-sparing benefit [67] although expert opinion has challenged the design of the studies and personal experience suggests that, like other agents, it is helpful in some but not all MG patients. The maintenance dose is typically 1 g twice a day. Common adverse effects are dyspepsia and bone marrow suppression. Regular blood monitoring is required.

Methotrexate acts through interference with DNA synthesis, which leads to impaired T-cell function. Compared with other autoimmune conditions, there is little good evidence to support its use in MG, although a recent small randomized controlled study has demonstrated a comparable effect to azathioprine [68], and personal experience supports its role in MG. A maximum dose of 20 mg weekly is recommended, along with folic acid supplementation. Common adverse effects include nausea, vomiting, bone marrow suppression, and hepatic and respiratory complications. Regular blood test monitoring is required.

Ciclosporin inhibits T-cell function through alterations in calcineurin signalling pathways. It was shown to be effective in a randomized controlled trial [69] and is thought to be as effective as azathioprine, but more rapidly acting. The typical dose is 2.5 mg kg^{-1}. Common adverse effects include nausea, vomiting, hirsuitism, hypertension, and renal impairment. It is necessary to monitor a patient's renal function and blood pressure whilst on treatment.

Tacrolimus (FK506) also inhibits T-cell proliferation via the calcium–calcineurin pathway, but also causes RyR-mediated calcium release from the sarcoplasmic reticulum, thereby potentiating excitation–contraction coupling in skeletal muscle [70]. This mechanism offers a theoretical benefit in those cases of MG where RyR antibodies are detected. Observational studies have shown a useful benefit [71], but a recent randomized study failed to show a significant steroid-sparing benefit at 6 months [72]. The typical daily dose is 50 µg kg^{-1}. Common adverse effects include nausea, vomiting, hypertension, bone marrow suppression, glucose intolerance, and renal and hepatic dysfunction. Patients must have regular blood pressure monitoring, and blood tests including tacrolimus levels are required.

Cyclophosphamide is a strong alkylating agent capable of suppressing B-cell function and antibody synthesis. In severe MG, a randomized trial with pulsed cyclophosphamide confirmed a steroid-sparing benefit [73]. Common adverse effects include nausea, vomiting, diarrhoea, haemorrhagic cystitis, and bone marrow suppression. There is also an increased incidence of cancer in the long term. Regular blood monitoring before and after treatment is necessary.

Newer biological agents include rituximab, a human/mouse chimeric anti-CD20 monoclonal antibody, which induces complement-dependent cytotoxicity against CD20-positive plasma cells. Retrospective studies suggest that it leads to improvement in a proportion of refractory AChR MG and MuSK MG cases [74–76]. Anti-tumour necrosis factor alpha (anti-TNFα) therapy has also been studied in a prospective study, with mixed outcomes [77].

Eculizimab, a monoclonal antibody directed against the complement protein C5, is currently (early 2014) undergoing clinical trials.

The principles of treatment for MG can be summarized as follows:

1. Treatment strategies should be individualized since no one regimen is perfect for all patients.

2. The immunosuppressive effects may not persist if treatment is discontinued and most patients will require treatment in the medium and long term.

3. Once pharmacological remission is achieved, the drugs should be slowly reduced starting first with pyridostigmine, then prednisolone, and finally the steroid-sparing agent.

4. Patients who do not achieve pharmacological remission are susceptible to acute deteriorations precipitated by intercurrent illness, surgery, or new medications.

5. If left untreated, myasthenic weakness may become fixed.

Treatment of myasthenic crisis

Myasthenic crisis is best managed in either an intensive therapy unit or high-dependency unit. Non-invasive ventilation (BiPAP, bilevel positive airway pressure) has been employed with some success [78], but mechanical ventilation is still required in the majority of cases. Most patients require ventilation for less than 2 weeks, thereby avoiding tracheostomy [58]. Complications related to mechanical ventilation include atelectasis and pneumonia. Supporting nutritional requirements, typically with nasogastric feeding, is also critical in the intensive care setting.

Both plasma exchange (PE) and intravenous immunoglobulin (IVIg) are employed in treating myasthenic exacerbations and crisis. They are also useful if the patient has significant generalized weakness in preparation for forthcoming surgery, including thymectomy.

PE allows for the removal of antibodies by membrane filtration or centrifugation. Traditionally 2–3 L are exchanged on five occasions. Improvement, which occurs in 75% of patients [79], is often seen within a week and the effect may last for 1–3 months. The short-term benefits are undisputed, but its long-term use appears to not confer any advantage over standard immunosuppressive treatment [80]. Complications related to PE include catheter-related venous thrombosis, infection, bleeding, hypotension, cardiac arrythmias, and pneumothorax.

The immunomodulatory effects of IVIg are thought to include interference with complement activation and production of cytokines, providing anti-idiotype antibodies and influencing the activation and effector functions of T and B cells [81,82]. The typical dose is 2 g kg^{-1} given over 5 days. Non-randomized evidence suggests that IVIg and PE are equally as effective [80]. Improvement may take 1–2 weeks to manifest, with the effects lasting between 2 and 3 months. Adverse effects include fever, rigors, rash, headache, venous and arterial thrombosis, and cardiac and renal dysfunction, but it is usually well tolerated.

Thymectomy

Thymectomy may be indicated in MG for two reasons. Firstly, in those patients without thymoma to try and achieve either clinical remission or improvement leading to a reduced requirement for immunosuppressive therapy. Secondly, in patients of any age with thymoma. This is to prevent local spread and invasion of vital structures and reduce the risk of seeding of the tumour within the pleural space. Most evidence suggests that removal of a thymoma does not in itself improve the myasthenia. The prognosis and need for additional treatment (radiotherapy, chemotherapy) depends on the surgical staging and the histological subtype [83].

Thymectomy for disease control should be considered in those patients with generalized MG who are younger than 45 years and who are AChR antibody positive. Despite its widespread use, the evidence for efficacy has not been demonstrated in adequate formal trials, which has recently led to the establishment of an international thymectomy trial to try to answer some of the uncertainties (<http://clinicaltrials.gov/show/NCT00294658>). One rather dated study demonstrated a remission rate of 34% and an improvement rate of 32% compared with 8% and 16%, respectively, in matched controls [84], but arguably there have been significant advances in immunosuppressive therapy since then which have altered the approaches to management. However, there is likely to remain a view that thymectomy is the only treatment that offers the possibility of remission, and thus avoidance of potentially toxic immunosuppressive therapies, perhaps strengthened by the increasing popularity of more minimally invasive approaches than conventional sternal-splitting surgery. Preoperatively, medical stabilization of MG should be undertaken, employing IVIg or PE if necessary. Preoperative bulbar dysfunction, myasthenic crisis, and high AChR antibody levels are associated with postoperative crisis [85]. The perioperative use of corticosteroids may be associated with complications related to wound healing [86], especially at higher doses. The anaesthetist must have suitable experience of dealing with MG, particularly in the appropriate use and monitoring of muscle relaxant drugs.

Different surgical approaches include transsternal, transcervical, and videoscopic [87] thymectomy. It has been argued that the transsternal approach offers the best chance of complete resection, but it has major cosmetic implications. The transcervical approach increases the chance of a suboptimal resection, but has cosmetic advantages. Videoscopic thymectomy is technically the most challenging, but is a bilateral approach, uses an operative robot, and may be as effective as conventional surgical approaches with better cosmetic outcomes and shorter hospital stays. Many patients (especially young women), will accept this but not the transsternal approach. Postoperative complications include infections, recurrent laryngeal nerve palsies, haemothorax, or chylothorax. The reported mortality of transsternal thymectomy is 0–2% [88].

Prognosis

With prompt diagnosis and effective treatment, most patients lead a normal or near normal life. Natural history studies have shown that approximately 20–35% of patients achieve complete remission on long-term follow-up [89,90]. Early and milder onset of symptoms, with shorter disease duration at diagnosis, are considered to be good prognostic factors [89,90]. Thymectomy has been shown to be associated with complete stable remission [91], although the on-going randomized controlled trial (see section on Thymectomy) may provide clearer evidence.

Conclusion

Myasthenia gravis is the prototypical autoimmune disease affecting the NMJ. The diagnosis can be established by an accurate history, with optimum use of neurophysiological and immunological tests.

With therapeutic advances in neuroimmunology its prognosis is improving, and patients often lead a near normal life.

MG: a summary

+ MG is the most common autoimmune disorder affecting the NMJ.

+ MG causes fatigable muscle weakness, which is typically worse after exercise or towards the end of the day.

+ Initial symptoms usually involve the extraocular muscles with ptosis and ophthalmoplegia being common.

+ MG has a bimodal incidence with early disease occurring more often in young women and later onset in older men.

+ AChR antibodies are seen in approximately 50% of OMG patients and in 85% of patients with generalized MG. Approximately 5% of patients have antibodies against clustered AChRs detected by a more sensitive immunocytofluorescent assay.

+ MuSK antibodies are seen in about 5–8% of patients with generalized MG and are very rarely found in purely ocular MG. MuSK MG is predominantly oculobulbar, is more likely to have myasthenic crisis, and can be resistant to conventional treatment with acetylcholinesterase inhibitors and immunosuppression.

+ Decremental response on repetitive nerve stimulation and prolonged jitter on single-fibre EMG examination are the neurophysiological hallmarks of MG.

+ Factors that worsen myasthenia and lead to crisis include infections, recent surgery, and drugs.

+ Monitoring of FVC is crucial in the management of bulbar dysfunction in myasthenia.

+ Treatment includes pyridostigmine, corticosteroids, and immunosuppressive drugs. Myasthenic crisis is often managed by PE or IVIg.

+ Thymoma should be excluded in all patients with myasthenia. Thymectomy is indicated in early onset myasthenia having AChR antibodies, with mild to moderate disease.

Botulism

The bacterium *Clostridium botulinum* produces a highly potent neurotoxin affecting neuromuscular transmission, with consequent paralysis. Botulinum toxin occurs in seven different serotypes (A to G) and act on different synaptic vesicular proteins. Human diseases are mostly caused by toxin types A, B, and E (rarely F).

The clinical syndrome of botulism can be caused by the ingestion of contaminated food (the usual source is home-canned food), wound infection (commonly in intravenous drug users and infected war wounds), or by inhalation of aerosolized toxin (a potent biological toxin threat). Infant botulism, in children below the age of 1, is caused by colonization of the intestine by the bacterium due to the lack of normal bowel flora. A proportion (up to 20%) of infant botulism has been reported to occur after consumption of honey. Adult intestinal botulism is extremely rare compared with infant botulism and tends to occur in patients with anatomical gastrointestinal abnormalities or with prolonged antibiotic usage. Patients present with acute flaccid neuromuscular paralysis, starting symmetrically in the cranial nerves (ptosis, ophthalmoplegia, dysphagia, and dysarthria) and descending down to other voluntary muscles. Hence the syndrome is very similar to myasthenia and can lead to respiratory paralysis and death. An important difference from myasthenia is the involvement of the pupils in botulism; they are typically dilated and fixed. Higher mental function and sensory systems are unaffected. Examination of the cerebrospinal fluid is usually normal. (In contrast, Guillain–Barré syndrome produces ascending paralysis with albumino-cytological dissociation in the cerebrospinal fluid.)

The diagnosis is established by demonstration of toxin in the food, serum, stool, or wound swabs. Botulism is a notifiable disease in most countries. Treatment involves administration of specific botulinum antitoxin with supportive care in an intensive care setting, often requiring mechanical ventilation.

Acknowledgements

The authors would like to acknowledge Dr Robin Kennett, Consultant Neurophysiologist, John Radcliffe Hospital, Oxford for providing the single-fibre EMG illustrations.

References

1. Oosterhuis HJ. Clinical aspects and epidemiology. In: Oosterhuis HJ (ed) *Myasthenia Gravis*, pp. 17–48. Groningen: Groningen Neurological Press, 1997.

2. Carr AS, Cardwell CR, McCarron PO, McConville J. A systematic review of population based epidemiological studies in myasthenia gravis. *BMC Neurol* 2010; **10**: 46.

3. Vincent A, Palace J, Hilton-Jones D. Myasthenia gravis. *Lancet* 2001; **357**: 2122–8.

4. Vincent A, Clover L, Buckley C, Grimley Evans J, Rothwell PM. Evidence of underdiagnosis of myasthenia gravis in older people. *J Neurol Neurosurg Psychiatry* 2003; **74**: 1105–8.

5. Compston DA, Vincent A, Newsom-Davis J, Batchelor JR. Clinical, pathological, HLA antigen and immunological evidence for disease heterogeneity in myasthenia gravis. *Brain* 1980; **103**: 579–601.

6. Niks EH, Kuks JB, Roep BO, et al. Strong association of MuSK antibody-positive myasthenia gravis and HLA-DR14-DQ5. *Neurology* 2006; **66**: 1772–4.

7. Bartoccioni E, Scuderi F, Augugliaro A, et al. HLA class II allele analysis in MuSK-positive myasthenia gravis suggests a role for DQ5. *Neurology* 2009; **72**: 195–7.

8. Ramanujam R, Pirskanen R, Ramanujam S, Hammarstrom L. Utilizing twins concordance rates to infer the predisposition to myasthenia gravis. *Twin Res Hum Genet* 2011; **14**: 129–36.

9. Toyka KV, Drachman DB, Pestronk A, Kao I. Myasthenia gravis: passive transfer from man to mouse. *Science* 1975; **190**: 397–9.

10. Cole RN, Reddel SW, Gervasio OL, Phillips WD. Anti-MuSK patient antibodies disrupt the mouse neuromuscular junction. *Ann Neurol* 2008; **63**: 782–9.

11. Osserman KE, Teng P. Studies in myasthenia gravis: neonatal and juvenile types. *J Mt Sinai Hosp NY* 1956; **23**: 711–27.

12. Niks EH, Verrips A, Semmekrot BA, et al. A transient neonatal myasthenic syndrome with anti-musk antibodies. *Neurology* 2008; **70**: 1215–16.

13. Patrick J, Lindstrom J. Autoimmune response to acetylcholine receptor. *Science* 1973; **180**: 871–2.

14. Shigemoto K, Kubo S, Maruyama N, et al. Induction of myasthenia by immunization against muscle-specific kinase. *J Clin Invest* 2006; **116**: 1016–24.

15. Newsom-Davis J, Vincent A, Wilson SG, Ward CD, Pinching AJ, Hawkey C. [Plasmapheresis for myasthenia gravis]. *N Engl J Med* 1978; **298**: 456–7.

16. Evoli A, Tonali PA, Padua L, et al. Clinical correlates with anti-MuSK antibodies in generalized seronegative myasthenia gravis. *Brain* 2003; **126**: 2304–11.

17. Engel AG, Arahata K. The membrane attack complex of complement at the endplate in myasthenia gravis. *Ann NY Acad Sci* 1987; **505**: 326–32.

18. Rodgaard A, Nielsen FC, Djurup R, Somnier F, Gammeltoft S. Acetylcholine receptor antibody in myasthenia gravis: predominance of IgG subclasses 1 and 3. *Clin Exp Immunol* 1987; **67**: 82–8.

19. Drachman DB, Angus CW, Adams RN, Michelson JD, Hoffman GJ. Myasthenic antibodies cross-link acetylcholine receptors to accelerate degradation. *N Engl J Med* 1978; **298**: 1116–22.

20. Lindstrom JM. Acetylcholine receptors and myasthenia. *Muscle Nerve* 2000; **23**: 453–77.

21. McConville J, Farrugia ME, Beeson D, et al. Detection and characterization of MuSK antibodies in seronegative myasthenia gravis. *Ann Neurol* 2004; **55**: 580–4.

22. van der Zee JS, van Swieten P, Aalberse RC. Serologic aspects of IgG4 antibodies. II. IgG4 antibodies form small, nonprecipitating immune complexes due to functional monovalency. *J Immunol* 1986; **137**: 3566–71.

23. Shiraishi H, Motomura M, Yoshimura T, et al. Acetylcholine receptors loss and postsynaptic damage in MuSK antibody-positive myasthenia gravis. *Ann Neurol* 2005; **57**: 289–93.

24. Leite MI, Jacob S, Viegas S, et al. IgG1 antibodies to acetylcholine receptors in 'seronegative' myasthenia gravis. *Brain* 2008; **131**: 1940–52.

25. Punga AR, Lin S, Oliveri F, Meinen S, Ruegg MA. Muscle-selective synaptic disassembly and reorganization in MuSK antibody positive MG mice. *Exp Neurol* 2011; **230**: 207–17.

26. DeChiara TM, Bowen DC, Valenzuela DM, et al. The receptor tyrosine kinase MuSK is required for neuromuscular junction formation *in vivo*. *Cell* 1996; **85**: 501–12.

27. Kong XC, Barzaghi P, Ruegg MA. Inhibition of synapse assembly in mammalian muscle *in vivo* by RNA interference. *EMBO Rep* 2004; **5**: 183–8.

28. Higuchi O, Hamuro J, Motomura M, Yamanashi Y. Autoantibodies to low-density lipoprotein receptor-related protein 4 in myasthenia gravis. *Ann Neurol* 2011; **69**: 418–22.

29. Pevzner A, Schoser B, Peters K, et al. Anti-LRP4 autoantibodies in AChR- and MuSK-antibody-negative myasthenia gravis. *J Neurol* 2012; **259**: 427–35.

30. Shen C, Lu Y, Zhang B, et al. Antibodies against low-density lipoprotein receptor-related protein 4 induce myasthenia gravis. *J Clin Invest* 2013; **123**: 5190–202.

31. Scadding GK, Vincent A, Newsom-Davis J, Henry K. Acetylcholine receptor antibody synthesis by thymic lymphocytes: correlation with thymic histology. *Neurology* 1981; **31**: 935–43.

32. Leite MI, Strobel P, Jones M, et al. Fewer thymic changes in MuSK antibody-positive than in MuSK antibody-negative MG. *Ann Neurol* 2005; **57**: 444–8.

33. Willis T. In: *De Anima Brutorum*, pp. 404–7. Oxford, 1672.

34. Erb WH. Zur Casuistick der bulbären Lähmungen. *Arch Psychiat Nervenkrankheit* 1879; **9**: 325–50.

35. Erb WH. Ueber einen eigenthümlichen bulbären? Symptomenkomplex. *Arch Psychiat Nervenkrankheit* 1879; **9**: 172–3.

36. Goldflam SV. Über einen scheinbar heilbaren bulbärparalytischen Symptomen-complex mit Betheiligung der Extremitäten. *Deutsch Z Nervenheilkunde* 1893; **4**: 312–52.

37. Gowers WR. *A Manual of Diseases of the Nervous System*, Vol. 1. London: J&A Churchill, 1886.

38. Jolly F. Ueber Myasthenia Gravis pseudoparalytica. *Berl Klin Wochenschr* 1895; **32**: 1–7.

39. Campbell H, Bramwell E. Myasthenia gravis. *Brain* 1900; **23**: 277–336.

40. Bever CT, Jr, Aquino AV, Penn AS, Lovelace RE, Rowland LP. Prognosis of ocular myasthenia. *Ann Neurol* 1983; **14**: 516–19.

41. Oosterhuis HJ. The natural course of myasthenia gravis: a long term follow up study. *J Neurol Neurosurg Psychiatry* 1989; **52**: 1121–7.

42. Grob D, Brunner NG, Namba T. The natural course of myasthenia gravis and effect of therapeutic measures. *Ann NY Acad Sci* 1981; **377**: 652–69.

43. MacDonald BK, Cockerell OC, Sander JW, Shorvon SD. The incidence and lifetime prevalence of neurological disorders in a prospective community-based study in the UK. *Brain* 2000; **123**: 665–76.

44. Phillips LH, 2nd, Torner JC. Epidemiologic evidence for a changing natural history of myasthenia gravis. *Neurology* 1996; **47**: 1233–8.

45. Chiu HC, Vincent A, Newsom-Davis J, Hsieh KH, Hung T. Myasthenia gravis: population differences in disease expression and acetylcholine receptor antibody titers between Chinese and Caucasians. *Neurology* 1987; **37**: 1854–7.

46. Zhang X, Yang M, Xu J, et al. Clinical and serological study of myasthenia gravis in HuBei Province, China. *J Neurol Neurosurg Psychiatry* 2007; **78**: 386–90.

47. Sommer N, Melms A, Weller M, Dichgans J. Ocular myasthenia gravis. A critical review of clinical and pathophysiological aspects. *Doc Ophthalmol* 1993; **84**: 309–33.

48. Barton JJ, Fouladvand M. Ocular aspects of myasthenia gravis. *Semin Neurol* 2000; **20**: 7–20.

49. Evoli A, Tonali P, Bartoccioni E, Lo Monaco M. Ocular myasthenia: diagnostic and therapeutic problems. *Acta Neurol Scand* 1988; **77**: 31–5.

50. Sanders DB, Stalberg EV. AAEM minimonograph #25: single-fiber electromyography. *Muscle Nerve* 1996; **19**: 1069–83.

51. Kupersmith MJ, Moster M, Bhuiyan S, Warren F, Weinberg H. Beneficial effects of corticosteroids on ocular myasthenia gravis. *Arch Neurol* 1996; **53**: 802–4.

52. Kaminski HJ, Li Z, Richmonds C, Ruff RL, Kusner L. Susceptibility of ocular tissues to autoimmune diseases. *Ann NY Acad Sci* 2003; **998**: 362–74.

53. Elrod RD, Weinberg DA. Ocular myasthenia gravis. *Ophthalmol Clin North Am* 2004; **17**: 275–309, v.

54. Kusner LL, Puwanant A, Kaminski HJ. Ocular myasthenia: diagnosis, treatment, and pathogenesis. *Neurologist* 2006; **12**: 231–9.

55. Osserman KE, Genkins G. Studies in myasthenia gravis: review of a twenty-year experience in over 1200 patients. *Mt Sinai J Med* 1971; **38**: 497–537.

56. Jaretzki A, 3rd, Barohn RJ, Ernstoff RM, et al. Myasthenia gravis: recommendations for clinical research standards. Task Force of the Medical Scientific Advisory Board of the Myasthenia Gravis Foundation of America. *Neurology* 2000; **55**: 16–23.

57. Cohen MS, Younger D. Aspects of the natural history of myasthenia gravis: crisis and death. *Ann NY Acad Sci* 1981; **377**: 670–7.

58. Thomas CE, Mayer SA, Gungor Y, et al. Myasthenic crisis: clinical features, mortality, complications, and risk factors for prolonged intubation. *Neurology* 1997; **48**: 1253–60.

59. Phillips LH, 2nd. The epidemiology of myasthenia gravis. *Neurol Clin* 1994; **12**: 263–71.

60. AAEM Quality Assurance Committee. American Association of Electrodiagnostic Medicine. Literature review of the usefulness of repetitive nerve stimulation and single fiber EMG in the electrodiagnostic evaluation of patients with suspected myasthenia gravis or Lambert–Eaton myasthenic syndrome. *Muscle Nerve* 2001; **24**: 1239–47.

61. Weatherbee SD, Anderson KV, Niswander LA. LDL-receptor-related protein 4 is crucial for formation of the neuromuscular junction. *Development* 2006; **133**: 4993–5000.

62. Zhang B, Tzartos JS, Belimezi M, et al. Autoantibodies to lipoprotein-related protein 4 in patients with double-seronegative myasthenia gravis. *Arch Neurol* 2012; **69**: 445–51.

63. Willcox N. Myasthenia gravis. *Curr Opin Immunol* 1993; **5**: 910–17.

64. Strobel P, Rosenwald A, Beyersdorf N, et al. Selective loss of regulatory T cells in thymomas. *Ann Neurol* 2004; **56**: 901–4.

65. Palace J, Newsom-Davis J, Lecky B. A randomized double-blind trial of prednisolone alone or with azathioprine in myasthenia gravis. Myasthenia Gravis Study Group. *Neurology* 1998; **50**: 1778–83.

66. Meriggioli MN, Ciafaloni E, Al-Hayk KA, et al. Mycophenolate mofetil for myasthenia gravis: an analysis of efficacy, safety, and tolerability. *Neurology* 2003; **61**: 1438–40.

67. Wolfe GI, Barohn RJ, Sanders DB, McDermott MP. Comparison of outcome measures from a trial of mycophenolate mofetil in myasthenia gravis. *Muscle Nerve* 2008; **38**: 1429–33.

68. Heckmann JM, Rawoot A, Bateman K, Renison R, Badri M. A single-blinded trial of methotrexate versus azathioprine as steroid-sparing agents in generalized myasthenia gravis. *BMC Neurol* 2011; **11**: 97.

69. Tindall RS, Rollins JA, Phillips JT, Greenlee RG, Wells L, Belendiuk G. Preliminary results of a double-blind, randomized, placebo-controlled trial of cyclosporine in myasthenia gravis. *N Engl J Med* 1987; **316**: 719–24.

70. Timerman AP, Ogunbumni E, Freund E, Wiederrecht G, Marks AR, Fleischer S. The calcium release channel of sarcoplasmic reticulum is modulated by FK-506-binding protein. Dissociation and reconstitution of FKBP-12 to the calcium release channel of skeletal muscle sarcoplasmic reticulum. *J Biol Chem* 1993; **268**: 22992–9.

71. Konishi T, Yoshiyama Y, Takamori M, Yagi K, Mukai E, Saida T. Clinical study of FK506 in patients with myasthenia gravis. *Muscle Nerve* 2003; **28**: 570–4.

72. Yoshikawa H, Kiuchi T, Saida T, Takamori M. Randomised, double-blind, placebo-controlled study of tacrolimus in myasthenia gravis. *J Neurol Neurosurg Psychiatry* 2011; **82**: 970–7.

73. De Feo LG, Schottlender J, Martelli NA, Molfino NA. Use of intravenous pulsed cyclophosphamide in severe, generalized myasthenia gravis. *Muscle Nerve* 2002; **26**: 31–6.

74. Maddison P, McConville J, Farrugia ME, et al. The use of rituximab in myasthenia gravis and Lambert–Eaton myasthenic syndrome. *J Neurol Neurosurg Psychiatry* 2011; **82**: 671–3.

75. Zebardast N, Patwa HS, Novella SP, Goldstein JM. Rituximab in the management of refractory myasthenia gravis. *Muscle Nerve* 2010; **41**: 375–8.

76. Benveniste O, Hilton-Jones D. The role of rituximab in the treatment of myasthenia gravis. *Eur Neurol Rev* 2010; **5**: 95–100.

77. Rowin J, Meriggioli MN, Tuzun E, Leurgans S, Christadoss P. Etanercept treatment in corticosteroid-dependent myasthenia gravis. *Neurology* 2004; **63**: 2390–2.

78. Rabinstein A, Wijdicks EF. BiPAP in acute respiratory failure due to myasthenic crisis may prevent intubation. *Neurology* 2002; **59**: 1647–9.

79. Mayer SA. Intensive care of the myasthenic patient. *Neurology* 1997; **48** (Suppl): 70S–75S.

80. Gajdos P, Simon N, de Rohan-Chabot P, Raphael JC, Goulon M. [Long-term effects of plasma exchange in myasthenia. Results of a randomized study]. *Presse Med* 1983; **12**: 939–42.

81. Dalakas MC. Intravenous immunoglobulin in autoimmune neuromuscular diseases. *J Am Med Assoc* 2004; **291**: 2367–75.

82. Jacob S, Rajabally YA. Current proposed mechanisms of action of intravenous immunoglobulins in inflammatory neuropathies. *Curr Neuropharmacol* 2009; **7**: 337–42.

83. Chen G, Marx A, Chen WH, et al. New WHO histologic classification predicts prognosis of thymic epithelial tumors: a clinicopathologic study of 200 thymoma cases from China. *Cancer* 2002; **95**: 420–9.

84. Buckingham JM, Howard FM, Jr, Bernatz PE, et al. The value of thymectomy in myasthenia gravis: a computer-assisted matched study. *Ann Surg* 1976; **184**: 453–8.

85. Watanabe A, Watanabe T, Obama T, et al. Prognostic factors for myasthenic crisis after transsternal thymectomy in patients with myasthenia gravis. *J Thorac Cardiovasc Surg* 2004; **127**: 868–76.

86. Huang CS, Hsu HS, Huang BS, et al. Factors influencing the outcome of transsternal thymectomy for myasthenia gravis. *Acta Neurol Scand* 2005; **112**: 108–14.

87. Jaretzki A, 3rd, Barohn RJ, Ernstoff RM, et al. Myasthenia gravis: recommendations for clinical research standards. Task Force of the Medical Scientific Advisory Board of the Myasthenia Gravis Foundation of America. *Ann Thorac Surg* 2000; **70**: 327–34.

88. Jaretzki A, 3rd, Aarli JA, Kaminski HJ, Phillips LH, 2nd, Sanders DB. Thymectomy for myasthenia gravis: evaluation requires controlled prospective studies. *Ann Thorac Surg* 2003; **76**: 1–3.

89. Mantegazza R, Beghi E, Pareyson D, et al. A multicentre follow-up study of 1152 patients with myasthenia gravis in Italy. *J Neurol* 1990; **237**: 339–44.

90. Beghi E, Antozzi C, Batocchi AP, et al. Prognosis of myasthenia gravis: a multicenter follow-up study of 844 patients. *J Neurol Sci* 1991; **106**: 213–20.

91. Mantegazza R, Baggi F, Antozzi C, et al. Myasthenia gravis (MG): epidemiological data and prognostic factors. *Ann NY Acad Sci* 2003; **998**: 413–23.

CHAPTER 21

The Lambert–Eaton myasthenic syndrome

Maarten J. Titulaer and Jan J. G. M. Verschuuren

Introduction

In 1953 Anderson and colleagues described a 47-year-old man with progressive muscle weakness and diminished tendon reflexes who improved dramatically after removal of a small-cell lung carcinoma (SCLC) [1]. A few years later, the American neurologists Lambert, Eaton, and Rooke described similar cases. They described in six patients repetitive nerve stimulation (RNS) that showed a distinctive electrophysiological pattern [2]. This syndrome, with or without SCLC, has become known as the Lambert–Eaton myasthenic syndrome (LEMS) and these electrophysiological features are still part of the diagnostic criteria.

Over the years, our knowledge about the epidemiological and clinical characteristics of LEMS has expanded. Improved awareness and knowledge of the disease has shortened the diagnostic delay, diminished misdiagnosis, and caused an apparent increase in frequency. The pathophysiological mechanisms leading to LEMS have been unravelled by the discovery of autoantibodies to voltage-gated calcium channels (VGCCs), which has facilitated diagnosis and improved our understanding of the pathogenesis. The presence of functional VGCCs on SCLC has linked these tumours to LEMS and provided an aetiological basis for the disorder. Clinical, genetic, and serological markers discriminate non-tumour LEMS (NT-LEMS) from SCLC-related LEMS (SCLC-LEMS). Recently, the DELTA-P score has offered a validated tool to adequately predict the presence of SCLC in LEMS patients at the moment of diagnosis [3]. Early diagnosis enables effective treatment (symptomatic or immunosuppressive), or an early start to oncological treatment.

Clinical diagnosis

The diagnosis is based on clinical signs and symptoms, antibody testing, and electrophysiological studies (Table 21.1). The typical clinical triad consists of proximal muscle weakness, autonomic features, and areflexia [4]. In 80% of cases the first symptom noted by the patient is proximal leg muscle weakness [5]. Weakness of the arms is present, or will also develop quickly [5,6]. In contrast to myasthenia gravis (MG) the weakness spreads caudally to cranially, finally reaching the oculobulbar region, and proximally to distally, involving the feet and hands (Fig. 21.1). The symptoms spread far more rapidly in SCLC-LEMS than in NT-LEMS [5]. The prevalence of ocular symptoms has been a matter of debate for years, occurring in 0–80% of cases; bulbar symptoms occur in 5–80% [5,7–12]. This enormous range in the literature is most likely due to inconsistency in the timing of assessment from presentation. In 234 patients, the frequency of

ocular and bulbar symptoms rose from 30% and 32% within 3 months to 49% and 52% within 12 months of onset, especially in SCLC-LEMS patients (Fig. 21.1) [13]. However, almost all patients with ocular symptoms or respiratory failure early in the disease also had generalized weakness [11,14], although isolated cases with purely ocular muscle weakness have been reported [11,15,16]. In sharp contrast to MG, it remains very rare to see isolated weakness of the external eye muscles. Cerebellar degeneration, with associated symptoms, is also found in a minority of patients with LEMS, especially in SCLC-LEMS [5]. This is likely to be explained by the presence of the target antigen, the P-/Q-type VGCC, in Purkinje cells in the cerebellum.

Autonomic dysfunction

Autonomic dysfunction is the second clinical clue for diagnosing LEMS. It can be very diverse, but usually is not very debilitating. It is found in 80–96% of patients [3–5,8,10]. The lower frequency in a Japanese cohort (37%) might present a real, still unknown, difference, although under-reporting is also a possible explanation [9]. The presence of autonomic symptoms also depends on the timing of assessment, as for muscular symptoms, rising from 66% within 3 months of onset to 91% at any stage [13]. Dry mouth and erectile dysfunction in males are the most common symptoms, followed by constipation and orthostatic dysfunction. Micturition difficulties, dry eyes, and altered perspiration are less frequent [13].

Tendon reflexes

Examination of the patient may reveal decreased or absent tendon reflexes, the third clinical clue. A characteristic phenomenon is 'post-exercise facilitation', a short-lasting return of tendon reflexes and muscle strength towards the normal range after muscle contraction. However, it is not a very sensitive sign as it is only present in 40% of patients [17,18]. As this phenomenon can mask the reduced tendon reflexes, tendon reflexes should be tested after a period of rest if a diagnosis of LEMS is suspected.

Misdiagnosis and differential diagnosis

Onset in LEMS patients often consists of mild upper leg weakness, in contrast to patients with MG in whom ptosis and diplopia usually dominate the clinical presentation. This LEMS pattern is less specific and can be difficult to recognize. Therefore, diagnostic delay (both patient- and physician-related) can be long, particularly in patients with NT-LEMS. In SCLC-LEMS median time to diagnosis was 4 months, but in NT-LEMS median delay ranged from 12 to 19 months [3,10]. Explanations for these difficulties

Table 21.1 Diagnosis and differential diagnosis of Lambert–Eaton myasthenic syndrome (LEMS) [13]

Criteria required for diagnosis

1. Clinical features:
   - proximal muscle weakness
   - autonomic symptoms
   - reduced tendon reflexes

2. Voltage-gated calcium channel antibodies

3. Repetitive nerve stimulation abnormalities:
   - low compound muscle action potential
   - AND decrement >10% at low frequency (1–5 Hz)
   - AND increment >100% after maximal voluntary contraction or at high frequency (50 Hz)

Criterion 1 should be present (proximal muscle weakness is required), with one or both of criteria 2 and 3.

Differential diagnosis

- Myasthenia gravis
- Myopathy (inclusion body myositis, polymyositis, myopathy associated with systemic autoimmune diseases, muscular dystrophy, polymyalgia rheumatica)
- Polyneuropathy (Guillain–Barré syndrome, chronic inflammatory demyelinating neuropathy, axonal)
- Amyotrophic lateral sclerosis
- Spinal disease (lumbar canal stenosis, cervical myelopathy)
- Cranial (cerebellar degeneration, multiple sclerosis, Parkinson disease, metastases)
- Other (depression, psychosomatic)

include the rather non-specific onset in most patients with symmetric, often mild, proximal weakness, and the slow progression of symptoms in a significant number of patients. To emphasize that diagnosis of LEMS can be challenging, 58% of patients were initially misdiagnosed (Table 21.1) [13]. The diagnosis of LEMS is most often confused with MG, especially if the oculobulbar muscles are involved [11]. However, 90% of MG patients start with oculobulbar symptoms, as opposed to only 5% in LEMS [12]. Generally, muscle weakness in MG evolves in a craniocaudal direction, as opposed to the reverse in LEMS [12], and patients with MG lack autonomic dysfunction and reduced tendon reflexes.

Proximal, symmetric muscle weakness is the most common presentation of a wide range of myopathies, including inclusion body myositis which is particularly common in older patients and typically presents with quadriceps weakness. Creatine kinase (CK) is substantially elevated in many myopathies, but is rarely more than two to three times the upper limit of normal in LEMS. Again, in this differential diagnosis, autonomic symptoms point towards LEMS. Lumbar canal stenosis can present with fatigability of leg muscles, but a detailed clinical history will help lead to the correct diagnosis. Many LEMS patients complain about 'starting problems', e.g. getting out of their chair or initiating walking. This can resemble an early phase of Parkinson disease or lower body Parkinsonism. As the patient's symptoms often sound disproportionate to the often rather limited signs on examination, a depressive or psychosomatic disorder is sometimes considered.

In some patients, a more subacute development of symptoms is seen: particularly if the subsequent electrophysiological examination is suboptimal, the low compound action potential (CMAP) can be mistaken for an axonal neuropathy or amyotrophic lateral sclerosis (ALS). Some patients may wrongly be diagnosed with Guillain–Barré syndrome (GBS), although sensory symptoms or radicular pain are not associated with LEMS and in GBS the cerebrospinal fluid will show typical abnormalities [19]. In ALS, fasciculations, atrophy, asymmetry, and onset in the upper extremities contrast with the signs and symptoms in LEMS.[20]

VGCC antibodies

LEMS is caused by antibodies to P-/Q-type VGCC. VGCC is a complex protein consisting of multiple subunits with a pore-forming α_1 subunit that also contains the voltage sensor, which regulates opening of the channel. VGCC antibodies have been detected in 85–90% of LEMS patients without tumour, while in LEMS patients with SCLC this may approach 100% [21–24]. In addition to these P-/Q-type VGCC antibodies some patients also have antibodies to N- and L-type VGCC [22,25].

The specificity of P-/Q-type VGCC antibodies is very high, although in patients with SCLC without neurological dysfunction these antibodies have been detected in 1–4%.

There is clear evidence that P-/Q-type VGCC antibodies are responsible for the clinical symptoms of LEMS. The antigen is present in SCLC and at the presynaptic nerve terminals of the neuromuscular junction and the autonomic nervous system.

Passive transfer of the disease has been described from an affected mother to her baby, resulting in transient neonatal weakness [26,27]. Passive transfer of human autoantibodies to mice induces disease [28,29]. LEMS immunoglobulin G (IgG) was equally effective in C5-deficient mice, indicating that late complement components are not required [30], which is in line with the lack of complement deposition observed in human biopsied material. Active immunization with VGCC peptides results in a mild LEMS-like disease in rats [31]. Mice with mutations in the P-/Q-type VGCC gene *CACNA1A* show the characteristic electrophysiological abnormalities of LEMS [32]. The weakness in patients responds well to immunomodulation therapy [33,34].

Electromyography

Next to antibody testing, additional diagnostic examinations consist of RNS, the electrophysiological study of choice to diagnose LEMS (Table 21.1). The first CMAP amplitude is small, and becomes even smaller with low stimulation frequencies (2–5 Hz) [35]. Interestingly, in patients with LEMS a decrement can be present at frequencies as low as 0.1 Hz. A decrement (decrease in the CMAP amplitude) of at least 10% is considered abnormal [35]. A significant decrement is very common in LEMS patients (94–98%) [18,36], but as MG patients also have a comparable decrement this is not specific. High-frequency stimulation (50 Hz), or preferably post-exercise stimulation, is performed to discriminate between LEMS and MG. In LEMS patients, an increase of the CMAP amplitude (increment) is seen. An increment over 100% after post-exercise stimulation has a diagnostic sensitivity of 84–96% [18,36,37], while also being highly specific for LEMS. High-frequency stimulation, although having comparable sensitivity, should be avoided if possible as it is very painful. A cut-off of 60% to consider an increment significant has been proposed,

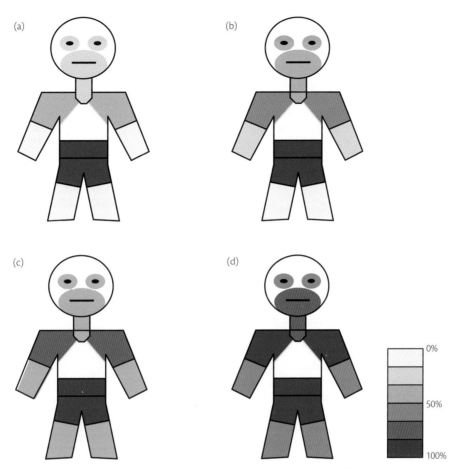

Fig. 21.1 Spreading of symptoms within 3 or 12 months, for non-tumour Lambert–Eaton myasthenic syndrome (NT-LEMS) and small-cell lung cancer LEMS (SCLC-LEMS) patients [13]. Frequency of symptoms at 3 months (a) and 12 months (b) in NT-LEMS patients, and frequency of symptoms at 3 months (c) and 12 months (d) in patients with SCLC-LEMS. The percentage of patients suffering from the specific symptoms, within the given time frame, is indicated in various shades of green colour.

as sensitivity rose to 97%, while the specificity (to exclude MG) remained excellent (99%) [18].

Single-fibre electromyography (SFEMG) might be slightly more sensitive than RNS, but specificity is only moderate. It doesn't distinguish between MG and LEMS and requires a degree of technical expertise [35]. RNS, on the contrary, if performed properly, is technically easier and both sensitive and specific. The sensitivity of RNS is increased by the withdrawal of symptomatic medication 12 h before the examination and ensuring that the examined muscles are warm (over 32°C) [35]. Patience is important when performing RNS, as the decrement is often present at stimulus frequencies as low as 0.1 Hz. If the physician is impatient, the first CMAP of a RNS train might actually still be decremented from the single stimulus before. For the best and most sensitive assessment of increment, the stimulus should follow as soon as possible after cessation of the muscle exercise as the increase in CMAP amplitude is very short-lived. Auditory control of contraction of the specific muscle and of cessation of muscle contraction will help the physician to time the post-exercise stimulus adequately.

Epidemiology of LEMS

LEMS is a rare disease and the estimated incidence is reported to be 0.48 per million per year [38]. In the Netherlands, incidence rose to 0.75 per million per year while prevalence rose to 3.42 per million after the start of a nationwide research programme, most probably due to improved recognition. The original description of LEMS as being a disease of older, male patients [4,39] is only valid for the paraneoplastic form, i.e. SCLC-LEMS. In this group, median age at onset was 60 years and 65% of patients were male, accounted for by the smoking habits of that generation [3]. NT-LEMS, however, is seen in all ages, with two peaks in age of onset, one around 35 and a second, larger, peak at the age of 60 [3]. In the early onset NT-LEMS group, females were slightly over-represented, but overall 52% of 115 NT-LEMS patients were female [3], similar to historic data (52%) [40]. Interestingly, the age and sex distribution in NT-LEMS is similar to that of MG [41], as is the genetic association with the HLA-B8-DR3 haplotype. This autoimmune prone HLA haplotype is present in around 65% of NT-LEMS patients [42]. However, the predominance is restricted to patients with young onset, again similar to MG [43]. Common genetic immunological risk factors might be important for the onset of LEMS or MG in this early onset non-tumour group. Interestingly, in NT-LEMS patients and their family members susceptibility to autoimmune diseases is also increased [44,45].

Tumour association

A tumour is found in 50–60% of patients with LEMS [3]. Most often this is a SCLC, a smoking-related lung carcinoma with neuroendocrine characteristics [4,9,46–49], although non-small-cell carcinoma and mixed lung carcinomas have been reported infrequently.

Associations with tumours other than lung cancer have been suggested [40]. It is likely that chance is responsible for many of these associations, but for some of these tumours, like prostate carcinoma or thymoma, the aetiology may be paraneoplastic. This is based on the observation that the clinical symptoms of LEMS correlated with tumour activity and in some cases remission of LEMS symptoms occurred after surgical removal of the tumour [13]. It remains impossible to demonstrate the validity of an association between lymphoproliferative disorders and LEMS, as in the 15 patients described the time frames of clinical symptoms of LEMS and lymphoproliferative disorders were less well connected [13,50].

Prediction and screening for SCLC

Screening for a SCLC is very important, as it has major impact on treatment and prognosis. Patients with SCLC-LEMS have more limited SCLC disease than patients with SCLC without LEMS (65% versus 39%), probably due to early detection or to a beneficial effect of the immune response against calcium channels or other antigens on the tumour [48]. The clinical symptoms of LEMS are nearly always present before SCLC is detected, although they are sometimes mild and non-specific. In only 6% of patents did the diagnosis of SCLC precede recognition of LEMS [48].

In most patients, however, diagnosis of LEMS alerts the physician to look for a SCLC [48]. Using different imaging modalities, a SCLC was detected in 91% of all SCLC-LEMS patients within 3 months and in 96% within 1 year of diagnosis of LEMS [48]. Patients in whom a SCLC was detected more than 2 years from diagnosis of LEMS had undergone screening that is nowadays regarded as inferior [4,48,51,52]. Factors that impose a raised or lowered risk for SCLC include older age, male gender, weight loss, and being a (former) smoker. All these factors point towards an underlying SCLC [3,4,39,40,42,48]. Rapid progression after the onset of the first symptoms is also a red flag for SCLC-LEMS [3,5,6] as well as a Karnofsky performance status under 70 (i.e. patients need at least some assistance with their activities of daily living) [3]. A raised erythrocyte sedimentation rate (ESR) [3,4], abnormal leucocyte cell count [3], and SOX1 antibodies [24,53] are serological markers for SCLC-LEMS, while HLA-B8 and HLA-DR3 are markers for NT-LEMS [3,42]. The presence of SOX1 antibodies had a specificity of 95% but sensitivity of only 65% [24]. Another tumour prediction algorithm, based on smoking behaviour and HLA-B8, had both good sensitivity and specificity (83% and 86%, respectively) [42]. However, none of these items offered a sufficient basis for screening guidelines. Recently, a multivariate analysis was performed using two cohorts of over 100 LEMS patients to create and independently validate a new prediction model [3]. The simple Dutch–English LEMS Tumor Association Prediction Score (DELTA-P score; Fig. 21.2) proved to be easy, sensitive, specific, and reproducible. The probability for SCLC in a LEMS patient can be calculated as early as 3 months from onset of LEMS using only clinically defined signs and symptoms. A DELTA-P score of 0–1 gives a risk of 0–2.6%, rising steeply to up to 83.9% and 100%, respectively, with a DELTA-P score of 3–6 (Fig. 21.2).

All patients, even those with a low chance of SCLC as calculated with the DELTA-P score, should be screened, as previously proposed [48,54], by computed tomography of the thorax (CT-thorax) and [18F]fluorodeoxyglucose positron emission tomography (FDG-PET) or by integrated FDG-PET/CT. Chest X-ray should

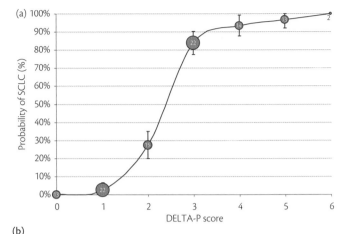

(b)

	Categories	<3 months of onset	Score
D	**D**ysarthria, dysphagia, chewing, neck weakness: bulbar weakness	absent	0
		present	1
E	**E**rectile dysfunction	female	0
		male: absent	0
		male: present	1
L	**L**oss of Weight	absent or <5%	0
		≥5 %	1
T	**T**obacco use at onset	absent	0
		present	1
A	**A**ge of onset	<50 years	0
		≥50 years	1
P	Karnofsky **P**erformance Score	70–100	0
		0–60	1
	DELTA-P score		0–6

Fig. 21.2 (a) Predicted percentage of small-cell lung cancer (SCLC) in patients with Lambert–Eaton myasthenic syndrome (LEMS), based on the Dutch–English LEMS Tumour Association Prediction (DELTA-P) score [3]. (b) The DELTA-P score is calculated as a sum score according to the different categories listed. The DELTA-P score can vary from 0 to 6. Point sizes in (a) are proportional to the number of patients with a specific score, also represented by the percentage inside the circle. Vertical bars indicate the standard error of the mean.

not be used as a screening tool as it has insufficient sensitivity. If negative, a second screening by CT-thorax or FDG-PET should be performed after 3 or 6 months, depending on the DELTA-P score (Fig. 21.3) [3,48,54].

Treatment

The treatment of LEMS is based on three modalities: symptomatic treatment to improve the function of neuromuscular transmission, immunosuppressive treatment, or tumour treatment.

The first choice is symptomatic treatment with drugs that increase the release of acetylcholine from the presynaptic nerve ending, as well as drugs that prolong the action of acetylcholine by blocking acetylcholinesterase.

Guanidine, 4-aminopyridine, or 3,4-diaminopyridine (3,4-DAP) have all been used to increase presynaptic release of acetylcholine. Guanidine has long been a standard drug for treatment, although

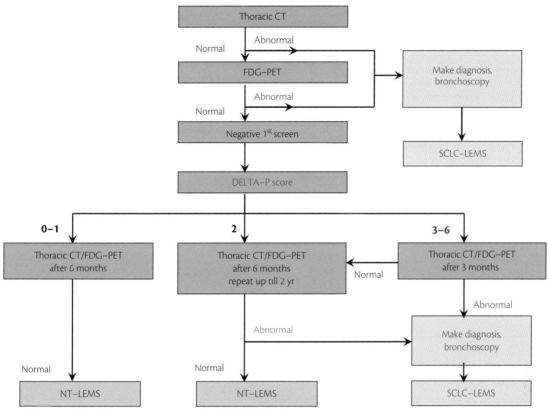

Fig. 21.3 Flowchart of recommended screening for small-cell lung cancer (SCLC) in patients with Lambert–Eaton myasthenic syndrome (LEMS) (FDG-PET, [^{18}F] fluorodeoxyglucose positron emission tomography; NT, non-tumour) [3,13,16,69].

results from well-designed trials are lacking. The most common side effects are gastrointestinal symptoms and distal paraesthesiae. Rare, but more serious, side effects that limit its use are bone marrow suppression and renal failure. Epigastric distress and perioral and distal paraesthesiae are also described as side effects of both the aminopyridine drugs. However, 4-aminopyridine penetrates more easily into the brain, which explains the higher prevalence of central nervous system side effects, especially epileptic seizures. The seizure risk in 3,4-DAP appears to be dose-dependent and can probably be avoided if the daily dose is kept below 100 mg [55,56]. There are some reports of cardiac side effects, but in the normal range of dosing these do not pose a major issue. After iatrogenic intoxication (360 mg 3,4-DAP), supraventricular tachycardia has been described [57]. One patient using 3,4-DAP died due to a myocardial infarction, but a causal relationship remained unclear [58]. In 25 patients, no evidence of prolongation of the QT-interval (a predicted possible side effect of the drug) was seen [56].

A recent Cochrane review described the results of four clinical trials with 3,4-DAP in 54 patients with LEMS [56,59–62]. Muscle strength score, myometric limb measurement, or CMAP amplitude improved significantly after treatment. Overall, 3,4-DAP is generally well tolerated and clinical trials showed a significant beneficial effect in LEMS.

The use of acetylcholinesterase inhibitors is well known in the treatment of MG. The use of acetylcholinesterase inhibitors, like pyridostigmine or neostigmine, as monotherapy for LEMS has been described in several case reports. In contrast to the generally beneficial therapeutic effect in MG, most papers describe a minimal or only modest improvement in the clinical weakness in LEMS. Some suggest that there might be a potentiation of the therapeutic effect of 3,4-DAP if both drugs are used together [47,60]. A small cross-over trial using intravenous pyridostigmine found no additional benefit of this drug [62].

An algorithm for the treatment of LEMS is proposed in Fig. 21.4.

Many patients need immunosuppressive treatment over and above symptomatic treatment. The drug choice and dosage are similar to MG. Prednisolone is the first choice, most often combined with azathioprine. In LEMS patients without tumour this was used in 80 of 114 (70%), whilst 46 of 104 (44%) of patients with SCLC-LEMS required these drugs [13]. Effectiveness of this combination therapy has only been demonstrated in a retrospective study [34], but is supported by the positive results of the combined treatment in MG which is a closely related disorder [63]. As in MG, other immunosuppressive drugs like ciclosporin or methotrexate can be used [64]. In LEMS one cross-over trial reported significant improvement in limb strength after treatment with intravenous immunoglobulin [33]. The improvement peaked at 2–4 weeks and was associated with a significant decline in serum VGCC antibody titres.

Rituximab was an effective treatment in three LEMS patients with severe myasthenic weakness who were resistant to treatment with several different immunosuppressive drugs [65,66].

The third treatment option—in those with SCLC-LEMS—is tumour therapy. Patients with a SCLC are usually treated with chemotherapy, like cisplatinum and etoposide [67]. This therapy aims to achieve tumour control, and improve the condition and

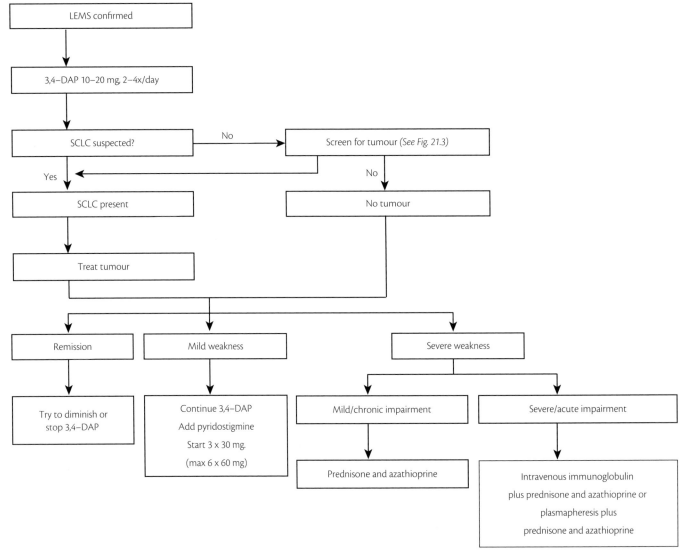

Fig. 21.4 Treatment scheme for Lambert–Eaton myasthenic syndrome (LEMS) (DAP, diaminopyridine; SCLC, small-cell lung cancer) [13].

survival of the patient. Chemotherapy has two beneficial effects on the signs and symptoms of LEMS. The drugs have a powerful immunosuppressive effect, which will contribute to the remission of LEMS. Secondly, tumour treatment removes an important antigenic stimulus for the immune system, ameliorating the symptoms of LEMS. In a series of 11 LEMS patients with SCLC, ten patients improved neurologically after treatment for their SCLC, followed by relapse in three. Only one patient showed no improvement, despite response of the SCLC to tumour treatment [68].

If remission of symptoms is incomplete after chemotherapy, additional immunosuppressive treatment may induce improvement. There are indications that the immune response against VGCC helps to control tumour growth [69], and consequently immunosuppressive treatment of LEMS patients with SCLC could potentially allow the tumour to escape immune-mediated suppression and enhance its growth. Clinical follow-up studies of these patients, however, did not indicate that immunosuppressive treatment is contraindicated [68]. It should also be taken into account

that although the presence of LEMS improves median survival in LEMS patients with SCLC, the majority still die from tumour complications. If myasthenic weakness severely impairs daily function, the evidence favours trying to achieve short-term symptomatic benefits and not be afraid of a theoretically disadvantageous influence of immunosuppressive treatment on tumour growth.

In general, most patients can be treated effectively with symptomatic treatment or a combination of prednisone and azathioprine, besides chemotherapy. Tumour treatment should be used as appropriate for the tumour involved. Acute treatments with intravenous immunoglobulin, plasmapheresis [47], or additional immunosuppressive agents can be used, but are rarely needed.

Conflicts of interest

The Neurology Department of the Leiden University Medical Center received fees from BioMarin Ltd in 2009–2010, because of consultancies by JJGMV. JJGMV did not receive any personal payments from BioMarin Ltd.

Acknowledgements

MJT is supported by a fellowship 2009-4451 of the Dutch Cancer Society.

References

1. Anderson HJ, Churchill-Davidson HC, Richardson AT. Bronchial neoplasm with myasthenia—prolonged apnoea after administration of succinylcholine. *Lancet* 1953; **265**: 1291–3.

2. Lambert EH, Eaton LM, Rooke ED. Defect of neuromuscular conduction associated with malignant neoplasms. *Am J Physiol* 1956; **187**: 612–13.

3. Titulaer MJ, Maddison P, Sont JK, et al. Clinical Dutch–English Lambert–Eaton Myasthenic Syndrome (LEMS) Tumor Association Prediction score accurately predicts small-cell lung cancer in the LEMS. *J Clin Oncol* 2011; **29**: 902–8.

4. O'Neill JH, Murray NMF, Newsom-Davis J. The Lambert–Eaton myasthenic syndrome—a review of 50 cases. *Brain* 1988; **111**: 577–96.

5. Titulaer MJ, Wirtz PW, Kuks JB, et al. The Lambert–Eaton myasthenic syndrome 1988–2008: a clinical picture in 97 patients. *J Neuroimmunol* 2008; **201–202**: 153–8.

6. Wirtz PW, Wintzen AR, Verschuuren JJ. Lambert–Eaton myasthenic syndrome has a more progressive course in patients with lung cancer. *Muscle Nerve* 2005; **32**: 226–9.

7. Burns TM, Russell JA, LaChance DH, Jones HR. Oculobulbar involvement is typical with Lambert–Eaton myasthenic syndrome. *Ann Neurol* 2003; **53**: 270–3.

8. Lorenzoni PJ, Scola RH, Kay CS, Parolin SF, Werneck LC. Non-paraneoplastic Lambert–Eaton myasthenic syndrome: a brief review of 10 cases. *Arq Neuropsiquiatr* 2010; **68**: 849–54.

9. Nakao YK, Motomura M, Fukudome T, et al. Seronegative Lambert–Eaton myasthenic syndrome. *Neurology* 2002; **59**: 1773–5.

10. Pellkofer HL, Armbruster L, Linke R, Schumm F, Voltz R. Managing non-paraneoplastic Lambert–Eaton myasthenic syndrome: clinical characteristics in 25 German patients. *J Neuroimmunol* 2009; **217**: 90–4.

11. Titulaer MJ, Wirtz PW, Wintzen AR, Verschuuren JJGM. Lambert–Eaton myasthenic syndrome with pure ocular weakness. *Neurology* 2008; **70**: 86.

12. Wirtz PW, Sotodeh M, Nijnuis M, et al. Difference in distribution of muscle weakness between myasthenia gravis and the Lambert–Eaton myasthenic syndrome. *J Neurol Neurosurg Psychiatry* 2002; **73**: 766–8.

13. Titulaer MJ, Lang B, Verschuuren JJ. Lambert–Eaton myasthenic syndrome: from clinical characteristics to therapeutic strategies. *Lancet Neurol* 2011; **10**: 1098–107.

14. Smith AG, Wald J. Acute ventilatory failure in Lambert–Eaton myasthenic syndrome and its response to 3,4-diaminopyridine. *Neurology* 1996; **46**: 1143–5.

15. Oh SJ. The Eaton–Lambert syndrome in ocular myasthenia gravis. *Arch Neurol* 1974; **31**: 183–6.

16. Rudnicki SA. Lambert–Eaton myasthenic syndrome with pure ocular weakness. *Neurology* 2007; **68**: 1863–4.

17. Odabasi Z, Demirci M, Kim DS, et al. Postexercise facilitation of reflexes is not common in Lambert–Eaton myasthenic syndrome. *Neurology* 2002; **59**: 1085–7.

18. Oh SJ, Kurokawa K, Claussen GC, Ryan HF, Jr. Electrophysiological diagnostic criteria of Lambert–Eaton myasthenic syndrome. *Muscle Nerve* 2005; **32**: 515–20.

19. van Doorn PA, Ruts L, Jacobs BC. Clinical features, pathogenesis, and treatment of Guillain–Barré syndrome. *Lancet Neurol* 2008; **7**: 939–50.

20. Kiernan MC, Vucic S, Cheah BC, et al. Amyotrophic lateral sclerosis. *Lancet* 2011; **377**: 942–55.

21. Lennon VA, Kryzer TJ, Griesmann GE, et al. Calcium-channel antibodies in the Lambert–Eaton syndrome and other paraneoplastic syndromes. *N Engl J Med* 1995; **332**: 1467–74.

22. Motomura M, Lang B, Johnston I, Palace J, Vincent A, Newsom-Davis J. Incidence of serum anti-P/Q-type and anti-N-type calcium channel autoantibodies in the Lambert–Eaton myasthenic syndrome. *J Neurol Sci* 1997; **147**: 35–42.

23. Takamori M, Takahashi M, Yasukawa Y, et al. Antibodies to recombinant synaptotagmin and calcium channel subtypes in Lambert–Eaton myasthenic syndrome. *J Neurol Sci* 1995; **133**: 95–101.

24. Titulaer MJ, Klooster R, Potman M, et al. SOX antibodies in small-cell lung cancer and Lambert–Eaton myasthenic syndrome: frequency and relation with survival. *J Clin Oncol* 2009; **27**: 4260–7.

25. Johnston I, Lang B, Leys K, Newsom-Davis J. Heterogeneity of calcium channel autoantibodies detected using a small-cell lung cancer line derived from a Lambert–Eaton myasthenic syndrome patient. *Neurology* 1994; **44**: 334–8.

26. Lecky BR. Transient neonatal Lambert–Eaton syndrome. *J Neurol Neurosurg Psychiatry* 2006; **77**: 1094.

27. Reuner U, Kamin G, Ramantani G, Reichmann H, Dinger J. Transient neonatal Lambert–Eaton syndrome. *J Neurol* 2008; **255**: 1827–8.

28. Lang B, Newsom-Davis J, Peers C, Wray DW. Selective action of Lambert–Eaton Myasthenic syndrome antibodies on Ca-2+ channels in the neuroblastoma × glioma hybrid cell-line Ng108–15. *J Physiol Lond* 1987; **394**: 43.

29. Fukunaga H, Engel AG, Lang B, Newsom-Davis J, Vincent A. Passive transfer of Lambert–Eaton myasthenic syndrome with IgG from man to mouse depletes the presynaptic membrane active zones. *Proc Natl Acad Sci USA* 1983; **80**: 7636–40.

30. Prior C, Lang B, Wray D, Newsom-Davis J. Action of Lambert–Eaton myasthenic syndrome IgG at mouse motor nerve terminals. *Ann Neurol* 1985; **17**: 587–92.

31. Komai K, Iwasa K, Takamori M. Calcium channel peptide can cause an autoimmune-mediated model of Lambert–Eaton myasthenic syndrome in rats. *J Neurol Sci* 1999; **166**: 126–30.

32. Kaja S, Van de Ven RC, van Dijk JG, et al. Severely impaired neuromuscular synaptic transmission causes muscle weakness in the Cacna1a-mutant mouse rolling Nagoya. *Eur J Neurosci* 2007; **25**: 2009–20.

33. Bain PG, Motomura M, Newsom-Davis J, et al. Effects of intravenous immunoglobulin on muscle weakness and calcium-channel autoantibodies in the Lambert–Eaton myasthenic syndrome. *Neurology* 1996; **47**: 678–83.

34. Newsom-Davis J, Murray NM. Plasma exchange and immunosuppressive drug treatment in the Lambert–Eaton myasthenic syndrome. *Neurology* 1984; **34**: 480–5.

35. AAEM Quality Assurance Committee. American Association of Electrodiagnostic Medicine. Practice parameter for repetitive nerve stimulation and single fiber EMG evaluation of adults with suspected myasthenia gravis or Lambert–Eaton myasthenic syndrome: summary statement. *Muscle Nerve* 2001; **24**: 1236–8.

36. Tim RW, Massey JM, Sanders DB. Lambert–Eaton myasthenic syndrome (LEMS)—clinical and electrodiagnostic features and response to therapy in 59 patients. *Ann NY Acad Sci* 1998; **841**: 823–6.

37. Hatanaka Y, Oh SJ. Ten-second exercise is superior to 30-second exercise for post-exercise facilitation in diagnosing Lambert–Eaton myasthenic syndrome. *Muscle Nerve* 2008; **37**: 572–5.

38. Wirtz PW, Nijnuis MG, Sotodeh M, et al. The epidemiology of myasthenia gravis, Lambert–Eaton myasthenic syndrome and their associated tumours in the northern part of the province of South Holland. *J Neurol* 2003; **250**: 698–701.

39. Sanders DB. Lambert–Eaton myasthenic syndrome: clinical diagnosis, immune-mediated mechanisms, and update on therapies. *Ann Neurol* 1995; **37** (Suppl 1): S63–S73.

40. Wirtz PW, Smallegange TM, Wintzen AR, Verschuuren JJ. Differences in clinical features between the Lambert–Eaton myasthenic syndrome with and without cancer: an analysis of 227 published cases. *Clin Neurol Neurosurg* 2002; **104**: 359–63.

41. Vincent A, Clover L, Buckley C, Grimley EJ, Rothwell PM. Evidence of underdiagnosis of myasthenia gravis in older people. *J Neurol Neurosurg Psychiatry* 2003; **74**: 1105–8.

42. Wirtz PW, Willcox N, van der Slik AR, et al. HLA and smoking in prediction and prognosis of small cell lung cancer in autoimmune Lambert–Eaton myasthenic syndrome. *J Neuroimmunol* 2005; **159**: 230–7.

43. Giraud M, Beaurain G, Yamamoto AM, et al. Linkage of HLA to myasthenia gravis and genetic heterogeneity depending on anti-titin antibodies. *Neurology* 2001; **57**: 1555–60.

44. Gutmann L, Crosby TW, Takamori M, Martin JD. The Eaton–Lambert syndrome and autoimmune disorders. *Am J Med* 1972; **53**: 354–6.

45. Wirtz PW, Bradshaw J, Wintzen AR, Verschuuren JJ. Associated autoimmune diseases in patients with the Lambert–Eaton myasthenic syndrome and their families. *J Neurol* 2004; **251**: 1255–9.

46. Elmqvist D, Lambert EH. Detailed analysis of neuromuscular transmission in a patient with myasthenic syndrome sometimes associated with bronchogenic carcinoma. *Mayo Clin Proc* 1968; **43**: 689–713.

47. Tim RW, Massey JM, Sanders DB. Lambert–Eaton myasthenic syndrome: electrodiagnostic finding and response to treatment. *Neurology* 2000; **54**: 2176–8.

48. Titulaer MJ, Wirtz PW, Willems LN, van Kralingen KW, Smitt PA, Verschuuren JJ. Screening for small-cell lung cancer: a follow-up study of patients with Lambert–Eaton myasthenic syndrome. *J Clin Oncol* 2008; **26**: 4276–81.

49. Wirtz PW, van Dijk JG, van Doorn PA, et al. The epidemiology of the Lambert–Eaton myasthenic syndrome in the Netherlands. *Neurology* 2004; **63**: 397–8.

50. Argov Z, Shapira Y, Averbuch-Heller L, Wirguin I. Lambert–Eaton myasthenic syndrome (LEMS) in association with lymphoproliferative disorders. *Muscle Nerve* 1995; **18**: 715–19.

51. Dongradi G, Poisson M, Beuve-Mery P, Fendler JP, Buge A, Fritel D. [Association of a lung cancer and several paraneoplastic syndromes (Lambert–Eaton syndrome, polymyositis and Schwartz–Bartter syndrome)]. *Ann Med Interne (Paris)* 1971; **122**: 959–64.

52. Ramos-Yeo YL, Reyes CV. Myasthenic syndrome (Eaton–Lambert syndrome) associated with pulmonary adenocarcinoma. *J Surg Oncol* 1987; **34**: 239–42.

53. Sabater L, Titulaer M, Saiz A, Verschuuren J, Gure AO, Graus F. SOX1 antibodies are markers of paraneoplastic Lambert–Eaton syndrome. *Neurology* 2008; **70**: 924–8.

54. Titulaer MJ, Soffietti R, Dalmau J, et al. Screening for tumours in paraneoplastic syndromes: report of an EFNS task force. *Eur J Neurol* 2011; **18**: 19–e3.

55. Lindquist S, Stangel M. Update on treatment options for Lambert–Eaton myasthenic syndrome: focus on use of amifampridine. *Neuropsychiatr Dis Treat* 2011; **7**: 341–9.

56. Sanders DB, Massey JM, Sanders LL, Edwards LJ. A randomized trial of 3,4-diaminopyridine in Lambert–Eaton myasthenic syndrome. *Neurology* 2000; **54**: 603–7.

57. Boerma CE, Rommes JH, van Leeuwen RB, Bakker J. Cardiac arrest following an iatrogenic 3,4-diaminopyridine intoxication in a patient with Lambert–Eaton myasthenic syndrome. *J Toxicol Clin Toxicol* 1995; **33**: 249–51.

58. Lundh H, Nilsson O, Rosen I, Johansson S. Practical aspects of 3,4-diaminopyridine treatment of the Lambert–Eaton myasthenic syndrome. *Acta Neurol Scand* 1993; **88**: 136–40.

59. Keogh M, Sedehizadeh S, Maddison P. Treatment for Lambert–Eaton myasthenic syndrome. *Cochrane Database Syst Rev* 2011; CD003279.

60. McEvoy KM, Windebank AJ, Daube JR, Low PA. 3,4-Diaminopyridine in the treatment of Lambert–Eaton myasthenic syndrome. *N Engl J Med* 1989; **321**: 1567–71.

61. Oh SJ, Claussen GG, Hatanaka Y, Morgan MB. 3,4-Diaminopyridine is more effective than placebo in a randomized, double-blind, cross-over drug study in LEMS. *Muscle Nerve* 2009; **40**: 795–800.

62. Wirtz PW, Verschuuren JJ, van Dijk JG, et al. Efficacy of 3,4-diaminopyridine and pyridostigmine in the treatment of Lambert–Eaton myasthenic syndrome: a randomized, double-blind, placebo-controlled, crossover study. *Clin Pharmacol Ther* 2009; **86**: 44–8.

63. Palace J, Newsom-Davis J, Lecky B. A randomized double-blind trial of prednisolone alone or with azathioprine in myasthenia gravis. Myasthenia Gravis Study Group. *Neurology* 1998; **50**: 1778–83.

64. Maddison P, Lang B, Mills K, Newsom-Davis J. Long term outcome in Lambert–Eaton myasthenic syndrome without lung cancer. *J Neurol Neurosurg Psychiatry* 2001; **70**: 212–17.

65. Maddison P, McConville J, Farrugia ME, et al. The use of rituximab in myasthenia gravis and Lambert–Eaton myasthenic syndrome. *J Neurol Neurosurg Psychiatry* 2011; **82**: 671–3.

66. Pellkofer HL, Voltz R, Kuempfel T. Favorable response to rituximab in a patient with anti-VGCC-positive Lambert–Eaton myasthenic syndrome and cerebellar dysfunction. *Muscle Nerve* 2009; **40**: 305–8.

67. Janssen-Heijnen ML, Maas HA, Siesling S, Koning CC, Coebergh JW, Groen HJ. Treatment and survival of patients with small-cell lung cancer: small steps forward, but not for patients >80. *Ann Oncol* 2012; **23**: 954–60.

68. Chalk CH, Murray NM, Newsom-Davis J, O'Neill JH, Spiro SG. Response of the Lambert–Eaton myasthenic syndrome to treatment of associated small-cell lung carcinoma. *Neurology* 1990; **40**: 1552–6.

69. Maddison P, Newsom-Davis J, Mills KR, Souhami RL. Favourable prognosis in Lambert–Eaton myasthenic syndrome and small-cell lung carcinoma. *Lancet* 1999; **353**: 117–18.

SECTION 6

Muscle

CHAPTER 22

The dystrophinopathies

Kevin M. Flanigan

Introduction

The dystrophinopathies are X-linked recessive disorders that are due to the absence or alteration of the dystrophin protein (see Fig. 22.1), encoded by the *DMD* gene on chromosome Xp21. The most common of the dystrophinopathies is Duchenne muscular dystrophy (DMD), in which dystrophin is in most cases entirely absent from its position on the subsarcolemmal surface of the muscle fibre. DMD has a commonly cited, yet estimated, incidence of 1 in 3500 male births [1], whereas the incidence in population-based studies ranges from 1 in 3802 to 1 in 6291 [2]. The milder allelic disorder Becker muscular dystrophy (BMD) is less common, with an incidence of around 1 in 18 450 male births, generally estimated as about one-third as frequent as DMD [1,3]. BMD is usually associated with the presence of significant amounts of a partially functional protein; as a result, the BMD phenotype varies widely in symptom onset and severity. X-linked dilated cardiomyopathy (XLDC) is yet another dystrophinopathy phenotype in which skeletal myopathy may be minimal or symptomatically absent. Female carriers of *DMD* mutations may occasionally show skeletal and cardiac muscle manifestations, which may present particular diagnostic difficulties if there are no known affected male family members.

The dystrophinopathies, and in particular DMD, have a special historical place in the fields of both neurology and molecular genetics. The identification of the *DMD* gene nearly three decades ago represented the first triumph of what was at the time considered 'reverse genetics', in which positional cloning led to the identification of a protein of unknown function. Today, the dystrophinopathies promise to hold a seminal position in the field of molecular genetics and gene therapies. A thorough understanding of the clinical syndromes, molecular diagnostics, and therapeutic approaches to the dystrophinopathies is useful to all neurologists.

Duchenne muscular dystrophy

History

This syndrome bears the name of the French neurologist Guillaume Duchenne de Boulogne, who provided a detailed description of both the clinical and microscopic features in publications of 1861 and 1868 [4,5], terming it *paralysie musculaire pseudohypertrophique ou paralysie myosclérosique*. Although most commonly associated with Duchenne, a compelling argument has been made for the primacy of a description by the English physician Edward Meryon [6,7], who provided a detailed description of a syndrome of 'granular and fatty degeneration of the voluntary muscles' in eight boys in 1852 [8]. An even earlier description is probably that of Gaetono Conte in Naples, who described affected brothers in 1836 [9]. Nevertheless, it is Duchenne's name by which the syndrome is known today, following the early adoption of the eponym by Charcot, Gowers, and Erb [10].

Clinical features

The clinical course of DMD is stereotyped. Boys present with symptoms between the ages of 3 and 5 years. The most common presenting symptom is abnormal gait, which often presents as toe walking early after gait acquisition. Affected boys often have delayed gait onset. Earlier motor findings may also be seen, and recent data support measurable differences in motor function in the infantile phase. However, these features may sometimes be obvious to parents only in retrospect, particularly if the affected boy is their first born, but delayed motor and developmental function can be demonstrated in boys with DMD in the first years of life [11].

Cognitive impairment is common, with IQ diminished by one standard deviation in populations of boys with DMD compared with normal controls [12]. Full-scale and performance IQ does not change with age, and although language development is delayed

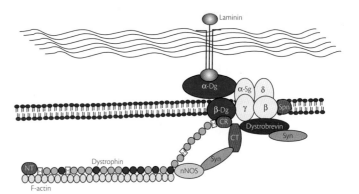

Fig. 22.1 Dystrophin and the dystrophin-glycoprotein complex. Dystrophin is found at the subsarcolemmal membrane, where it links the intracellular actin cytoskeleton to the extracellular matrix ligand laminin via the dystrophin glycoprotein complex. Dystrophin consists of the N-terminal (NT) actin-binding domain ABD1; a central rod domain made up of 24 spectrin-like repeats separated by four hinges (H) and containing a second actin-binding domain (marked as dark green spectrin repeats); a cysteine-rich (CR) region; and a C-terminal dimeric coiled-coil region (CT). Dystrophin binds to the intracellular portion of the β-dystroglycan (β-Dg) protein via the CR domain; β-Dg binds to α-dystroglycan (α-Dg), which in turns binds to laminin-α2 within the extracellular matrix. The complex includes the α-, β-, γ-, and δ-sarcoglycans, mutations of which each cause a limb-girdle muscular dystrophy. Other dystrophin-binding partners include neuronal nitric oxide synthase (nNOS), α1- and β1-syntrophin (Syn), and α-dystrobrevin. (Modified from Konieczny P et al., Gene and cell-mediated therapies for muscular dystrophy. *Muscle Nerve* 2013 May; **47**(5): 649–63.)

[13] the verbal IQ improves somewhat [14]. Nevertheless, difficulties with expression may occur [15], and this combined with dysarthria due to tongue hypertrophy may make communication challenging as boys get older. In addition, boys with DMD are at increased risk of autism, attention deficit hyperactivity disorder, and obsessive–compulsive disorder [16].

At the time of presentation, proximal weakness is typically evident. Even at a young age, where isolated muscle strength testing may be unreliable, an examiner can see proximal weakness as a difficulty in climbing stairs, hopping, or arising from the floor. The latter is typically exemplified by the Gowers manoeuvre, which is always seen in DMD. The boy rolls over, raises his bottom into the air first, and places a hand or both hands on his knees, walking his hands up his thighs to reach an upright position. Although the presence of the Gowers manoeuvre is often all that medical students recall from their single lecture regarding DMD, it is not specific for DMD but is rather a sign that may be seen in any syndrome with pelvic-girdle weakness including limb-girdle muscular dystrophy and spinal muscular atrophy. Other signs of DMD at presentation include muscle enlargement, first termed 'pseudohypertrophy' by Duchenne who attributed the enlargement to increased fibrosis and fatty replacement rather than muscle fibre hypertrophy, although true hypertrophy of contractile mass also occurs [17]. The heel cords are typically tight, resulting in toe walking. Mild lordosis is common. Pelvic- and shoulder-girdle weakness relative to age is common, and neck flexors are particularly weak. Given these signs, boys are often referred first to orthopaedic physicians or physical therapists prior to their diagnosis.

The clinical course has been well described [18–21]. In the years following presentation, strength may generally continue to improve, with continued gains in motor function into the sixth or seventh year, at which time a plateau in motor function is reached that tends to last some 12 to 18 months prior to decline. Weakness progresses, leading eventually to wheelchair dependence. Prior to the widespread use of corticosteroid treatment, wheelchair dependence (the loss of the ability to walk independently) occurred by the age of 12. Once boys are in a wheelchair, further disease progression is marked not only by progressive loss of arm movements, but by increasing incidence of respiratory insufficiency and scoliosis. Cardiomyopathy occurs, increasing in frequency with age, and death without supportive ventilation typically occurs by the age of 20, although (as discussed in some detail in the section Therapies) this natural history is altered by the use of corticosteroids. The best predictor of disease severity in an individual patient is that of any affected male relative carrying the same mutation, although this must be evaluated in the light of different treatment practices (and with the knowledge that there are rare families with significant differences between affected individuals). In the absence of this historical information, there is little on which to base a prognosis. Regarding disease progression, the 10-m walk test (i.e. the time taken to walk 10 m) is one of the few tests that have been correlated with time to wheelchair use, with a time of more than 12 seconds predicting wheelchair use within 1 year in 100% of patients [20].

Becker muscular dystrophy

A milder X-linked muscular dystrophy, with later onset and slower disease progression than DMD, was described by the German neurologist Peter Becker, who proposed it as a 'benign variant' [22,23]. The identification of the *DMD* gene locus, and subsequently the gene, led to the recognition that BMD and DMD were allelic disorders, differing in the degree of functionality of the dystrophin protein, as discussed in some detail in the section Genotype–phenotype correlations.

Clinically, BMD is associated with a widely variable phenotype. The presentation may appear as a 'mild DMD', with limb-girdle weakness and calf hypertrophy that presents somewhat later than DMD, with half of BMD patients demonstrating symptoms by the age of 10 [24]. However, BMD may present with much milder weakness, often with prominent quadriceps involvement [25], and symptoms may not occur until well into mid- or late adulthood [26,27]. Milder variants included cramp-myalgia syndromes [24,28], exercise-induced myoglobinuria [29], and asymptomatic hyperCKaemia [30], and the only North American founder allele yet reported in the *DMD* gene results in each of these relatively mild symptoms in different family members, with others entirely asymptomatic in their eighth decade [31]. In contrast to DMD, patients with BMD have a normal IQ distribution [32], even though isolated cognitive impairment has rarely been reported as the predominant presenting feature of BMD [33]. Clinically relevant behavioural problems are common (found in 67% of BMD children assessed by the Child Behavior Checklist), and the frequency of autism and attention deficit disorder is also increased [32].

Despite the wide variability in phenotype associated with BMD, those at the most severe end of the spectrum appear with limb-girdle weakness in childhood but are distinct from DMD patients in that they do not lose ambulation until after the age of 13 years. Many clinicians find useful the idea of an 'intermediate muscular dystrophy' phenotype to categorize patients who walk past the age of 12 but stop walking by 15, reserving the term BMD for patients who lose ambulation after 15. This distinction encompasses patients who are less severe than is typical for DMD but more severe than the typical BMD [21,34].

X-linked dilated cardiomyopathy (XLDC)

Cardiomyopathy is a common feature of both DMD and BMD. However, absence of dystrophin in the heart, with expression of minimum protective levels of dystrophin in skeletal muscle [35] results in isolated or X-linked cardiomyopathy associated with specific mutational mechanisms [35–42].

Laboratory features

Both DMD and BMD are associated with elevations of serum creatine kinase (CK), generally considered to be due to increased permeability of the muscle sarcolemmal membrane. In suspected dystrophinopathies, serum CK is typically the initial diagnostic test performed. In the case of DMD it is often 50–100 times the normal value at presentation. In BMD, serum CK levels are generally lower than in DMD, and reach a maximum at 10–15 years of age, probably reflecting both preservation of muscle mass and activity in comparison with DMD [43]. Cases of episodic extreme elevations leading to myoglobinuria or even a diagnosis of rhabdomyolysis have been described in BMD patients, often in those at the very mild end of the phenotypic spectrum [29,31,44–46]. Presumably, this is due to the fact that patients with very mild BMD phenotypes are able to perform much more vigorous physical activity, leading to these episodic elevations [29,45].

Although no other clinical laboratory values are useful for aiding diagnosis, it is important for clinicians be aware that the serum transaminases aspartate aminotransferase (AST) and alanine aminotransferase (ALT) are also reliably elevated in the dystrophinopathies [47–51]. They do not reflect liver damage, but are derived from muscle. Primary-care physicians should be encouraged to check a serum CK in the setting of unexplained transaminase elevations in order to avoid unnecessary liver biopsies, which are not infrequently reported in the DMD population. The gamma-glutamyl transferase (GGT) level has instead proven to be a useful marker of liver injury in patients with dystrophinopathy [52]. Assessment of renal function is similarly liable to misinterpretation if serum creatinine or creatinine clearance are assessed, as both are decreased in DMD due to diminished muscle mass; serum cystatin C is a more appropriate clinical marker of renal dysfunction in DMD patients [53].

Neonatal screening

Because serum CK is elevated at birth, it can been used as the basis for screening newborns [54–59]. CK testing can be performed via a fluorometric assay on a dried blood spot, with diagnosis confirmed by subsequent follow-up serum CK testing and genomic mutational analysis. However, the recently described two-tiered system makes use of advances in genetic technologies to allow both CK determination and mutational analysis of DNA extracted from the same Guthrie card, making newborn screening much more feasible [2].

Pathology

The dystrophin protein

The *DMD* gene consists of 79 exons, encoding at least seven isoforms of the dystrophin protein by use of different promoters that are expressed in different tissues. (An eighth isoform, making use of a putative lymphocyte-specific promoter, has only been described once.) A nearly 14 kilobase (kb) nucleotide [60] encodes the major full-length isoform in muscle (Dp427m), which weighs 427 kilodaltons (kDa) and consists of: an N-terminal actin-binding domain (ABD1); a central rod domain made up of 24 spectrin-like repeats separated by four hinges and containing a second actin-binding domain (ABD2); a cysteine-rich (CR) region; and a C-terminal dimeric coiled-coil region (CT) (Fig. 22.1). The CR region—consisting of three distinct domains: the WW domain (named after two conserved tryptophan residues), the EF hand domain, and the ZZ domain—is critical for binding to the intracellular portion of the β-dystroglycan (βDG) protein. βDG binds to αDG as part of the transmembrane dystrophin-associated glycoprotein complex, and αDG binds (in a glycosylation-dependent fashion) to laminin-α2 and other proteins of the extracellular matrix (ECM). Dystrophin thus forms an important link between the actin cytoskeleton and the ECM, stabilizing the muscle membrane in the highly distortable muscle fibres. In addition, a variety of other binding partners for dystrophin have been defined, which together suggest an important role for dystrophin in cell signalling pathways; these include neuronal nitric oxide synthase (nNOS), α1- and β1-syntrophin, α-dystrobrevin, and microtubules [61–66].

Muscle histopathology

Deficiency of dystrophin leads to failure of muscle fibre integrity and to a degenerative process marked by myofibre necrosis, muscle fibrosis, and failure of regenerative capacity. The result is the pathology first described by Duchenne and Meryon. Muscle histopathology, best ascertained on muscle specimens snap-frozen and evaluated via standardized methods [67], reveals chronic and severe myopathic changes that lead to the use of the term 'dystrophic' (Fig. 22.2). These include a wide variation in myofibre diameter, with both atrophic and hypertrophic fibres. Some of the latter may stain intensely with haematoxylin and eosin (H&E) or other stains, and are often considered 'hypercontracted' fibres. There are typical degenerating myofibres, as well as necrotic fibres that are often seen undergoing phagocytosis. Regenerating fibres are present, but are less frequent as severity progresses. Centralized nuclei are a common feature, and are interpreted as evidence of past regeneration. Fibrosis and fatty replacement—two of the classic components of descriptions of dystrophic muscle—increase over time. Endomysial fibrosis is easily detected with standard stains, including H&E and the modified Gomori trichrome (GT) stain. As regenerative capacity declines, fatty replacement of myofibres occurs, leading eventually to end-stage myopathic change.

Histopathological alterations in BMD may vary, depending upon the severity of weakness. In more severely affected muscles or cases, biopsy may reveal all of the features of DMD muscle. In less affected muscles, pathology may be much less severe, with evidence for chronic myopathic alterations including variation in fibre size and fibrosis, with varying degrees of degeneration or necrosis.

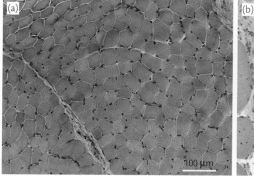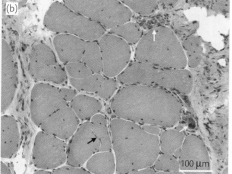

Fig. 22.2 Histopathology in DMD muscle. Haematoxylin and eosin stained sections of (a) normal muscle and (b) Duchenne muscular dystrophy (DMD) muscle. DMD muscle fibres show chronic and severe myopathic changes (dystrophic changes), including variability in fibre size, with both atrophic and more pronounced hypertrophic muscle fibres; necrotic fibres undergoing phagocytosis (white arrows); fibre splitting (black arrow); endomysial and perimysial fibrosis; and fatty infiltration. (See also figure in colour plate section)

Ultrastructural examination has little place in the diagnosis of dystrophinopathy, but is of historical significance because it demonstrated that loss of integrity of the sarcolemmal membrane is a critical early step in the disease process [68–70].

Immunohistochemical studies

The histopathology of DMD is not specific, and in fact the chronic myopathic features may be seen in many muscular dystrophies. In particular, the limb-girdle muscular dystrophies that are associated with mutations in the sarcoglycan genes, encoding members of the dystrophin-associated glycoprotein complex, demonstrate very similar histological alterations. Pathological diagnosis of the dystrophinopathies therefore relies upon the analysis of dystrophin expression, either by immunohistochemical (IHC) or immunofluorescent (IF) analysis of muscle sections, or by immunoblot (IB). Clinically, such analysis makes use of several antibodies, each directed at a different region of the dystrophin protein; most commonly, antibodies are used that target the N-terminal, central rod, and C-terminal domains. This is essential, because the presence of an internally truncated yet functional BMD-associated protein could be misinterpreted as absent if the underlying mutation deletes the coding region for the relevant epitope. An example of this is shown in Fig. 22.3, where staining is entirely absent using an antibody directed against a rod domain epitope but nearly normal with antibodies against N- and C-terminal domains in a patient with BMD. With the use of multiple antibodies, the complete absence of dystrophin protein staining by IF or IHC reliably predicts a DMD phenotype, whereas in BMD dystrophin staining is typically patchy and less intense.

DMD muscle biopsies frequently show, however, the presence of fibres that stain relatively intensely and often appear in small foci. These fibres, termed revertant fibres, are ones in which secondary alterations in the gene message allow expression of some amount of dystrophin (e.g. by altered splicing of pre-mRNA that restores the open reading frame, as discussed in greater detail in the section Reading frame rule). Revertant fibres are relatively common, occurring in up to 50% of patient biopsies [71–75]. Their frequency has not been demonstrated to be associated with the severity of dystrophinopathic symptoms. In addition, conditions intended to increase the sensitivity of IF detection reveal some fibres with very low levels of staining, described by some as 'traces', on a significant number of fibres [76]. Robust quantification of dystrophin IF images should ideally take into account not only the intensity of staining but the number of fibres expressing dystrophin, but one of the challenges in comparing these reports is that methods of reporting are not standardized. Several methods have been proposed for improved quantification, using both standard and confocal IF microscopy [77–80].

Unlike IF or IHC analysis, which are in widespread use in pathology laboratories, IB analysis can not only demonstrate the presence or absence of dystrophin but can provide information on dystrophin size. BMD muscle from patients with in-frame deletions resulting in internally truncated proteins typically demonstrates significant (yet diminished) amounts of dystrophin, but of diminished size (Fig. 22.4). IB analysis also provides a robust method of quantification, and it was suggested early on that dystrophin levels of less than 3% were consistent with DMD whereas levels of greater than 20% were consistent with mild BMD [81]. These values, although still reported as predictive by some major North American diagnostic laboratories, cannot be considered absolute. In part this is because of significant differences in methodology, making standardized reporting between labs unreliable. However, other examples of the challenges of quantification as a predictor are the rare patients in whom dystrophin expression is essentially absent yet

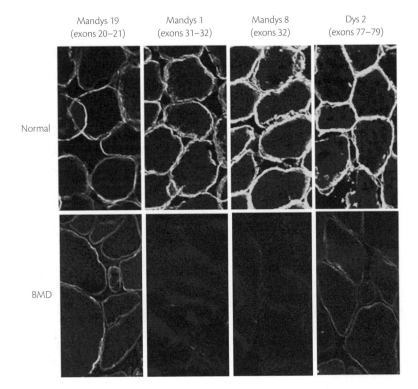

Mandys 19 (exons 20–21) Mandys 1 (exons 31–32) Mandys 8 (exons 32) Dys 2 (exons 77–79)

Normal

BMD

Fig. 22.3 Epitope mapping demonstrates internally truncated dystrophin in Becker muscular dystrophy (BMD) muscle, consistent with the reading frame rule. Immunofluorescent analysis of muscle from a normal (upper) and BMD (lower) muscle sample reveals the presence of both N-terminal and C-terminal dystrophin at the muscle membrane in the BMD patient, although in diminished amounts. In contrast, staining is absent with antibodies directed at peptides encoded by exons excluded from the *DMD* messenger RNA. (See also figure in colour plate section)

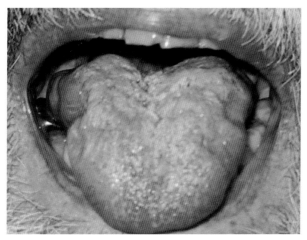

Fig. 4.2 Wasting of the tongue in amyotrophic lateral sclerosis. Typically dysarthria precedes dysphagia, and the lateral borders of the tongue tend to waste first and symmetrically. Reduced movement may exacerbate coating of the tongue surface as seen, which requires focused oral hygiene measures.

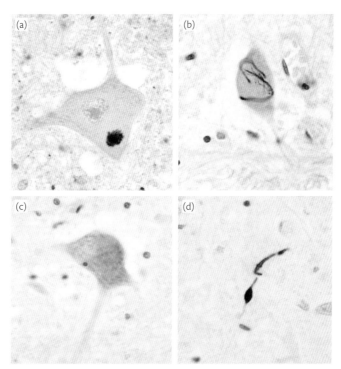

Fig. 4.7 Jean-Martin Charcot observed cellular 'debris' in his histopathological descriptions of amyotrophic lateral sclerosis (ALS). Mislocalized cytoplasmic inclusions of ubiquitinated protein (here stained with antibodies against p62) which contain TDP-43 are the pathological hallmark of nearly all cases of ALS (a), though not found in clinically identical cases associated with mutations in *SOD1*. Skein-like inclusions may also be seen (b). The Bunina body is highly specific for ALS but harder to spot (c, small brown inclusion). Dystrophic neurites are a more non-specific pathological observation (d). (Courtesy of Dr Olaf Ansorge, Department of Neuropathology, John Radcliffe Hospital, Oxford, UK.)

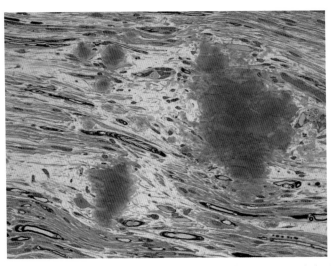

Fig. 10.1 Superficial peroneal nerve biopsy specimen to show massive endoneurial amyloid deposits from a patient with the Tyr77 mutation. One micron thick plastic section with thionin staining. With acknowledgement to Professor Said.

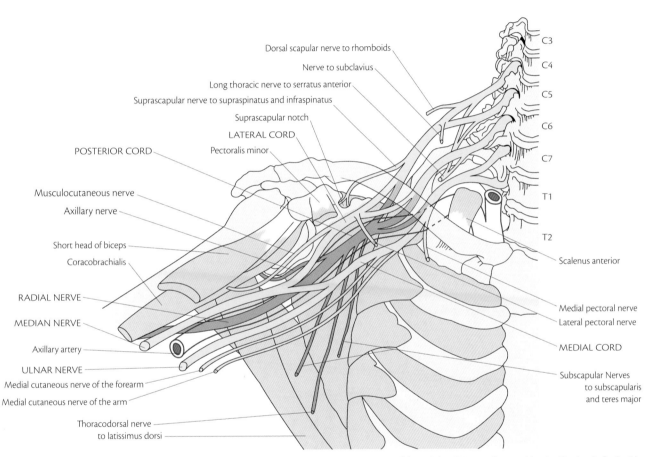

Fig. 12.1 Anatomy of the brachial plexus. (Adapted from O'Brien MD (2000). *Aids to the Examination of the Peripheral Nervous System*, 4th edn. Elsevier, Oxford, with kind permission of Elsevier.)

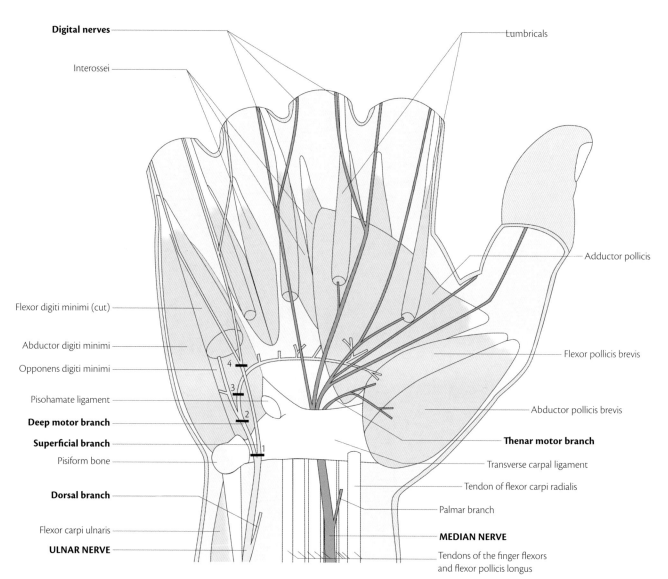

Digital nerves

Lumbricals

Interossei

Adductor pollicis

Flexor digiti minimi (cut)

Abductor digiti minimi

Opponens digiti minimi

Flexor pollicis brevis

4

Pisohamate ligament

3

Deep motor branch

2

Abductor pollicis brevis

Superficial branch

Pisiform bone

1

Thenar motor branch

Transverse carpal ligament

Dorsal branch

Tendon of flexor carpi radialis

Palmar branch

Flexor carpi ulnaris

MEDIAN NERVE

ULNAR NERVE

Tendons of the finger flexors
and flexor pollicis longus

Fig. 12.2 The median and ulnar nerves in the wrist and hand. Patterns of ulnar nerve injury are indicated by numbers: (1) deep and superficial branches; (2) deep branch proximal to the origin of branches to the hypothenar muscles; (3) deep branch distal to the origin of branches to the hypothenar muscles; (4) superficial branch only.

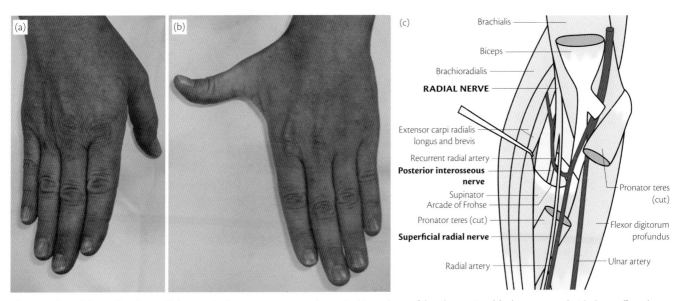

Fig. 12.5 The radial tunnel syndrome. Right posterior interosseous neuropathy resulted in weakness of thumb extension (a) when compared with the unaffected hand (b). The anatomy of the radial tunnel is illustrated (c), demonstrating the relationship of the posterior interosseous nerve to supinator.

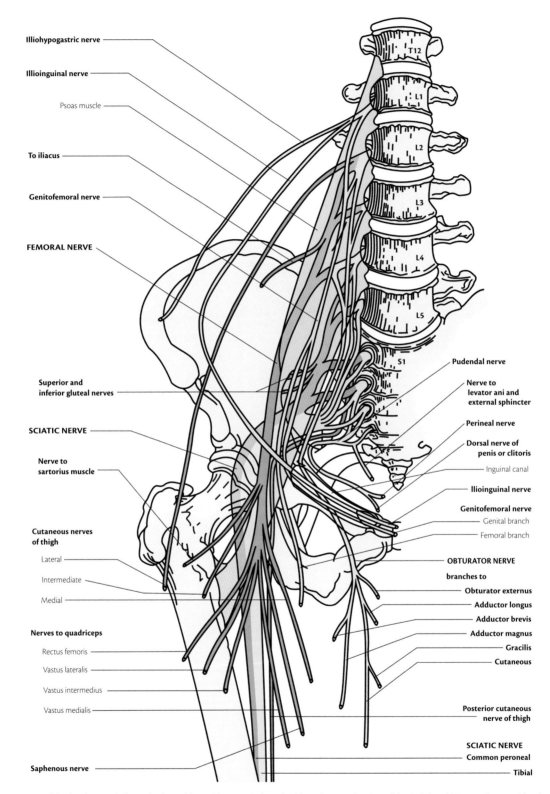

Fig. 12.6 The anatomy of the lumbosacral plexus. (Adapted from O'Brien MD (2000). *Aids to the Examination of the Peripheral Nervous System*, 4th edn. Elsevier, Oxford, with kind permission of Elsevier.)

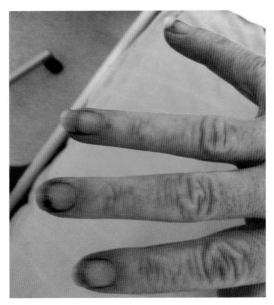

Fig. 13.1 Digital infarcts in a patient with antineutrophil cytoplasmic antibodies (ANCA)-negative vasculitis.

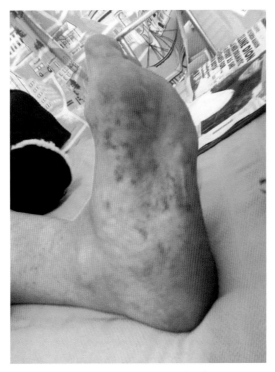

Fig. 13.2 Dusky discoloration with livedo rash of the foot (same patient as Fig. 13.1).

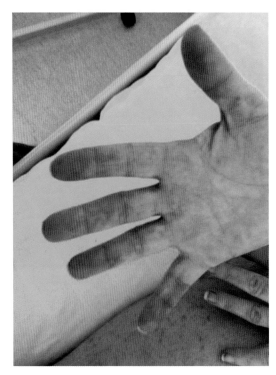

Fig. 13.3 Dusky discoloration with livedo rash of the hand (same patient as Fig. 13.1).

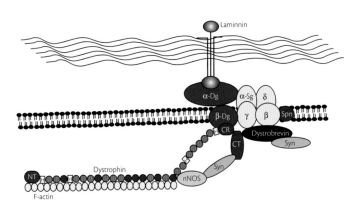

Fig. 22.1 Dystrophin and the dystrophin-glycoprotein complex. Dystrophin is found at the subsarcolemmal membrane, where it links the intracellular actin cytoskeleton to the extracellular matrix ligand laminin via the dystrophin glycoprotein complex. Dystrophin consists of the N-terminal (NT) actin-binding domain ABD1; a central rod domain made up of 24 spectrin-like repeats separated by four hinges (H) and containing a second actin-binding domain (marked as blue spectrin repeats); a cysteine-rich (CR) region; and a C-terminal dimeric coiled-coil region (CT). Dystrophin binds to the intracellular portion of the β-dystroglycan (β-Dg) protein via the CR domain; β-Dg binds to α-dystroglycan (α-Dg), which in turns binds to laminin-α2 within the extracellular matrix. The complex includes the α-, β-, γ-, and δ-sarcoglycans, mutations of which each cause a limb-girdle muscular dystrophy. Other dystrophin-binding partners include neuronal nitric oxide synthase (nNOS), α1- and β1-syntrophin (Syn), and α-dystrobrevin. (Modified from Konieczny P et al., Gene and cell-mediated therapies for muscular dystrophy. *Muscle Nerve* 2013 May; **47**(5): 649–63.)

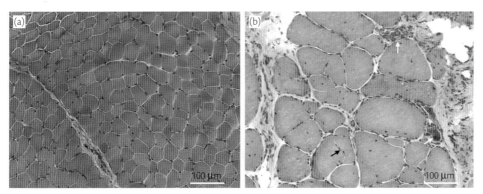

Fig. 22.2 Histopathology in DMD muscle. Haematoxylin and eosin stained sections of (a) normal muscle and (b) Duchenne muscular dystrophy (DMD) muscle. DMD muscle fibres show chronic and severe myopathic changes (dystrophic changes), including variability in fibre size, with both atrophic and more pronounced hypertrophic muscle fibres; necrotic fibres undergoing phagocytosis (white arrows); fibre splitting (black arrow); endomysial and perimysial fibrosis; and fatty infiltration.

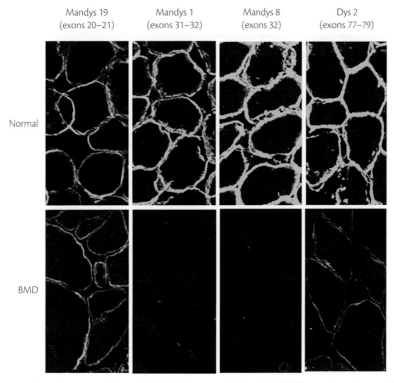

Fig. 22.3 Epitope mapping demonstrates internally truncated dystrophin in Becker muscular dystrophy (BMD) muscle, consistent with the reading frame rule. Immunofluorescent analysis of muscle from a normal (upper) and BMD (lower) muscle sample reveals the presence of both N-terminal and C-terminal dystrophin at the muscle membrane in the BMD patient, although in diminished amounts. In contrast, staining is absent with antibodies directed at peptides encoded by exons excluded from the *DMD* messenger RNA.

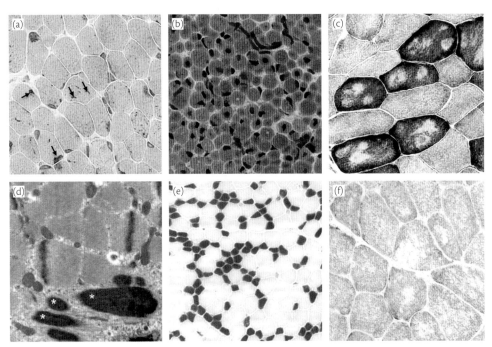

Fig. 28.2 The main histological features of common congenital myopathies. (a), (d) Nemaline myopathy. Intensely staining inclusions (arrows) on the Gomori trichrome stain (a) represent clumps of nemaline bodies, which appear as electron-dense rods (*) on electron microscopy (d). (b) *MTM1*-related centronuclear myopathy. There are numerous internalized nuclei, many of which occupy central positions, on haematoxylin and eosin staining. (c) Central core disease (CCD). Nicotinamide adenine dinucleotide tetrazolium reductase (NADH-TR) staining shows large cores limited to Type 1 (dark) fibres. Many CCD muscle biopsies also show complete Type 1 fibre predominance, not present here. (e) Congenital fibre-type disproportion due to a heterozygous mutation in *TPM3*. An ATPase 4.3 stain shows marked consistent smallness of Type 1 (dark staining) fibres compared with Type 2 (pale) fibres. (f) Succinate dehydrogenase stain showing multiminicores in most fibres.

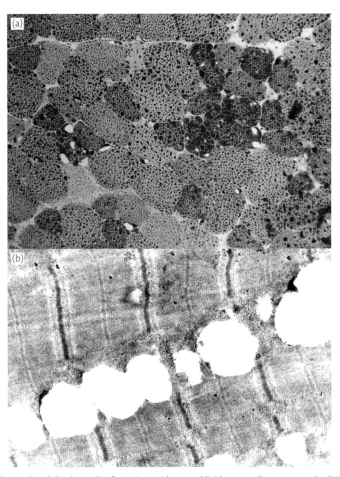

Fig. 29.5 Massive lipid accumulation is observed in skeletal muscle of a patient with neutral lipid storage disease myopathy (NLSDM) with optic oil red O (a) and electronic microscopy (b).

Reprinted from Neuromuscular Disorders, 20, Pascal Laforêt, Christine Vianey-Saban, Disorders of muscle lipid metabolism: Diagnostic and therapeutic challenges, 693–700, Copyright (2010), with permission from Elsevier. Histological and electron microscopy photos were provided by courtesy of Drs P. Laforêt[1], B. Eymard[1], and N. B. Romero[2] ([1]Centre de Référence de Pathologie Neuromusculaire Paris-Est, Groupe Hospitalier Pitié-Salpêtrière, Assistance Publique-Hôpitaux de Paris, Paris, France, [2]Département de Neurologie, Hôpitaux Universitaires, Strasbourg, France).

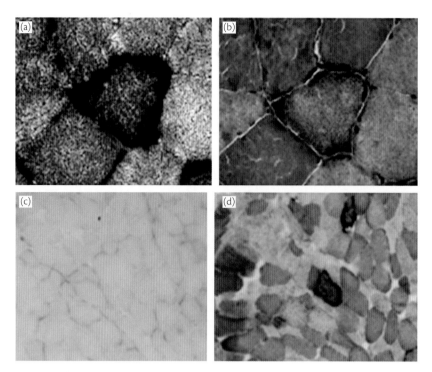

Fig. 30.1 (a) Succinate dehydrogenase (SDH) histochemistry and (b) Gomori trichrome histochemistry, both demonstrating subsarcolemmal accumulation of mitochondria in a 'ragged red fibre'. Cytochrome *c* oxidase (COX) histochemistry demonstrates diffusely COX-negative fibres in a nuclear gene defect (c) and serial COX/SDH assay reveals mosaic pattern of COX deficiency in a heteroplasmic mitochondrial DNA disorder (d).

Adapted from Chinnery PF, Betts J, Jaros E, Turnbull DM, DiMauro S, Perry R. Mitochondrial diseases. Chapter 8. *Greenfields Neuropathology*, 8th Edition, 2008. Editors: Love S, Louis DN, Ellison BW. pp. 601–642. With thanks to Prof Robert Taylor..

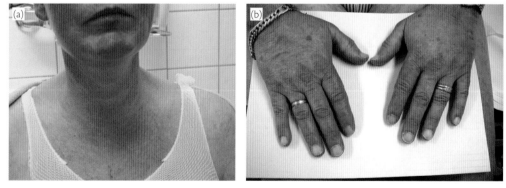

Fig. 32.2 (a) Characteristic skin feature in a patient with dermatomyositis: erythematous dermatitis over the dorsum of the hands (Gottron papules or macules). (b) Characteristic skin feature in a patient with dermatomyositis: erythematous rash on the face, neck, and anterior chest (V sign).

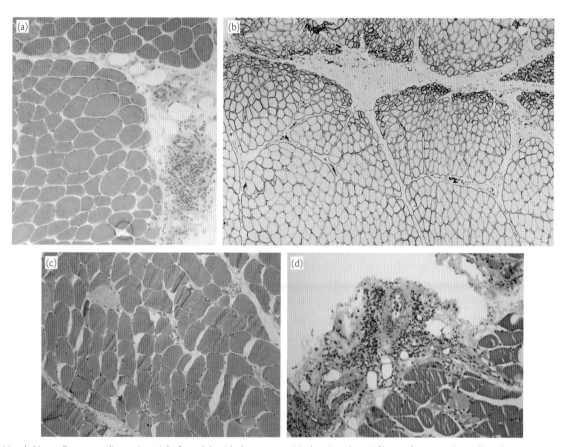

Fig. 32.4 (a) Muscle biopsy (haematoxylin–eosin stain) of an adult with dermatomyositis showing a large infiltrate of mononuclear cells in the perimysium and around the microvasculature. (b) Muscle biopsy (spectrin stain) from a child with dermatomyositis showing perifascicular muscle fibre atrophy. (c) Muscle biopsy (haematoxylin–eosin stain) of an adult with necrotizing autoimmune myopathy showing scattered necrotic muscle fibres sometimes undergoing phagocytosis. (d) Muscle biopsy of a patient with the antisynthetase syndrome showing a histological picture similar to that of dermatomyositis with mononuclear cell infiltrates at the perimysial site and surrounding blood vessels. In the perifascicular region necrotizing and regenerating muscle fibres are present.

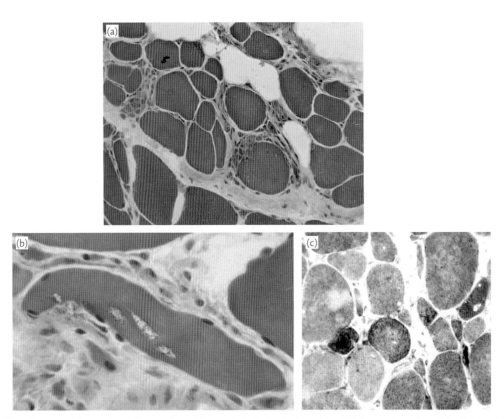

Fig. 32.7 (a) Muscle biopsy (haematoxylin–eosin stain) of a patient with sporadic inclusion body myositis (sIBM) showing endomysial collections of mononuclear cells surrounding and sometimes invading non-necrotic muscle fibres. (b) Muscle biopsy of a patient with IBM showing a muscle fibre with rimmed vacuoles. (c) Muscle bopsy (succinate dehydrogenase–cytochrome *c* oxidase stain) of a patient with sIBM showing an increased number of cytochrome *c* oxidase-negative muscle fibres which stain blue.

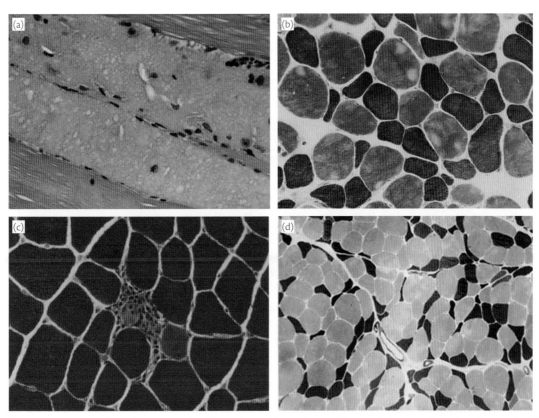

Fig. 34.2 (a) Myofibre necrosis in a case of hypothyroid myopathy. (b) Cores in myofibres and Type 2 fibre atrophy in a case of hypothyroid myopathy (ATPase, 9.4). (c) Single myofibre necrosis and inflammatory infiltrate in a case of hyperthyroid myopathy (haematoxylin and eosin). (d) Type 2 fibre atrophy in a case of corticosteroid myopathy (ATPase, 9.4).

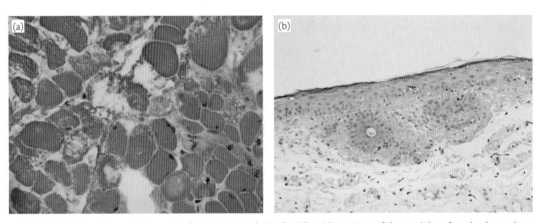

Fig. 36.3 (a) A case of paraneoplastic acute necrotizing myopathy in a patient admitted to ICU with respiratory failure and there found to have a breast tumour; muscle tissue from the pectorals was obtained at mastectomy. (b) A biopsy from a skin rash confirming dermatomyositis in a patient with respiratory failure, coagulopathy, and septic shock unable to undergo muscle biopsy. (Courtesy Dr D. O'Donovan and Dr E. Rytina, Cambridge University Hospitals, Cambridge, UK.)

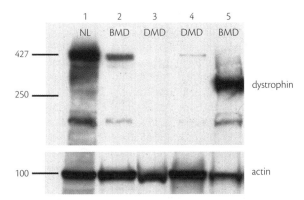

Fig. 22.4 Immunoblot analysis of dystrophin in Duchenne muscular dystrophy (DMD) and Becker muscular dystrophy (BMD). Immunoblot of muscle lysate from normal muscle (NL; lane 1) shows a 427 kDa isoform. This isoform is either absent (lane 3) or nearly absent (lane 4) in muscle from patients with DMD. In contrast, BMD patients (lanes 2 and 5) typically show diminished but still significant amounts of dystrophin of either slightly (lane 2) or markedly diminished size (lane 5). In this example, the BMD sample in lane 5 results from an in-frame deletion of exons 3–27, whereas the BMD sample in lane 2 results from an alternative translational initiation within exon 6, as discussed in the text. The dystrophin antibody is the polyclonal Ab15277 (Abcam, Cambridge, MA, USA), directed at the C-terminus. The lower panel is a pan-actin antibody (Neomarkers, Kalamazoo, MI, USA) used as a loading control on the same blot.

the disease is quite mild, and patients with relatively abundant dystrophin of small size but with evidently non-functional dystrophin based upon clinical phenotype [80]. Such patients, however, are clearly the exception. Efforts to standardize quantification assays by both IF/IHC and IB are under way, largely driven by the need for qualified biomarkers for trials of therapies directed at restoring dystrophin to the sarcolemmal membrane.

Molecular diagnosis

The *DMD* gene historically presented challenges for molecular diagnosis, primarily because of its size. Its 79 exons are spread over 2.2 million bases, representing the largest known gene. Early studies demonstrated that deletions of one or more exons accounted for nearly two-thirds of mutations, and since males are hemizygous for the *DMD* locus, a polymerase chain reaction (PCR)-based test with exon-specific primers can readily and relatively cheaply detect the presence or absence of a given exon. The observation that exon deletions were clustered around two 'hot-spots' within the gene led to the widespread use of the economical multiplex PCR test, by which around 25 exons were tested by using multiple primer sets in each reaction [82,83]. Using this method permitted identification of the presence of a deletion in up to 98% of deletion-positive patients [82,83]. However, because increases in copy number could not be reliably detected, this method could not detect exon duplications nor be reliably used for carrier testing. It also does not test every exon, so that the limits of exonic deletions were frequently not defined—an important consideration now that novel therapies dependent upon specific mutations are entering clinical trials.

With advances in molecular genetic methodology, multiplex PCR has now been superseded by methods that test for copy number in every exon, allowing characterization of the extent of exon deletions or duplications as well as identifying female carriers of these mutations. Several methods robustly identify DMD exon copy number variations, including multiplex ligation-dependent probe amplification (MLPA) as well as comparative genomic hybridization (CGH) using either custom or commercial microarrays. Because these methods interrogate all exons, they have the additional advantage of identifying those rare patients with complex exon duplications or deletions (i.e. affecting non-contiguous blocks of exons) [34,84,85]. For patients without exon copy number variations, sequencing of the *DMD* gene may be performed to detect point mutations, including nonsense, small subexonic insertions or deletions, or splice site mutations. Because nearly all point mutations are 'private' mutations, and do not occur in hot-spots, sequencing must be performed across the entire coding region. Several methods robustly do this, including both the semiautomated PCR-based single-condition amplification/internal primer (SCAIP) sequencing method [86] and high-throughput genomic approaches.

Using such methods, the sensitivity of mutation detection in lymphocyte-derived genomic DNA samples reaches 93–95% [34,87]. The distribution of *DMD* mutation classes varies slightly depending upon the sample tested. In an unselected clinic cohort of 68 index cases [88], exonic deletions accounted for 65% of mutations and exonic duplications for 6%; nonsense mutations for 13%; missense mutations for 4%; and small insertions/deletions for 3%. These numbers differ slightly for reports from referral laboratory settings, particularly those in which a referral bias exists for a specific diagnostic test for one mutation class exists [34], but are similar in large aggregate collections of patients [89].

Patients with no detectable mutation on genomic DNA analysis require muscle biopsy, both to confirm the diagnosis of a dystrophinopathy (by IHC, IF, or IB) and to provide muscle tissue for mRNA extraction for further analysis. Standard mutational methods result in sequencing of the coding regions (exons) and flanking intronic sequence, and many dystrophinopathy patients without mutations detectable by these methods turn out to have deep intronic mutations that result in the creation or activation of a cryptic splice site, resulting in the inclusion of an intronic sequence as a pseudoexon within the mature mRNA [90,91]. Such mutations require reverse transcription of the *DMD* mRNA, and sequencing of the subsequent cDNA, for detection. cDNA sequencing can also help to clarify unusual mutations such as exon inversions, for which standard mutational analyses may provide an incomplete picture [84,92–94].

Characterization of the *DMD* mutation represents the current standard of care, both for confirmation of the diagnosis and because several molecular therapies reaching clinical trials are directed toward treating only certain classes of mutation. Carrier testing is not required in the setting of a clear X-linked history revealing an obligate carrier status. However, consistent with the Haldane rule for an X-linked lethal disorder, one-third of DMD cases are *de novo*. Genetic counselling should be considered an essential part of clinical care, and must address the risk of germline mosaicism in mothers whose lymphocyte DNA analysis was negative, which may be as high as 10% [95,96]; such germline mosaicism carriers are often only detected after the birth of a second affected boy to a mother who had a negative lymphocyte DNA test.

Genotype–phenotype correlations
The reading frame rule

The reading frame rule was first proposed by Monaco *et al* as an explanation for the phenotypic difference between DMD and BMD in patients with deletions in the *DMD* gene [97]. Briefly, it stated that the primary determinant of severity was not the size of the deletion, i.e. the number of exons deleted, but whether the resultant mRNA maintained an open reading frame (ORF) such that functional N- and C-terminal domains were translated. Patients with quite large deletions, particularly of the spectrin repeat-containing central rod domain, can have relatively mild disease. This rule has proven useful in understanding phenotypic differences, with a sensitivity of 93–96% in predicting DMD in large series [34,89]. It also has helped to serve as a template for therapeutic approaches for DMD. As examples, both virally mediated microdystrophin gene therapy and antisense oligonucleotide (AON) exon-skipping therapies (discussed in detail in the section Novel therapies) are directed toward expression of internally truncated dystrophin proteins from in-frame 'BMD-like' transcripts.

Exceptions to the reading frame rule

As useful as the reading frame rule is, it is important for clinicians to recognize that exceptions to it are not uncommon. One example is large in-frame deletions that encompass all or a large portion of the dystrophin ABD1 and extend into the central rod domain, which often result in DMD [98,99]. Another important exception is in the category of nonsense mutations. By definition, all nonsense mutations are predicted to interrupt the reading frame, resulting in no dystrophin expression and hence DMD. However, 14% of nonsense mutations are instead associated with BMD [100], and nearly all of these are associated with altered pre-mRNA splicing [100–102]. The nucleotide change alters splicing signals (frequently ablating an exon splice enhancer or creating an exon splice suppressor sequence); as a result, the mature mRNA does not contain a premature stop codon. This mechanism requires that the mutation be present in a 'zero-frame' exon, i.e. one in which the flanking exons would maintain an ORF, and most are BMD-associated nonsense mutations are found in such a region spanning exons 23–42. Although overall not terribly common, this mechanism is frequent enough that in the absence of a family history to offer guidance, prognosis based upon a predicted nonsense mutation in this region should be offered with caution, despite genetic reports that frequently predict a DMD phenotype.

Other genotype–phenotype correlations; particular illustrative mutations

The accumulation of large patient data sets provides more information for studying phenotype/genotype correlations. Most of the effects described relate to the underlying *DMD* mutation itself, and the effect on the ORF of the mature mRNA as described by the reading frame rule. In the complete absence of dystrophin, as is the case with most frame-truncating mutations, it is not surprising that the specifics of the mutation do not significantly influence skeletal muscle phenotype. However, there is growing evidence that altered expression of other tissue isoforms may result in variation in non-muscle manifestations. Specifically, mutations that ablate expression of the shorter dystrophin isoforms that are expressed in the brain (Dp140, Dp71) result in a higher frequency of cognitive impairment [103–106]. In cases of DMD or BMD where an ORF allows expression of a partially functional dystrophin, variations in phenotype are much more likely to be related to the absence or dysfunction of specific functional domains. An example is the observation that in BMD patients with in-frame rod domain mutations, the age at onset of cardiomyopathy is younger if the deletion affects the

N-terminal domain (mid-20s) as opposed to deletions affecting the latter part of the rod domain [107].

Several particular examples of mutations or mutational mechanisms merit special comment because they demonstrate molecular mechanisms. One example is the out-of-frame deletion of exons 3–7, which is relatively common and has long been described as being associated with both DMD and the milder BMD phenotypes [108,109]. In this case, epitope mapping reveals initiation of translation in exon 8, with variable efficiency apparently accounting for the variable phenotype. A second is c.9G>A (p.Trp3X), the only *DMD* founder allele mutation described in North American families. This mutation results in a predicted nonsense mutation in exon 1 of the Dp427m isoform, and might be predicted to be a null allele resulting in no dystrophin expression and DMD. Instead, it is associated with a very mild BMD phenotype; although the proband took to a wheelchair permanently in his seventh decade, other family members were asymptomatic in their eighth; children examined have only mild cramp/myalgias or exertional myoglobinuria [31]. The mechanism of phenotypic rescue is explained by alternative translational initiation from one of two methionines encoded within exon 6 [110], a mechanism which may be generalizable to truncating mutations within the first few exons. The resultant protein is abundant and highly functional despite the absence of the first calponin homology domain within ABD1, an observation that has yet to be fully explained.

Other examples include the large central rod domain deletions that have directly informed therapeutic approaches. Perhaps the most famous is that of a BMD patient with a deletion of exons 17–48, leading to a deletion of 46% of the coding sequence yet a very mild phenotype of walking past the age of 60 [60]. The identification of this and similar patients has led directly to the concept of mini- or microdystrophin approaches to transgene design for viral gene therapies [111]. The in-frame deletion of exons 45–55 can result in XLDC without significant limb weakness [112,113] or with only relatively mild BMD [26,40]. A multiexon skipping therapeutic approach directed at creating this mRNA would be predicted to be beneficial to 63% of patients [114].

A final example is provided by missense mutations, which are relatively uncommon but can elucidate the principles of dystrophin function. Missense mutations in the actin-binding domain typically result in BMD; this was attributed to effects on actin binding, but more recent work has shown that this is due to alteration of protein stability, rather than direct effects on binding [115]. Missense mutations in the C-terminal region are often associated with severe DMD, suggesting a role for critical domains into DG binding [116,117].

Genetic modifiers

Although the largest determinant of phenotype is the *DMD* genotype, and the reading frame that ultimately results from it, it is reasonable to predict that other genes may modify the disease course. Two such candidates have recently been identified. One is the *SPP1* gene, encoding osteopontin, a cytokine important in cell migration and survival that influences fibrosis in dystrophic muscle via the transforming growth factor β (TGFβ) pathway [118]. A polymorphism in *SPP1* has been associated with prolonged ambulation in DMD patients [119,120]. The TGFβ pathway was also implicated by the identification of a variation in the latent TGFβ binding protein 4 (LTBP4) responsible for differences in muscle leakiness and fibrosis in a mouse model of sarcoglycanopathy [121]. In a large cohort of patients (in whom the effect of *SPP1* polymorphisms were not confirmed), polymorphisms in the *LTBP4* gene were shown to both have a functional effect on TGFβ signalling in human cell culture and to significantly affect the severity of DMD; patients homozygous for the minor, protective allele walked for a mean of 1.8 years longer than patients with the major allele [122]. The identification of such significant genetic modifiers raises issues of stratification for clinical trials, and suggests new therapeutic pathways.

Differential diagnosis

In the presence of an X-linked family history, the diagnosis of DMD can essentially be made on clinical grounds with nearly complete certainly (although confirmation by genetic testing represents the standard of care). Even in the absence of an X-linked family history it can be made on presentation alone with reasonable reliability. The most common syndromes in the differential diagnosis of DMD include the autosomal recessive limb-girdle muscular dystrophies (LGMD2s) which occur due to mutations in the genes encoding α-sarcoglycan (*SGCA*; LGMD2D), β-sarcoglycan (*SGCB*; LGMD2E), γ-sarcoglycan (*SGCG*; LGMD2C), and δ-sarcoglycan (*SGCD*; LGMD2F). Although each of these is associated with a spectrum of severity, in their severe form they may be nearly indistinguishable from DMD except for the pattern of inheritance, a phenotype historically called severe childhood autosomal recessive muscular dystrophy (SCAR-MD) [123,124]. In addition to the sarcoglycanopathies, mutations in the *FKRP* gene can also result a limb-girdle muscular dystrophy (LGMD2I) with either a Duchenne- or Becker-like phenotype, notably including cardiomyopathy [125,126]. In the clinical setting of a dystrophinopathy phenotype but negative genomic mutational analysis, muscle biopsy assessment of sarcoglycan expression and glycosylation of α-DG is informative, although mutational analysis of all of these genes can be undertaken after a negative *DMD* analysis instead of muscle biopsy.

Carriers

Most heterozygous female carriers of *DMD* mutations are asymptomatic. Myalgias are common, particularly with exertion [127,128], but between 2.5 and 17% of carriers show a signs of muscle dysfunction, ranging from mild muscle weakness to a DMD-like muscular dystrophy, and are termed manifesting carriers [127–133]. Weakness may be, but is not always [127,128,132], asymmetric and may rarely involve more focal weakness, such as of the paraspinal muscles [134]. In addition there is significant risk of cardiomyopathy in carriers, with dilated cardiomyopathy found in 36–38% [128,135], and a decline in cardiac function may happen relatively acutely, or related to pregnancy [128]. Screening of carriers by echocardiogram at intervals is warranted.

Therapies

It has become increasingly evident that the care of DMD requires not only pharmacological intervention but also attention to the multiple systems affected within the patient, and to the psychosocial and economic issues that affect the patient's family. In practice, care standards have historically varied very widely. The practising clinician can benefit from reviewing recent transnational efforts to define universal care standards in the dystrophinopathies [136,137].

Corticosteroids

The corticosteroids prednisone/prednisolone and deflazacort are the only medications that have been shown to alter the course of DMD. The mechanism of action of corticosteroids is unclear, but they apparently play a role in membrane stabilization as well as in interrupting inflammatory and fibrotic responses within degenerating muscle. Prednisone was first used in DMD in the early 1970s by Siegel [138] and by Drachman [139], who suggested conflicting results regarding a potential therapeutic benefit. The definitive trial, however, was the randomized, double-blind, placebo-controlled trial performed by the Cooperative Investigation in Duchenne Dystrophy (CIDD) consortium in 1989 [140]. This landmark study showed that treatment with prednisone at 0.75 mg kg^{-1} day^{-1} resulted in improvements in muscle strength at 6 months as measured by manual muscle testing. Treatment with 1.5 mg kg^{-1} day^{-1} showed a similar degree of improvement, but with significantly greater side effects, whereas treatment with an every other day regimen showed no significant improvement. Deflazacort at a dose of 0.9 mg kg^{-1} day^{-1} is an alternative corticosteroid used in DMD that has potentially greater immunosuppressive effects than prednisone in some experimental settings [141,142]. It is in widespread use, including in the United States where it has not been approved.

Multiple trials have now confirmed a beneficial effect of corticosteroids on strength, and although the effect on ambulation has not been studied in a randomized placebo-controlled trial, early steroid treatment is estimated to prolonged ambulation for up to 1–3 years or more [140,143–149]. Deflazacort and prednisone have nearly equal efficacy, with some difference in their side effect profile—weight gain in particular is less with deflazacort [150]. Treatment with either prednisone or deflazacort is marked by diminished height, weight gain, increased appetite, increased osteoporosis, an increased risk of cataracts, and a tendency toward behavioural disturbances, and it is important for both clinicians and parents to recognize that deflazacort is not free from these side effects. A number of alternative regimens have been used, primarily with prednisone, in order to minimize the side effects. The most common are prednisone given 0.75 mg kg^{-1} on the first 10 days of each month, or the same dose taken alternating 10 days on and 10 days off. Dosing every other day was tested in the earliest randomized trials, and although not shown to be significantly beneficial is still in use in some clinics. Recent data suggest that weekend dosing, in which 10 mg kg^{-1} week^{-1} is divided between a Saturday and Sunday dose (i.e. 5 mg kg^{-1} each weekend day), has nearly equal efficacy to daily treatment with a similar side effect profile [151].

One of the significant challenges for a clinician is to know when to initiate and when to stop treatment with corticosteroids. Current care recommendations are ambiguous, and one consensus document suggest initiation during the phase of functional motor plateau, generally between the ages of 4 and 8 years [136]. However, anecdotal reports suggest that very early treatment with steroids provides an additional long-term benefit [152,153], and in many clinics initiation of treatment by the age of 5 years is standard. The issue of when to cease steroid therapy is also unclear; in many clinics, it is stopped at the time of loss of ambulation. A variety of retrospective studies suggest that scoliosis is minimized, and ventilation is preserved, with continued low-dose steroid therapy in a wheelchair [149]. The effect of corticosteroids on cardiomyopathy is entirely unclear, with only very limited retrospective data to support this hypothesis.

Pulmonary care and ventilatory support

Ventilatory insufficiency is a common feature of DMD, resulting in significant morbidity and ultimately mortality [154]. It becomes clinically significant in the second decade, as the percentage predicted forced vital capacity (FVC%) begins to decline after loss of ambulation due to both progression of weakness of the diaphragm and accessory muscles and diminished thoracic capacity. Insufficiency increases in frequency through the second decade, and ventilatory insufficiency resulting in pneumonia as a frequent proximate cause of death; integration of a pulmonologist into the multidisciplinary clinical care role is therefore critical. Importantly, respiratory infections can be decreased in frequency by the use of an insufflator/exsufflator device, and early evaluation and training for this device should be considered standard for boys with DMD, particularly once they are in a wheelchair.

Nocturnal ventilatory support clearly has an impact on morbidity and mortality, and early recognition and treatment by appropriate nocturnal ventilation have been attributed with increasing survival at age 25 years to 53% of patients in one large clinic population [155]. Diagnosis of nocturnal ventilatory insufficiency depends upon recognition of symptoms as well as ancillary testing. Symptoms of snoring, morning headaches, or excessive daytime sleepiness should automatically lead to a polysomnogram. Obstructive sleep apnoea may also occur, often accentuated by a weight gain associated with steroid therapy. Bilevel continuous positive airway pressure ventilation (BiPAP) is typically the treatment of choice [154]. As weakness progresses, tracheostomy may be considered, for either nocturnal or full-time ventilation.

Scoliosis

Scoliosis is typically not a feature of DMD until the boy reaches a wheelchair, at which point the risk of scoliosis increases. Proper wheelchair fitting may delay scoliosis, as may steroid use [156,157], but ultimately up to 77% of boys may develop it [157]. It is difficult to assess the benefit of scoliosis surgery, as data are largely retrospective [158]. Scoliosis surgery may have little impact on short-term survival (by age 17 years) [159], but may have significant impact in the longer term in those with severe scoliosis, where combined with ventilator support it increased survival by nearly 8 years in one clinic's experience [160].

Cardiac care

It is generally assumed that all DMD patients develop a cardiomyopathy if they live long enough [161]. The older literature estimates the incidence as 25% by age 6 years, and 59% by age 10 years [162], which may be high [163,164]; other studies suggest the median age of onset is around 14–15 years [164,165]. One challenge is in defining the onset of cardiomyopathy; cardiac fibrosis and diastolic dysfunction may precede systolic dysfunction [166–168], and cardiac MRI may show the early changes, but it is nevertheless primarily systolic dysfunction that is readily detectable on standard clinical echocardiogram and that alerts the clinician to dysfunction. For this reason, screening echocardiograms are recommended at diagnosis or by the age of 6 years; every 2 years up to age 8; and yearly after age 10 [137]. Additional cardiac abnormalities include electrocardiogram changes [169,170] and conduction disturbances including

ventricular arrhythmias [169,171]; a low threshold for Holter monitoring is warranted. Treatment of cardiomyopathy usually makes use of angiotensin-converting enzyme (ACE) inhibitors such as lisinopril or enalapril and angiotensin receptor blockers (ARBs) such as losartan for afterload reduction. One area of significant debate is whether these drugs should be used prior to the diagnosis of clinical systolic dysfunction, with some limited evidence that this approach offers long-term protection [172]; further prospective studies are needed.

Novel therapies

A variety of therapies have recently entered clinical trials, and other emerging routes to therapeutics are derived from promising preclinical work in the standard *mdx* mouse model. These include both gene corrective therapies and gene transfer studies that are directed toward inducing expression of an at least partially functional dystrophin protein, as well as a variety of other approaches.

Nonsense suppression

Nonsense suppression therapies are directed toward inducing the cell's translational machinery to ignore (or 'readthrough') nonsense mutations, allowing continued translation of the gene's ORF. This has been best described in the case of aminoglycoside antibiotics, which alter the fidelity of mammalian ribosomal translation such that near-cognate codon–anticodon pairings are accepted in place of perfect cognate pairings; as a result, an amino acid is inserted into the nascent peptide chain and translation continues [173,174]. The potential of this serving as a therapy for DMD was suggested by studies in the *mdx* mouse, which carries a nonsense mutation within exon 23; treatment with gentamicin resulted in the expression of significant amounts of dystrophin [175]. Treatment of boys with DMD with gentamicin results in measurable changes in dystrophin expression [79], but the risks of ototoxicity and nephrotoxicity, along with the burden of intravenous treatment, makes this difficult to pursue as a long-term therapy. Screens for orally available compounds that similarly induce readthrough have led to the development of an orally available agent now in clinical trials for DMD (ataluren) [176], with other agents in preclinical studies [177,178].

Exon skipping

The concept of exon skipping therapy relies on the reading frame rule: the goal is to affect splicing of the pre-mRNA in a way that exons are left out of the mature mRNA, allowing translation of an internally truncated protein. Targeting a single exon would theoretically be beneficial for multiple deletion mutations; e.g. skipping of exon 51 will restore the reading frame for patients with deletions of the following exons: 13–50, 29–50, 43–50, 45–50, 47–50, 48–50, 49–50, 50 alone, 52 alone, and 52–63. Furthermore, because of the clustering of exon deletions around the central rod domain deletion hot-spot, targeting a limited number of exons will allow restoration of an ORF for a relatively large number of patients. Skipping of only four exons would be thus be beneficial to around 35% of patients: these include exon 51 (13.0% of patients), exon 45 (8.1%), exon 53 (7.7%), and exon 44 (6.2%) [179]. By skipping up to two exons, this treatment could theoretically be extended to 83% of all DMD mutations [179].

Exon skipping may be achieved by the use of AONs directed at a specific exon definition element, such as the splice donor or acceptor sites, or exon splice enhancer sites [180]. Binding of the AON to the single-stranded pre-mRNA results in the spliceosome ignoring the exon, to varying degrees of efficiency. To date, two different AON chemistries have reached clinical trials: 2'O-methyl phosphothiorate (2OMe) AONs and phosphorodiamidate morpholino oligomers (PMOs). Following success in animal models, each has been delivered by intramuscular injection and by systemic delivery, with promising results for dystrophin expression [78,181–183]. Trials that will presumably be definitive are under way with each chemistry. A second approach makes use of viral delivery of the small nuclear RNA (snRNA) U7 to an exonic target sequence [184,185]. U7 interferes with spliceosome assembly, resulting in exclusion of the targeted exon. The U7 sequence and the targeting sequence can be included in the same cistron delivered via a viral targeting vector—generally, an adeno-associated virus (AAV). This approach has the theoretical benefit of sustained expression following a single dose, and has proven efficacious in a dog model of DMD [186].

Although currently in trials for exonic duplications, other mutations are amenable to exon skipping. These include nonsense-containing exons in the 'zero-frame' context, single exon duplication mutations (with titration to skip a single copy of the duplicated exon, which would result in a wild type rather than a BMD transcript), and pseudo-exon mutations due to deep intronic point mutations [90]. Notably, in these last two, skipping would result in a full-length dystrophin protein, unlike exon skipping of deletions which will results in an internally truncated 'BMD' protein.

Gene transfer

Transfer of a naked plasmid containing the full-length *DMD* gene has been carried out in a human trial of intramuscular injection, with little success [187]. Current approaches to gene therapy make use of AAVs to deliver therapeutic transgenes to muscle. Several AAV serotypes show significant muscle tropism, and these viruses are not associated with illness. One challenge is that the size of the *DMD* coding region precludes packaging of a full-length *DMD* transgene into AAVs, which have a transgene size limit of around 5 kb. This has led to the development of micro- or mini-dystrophin constructs in which portions of the dystrophin central rod domain (and frequently the C-terminus) are missing from the transgene [188]; trials of refined vectors should occur in the near future.

Other emerging therapeutics

A variety of other therapeutic approaches have shown significant preclinical promise, and several are likely to reach clinical trials in the near term. These include overexpression of surrogate gene products in place of the missing dystrophin. One example is utrophin, which shares significant homology to dystrophin and is expressed at the sarcolemmal membrane in embryonic development but disappears postnatally except at the neuromuscular junction. Upregulation of utrophin via transgenic or viral approaches leads to significant rescue of the *mdx* phenotype, and preclinical studies of utrophin gene upregulation or protein delivery are under way [189–192]. Another example of surrogate gene therapy is found in AAV-mediated delivery of the *GALGT2* gene encoding the cytotoxic T cell (CT) GalNAc transferase [193], which results in significant expression of utrophin throughout the sarcolemma and correction of muscle defects in *mdx* mice.

References

1. Emery AE. Population frequencies of neuromuscular diseases—a world survey. *Neuromuscul Disord* 1991; **1**: 19–29.
2. Mendell JR, Shilling C, Leslie ND, et al. Evidence-based path to newborn screening for Duchenne muscular dystrophy. *Ann Neurol* 2012; **71**: 304–13.
3. Bushby KM, Thambyayah M, Gardner-Medwin D. Prevalence and incidence of Becker muscular dystrophy. *Lancet* 1991; **337**: 1022–4.
4. Duchenne GBA. *De l'Électrisation Localisée et son Application à la Pathologie et à la Thérapeutique*, 2nd edn. Paris: Ballière, 1861.
5. Duchenne GBA. Récherches sur la paralysie musculaire pseudohypertrophique, ou paralysie myosclérosique. *Arch Gén Méd* 1868; **11**(5).
6. Emery AE. Duchenne muscular dystrophy—Meryon's disease. *Neuromuscul Disord* 1993; **3**: 263–6.
7. Emery AEH, Emery MLH. *The History of a Genetic Disease: Duchenne Muscular Dystrophy or Meryon's Disease*, 2nd edn. Oxford: Oxford University Press, 2011.
8. Meryon E. On granular and fatty degeneration of the voluntary muscles. *Medico-Chirurg Trans* 1852; **35**: 73–84.1.
9. Nigro G. One-hundred-seventy-five years of Neapolitan contributions to the fight against the muscular diseases. *Acta Myol* 2010; **29**: 369–91.
10. Fardeau M. Duchenne de Boulogne: sa vie et son oeuvre. *Cahiers Myol* 2009; **1**: 6–11.
11. Pane M, Scalise R, Berardinelli A, et al. Early neurodevelopmental assessment in Duchenne muscular dystrophy. *Neuromuscul Disord* 2013; **23**: 451–5.
12. Cotton S, Voudouris NJ, Greenwood KM. Intelligence and Duchenne muscular dystrophy: full-scale, verbal, and performance intelligence quotients. *Dev Med Child Neurol* 2001; **43**: 497–501.
13. Cyrulnik SE, Fee RJ, De Vivo DC, Goldstein E, Hinton VJ. Delayed developmental language milestones in children with Duchenne's muscular dystrophy. *J Pediatr* 2007; **150**: 474–8.
14. Cotton SM, Voudouris NJ, Greenwood KM. Association between intellectual functioning and age in children and young adults with Duchenne muscular dystrophy: further results from a meta-analysis. *Dev Med Child Neurol* 2005; **47**: 257–65.
15. Marini A, Lorusso ML, D'Angelo MG, et al. Evaluation of narrative abilities in patients suffering from Duchenne Muscular Dystrophy. *Brain Language* 2007; **102**: 1–12.
16. Hendriksen JG, Vles JS. Neuropsychiatric disorders in males with Duchenne muscular dystrophy: frequency rate of attention-deficit hyperactivity disorder (ADHD), autism spectrum disorder, and obsessive–compulsive disorder. *J Child Neurol* 2008; **23**: 477–81.
17. Kornegay JN, Childers MK, Bogan DJ, et al. The paradox of muscle hypertrophy in muscular dystrophy. *Phys Med Rehabil Clin N Am* 2012; **23**: 149–72, xii.
18. Brooke MH, Fenichel GM, Griggs RC, et al. Clinical investigation in Duchenne dystrophy: 2. Determination of the 'power' of therapeutic trials based on the natural history. *Muscle Nerve* 1983; **6**: 91–103.
19. Brooke MH, Griggs RC, Mendell JR, Fenichel GM, Shumate JB. The natural history of Duchenne muscular dystrophy: a caveat for therapeutic trials. *Trans Am Neurol Assoc* 1981; **106**: 195–9.
20. McDonald CM, Abresch RT, Carter GT, et al. Profiles of neuromuscular diseases. Duchenne muscular dystrophy. *Am J Phys Med Rehabil* 1995; **74** (5 Suppl): S70–S92.
21. Nicholson LV, Johnson MA, Bushby KM, et al. Integrated study of 100 patients with Xp21 linked muscular dystrophy using clinical, genetic, immunochemical, and histopathological data. Part 1. Trends across the clinical groups. *J Med Genet* 1993; **30**: 728–36.
22. Becker PE. *Dystrophia Musculorum Progressiva. Eine genetische und klinische Untersuchung der Muskeldystrophien*. Stuttgart: Thieme, 1953.
23. Becker PE. Two families of benign sex-linked recessive muscular dystrophy. *Rev Can Biol* 1962; **21**: 551–66.

24. Bushby KM, Gardner-Medwin D. The clinical, genetic and dystrophin characteristics of Becker muscular dystrophy. I. Natural history. *J Neurol* 1993; **240**: 98–104.

25. Sunohara N, Arahata K, Hoffman EP, et al. Quadriceps myopathy: forme fruste of Becker muscular dystrophy. *Ann Neurol* 1990; **28**: 634–9.

26. Yazaki M, Yoshida K, Nakamura A, et al. Clinical characteristics of aged Becker muscular dystrophy patients with onset after 30 years. *Eur Neurol* 1999; **42**: 145–9.

27. Heald A, Anderson LV, Bushby KM, Shaw PJ. Becker muscular dystrophy with onset after 60 years. *Neurology* 1994; **44**: 2388–90.

28. Bushby KM, Cleghorn NJ, Curtis A, et al. Identification of a mutation in the promoter region of the dystrophin gene in a patient with atypical Becker muscular dystrophy. *Hum Genet* 1991; **88**: 195–9.

29. Minetti C, Tanji K, Chang HW, et al. Dystrophinopathy in two young boys with exercise-induced cramps and myoglobinuria. *Eur J Pediatr* 1993; **152**: 848–51.

30. Melis MA, Cau M, Muntoni F, et al. Elevation of serum creatine kinase as the only manifestation of an intragenic deletion of the dystrophin gene in three unrelated families. *Eur J Paediatr Neurol* 1998; **2**: 255–61.

31. Flanigan KM, Dunn DM, von Niederhausern A, et al. DMD Trp3X nonsense mutation associated with a founder effect in North American families with mild Becker muscular dystrophy. *Neuromuscul Disord* 2009; **19**: 743–8.

32. Young HK, Barton BA, Waisbren S, et al. Cognitive and psychological profile of males with Becker muscular dystrophy. *J Child Neurol* 2008; **23**: 155–62.

33. North KN, Miller G, Iannaccone ST, et al. Cognitive dysfunction as the major presenting feature of Becker's muscular dystrophy. *Neurology* 1996; **46**: 461–5.

34. Flanigan KM, Dunn DM, von Niederhausern A, et al. Mutational spectrum of DMD mutations in dystrophinopathy patients: application of modern diagnostic techniques to a large cohort. *Hum Mutat* 2009; **30**: 1657–66.

35. Neri M, Torelli S, Brown S, et al. Dystrophin levels as low as 30% are sufficient to avoid muscular dystrophy in the human. *Neuromuscul Disord* 2007; **17**: 913–18.

36. Ferlini A, Sewry C, Melis MA, Mateddu A, Muntoni F. X-linked dilated cardiomyopathy and the dystrophin gene. *Neuromuscul Disord* 1999; **9**: 339–46.

37. Juan-Mateu J, Paradas C, Olive M, et al. Isolated cardiomyopathy caused by a DMD nonsense mutation in somatic mosaicism: genetic normalization in skeletal muscle. *Clin Genet* 2012; **82**: 574–8.

38. Klamut HJ, Bosnoyan-Collins LO, Worton RG, Ray PN, Davis HL. Identification of a transcriptional enhancer within muscle intron 1 of the human dystrophin gene. *Hum Molec Genet* 1996; **5**: 1599–606.

39. Milasin J, Muntoni F, Severini GM, et al. A point mutation in the 5′ splice site of the dystrophin gene first intron responsible for X-linked dilated cardiomyopathy. *Hum Molec Genet* 1996; **5**: 73–9.

40. Miyazaki D, Yoshida K, Fukushima K, et al. Characterization of deletion breakpoints in patients with dystrophinopathy carrying a deletion of exons 45–55 of the Duchenne muscular dystrophy (DMD) gene. *J Hum Genet* 2009; **54**: 127–30.

41. Rimessi P, Fabris M, Bovolenta M, et al. Antisense modulation of both exonic and intronic splicing motifs induces skipping of a DMD pseudo-exon responsible for X-linked dilated cardiomyopathy. *Hum Gene Ther* 2010; **21**: 1137–46.

42. Towbin JA, Hejtmancik JF, Brink P, et al. X-linked dilated cardiomyopathy. Molecular genetic evidence of linkage to the Duchenne muscular dystrophy (dystrophin) gene at the Xp21 locus. *Circulation* 1993; **87**: 1854–65.

43. Zatz M, Rapaport D, Vainzof M, et al. Serum creatine-kinase (CK) and pyruvate-kinase (PK) activities in Duchenne (DMD) as compared with Becker (BMD) muscular dystrophy. *J Neurol Sci* 1991; **102**: 190–6.

44. Thakker PB, Sharma A. Becker muscular dystrophy: an unusual presentation. *Arch Dis Child* 1993; **69**: 158–9.

45. Doriguzzi C, Palmucci L, Mongini T, Chiado-Piat L, Restagno G, Ferrone M. Exercise intolerance and recurrent myoglobinuria as the only expression of Xp21 Becker type muscular dystrophy. *J Neurol* 1993; **240**: 269–71.

46. Shoji T, Nishikawa Y, Saito N, et al. A case of Becker muscular dystrophy and massive myoglobinuria with minimal renal manifestations. *Nephrol Dialysis Transplant* 1998; **13**: 759–60.

47. Morse RP, Rosman NP. Diagnosis of occult muscular dystrophy: importance of the 'chance' finding of elevated serum aminotransferase activities. *J Pediatr* 1993; **122**: 254–6.

48. Zamora S, Adams C, Butzner JD, Machida H, Scott RB. Elevated aminotransferase activity as an indication of muscular dystrophy: case reports and review of the literature. *Can J Gastroenterol/J Can Gastroenterol* 1996; **10**: 389–93.

49. Vajro P, Del Giudice E, Veropalumbo C. Muscular dystrophy revealed by incidentally discovered elevated aminotransferase levels. *J Pediatr* 2010; **156**: 689.

50. Veropalumbo C, Del Giudice E, Esposito G, Maddaluno S, Ruggiero L, Vajro P. Aminotransferases and muscular diseases: a disregarded lesson. Case reports and review of the literature. *J Paediatr Child Health* 2012; **48**: 886–90.

51. McMillan HJ, Gregas M, Darras BT, Kang PB. Serum transaminase levels in boys with Duchenne and Becker muscular dystrophy. *Pediatrics* 2011; **127**: e132–e136.

52. Rosales XQ, Chu ML, Shilling C, Wall C, Pastores GM, Mendell JR. Fidelity of gamma-glutamyl transferase (GGT) in differentiating skeletal muscle from liver damage. *J Child Neurol* 2008; **23**: 748–51.

53. Viollet L, Gailey S, Thornton DJ, et al. Utility of cystatin C to monitor renal function in Duchenne muscular dystrophy. *Muscle Nerve* 2009; **40**: 438–42.

54. Drummond LM. Creatine phosphokinase levels in the newborn and their use in screening for Duchenne muscular dystrophy. *Arch Dis Child* 1979; **54**: 362–6.

55. Pearce JM, Pennington RJ, Walton JN. Serum enzyme studies in muscle disease. III. Serum creatine kinase activity in relatives of patients with the Duchenne type of muscular dystrophy. *J Neurol Neurosurg Psychiatry* 1964; **27**: 181–5.

56. Drousiotou A, Ioannou P, Georgiou T, et al. Neonatal screening for Duchenne muscular dystrophy: a novel semiquantitative application of the bioluminescence test for creatine kinase in a pilot national program in Cyprus. *Genet Test* 1998; **2**: 55–60.

57. Bradley DM, Parsons EP, Clarke AJ. Experience with screening newborns for Duchenne muscular dystrophy in Wales. *Br Med J* 1993; **306**: 357–60.

58. Plauchu H, Dorche C, Cordier MP, Guibaud P, Robert JM. Duchenne muscular dystrophy: neonatal screening and prenatal diagnosis. *Lancet* 1989; **1**(8639): 669.

59. Skinner R, Emery AE, Scheuerbrandt G, Syme J. Feasibility of neonatal screening for Duchenne muscular dystrophy. *J Med Genet* 1982; **19**: 1–3.

60. England SB, Nicholson LV, Johnson MA, et al. Very mild muscular dystrophy associated with the deletion of 46% of dystrophin. *Nature* 1990; **343**: 180–2.

61. Tinsley JM, Blake DJ, Zuellig RA, Davies KE. Increasing complexity of the dystrophin-associated protein complex. *Proc Natl Acad Sci USA* 1994; **91**: 8307–13.

62. Suzuki A, Yoshida M, Ozawa E. Mammalian alpha 1- and beta 1-syntrophin bind to the alternative splice-prone region of the dystrophin COOH terminus. *J Cell Biol* 1995; **128**: 373–81.

63. Khairallah RJ, Shi G, Sbrana F, et al. Microtubules underlie dysfunction in Duchenne muscular dystrophy. *Sci Signal* 2012; **5**(236): ra56.

64. Fuentes-Mera L, Rodriguez-Munoz R, Gonzalez-Ramirez R, et al. Characterization of a novel Dp71 dystrophin-associated protein

complex (DAPC) present in the nucleus of HeLa cells: members of the nuclear DAPC associate with the nuclear matrix. *Exp Cell Res* 2006; **312**: 3023–35.

65. Campbell KP. Three muscular dystrophies: loss of cytoskeleton-extracellular matrix linkage. *Cell* 1995; **80**: 675–9.

66. Brenman JE, Chao DS, Xia H, Aldape K, Bredt DS. Nitric oxide synthase complexed with dystrophin and absent from skeletal muscle sarcolemma in Duchenne muscular dystrophy. *Cell* 1995; **82**: 743–52.

67. Dubowitz V. *Muscle Biopsy: a Practical Approach*, 2nd edn. London: Bailliere Tindall, 1985.

68. Carpenter S, Karpati G. Duchenne muscular dystrophy: plasma membrane loss initiates muscle cell necrosis unless it is repaired. *Brain* 1979; **102**: 147–61.

69. Mokri B, Engel AG. Duchenne dystrophy: electron microscopic findings pointing to a basic or early abnormality in the plasma membrane of the muscle fiber. *Neurology* 1975; **25**: 1111–20.

70. Cullen MJ, Fulthorpe JJ. Stages in fibre breakdown in Duchenne muscular dystrophy. An electron-microscopic study. *J Neurol Sci* 1975; **24**: 179–200.

71. Nicholson LV, Davison K, Johnson MA, et al. Dystrophin in skeletal muscle. II. Immunoreactivity in patients with Xp21 muscular dystrophy. *J Neurol Sci* 1989; **94**: 137–46.

72. Nicholson LV, Johnson MA, Gardner Medwin D, Bhattacharya S, Harris JB. Heterogeneity of dystrophin expression in patients with Duchenne and Becker muscular dystrophy. *Acta Neuropathol Berl* 1990; **80**: 239–50.

73. Klein CJ, Coovert DD, Bulman DE, Ray PN, Mendell JR, Burghes AH. Somatic reversion/suppression in Duchenne muscular dystrophy (DMD): evidence supporting a frame-restoring mechanism in rare dystrophin-positive fibers. *Am J Hum Genet* 1992; **50**: 950–9.

74. Fanin M, Danieli GA, Vitiello L, Senter L, Angelini C. Prevalence of dystrophin-positive fibers in 85 Duchenne muscular dystrophy patients. *Neuromuscul Disord* 1992; **2**: 41–5.

75. Burrow KL, Coovert DD, Klein CJ, et al. Dystrophin expression and somatic reversion in prednisone-treated and untreated Duchenne dystrophy. CIDD Study Group. *Neurology*; **41**: 661–6.

76. Arechavala-Gomeza V, Kinali M, Feng L, et al. Revertant fibres and dystrophin traces in Duchenne muscular dystrophy: implication for clinical trials. *Neuromuscul Disord* 2010; **20**: 295–301.

77. Arechavala-Gomeza V, Kinali M, Feng L, et al. Immunohistological intensity measurements as a tool to assess sarcolemma-associated protein expression. *Neuropathol Appl Neurobiol* 2010; **36**: 265–74.

78. Cirak S, Arechavala-Gomeza V, Guglieri M, et al. Exon skipping and dystrophin restoration in patients with Duchenne muscular dystrophy after systemic phosphorodiamidate morpholino oligomer treatment: an open-label, phase 2, dose-escalation study. *Lancet* 2011; **378**: 595–605.

79. Malik V, Rodino-Klapac LR, Viollet L, et al. Gentamicin-induced readthrough of stop codons in Duchenne muscular dystrophy. *Ann Neurol* 2010; **67**: 771–80.

80. Taylor LE, Kaminoh YJ, Rodesch CK, Flanigan KM. Quantification of dystrophin immunofluorescence in dystrophinopathy muscle specimens. *Neuropathol Appl Neurobiol* 2012; **38**: 591–601.

81. Hoffman EP, Kunkel LM, Angelini C, Clarke A, Johnson M, Harris JB. Improved diagnosis of Becker muscular dystrophy by dystrophin testing. *Neurology* 1989; **39**: 1011–17.

82. Beggs AH, Koenig M, Boyce FM, Kunkel LM. Detection of 98% of DMD/BMD gene deletions by polymerase chain reaction. *Hum Genet* 1990; **86**: 45–8.

83. Chamberlain JS, Gibbs RA, Ranier JE, Caskey CT. Multiplex PCR for the diagnosis of Duchenne muscular dystrophy. In: Innis MA, Gelfand DH, Sninsky JJ, White TJ (ed) *PCR Protocols: a Guide to Methods and Applications*, pp. 272–81. San Francisco, CA: Academic Press, 1990.

84. Madden HR, Fletcher S, Davis MR, Wilton SD. Characterization of a complex Duchenne muscular dystrophy-causing dystrophin gene inversion and restoration of the reading frame by induced exon skipping. *Hum Mutat* 2009; **30**: 22–8.

85. White SJ, Aartsma-Rus A, Flanigan KM, et al. Duplications in the DMD gene. *Hum Mutat* 2006; **27**: 938–45.

86. Flanigan KM, von Niederhausern A, Dunn DM, Alder J, Mendell JR, Weiss RB. Rapid direct sequence analysis of the dystrophin gene. *Am J Hum Genet* 2003; **72**: 931–9.

87. Yan J, Feng J, Buzin CH, et al. Three-tiered noninvasive diagnosis in 96% of patients with Duchenne muscular dystrophy (DMD). *Hum Mutat* 2004; **23**: 203–4.

88. Dent KM, Dunn DM, von Niederhausern AC, et al. Improved molecular diagnosis of dystrophinopathies in an unselected clinical cohort. *Am J Med Genet A* 2005; **134**: 295–8.

89. Tuffery-Giraud S, Beroud C, Leturcq F, et al. Genotype-phenotype analysis in 2,405 patients with a dystrophinopathy using the UMD-DMD database: a model of nationwide knowledgebase. *Hum Mutat* 2009; **30**: 934–45.

90. Gurvich OL, Tuohy TM, Howard MT, et al. DMD pseudoexon mutations: splicing efficiency, phenotype, and potential therapy. *Ann Neurol* 2008; **63**: 81–9.

91. Tuffery-Giraud S, Saquet C, Chambert S, Claustres M. Pseudoexon activation in the DMD gene as a novel mechanism for Becker muscular dystrophy. *Hum Mutat* 2003; **21**: 608–14.

92. Flanigan KM, Dunn D, Larsen CA, Medne L, Bonnemann CB, Weiss RB. Becker muscular dystrophy due to an inversion of exons 23 and 24 of the DMD gene. *Muscle Nerve* 2011; **44**: 822–5.

93. Cagliani R, Sironi M, Ciafaloni E, et al. An intragenic deletion/inversion event in the DMD gene determines a novel exon creation and results in a BMD phenotype. *Hum Genet* 2004; **115**: 13–18.

94. Bettecken T, Muller CR. Identification of a 220-kb insertion into the Duchenne gene in a family with an atypical course of muscular dystrophy. *Genomics* 1989; **4**: 592–6.

95. Grimm T, Muller B, Muller CR, Janka M. Theoretical considerations on germline mosaicism in Duchenne muscular dystrophy. *J Med Genet* 1990; **27**: 683–7.

96. Barbujani G, Russo A, Danieli GA, Spiegler AW, Borkowska J, Petrusewicz IH. Segregation analysis of 1885 DMD families: significant departure from the expected proportion of sporadic cases. *Hum Genet* 1990; **84**: 522–6.

97. Monaco AP, Bertelson CJ, Liechti-Gallati S, Moser H, Kunkel LM. An explanation for the phenotypic differences between patients bearing partial deletions of the DMD locus. *Genomics* 1988; **2**: 90–5.

98. Muntoni F, Gobbi P, Sewry C, et al. Deletions in the 5′ region of dystrophin and resulting phenotypes. *J Med Genet* 1994; **31**: 843–7.

99. Winnard AV, Klein CJ, Coovert DD, et al. Characterization of translational frame exception patients in Duchenne/Becker muscular dystrophy. *Hum Mol Genet* 1993; **2**: 737–44. [Erratum in *Hum Mol Genet* 1993; **2**: 1347.]

100. Flanigan KM, Dunn DM, von Niederhausern A, et al. Nonsense mutation-associated Becker muscular dystrophy: interplay between exon definition and splicing regulatory elements within the DMD gene. *Hum Mutat* 2011; **32**: 299–308.

101. Ginjaar IB, Kneppers AL, v d Meulen JD, et al. Dystrophin nonsense mutation induces different levels of exon 29 skipping and leads to variable phenotypes within one BMD family. *Eur J Hum Genet* 2000; **8**: 793–6.

102. Disset A, Bourgeois CF, Benmalek N, Claustres M, Stevenin J, Tuffery-Giraud S. An exon skipping-associated nonsense mutation in the dystrophin gene uncovers a complex interplay between multiple antagonistic splicing elements. *Hum Molec Genet* 2006; **15**: 999–1013.

103. Bardoni A, Felisari G, Sironi M, et al. Loss of Dp140 regulatory sequences is associated with cognitive impairment in dystrophinopathies. *Neuromuscul Disord* 2000; **10**: 194–9.

104. Moizard MP, Toutain A, Fournier D, et al. Severe cognitive impairment in DMD: obvious clinical indication for Dp71 isoform point mutation screening. *Eur J Hum Genet* 2000; **8**: 552–6.

105. Giliberto F, Ferreiro V, Dalamon V, Szijan I. Dystrophin deletions and cognitive impairment in Duchenne/Becker muscular dystrophy. *Neurol Res* 2004; **26**: 83–7.

106. Pane M, Lombardo ME, Alfieri P, et al. Attention deficit hyperactivity disorder and cognitive function in Duchenne muscular dystrophy: phenotype-genotype correlation. *J Pediatr* 2012; **161**: 705–9 e1.

107. Kaspar RW, Allen HD, Ray WC, et al. Analysis of dystrophin deletion mutations predicts age of cardiomyopathy onset in Becker muscular dystrophy. *Circ Cardiovasc Genet* 2009; **2**: 544–51.

108. Gangopadhyay SB, Sherratt TG, Heckmatt JZ, et al. Dystrophin in frameshift deletion patients with Becker muscular dystrophy. *Am J Hum Genet* 1992; **51**: 562–70.

109. Winnard AV, Mendell JR, Prior TW, Florence J, Burghes AH. Frameshift deletions of exons 3–7 and revertant fibers in Duchenne muscular dystrophy: mechanisms of dystrophin production. *Am J Hum Genet* 1995; **56**: 158–66.

110. Gurvich OL, Maiti B, Weiss RB, Aggarwal G, Howard MT, Flanigan KM. DMD exon 1 truncating point mutations: amelioration of phenotype by alternative translation initiation in exon 6. *Hum Mutat* 2009; **30**: 633–40.

111. Harper SQ, Hauser MA, DelloRusso C, et al. Modular flexibility of dystrophin: implications for gene therapy of Duchenne muscular dystrophy. *Nat Med* 2002; **8**: 253–61.

112. Nakamura A, Yoshida K, Fukushima K, et al. Follow-up of three patients with a large in-frame deletion of exons 45–55 in the Duchenne muscular dystrophy (DMD) gene. *J Clin Neurosci* 2008; **15**: 757–63.

113. Tasaki N, Yoshida K, Haruta SI, et al. X-linked dilated cardiomyopathy with a large hot-spot deletion in the dystrophin gene. *Intern Med (Tokyo, Japan)* 2001; **40**: 1215–21.

114. Beroud C, Tuffery-Giraud S, Matsuo M, et al. Multiexon skipping leading to an artificial DMD protein lacking amino acids from exons 45 through 55 could rescue up to 63% of patients with Duchenne muscular dystrophy. *Hum Mutat* 2007; **28**: 196–202.

115. Henderson DM, Lee A, Ervasti JM. Disease-causing missense mutations in actin binding domain 1 of dystrophin induce thermodynamic instability and protein aggregation. *Proc Natl Acad Sci USA* 2010; **107**: 9632–7.

116. Draviam RA, Wang B, Li J, Xiao X, Watkins SC. Mini-dystrophin efficiently incorporates into the dystrophin protein complex in living cells. *J Muscle Res Cell Motil* 2006; **27**: 53–67.

117. Ishikawa-Sakurai M, Yoshida M, Imamura M, Davies KE, Ozawa E. ZZ domain is essentially required for the physiological binding of dystrophin and utrophin to beta-dystroglycan. *Hum Molec Genet* 2004; **13**: 693–702.

118. Vetrone SA, Montecino-Rodriguez E, Kudryashova E, et al. Osteopontin promotes fibrosis in dystrophic mouse muscle by modulating immune cell subsets and intramuscular TGF-beta. *J Clin Invest* 2009; **119**: 1583–94.

119. Bello L, Piva L, Barp A, et al. Importance of SPP1 genotype as a covariate in clinical trials in Duchenne muscular dystrophy. *Neurology* 2012; **79**: 159–62.

120. Pegoraro E, Hoffman EP, Piva L, et al. SPP1 genotype is a determinant of disease severity in Duchenne muscular dystrophy. *Neurology* 2011; **76**: 219–26.

121. Heydemann A, Ceco E, Lim JE, et al. Latent TGF-beta-binding protein 4 modifies muscular dystrophy in mice. *J Clin Invest* 2009; **119**: 3703–12.

122. Flanigan KM, Ceco E, Lamar KM, et al. LTBP4 genotype predicts age of ambulatory loss in Duchenne muscular dystrophy. *Ann Neurol* 2013; **73**: 481–8.

123. Matsumura K, Tome FM, Collin H, et al. Deficiency of the 50K dystrophin-associated glycoprotein in severe childhood autosomal recessive muscular dystrophy. *Nature* 1992; **359**: 320–2.

124. Matsumura K, Campbell KP. Deficiency of dystrophin-associated proteins: a common mechanism leading to muscle cell necrosis in severe childhood muscular dystrophies. *Neuromuscul Disord* 1993; **3**: 109–18.

125. Brockington M, Blake DJ, Prandini P, et al. Mutations in the fukutin-related protein gene (FKRP) cause a form of congenital muscular dystrophy with secondary laminin alpha2 deficiency and abnormal glycosylation of alpha-dystroglycan. *Am J Hum Genet* 2001; **69**: 1198–209.

126. Schwartz M, Hertz JM, Sveen ML, Vissing J. LGMD2I presenting with a characteristic Duchenne or Becker muscular dystrophy phenotype. *Neurology* 2005; **64**: 1635–7.

127. Hoffman EP, Arahata K, Minetti C, Bonilla E, Rowland LP. Dystrophinopathy in isolated cases of myopathy in females. *Neurology* 1992; **42**: 967–75.

128. Soltanzadeh P, Friez MJ, Dunn D, et al. Clinical and genetic characterization of manifesting carriers of DMD mutations. *Neuromuscul Disord* 2010; **20**: 499–504.

129. Moser H, Emery AE. The manifesting carrier in Duchenne muscular dystrophy. *Clin Genet* 1974; **5**: 271–84.

130. Norman A, Harper P. A survey of manifesting carriers of Duchenne and Becker muscular dystrophy in Wales. *Clin Genet* 1989; **36**: 31–7.

131. Taylor PJ, Maroulis S, Mullan GL, et al. Measurement of the clinical utility of a combined mutation detection protocol in carriers of Duchenne and Becker muscular dystrophy. *J Med Genet* 2007; **44**: 368–72.

132. Hoogerwaard EM, Bakker E, Ippel PF, et al. Signs and symptoms of Duchenne muscular dystrophy and Becker muscular dystrophy among carriers in The Netherlands: a cohort study. *Lancet* 1999; **353**: 2116–19.

133. Bushby KM, Goodship JA, Nicholson LV, Johnson MA, Haggerty ID, Gardner-Medwin D. Variability in clinical, genetic and protein abnormalities in manifesting carriers of Duchenne and Becker muscular dystrophy. *Neuromuscul Disord* 1993; **3**: 57–64.

134. Findlay AR, Lewis S, Sahenk Z, Flanigan KM. Camptocormia as a late presentation in a manifesting carrier of Duchenne muscular dystrophy. *Muscle Nerve* 2013; **47**: 124–7.

135. Hoogerwaard EM, van der Wouw PA, Wilde AA, et al. Cardiac involvement in carriers of Duchenne and Becker muscular dystrophy. *Neuromuscul Disord* 1999; **9**: 347–51.

136. Bushby K, Finkel R, Birnkrant DJ, et al. Diagnosis and management of Duchenne muscular dystrophy, part 1: diagnosis, and pharmacological and psychosocial management. *Lancet Neurol* 2010; **9**: 77–93.

137. Bushby K, Finkel R, Birnkrant DJ, et al. Diagnosis and management of Duchenne muscular dystrophy, part 2: implementation of multidisciplinary care. *Lancet Neurol* 2010; **9**: 177–89.

138. Siegel IM, Miller JE, Ray RD. Failure of corticosteroid in the treatment of Duchenne (pseudo-hypertrophic) muscular dystrophy. Report of a clinically matched three year double-blind study. *Illinois Med J* 1974; **145**: 32–3 passim.

139. Drachman DB, Toyka KV, Myer E. Prednisone in Duchenne muscular dystrophy. *Lancet* 1974; **2**(7894): 1409–12.

140. Mendell JR, Moxley RT, Griggs RC, et al. Randomized, double-blind six-month trial of prednisone in Duchenne's muscular dystrophy. *N Engl J Med* 1989; **320**: 1592–7.

141. Scudeletti M, Piccardo C, Piovano P, Imbimbo B, Indiveri F. Effects of a new heterocyclic glucocorticoid, deflazacort (DFC), on the functions of lymphocytes from patients with rheumatoid arthritis (RA). *Int J Immunopharmacol* 1987; **9**: 133–9.

142. Omote M, Sakai K, Mizusawa H. Acute effects of deflazacort and its metabolite 21-desacetyl-deflazacort on allergic reactions. *Arzneimittelforschung* 1994; **44**: 149–53.

143. Fenichel GM, Florence JM, Pestronk A, et al. Long-term benefit from prednisone therapy in Duchenne muscular dystrophy. *Neurology* 1991; **41**: 1874–7.

144. Fenichel GM, Mendell JR, Moxley RT, 3rd, et al. A comparison of daily and alternate-day prednisone therapy in the treatment of Duchenne muscular dystrophy. *Arch Neurol* 1991; **48**: 575–9.

145. Griggs RC, Moxley RT, 3rd, Mendell JR, et al. Prednisone in Duchenne dystrophy. A randomized, controlled trial defining the time course and dose response. Clinical Investigation of Duchenne Dystrophy Group. *Arch Neurol* 1991; **48**: 383–8.

146. Griggs RC, Moxley RT, 3rd, Mendell JR, et al. Duchenne dystrophy: randomized, controlled trial of prednisone (18 months) and azathioprine (12 months). *Neurology* 1993; **43**: 520–7.

147. Manzur AY, Kuntzer T, Pike M, Swan A. Glucocorticoid corticosteroids for Duchenne muscular dystrophy. *Cochrane Database Syst Rev* 2008(1): CD003725.

148. Wong BL, Christopher C. Corticosteroids in Duchenne muscular dystrophy: a reappraisal. *J Child Neurol* 2002; **17**: 183–90.

149. Moxley RT, 3rd, Pandya S, Ciafaloni E, Fox DJ, Campbell K. Change in natural history of Duchenne muscular dystrophy with long-term corticosteroid treatment: implications for management. *J Child Neurol* 2010; **25**: 1116–29.

150. Bonifati MD, Ruzza G, Bonometto P, et al. A multicenter, double-blind, randomized trial of deflazacort versus prednisone in Duchenne muscular dystrophy. *Muscle Nerve* 2000; **23**: 1344–7.

151. Escolar DM, Hache LP, Clemens PR, et al. Randomized, blinded trial of weekend vs daily prednisone in Duchenne muscular dystrophy. *Neurology* 2011; **77**: 444–52.

152. Merlini L, Cicognani A, Malaspina E, et al. Early prednisone treatment in Duchenne muscular dystrophy. *Muscle Nerve* 2003; **27**: 222–7.

153. Merlini L, Gennari M, Malaspina E, et al. Early corticosteroid treatment in 4 Duchenne muscular dystrophy patients: 14-year follow-up. *Muscle Nerve* 2012; **45**: 796–802.

154. Birnkrant DJ, Bushby KM, Amin RS, et al. The respiratory management of patients with Duchenne muscular dystrophy: a DMD care considerations working group specialty article. *Pediatr Pulmonol* 2010; **45**: 739–48.

155. Eagle M, Baudouin SV, Chandler C, Giddings DR, Bullock R, Bushby K. Survival in Duchenne muscular dystrophy: improvements in life expectancy since 1967 and the impact of home nocturnal ventilation. *Neuromuscul Disord* 2002; **12**: 926–9.

156. King WM, Ruttencutter R, Nagaraja HN, et al. Orthopedic outcomes of long-term daily corticosteroid treatment in Duchenne muscular dystrophy. *Neurology* 2007; **68**: 1607–13.

157. Kinali M, Main M, Eliahoo J, et al. Predictive factors for the development of scoliosis in Duchenne muscular dystrophy. *Eur J Paediatr Neurol* 2007; **11**: 160–6.

158. Cheuk DK, Wong V, Wraige E, Baxter P, Cole A. Surgery for scoliosis in Duchenne muscular dystrophy. *Cochrane Database Syst Rev* 2013; **2**: CD005375.

159. Kinali M, Messina S, Mercuri E, et al. Management of scoliosis in Duchenne muscular dystrophy: a large 10-year retrospective study. *Dev Med Child Neurol* 2006; **48**: 513–18.

160. Eagle M, Bourke J, Bullock R, et al. Managing Duchenne muscular dystrophy–the additive effect of spinal surgery and home nocturnal ventilation in improving survival. *Neuromuscul Disord* 2007; **17**: 470–5.

161. Cox GF, Kunkel LM. Dystrophies and heart disease. *Curr Opin Cardiol* 1997; **12**: 329–43.

162. Nigro G, Comi LI, Politano L, Bain RJ. The incidence and evolution of cardiomyopathy in Duchenne muscular dystrophy. *Int J Cardiol* 1990; **26**: 271–7.

163. Allen HD, Thrush PT, Hoffman TM, Flanigan KM, Mendell JR. Cardiac management in neuromuscular diseases. *Phys Med Rehabil Clin N Am* 2012; **23**: 855–68.

164. Viollet L, Thrush PT, Flanigan KM, Mendell JR, Allen HD. Effects of angiotensin-converting enzyme inhibitors and/or beta blockers on the cardiomyopathy in Duchenne muscular dystrophy. *Am J Cardiol* 2012; **110**: 98–102.

165. Connuck DM, Sleeper LA, Colan SD, et al. Characteristics and outcomes of cardiomyopathy in children with Duchenne or Becker muscular dystrophy: a comparative study from the Pediatric Cardiomyopathy Registry. *Am Heart J* 2008; **155**: 998–1005.

166. Takenaka A, Yokota M, Iwase M, Miyaguchi K, Hayashi H, Saito H. Discrepancy between systolic and diastolic dysfunction of the left ventricle in patients with Duchenne muscular dystrophy. *Eur Heart J* 1993; **14**: 669–76.

167. Giglio V, Pasceri V, Messano L, et al. Ultrasound tissue characterization detects preclinical myocardial structural changes in children affected by Duchenne muscular dystrophy. *J Am Coll Cardiol* 2003; **42**: 309–16.

168. American Academy of Pediatrics Section on Cardiology and Cardiac Surgery. Cardiovascular health supervision for individuals affected by Duchenne or Becker muscular dystrophy. *Pediatrics* 2005; **116**: 1569–73.

169. Corrado G, Lissoni A, Beretta S, et al. Prognostic value of electrocardiograms, ventricular late potentials, ventricular arrhythmias, and left ventricular systolic dysfunction in patients with Duchenne muscular dystrophy. *Am J Cardiol* 2002; **89**: 838–41.

170. Thrush PT, Allen HD, Viollet L, Mendell JR. Re-examination of the electrocardiogram in boys with Duchenne muscular dystrophy and correlation with its dilated cardiomyopathy. *Am J Cardiol* 2009; **103**: 262–5.

171. Chenard AA, Becane HM, Tertrain F, de Kermadec JM, Weiss YA. Ventricular arrhythmia in Duchenne muscular dystrophy: prevalence, significance and prognosis. *Neuromuscul Disord* 1993; **3**: 201–6.

172. Duboc D, Meune C, Lerebours G, Devaux JY, Vaksmann G, Becane HM. Effect of perindopril on the onset and progression of left ventricular dysfunction in Duchenne muscular dystrophy. *J Am Coll Cardiol* 2005; **45**: 855–7.

173. Howard MT, Anderson CB, Fass U, et al. Readthrough of dystrophin stop codon mutations induced by aminoglycosides. *Ann Neurol* 2004; **55**: 422–6.

174. Howard MT, Shirts BH, Petros LM, Flanigan KM, Gesteland RF, Atkins JF. Sequence specificity of aminoglycoside-induced stop codon readthrough: potential implications for treatment of Duchenne muscular dystrophy. *Ann Neurol* 2000; **48**: 164–9.

175. Barton-Davis ER, Cordier L, Shoturma DI, Leland SE, Sweeney HL. Aminoglycoside antibiotics restore dystrophin function to skeletal muscles of mdx mice. *J Clin Invest* 1999; **104**: 375–81.

176. Welch EM, Barton ER, Zhuo J, et al. PTC124 targets genetic disorders caused by nonsense mutations. *Nature* 2007; **447**: 87–91.

177. Du L, Damoiseaux R, Nahas S, et al. Nonaminoglycoside compounds induce readthrough of nonsense mutations. *J Exp Med* 2009; **206**: 2285–97.

178. Kayali R, Ku JM, Khitrov G, Jung ME, Prikhodko O, Bertoni C. Read-through compound 13 restores dystrophin expression and improves muscle function in the mdx mouse model for Duchenne muscular dystrophy. *Hum Molec Genet* 2012; **21**: 4007–20.

179. Aartsma-Rus A, Fokkema I, Verschuuren J, et al. Theoretic applicability of antisense-mediated exon skipping for Duchenne muscular dystrophy mutations. *Hum Mutat* 2009; **30**: 293–9.

180. Aartsma-Rus A. Overview on DMD exon skipping. *Methods Mol Biol* 2012; **867**: 97–116.

181. Goemans NM, Tulinius M, van den Akker JT, et al. Systemic administration of PRO051 in Duchenne's muscular dystrophy. *N Engl J Med* 2011; **364**: 1513–22.

182. Kinali M, Arechavala-Gomeza V, Feng L, et al. Local restoration of dystrophin expression with the morpholino oligomer AVI-4658 in Duchenne muscular dystrophy: a single-blind, placebo-controlled, dose-escalation, proof-of-concept study. *Lancet Neurol* 2009; **8**: 918–28.

183. van Deutekom JC, Janson AA, Ginjaar IB, et al. Local dystrophin restoration with antisense oligonucleotide PRO051. *N Engl J Med* 2007; **357**: 2677–86.

184. Goyenvalle A, Babbs A, van Ommen GJ, Garcia L, Davies KE. Enhanced exon-skipping induced by U7 snRNA carrying a splicing silencer sequence: promising tool for DMD therapy. *Mol Ther* 2009; **17**: 1234–40.

185. Goyenvalle A, Vulin A, Fougerousse F, et al. Rescue of dystrophic muscle through U7 snRNA-mediated exon skipping. *Science* 2004; **306**: 1796–9.

186. Vulin A, Barthelemy I, Goyenvalle A, et al. Muscle function recovery in golden retriever muscular dystrophy after AAV1-U7 exon skipping. *Mol Ther* 2012; **20**: 2120–33.

187. Braun S. Naked plasmid DNA for the treatment of muscular dystrophy. *Curr Opin Mol Ther* 2004; **6**: 499–505.

188. Mendell JR, Campbell K, Rodino-Klapac L, et al. Dystrophin immunity in Duchenne's muscular dystrophy. *N Engl J Med* 2010; **363**: 1429–37.

189. Perkins KJ, Davies KE. The role of utrophin in the potential therapy of Duchenne muscular dystrophy. *Neuromuscul Disord* 2002; **12** (Suppl 1): S78–S89.

190. Sonnemann KJ, Heun-Johnson H, Turner AJ, Baltgalvis KA, Lowe DA, Ervasti JM. Functional substitution by TAT-utrophin in dystrophin-deficient mice. *PLoS Med* 2009; **6**(5): e1000083.

191. Amenta AR, Yilmaz A, Bogdanovich S, et al. Biglycan recruits utrophin to the sarcolemma and counters dystrophic pathology in mdx mice. *Proc Natl Acad Sci USA* 2011; **108**: 762–7.

192. Moorwood C, Lozynska O, Suri N, Napper AD, Diamond SL, Khurana TS. Drug discovery for Duchenne muscular dystrophy via utrophin promoter activation screening. *PLoS One* 2011; **6**: e26169.

193. Martin PT, Xu R, Rodino-Klapac LR, et al. Overexpression of Galgt2 in skeletal muscle prevents injury resulting from eccentric contractions in both mdx and wild-type mice. *Am J Physiol Cell Physiol* 2009; **296**: C476–C488.

CHAPTER 23

Limb-girdle muscular dystrophies

Fiona L.M. Norwood and Kate Bushby

Introduction

This chapter aims to set out an introduction to the group of conditions termed limb-girdle muscular dystrophies (LGMDs), combining a brief description of the main features of a number of the more common LGMDs with a suggested diagnostic approach.

Historical context

LGMDs were first defined as a group separate from other muscle conditions by Walton and Natrass in 1954 in their population study of part of northern England [1]. They realized that these conditions shared the feature of limb-girdle weakness but had variable involvement of other muscle groups. At that time, muscle diseases were described exclusively by their phenotypic characteristics, but the authors did appreciate a likely autosomal recessive inheritance pattern in the majority of families and the possible involvement of other organs such as the heart.

Little further progress was made in separating out the individual conditions until genetic studies in the 1990s allowed the identification of disease-causing genes and their protein products [2], a process of increasing genetic and allelic heterogeneity which continues to this day. It is now apparent that some conditions are much more common than others and that regional variations in frequency are striking. LGMD2A and LGMD2I were thought to be the most common [3], but now the more recently defined LGMD2L may be at least as frequent [4]. This is helpful diagnostically when choosing how to proceed through sequential testing of potential causative genes.

Current classification

The LGMDs are classified according to their mode of inheritance, with the less common autosomal dominant conditions named LGMD1 and the more common LGMD2 comprising those that are autosomal recessive. LGMD2 represents perhaps 90% of patients [3]. Within each group the conditions are named according to the chronological order in which their causative genes were defined. The current classification is set out in Table 23.1; it was developed via expert workshops at the European Neuromuscular Centre [5,6] and has been updated sequentially as new genes have been identified [7].

The range of LGMDs includes conditions with mainly proximal involvement, such as LGMD2I, and those which may present with either proximal or predominantly distal leg involvement, such as LGMD2B (Miyoshi phenotype). Some conditions include both proximal and distal weakness from the outset, and in others one distribution of weakness may slowly progress to affect other muscles. The age of onset and rate at which this occurs varies greatly. Other clinical findings may include muscle hypertrophy or atrophy, limb contractures, or scapular winging. The extraocular, facial, and bulbar muscles are usually spared. Cardiac and respiratory involvement may be an integral feature of some conditions such as LGMD1B and LGMD2I, whereas in others such as LGMD2A and LGMD2L it may be relatively unusual.

Making a precise diagnosis

Navigating this apparent complexity to achieve a diagnosis may seem daunting to those less familiar with muscle disorders, and indeed may prove greatly challenging even for the experienced myologist [8]. It is sometimes possible to suggest a likely diagnosis on the patient's first visit; this is through pattern recognition of specific features and can usually only be done through extensive practice. For those encountering the LGMDs infrequently, an intuitive approach is not recommended and can be highly misleading. By breaking down the diagnostic process into steps, however, it is possible to narrow down the number of possible conditions and eventually to refine these into a definite diagnosis. These steps are outlined in the rest of this section. Attempts at diagnostic algorithms have been made, and although potentially helpful they do need to be interpreted carefully and used in conjunction with clinical judgement [8,9].

Step 1: Exclude LGMD mimics

Limb-girdle muscle weakness is not limited to the LGMDs. In all patient series, dystrophinopathy [Duchenne muscular dystrophy (DMD), Becker muscular dystrophy (BMD), and manifesting carrier status] is more common than all forms of LGMD considered together and should be excluded. Other conditions such as Pompe disease and other metabolic myopathies, Bethlem myopathy, spinal muscular atrophy, facioscapulohumeral dystrophy (FSHD) and the inflammatory myopathies may also have prominent limb-girdle weakness as part of their phenotype, and often it is sensible to exclude these conditions through appropriate testing before proceeding to investigate other possibilities. Failure to do this at the beginning of the diagnostic process may lead to a complex but futile trail of time-consuming investigations to be set in motion,

Table 23.1 Current classification of the limb-girdle muscular dystrophies (LGMDs)

	Disorder	Gene location	Gene symbol; gene product
Autosomal dominant LGMDs (LGMD1)	LGMD1A	5q22-q34	*TTID*; myotilin
	LGMD1B	1q11-21	*LMNA*; lamin A/C
	LGMD1C	3p25	*CAV3*; caveolin-3
	LGMD1D	7q36	*DNAJB6*
	LGMD1E	6q23	
	LGMD1F	7q32	
	LGMD1G	4p21	
Autosomal recessive LGMDs (LGMD2)	LGMD2A	15q15.1–q21.1	*CAPN3*; calpain 3
	LGMD2B	2p13	*DYSF*; dysferlin
	LGMD2C	13q12	*SGCG*; γ-sarcoglycan
	LGMD2D	17q12–q21.33	*SGCA*; α-sarcoglycan
	LGMD2E	4q12	*SGCB*; β-sarcoglycan
	LGMD2F	5q33–q34	*SGCD*; δ-sarcoglycan
	LGMD2G	17q11–q12	*TCAP*; telethonin
	LGMD2H	9q31–q34.1	*TRIM32*
	LGMD2I	19q13.3	*FKRP*; Fukutin related protein
	LGMD2J	2q	*TTN*; titin
	LGMD2K	9q34	*POMT1*
	LGMD2L	11p14.3	*ANO5*; anoctamin 5
	LGMD2M	9q31	*FKTN*; Fukutin
	LGMD2N	14q24	*POMT2*
	LGMD2O	1p34.1	*POMGNT1*
	LGMD2Q	8q24	*PLEC1*; plectin 1

leading to frustration for both the neurologist and the patient, only for the true diagnosis to become apparent on review. If in doubt as to how to proceed, we would advise going back to the initial history and examination findings and consider whether the patient's presentation may represent a variant of one of the much more common conditions. Knowledge of the relative prevalence of the different forms of LGMDs, geographical, and family history aspects can be helpful here.

Step 2: Pattern recognition of specific clinical features

As mentioned at the start of this section (Making a precise diagnosis), this step relies on considerable experience: in such scenarios, it may be possible to recognize the distinctive clinical features which allow a diagnosis to be made promptly. Examples include the presence of rippling muscle movements, suggesting caveolin deficiency in LGMD1C, or an autosomal dominant family history of early cardiac rhythm disturbance, muscle weakness, and contracture formation, making laminopathy (LGMD1B) a strong possibility. The LGMD2 disorders may show both overlapping features and wide phenotypic variability, making this pattern-recognition approach

more tricky. Nonetheless, there are features which may help, such as prominent scapular winging and preserved forced vital capacity (FVC) in LGMD2A [10] and asymmetry as a striking finding in LGMD2L [4].

Step 3: Logical use of investigations

Serum creatine kinase measurement

The simple step of measuring the serum creatine kinase (CK) is very helpful. It may allow a number of possible diagnoses to be excluded immediately. Examples include the detection of a very high CK (over 5000 units) which then makes conditions such as LGMD1B or LGMD2I highly unlikely; conversely a normal or mildly raised CK eliminates LGMD2B. Guidelines for interpreting the CK levels are given in Table 23.2. We have seen many inappropriate requests for muscle immunohistochemistry or genetic tests, which could have been avoided if this initial test result had been interpreted correctly. We should mention the importance of establishing that the measurement is a true baseline and not affected by exercise or trauma, for example. There are also ethnic and gender factors that influence the expected normal ranges; these are reviewed by Kyriakides et al. [11].

Table 23.2 Serum creatine kinase (CK) measurements in the more common limb-girdle muscular dystrophies (LGMDs)*

Disorder	Approximate CK level
LGMD1B	N/+
LGMD1C	+++
LGMD2A	+++
LGMD2B	++++
LGMD2C-F	++++
LGMD2I	++/ +++
LGMD2L	++/ +++

*CK level: N, normal range for gender and ethnic background; +, up to 1000 units; ++, 1000–2499 units; +++, 2500–5000 units; ++++, above 5000 units.

Peripheral neurophysiology

Nerve conduction studies and electromyography (EMG) are often requested as part of the investigation sequence but have limited utility. They are most useful in excluding conditions such as a significant peripheral neuropathy, spinal muscular atrophy, myotonia, or a limb-girdle myasthenia, for example, rather than confirming the definite presence or further characterization of a degenerative muscle disease. EMG is an interpretative test and should be considered in the overall clinical context; it cannot be expected to produce a specific LGMD diagnosis on its own.

Limb muscle imaging

In the last few years, the use of limb muscle magnetic resonance imaging (MRI) and magnetic resonance spectroscopy (MRS) has greatly increased [12]. The advantage of MRI is that it allows a non-invasive view of many muscle groups simultaneously and so selective patterns of muscle involvement may be seen. If biopsy is required then the MRI can guide the best muscle to sample, namely one that appears involved but not to too great an extent. The use of muscle MRI is likely to increase further in the coming years and, together with the development of clear diagnostic algorithms, may help to expedite diagnoses and perhaps help to monitor serial muscle changes within a clinical trial context.

Attempts at diagnostic algorithms have been made [13] but these can be complex and, at present, interpretation of the patterns of

muscle involvement is not fully developed. However in certain conditions characteristic configurations of differential muscle involvement may be apparent and guide diagnosis.

However, caution is needed as matters are not straightforward, and it would be premature to think that, at present, muscle imaging will lead to a clear diagnosis in most or all cases. For example, a recent study of CT imaging in the LGMDs compared this with its use in the diagnosis of BMD and Bethlem myopathy [14]. Overall the identification of the individual LGMDs was much less successful than for BMD and Bethlem myopathy, mainly due to inter-observer variability and lack of distinctive findings in the LGMD patients. A recent TREAT-NMD workshop reviewed typical findings in several of the LGMDs [12]. Again, in certain conditions changes were diagnostic but in others the changes lacked the ability to differentiate disorders. LGMD2A was one of the first muscle disorders in which a distinctive pattern of muscle involvement became apparent [15]. The gluteal and posterior compartments of the thigh muscles are mainly involved. In LGMD2B, involvement may be more variable with no consistent pattern other than involvement of the calf muscles in both the proximal (LGMD2B) and distal (Miyoshi) presentations of the condition. In the thighs of LGMD2I patients, involvement of biceps femoris was most marked followed by semimembranosus and semitendinosus with sparing of the vastus lateralis. In the lower leg, gastrocnemii and soleus were more affected than tibialis anterior [13,16]. Data on LGMD2L patients showed lack of gluteal involvement but preferential changes in the posterior compartment of the thigh and severe atrophy of the medial gastrocnemius and soleus muscles [17,18]. Changes seen in the more common conditions are summarized in Table 23.3 and Fig. 23.1.

Muscle biopsy

The tests detailed in Step 3 can provide helpful information but remain, by their nature, indirect methods. Biopsy of a muscle allows the muscle fibres, intracellular structures, and associated features to be viewed directly. There is also an extensive range of immunohistochemistry techniques that may be applied to establish deficiency or aggregation of various proteins [19]. Interpretation of such biopsies is specialized and time-intensive but when diagnostic is rewarding.

Initial analysis of histology and histochemistry usually shows standard dystrophic features with variation in fibre size, increased internal nucleation, necrotic/regenerating fibres, and increased endomysial connective tissue. These are not specific for LGMDs and so immunohistochemistry to examine specific proteins is required.

Table 23.3 Muscle changes on magnetic resonance imaging in selected limb-girdle muscul dystrophies (LGMDs)

Disorder	Selective muscle involvement: thighs	Selective muscle involvement: lower legs
LGMD1B	Variable, may be normal	Medial gastrocnemius, soleus
LGMD2A	Gluteal, posterior compartment	Posterior compartment
LGMD2B	Adductor magnus but variable	Posterior compartment
LGMD2C-F	Anterior compartment	Little change seen
LGMD2I	Biceps femoris	Gastrocnemii, soleus
LGMD2J	No distinct pattern	Tibialis anterior (in heterozygotes)
LGMD2L	Posterior compartment	Posterior compartment

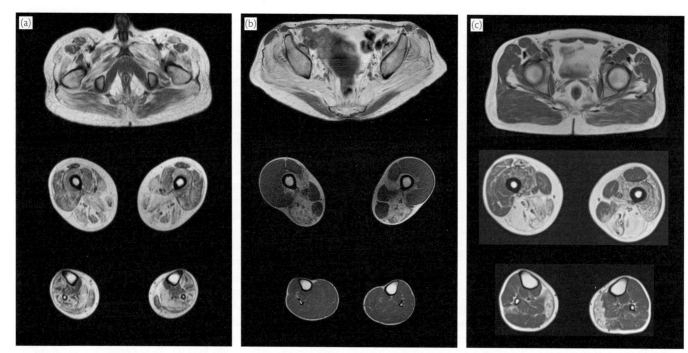

Fig. 23.1 Examples of magnetic resonance imaging scans of lower limb muscles. (a) LGMD2B in a 31-year-old patient. Upper leg: involvement of the pelvic girdle and thigh. Lower leg: prominent involvement of the muscles of the posterior compartment. (b) LGMD2D in a 47-year-old patient. Upper leg: marked involvement of the gluteal muscles. Lower leg: no evidence of muscle involvement, typical for the sarcoglycanopathies. (c) LGMD2L in a 47-year-old patient. Asymmetry of features. Upper leg: fairly well-preserved gluteal muscles and prominent involvement of the thigh. Lower leg: selective changes in medial gastrocnemius muscles.

The panel of antibodies now used is extensive. Both primary changes due to reduction in the expressed protein itself and secondary changes resulting from alterations in the levels of interacting proteins may be seen. Care in interpretation is required due to the increasing recognition of conditions that may show overlapping features, such as the myofibrillar myopathies (see section on Specific conditions). Primary changes are most reliable in LGMD1C, LGMD2B, and LGMD2C–2F but may be normal in LGMD1B, LGMD2A, LGMD2I, and LGMD2L. Secondary changes with reduction in linked proteins such as α-dystroglycan may be suggestive of LGMD2I, or more rarely LGMD2N (*POMT2*) or LGMD2O (*POMGNT1*). Muscle biopsy findings in the more common LGMDs are given in Table 23.4.

Genetic testing

Despite the progress in muscle imaging and biopsy interpretation techniques, demonstration of a mutation(s) within a gene is necessary to provide gold standard confirmation of the specific diagnosis. It enables the option of prenatal diagnosis if relevant to the family and also allows other family members to be tested quickly and easily without the need for invasive tests. The availability of such genetic tests varies according to the arrangements in individual countries; in the UK there is a nationally funded laboratory service that performs appropriate genetic tests (and/or muscle biopsy analysis) at the request of specialists in other centres.

In our practice, genetic testing may be the first investigation when a specific diagnosis is suspected on the basis of clinical assessment, thus obviating the need for a muscle biopsy, a point gratefully appreciated by patients. This has the dual benefit of direct confirmation of the diagnosis through demonstration of the genetic mutations(s) and removes the likely delay and distraction of a muscle biopsy which may be non-diagnostic. Thus our approach in individual patients depends on our suspicions following clinical assessment, and genetic testing would be the first step if lamin A/C, calpain-3, ANO5, or FKRP related disorders are suspected. The latter three tests are particularly useful for those patients who have a moderately high CK and limb-girdle weakness with or without distinctive clinical pointers.

In addition to its use in the proband, genetic screening is being used increasingly to test the partners of patients with autosomal recessive conditions to establish if subsequent offspring will be at risk of inheriting not just one gene from the affected parent but also another affected gene from a carrier parent. Requests for these tests are growing, despite the relatively low prevalence of the LGMD2s in most populations.

Next-generation sequencing technologies are already under development for heterogeneous groups of rare diseases such as the LGMDs and are being slowly introduced into service. The application of techniques such as exomic or whole genome sequencing certainly opens up the possibility of a more streamlined 'one stop' approach to diagnosis, apparently bypassing the need for muscle biopsy, MRI, and detailed clinical assessment. In practice, however, these skill sets are still likely to be required for the foreseeable future. The number of unclassified variants discovered during the application of these technologies can be daunting and the interpretation stage of such analyses presents a new challenge. This is in addition to the ethical and societal issues around undirected testing and the findings of incidental variants in other genes: a topic currently being addressed at many levels but not felt to be ready as yet for diagnostic testing in most settings.

Specific conditions

Specific LGMDs are covered in this section and a summary of defining clinical features is given in Table 23.5.

Table 23.4 Typical primary and secondary changes on immunohistochemical analysis of muscle biopsies in selected limb-girdle muscular dystrophies (LGMDs)

Disease	Protein	Histological features	Immunohistochemistry: primary changes	Secondary changes
LGMD1A	Myotilin	Dystrophic, inflammatory infiltrate, rimmed vacuoles	Myotilin normal, DGC intact	↓ Laminin γ1
LGMD1B	Lamin A/C	Dystrophic	Lamin A/C usually normal	↓ Laminin β1
LGMD1C	Caveolin-3	Myopathic or dystrophic	↓ Caveolin-3 labelling	↓ Dysferlin
LGMD2A	Calpain-3	Dystrophic	Normal	None, but absent, partial deficiency or normal calpain-3 on immunoblotting
LGMD2B	Dysferlin	Dystrophic, inflammatory	↓ Dysferlin	↓ Calpain-3 in half
LGMD2C	γ-Sarcoglycan	Dystrophic	↓ γ-Sarcoglycan	↓ Other SG, dystrophin
LGMD2D	α-Sarcoglycan	Dystrophic	↓ α-Sarcoglycan	↓ Other SG, dystrophin
LGMD2E	β-Sarcoglycan	Dystrophic	↓ β-Sarcoglycan	Severe ↓ other SG, dystrophin
LGMD2F	δ-Sarcoglycan	Dystrophic	↓ δ-Sarcoglycan	Severe ↓ other SG, dystrophin
LGMD2I	FKRP	Dystrophic	Often normal	↓ Laminin α2 and α-dystroglycan
LGMD2J	Titin	Myopathic, dystrophic, rimmed vacuoles	↓ Titin	↓ Calpain-3
LGMD2L	Anoctamin 5	Myopathic or dystrophic, occasional inflammatory cells	Normal with currently available antibodies	None [4] or reduced calpain/dystrophin [21]

SG, sarcoglycan
Adapted from [20].

Autosomal dominant LGMDs (LGMD1)

LGMD1A (myotilinopathy)

LGMD1A was described in 2000 [22] as a form of LGMD due to mutations within the myotilin gene. Both proximal and distal muscle involvement together with a distinctive dysarthria were described. Myotilin appears to have a role in the assembly of sarcomeres and hence altered function may disrupt the myofibrillar architecture [23]. In practice, this form of LGMD is very rare and mutations in myotilin are much more commonly encountered as a cause of late-onset distal weakness within the group of conditions called myofibrillar myopathies (MFMs).

Myofibrillar myopathies (MFM) are reviewed, for example, by Selcen [24] and are covered in more detail in Chapter 27. For

Table 23.5 Clinical features of the individual limb-girdle muscular dystrophies (LGMDs)

Condition	Average age of onset*	Distribution of weakness	Scapular winging	Contractures	Discriminating features	Respiratory involvement	Cardiac involvement
LGMD1A	c, d	Proximal/distal	No	No	Dysarthria	?	Yes?
LGMD1B	a, b	Proximal/distal	Yes	Yes: prominent	Rigid spine in some	Yes	Yes (arrhythmia, cardiomyopathy)
LGMD1C	a–d	Proximal/distal	No	No	Rippling muscles	No	No
LGMD2A	a–c	Proximal	Yes	Yes		No	No
LGMD2B	b, c	Proximal/distal	No	No		No	No
LGMB2C–F	a, b	Proximal	Yes	Yes	Childhood onset	Yes	Yes (cardiomyopathy)
LGMD2G	a, b	Proximal/distal		No	Brazil	?	No
LGMD2H	b, c	Proximal		No	Hutterites	?	No
LGMD2I	a–d	Proximal	Yes	No		Yes	Yes (cardiomyopathy)
LGMD2J	a, b	Proximal/distal	No	No	Finnish	?	No?
LGMD2L	35 years	Proximal/distal	In some	In some	Asymmetry, milder in females	No	No

*a, childhood; b, teens; c, early adult life; d, mid life and older.

context here, it has become clear in recent years that this group of conditions is also clinically and genetically heterogeneous. A number of causative genes in addition to myotilin have been identified, such as desmin, *ZASP*, αB-crystallin, filamin C, and *BAG3*, but in approximately half of cases no causative gene mutation has yet been found [24]. The majority are autosomal dominant. Progressive muscle weakness tends to begin from middle or later life and be slowly progressive. It is often distal but may evolve to become proximal as well, or be limb-girdle or scapuloperoneal at onset. Bag3opathy is the exception, and is of childhood onset with severe cardiorespiratory involvement and a rigid spine. The other MFMs may also involve cardiac muscle, in some cases of desminopathy leading to a severe cardiomyopathy requiring cardiac transplantation, and all patients should be screened for cardiac problems at intervals. Screening for respiratory muscle weakness and for peripheral neuropathy is also recommended. No doubt further elucidation of the genetic basis for this group of conditions will become apparent in the coming years.

LGMD1B (laminopathy)

LGMD1B is an important condition and is increasingly recognized in both neurological and cardiological practice [25]. There are a number of other potential features associated with mutations within the gene, including a form of Charcot–Marie–Tooth disease, partial lipodystrophy, and a progeria phenotype, but this discussion is limited to skeletal and cardiac muscle disease.

Limb involvement may be striking, with marked muscle atrophy, joint contractures, and a rigid spine from childhood or teenage years, although the range in severity of limb features is quite wide. Some patients have a wide neck with reduced lateral flexion.

However, it is the cardiac aspects that are life-threatening [26]. Rhythm disturbances commonly occur at a relatively early age (95% before 30 years) and there is uncertainty as to the best intervention. Sudden cardiac death may occur despite pacing, and so implantable defibrillators are used [27–30] although these are not failsafe and may result in other issues such as severe psychological problems if false shocks occur. Dilated cardiomyopathy may coexist and require cardiac transplantation.

Due to the inheritance pattern of LGMD1B, it is important to suspect and confirm the diagnosis in these patients to permit prompt screening of at-risk family members. There is phenotypic overlap with both autosomal dominant Emery–Dreifuss muscular dystrophy (AD-EDMD) and with X-EDMD, the original X-linked form [31]. Therefore those who do not have mutations within the lamin A/C gene should be tested for mutations in emerin, another nuclear membrane protein.

LGMD1C (caveolinopathy)

LGMD1C describes the manifestation of limb-girdle weakness due to mutations in the caveolin-3 gene [32,33]. Mutations in this gene also cause other clinical presentations including rippling muscle disease [34], distal myopathy, hyperCKaemia, myalgia [35], and familial hypertrophic cardiomyopathy [36]; these phenotypes may overlap [37]. LGMD1C is rare in clinical practice. A recessive form has also been described [38].

The remainder of the autosomal dominant LGMDs are less well-defined and not characterized sufficiently to be clinically distinguishable at present.

Autosomal recessive LGMDs (LGMD2)

LGMD2A (calpainopathy)

LGMD2A is the most common autosomal recessive LGMD, with quoted prevalences including 9.47 per million [39] and 0.60 per 100 000 [3]. Mutations in the gene for the cytoplasmic enzyme calpain-3 (*CAPN3*) were identified initially in the small island population of La Réunion in the mid-1990s [40]; subsequently many more mutations have been found almost throughout the gene and extensive series published [41–44]. The majority of pathogenic mutations, however, are found in only seven exons [42], allowing targeted gene screening.

The clinical presentation is fairly uniform among all the studies, e.g. [43,45]. The age of onset is typically in the teens, although there is a wide range from early childhood to the fifth decade. The mean age of wheelchair use is from the thirties. The phenotype is of early pelvic-girdle weakness with relative sparing of the hip abductors and scapular winging. Limb contractures are frequent features. Calf hypertrophy is not seen, but there is often atrophy here and sometimes of other muscles. Patients do not usually have facial or bulbar weakness. Cardiac problems are not reported and only mild respiratory involvement is found in the majority of patients.

CK is moderately raised to between 1500 and 3000 units. Muscle MRI shows particular involvement of the posterior thigh muscles [15]. Other thigh muscles can be involved but variably and depending on clinical severity. In keeping with the clinical features, hip adductors are more involved than abductors. In the lower legs, soleus and medial gastrocnemius are the most affected.

Muscle biopsy shows a dystrophic pattern but no diagnostic primary changes in immunohistochemistry. Quantification of calpain-3 protein through immunoblotting and immunoassay is helpful if there is marked reduction in calpain-3 levels, but normal levels do not exclude calpainopathy. There has been discussion as to the optimal method for the diagnosis of calpainopathy and whether this should focus first on the genetic analysis of a relatively large gene or on the protein expression level estimated from immunoblotting or assay [42]. Unfortunately there is not an absolute correlation between the two, and pathogenic mutations are found in patients with normal levels of calpain-3 expression, although the protein may be functionally defective. Thus current practice, made more straightforward due to ongoing technological advances, is towards genetic testing of all the exons as this provides a conclusive answer.

LGMD2B (dysferlinopathy)

This may present either as a limb-girdle or a distal phenotype; the former is known as LGMD2B and the latter as Miyoshi myopathy (MM). The disorders are allelic [46,47]. Thus weakness may begin either proximally or distally and then proceed to involve the other lower limb muscles. Marked upper limb, usually proximal, weakness is also seen later in the disease.

Investigations show a very high CK level of between 5000 and 10 000 units and changes on muscle imaging affecting the posterior compartment of the lower legs but more variable proximally. Muscle biopsy may show quite marked changes, both of myopathic/dystrophic features and also sometimes with striking inflammation. Primary changes in dysferlin immunostaining are helpful, although they have to be interpreted with care as more subtle staining alterations may be very non-specific.

The range of age of onset is quite tight around the late teens or early twenties. There is sometimes a history of preceding sporting achievement to a high level, followed by rapid decline of physical function. Muscles may be swollen and painful before the weakness becomes apparent. These factors, taken together with the high CK level and the presence of inflammation on the muscle biopsy, explain why a number of these patients have been treated for presumed inflammatory myopathy for years before the correct diagnosis is made. They tend to come to light due to the relentless progression of weakness despite immunosuppressive treatment, leading to a diagnostic review.

Cardiac and respiratory complications are infrequent although routine practice is to screen for them at intervals.

LGMD2C–F (sarcoglycanopathies)

These are generally severe conditions of childhood onset which resemble DMD [48–51]. Patients have marked limb-girdle weakness, prominent scapular winging, and cardiorespiratory involvement. These disorders are named according to which member of the transmembrane sarcoglycan complex (SGC) is lost. This complex of proteins is closely linked to a region near the C-terminal end of dystrophin and explains why loss of one member of the SGC results in deficiency of its partner molecules, to varying extents, and also a secondary reduction in dystrophin. These factors mean that diagnosis on muscle biopsy immunostaining with subsequent genetic confirmation is relatively straightforward. These of the more common autosomal recessive [3] but more frequent in The Netherlands [52] and in other areas such as North Africa.

LGMD2G

LGMD2G has been identified in Brazilian families [53] but there are no known cases elsewhere. The phenotype is that of a relatively mild proximal weakness.

LGMD2H

LGMD2H is also reported to be relatively mild and is limited to a particular geographical region and population, namely the Hutterite population of Canada [54]. A single mutation is responsible.

LGMD2I

LGMD2I results from mutations within the *FKRP* gene, in northern Europe usually the 'common' mutation C826A. *FKRP* mutations were originally identified in relation to a form of congenital muscular dystrophy termed MDC1C [55] which is not covered further here. It is important to recognize LGMD2I due to the severe respiratory and cardiac complications that may occur even at an early stage of limb muscle weakness. The pattern of muscle weakness, scapular winging, and calf hypertrophy is similar to BMD and a number of patients who were previously thought to have BMD, and therefore an X-linked pattern of inheritance, actually have autosomal recessive LGMD2I with altered consequences for genetic counselling of relatives. LGMD2I has emerged as one of the more common autosomal recessive LGMDs with an estimated prevalence of 0.43 per 100 000 [3]. The clinical presentation was described in detail initially in 16 patients [56]. Most showed some subtle or mild symptoms in childhood but marked, predominantly lower, limb-girdle muscle weakness did not manifest until early adulthood. Calf hypertrophy was prominent, and in some there was hypertrophy of other muscles, including the tongue in one case. Serial respiratory monitoring showed the progressive

fall in FVC over several years, often requiring support from nocturnal non-invasive ventilation. Cardiac involvement was also frequent and comprised both cardiomyopathy and dysrhythmia, treated with standard interventions. Notably both the respiratory and cardiac complications occurred in some patients who were still ambulant; therefore serial monitoring of these should occur in all LGMD2I patients from the outset.

CK was significantly raised but usually not to such an extent as in BMD. Muscle MRI revealed involvement of most of the proximal leg muscles although with sparing of the adductors, and in the lower leg mainly those muscles of the posterior compartment. Dystrophic features are evident on muscle biopsy but no specific primary changes could be seen on immunohistochemistry. Secondary changes were more helpful in that a reduction in laminin α2 labelling could be seen. A reduction in the α-dystroglycan band on immunoblotting was also helpful; later studies described this in more depth and it was shown that the severity of the phenotype was related to the amount of residual dystroglycan expression [57].

Proceeding to genetic analysis is therefore recommended in those patients with a suggestive phenotype who do not have a dystrophin mutation, and this can be done prior to performing a muscle biopsy.

LGMD2J

LGMD2J is one of the consequences of mutations in the large titin gene. Heterozygous mutations produce autosomal dominant tibial muscular dystrophy. This is a distal myopathy in which the anterior compartment of the lower leg is affected; weakness is very slowly progressive with some mild proximal involvement in old age. Homozygous titin mutations are rare (only having been described in Finnish patients) and are associated with autosomal recessive LGMD2J. Other mutations cause dilated cardiomyopathy without skeletal muscle involvement [58] and most recently heterozygous mutations have been demonstrated in cases of MFM especially with early respiratory failure [59,60].

LGMD2L

LGMD2L was defined only relatively recently [61] but it has already become apparent that it is one of the more common autosomal recessive subtypes [4]. The condition is due to mutations within the anoctamin 5 (*ANO5*) gene; a 'common' (c.191dupA) mutation within exon 5 exists and may be a founder mutation in northern Europe and particularly the UK. Developmental motor milestones are normal in all cases so far, age of onset is in the third decade or later, and progression is generally slow. There may be intrafamilial variation in severity. It appears that women display a milder phenotype.

Initially the reported clinical presentation was of calf hypertrophy and pain followed by distal weakness [62], but now the known range of presentations has expanded. Screening of a large series [4] of patients due to their phenotype being similar to LGMD2B/MM but without dysferlin mutations identified mainly proximal weakness, muscle atrophy, and asymmetry of muscle involvement. Wasting mainly affected vastus medialis and medial gastrocnemius. Onset was from the twenties to the fifties and was slowly progressive. Distal weakness was uncommon in this series. The arms were not markedly involved. Cardiorespiratory function was normal.

A further study [21] reported new mutations and a wider phenotypic range, including high hyperCKaemia (often without overt symptoms), exercise-related myalgia, calf hypertrophy, and proximal weakness. The phenotype again appeared markedly milder in women. Asymmetry of muscle involvement was a consistent feature and progression was slow. No respiratory or cardiac involvement was found.

CK values have been found to be moderately to significantly high, within the range of 3000–5000 units. Muscle MRI shows involvement of the posterior compartment of the thigh and calf, progressing to include the quadriceps later. Muscle biopsy shows myopathic or dystrophic changes, minor inflammation (in contrast to dysferlinopathy), and sarcolemmal membrane disruption on electron microscopy. However, extensive immunostaining with the full range of diagnostic antibodies is normal.

The combination of typical findings of raised CK, paucity of symptoms and signs, and normal findings on immunostaining in female patients may have implications for the further investigation of such patients who present to the clinic with apparent idiopathic raised CK or muscle pain.

Overall management needs

At present there is no treatment that can cure any of the LGMDs, although interventions can ameliorate some of the symptoms. Therefore current management should be supportive and active. It is particularly important to maintain vigilant monitoring in case cardiac and/or respiratory complications ensue. Some patients do become frustrated at the length of the diagnostic process; sometimes this is because the gene causing their particular condition has not yet been identified. It is good practice therefore periodically to review those patients without a specific genetic diagnosis to see if a new condition has come to light that may fit. Other patients may discontinue their attendance at the clinic due to a perception that 'nothing can be done'. This latter group should be encouraged to attend even if on an infrequent basis so that they can receive encouragement and physiotherapy review, for example, as well as monitoring for potentially manageable complications. Regardless of whether or not it is possible to apply a specific diagnostic label, patients should feel supported in their condition as the vast majority will unfortunately experience deteriorating mobility and/or function over years and decades.

Physiotherapy assessment

Physiotherapy assessment by a specialist neuromuscular physiotherapist is the ideal, allowing a tailored exercise programme to be developed. The purpose of physiotherapy is to maintain and enhance strength and range of movement through exercise and to prevent the formation of contractures. The specialist physiotherapist can liaise with locally based colleagues nearer to the patient's home to ensure that the correct programme is being followed. He or she can also link in with an orthotist and wheelchair services to provide suitable appliances where necessary. These aspects are covered in greater detail elsewhere, e.g. [63].

Cardiac monitoring

This is mandatory for all patients with LGMD, ideally in liaison with a cardiologist with a special interest in these disorders. Twelve-lead and 24-h electrocardiogram and transthoracic echocardiography should all be considered, with a frequency depending on the underlying diagnosis. For example, patients with LGMD1B (laminopathy) or LGMD2I (*FKRP*) should be watched very closely,

whereas those with LGMD2A (calpainopathy) do not (usually) need frequent surveillance, although any features suggestive of cardiac involvement should be pursued regardless of the diagnosis. In those in whom the diagnostic process is not yet complete, monitoring for a rhythm disturbance and/or cardiomyopathy at annual intervals is recommended.

Respiratory monitoring

This is similar to cardiac monitoring in that whilst particular attention should be directed at those who have a condition known to be associated with a high risk of developing respiratory muscle weakness, all patients with LGMD should be asked routinely about possibly relevant respiratory symptoms and have their FVC measured on routine clinic review. Patients most likely to develop respiratory compromise are those with LGMD1B, LGMD2I, and the sarcoglycanopathies.

Treatment

Treatment at present is limited to supportive measures. Creatine monohydrate produced only a 3% improvement in muscle strength in six patients with sarcoglcanopathy [64]. Case reports have appeared describing improvement with corticosteroids (e.g. [65]) but these have not translated to widespread use. Deflazacort was used in LGMD2B (dysferlinopathy) in a placebo-controlled trial; results reported very recently indicated that there was no improvement and even a small worsening in strength during the trial period on the drug [66].

Patient registries

Patient registries for a number of conditions have been or are in the process of being set up. This began with the more common conditions such as DMD and spinal muscular atrophy and is now extending to other disease groups, notably LGMD2I. The purpose of registries is to allow a ready source of patients who can be contacted in the event of a clinical trial being planned. The exact organization of these registries varies across different countries; ideally the registry data items should show concordance across countries to allow more meaningful data comparison, especially for the rarer conditions where numbers in an individual country may be too few. TREAT-NMD oversees the process for a number of registries internationally (<http://www.treat-nmd.eu/resources/patient-registries/what/>).

Acknowledgement

The authors are grateful to V. Straub for kindly supplying the images in Figure 23.1.

References

1. Walton JN, Nattrass FJ. On the classification, natural history and treatment of the myopathies. *Brain* 1954; **77**: 169–231.
2. Bushby KMD. Making sense of the limb-girdle muscular dystrophies. *Brain* 1999; **122**: 1403–20.
3. Norwood FLM, Harling C, Chinnery PF, Eagle M, Bushby K, Straub V. Prevalence of genetic muscle disease in Northern England: in-depth analysis of a muscle clinic population. *Brain* 2009; **132**: 3175–86.
4. Hicks D, Sarkozy A, Muelas N, et al. A founder mutation in Anoctamin 5 is a major cause of limb-girdle muscular dystrophy. *Brain* 2011; **134**: 171–82.

5. Beckmann JS, Brown RH, Muntoni F, Urtizberea A, Bonnemann C, Bushby KM. 66th/67th ENMC sponsored international workshop: The limb-girdle muscular dystrophies, 26–28 March 1999, Naarden, The Netherlands. *Neuromusc Disord* 1999; **9**: 436–45.

6. Bushby KMD, Beckmann JS. The 105th ENMC sponsored workshop: pathogenesis in the non-sarcoglycan limb-girdle muscular dystrophies, Naarden, April 12–14, 2002. *Neuromusc Disord* 2003; **13**: 80–90.

7. Kaplan JC. *World Muscle Society Genetable of Neuromuscular Disorders*, 2013. Available at: <http://www.musclegenetable.fr/>

8. Bushby K, Norwood F, Straub V. The limb-girdle muscular dystrophies—diagnostic strategies. *Biochem Biophys Acta* 2007; **1772**: 238–42.

9. Jain Foundation: <http://www.jain-foundation.org/>

10. Groen EJ, Charlton R, Barresi R, Anderson LV, Eagle M, Hudson J. Analysis of the UK diagnostic strategy for limb-girdle muscular dystrophy 2A. *Brain* 2007; **130**: 3237–49.

11. Kyriakides T, Angelini C, Schaefer J, Sacconi S, Vichez JJ, Hilton-Jones D. EFNS guidelines on the diagnostic approach to pauci- or asymptomatic hyperCKemia. *Eur J Neurol* 2010; **17**: 767–73.

12. Straub V, Carlier PG, Mercuri E. TREAT-NMD workshop: Pattern recognition in genetic muscle diseases using muscle MRI 25–26 February 2011, Rome, Italy. *Neuromusc Disord* 2012; **22**: S42–S53.

13. Udd B. 165th ENMC International Workshop: Distal myopathies. 6–8th February 2009 Naarden, The Netherlands. *Neuromusc Disord* 2009; **19**: 429–38.

14. ten Dam L, van der Kooi A, van Wattingen M, de Hann R, de Visser M. Reliability and accuracy of skeletal muscle imaging in limb-girdle muscular dystrophies. *Neurology* 2012; **79**: 1716–23.

15. Mercuri E, Bushby K, Ricci E, et al.. Muscle MRI findings in patients with limb-girdle muscular dystrophy with calpain 3 deficiency (LGMD2A) and early contractures. *Neuromuscul Disord* 2005; **15**: 164–71.

16. Poppe M, Cree L, Bourke J, et al. The phenotype of limb-girdle muscular dystrophy type 2I. *Neurology* 2003; **60**: 1246–51.

17. Sarkozy A, Deschauer M, Carlier R-Y, et al. Muscle MRI findings in limb-girdle muscular dystrophy type 2L. *Neuromusc Disord* 2012; **22**: S122–S129.

18. Mahjneh I, Bashir R, Kiuru-Enari S, Linssen W, Lamminen A, de Visser M. Selective pattern of muscle involvement seen in distal muscular dystrophy associated with anoctamin 5 mutations: a follow-up muscle MRI study. *Neuromusc Disord* 2012; **22**: S130–S136.

19. Dubowitz V, Sewry C. Muscular dystrophies and allied disorders II: Limb-girdle muscular dystrophies. In: *Muscle Biopsy: a Practical Approach*, pp. 325–47. Oxford: Saunders, Elsevier, 2007.

20. Norwood F, de Visser M, Eymard B, Lochmuller H, Bushby K. Limb-girdle muscular dystrophies. In: Gilhus NE, Brainin M, Barnes MP (eds) *European Handbook of Neurological Management: Vol.1*, pp. 363–71. Oxford: Blackwell, 2011.

21. Penttila S, Palmio J, Suominen T, et al. Eight new mutations and the expanding phenotype variability in muscular dystrophy caused by ANO5. *Neurology* 2012; **78**: 897–903.

22. Hauser MA, Horrigan SK, Salmikangas P, et al.. Myotilin is mutated in limb-girdle muscular dystrophy 1A. *Hum Mol Genet* 2000; **9**: 2141–7.

23. Salmikangas P, van der Ven PFM, Lalowski M, et al. Myotilin, the limb-girdle muscular dystrophy 1A (LGMD1A) protein, cross-links actin filaments and controls sarcomere assembly. *Hum Mol Genet* 2003; **12**: 189–203.

24. Selcen D. Myofibrillar myopathies. *Neuromusc Disord* 2011; **21**: 161–71.

25. Muchir A, Bonne G, van der Kooi AJ, et al. Identification of mutations in the gene encoding lamin A/C in autosomal dominant limb-girdle muscular dystrophy with atrioventricular conduction disturbances (LGMD1B). *Hum Mol Genet* 2000; **9**: 1453–9.

26. Bushby K, Muntoni F, Bourke JP. 107th ENMC International Workshop: the management of cardiac involvement in muscular dystrophy and myotonic dystrophy. 7th–9th June 2002, Naarden, the Netherlands. *Neuromusc Disord* 2003; **13**: 166–72.

27. van Berlo JH, de Voogt WG, van der Kooi AJ, et al. Meta-analysis of clinical characteristics of 299 carriers of LMNA gene mutations: do lamin A/C mutations portend a high risk of sudden death? *J Mol Med* 2005; **83**: 79–83.

28. Lu JT, Muchir A, Nagy PL, Worman HJ. LMNA cardiomyopathy: cell biology and genetics meet clinical medicine. *Dis Model Mech* 2011; **4**: 562–8.

29. van Rijsingen IA, Arbustini E, Elliott PM, et al. Risk factors for malignant ventricular arrhythmias in lamin A/C mutation carriers—a European cohort study. *J Am Coll Cardiol* 2012; **59**: 493–500.

30. van Rijsingen IA, Nannenberg EA, Arbustini E, et al. Gender-specific differences in major cardiac events and mortality in lamin A/C mutation carriers. *Eur J Heart Fail* 2013; **15**: 376–84.

31. Bonne G, Di Barletta MR, Varnous S, et al. Mutations in the gene encoding lamin A/C cause autosomal Emery–Dreifuss muscular dystrophy. *Nat Genet* 1999; **21**: 285–8.

32. McNally EM, de Sa Moreira, Duggan DJ, et al. Caveolin-3 in muscular dystrophy. *Hum Mol Genet* 1998; **7**: 871–7.

33. Minetti C, Sotgia F, Bruno C, et al. Mutations in the caveolin-3 gene cause autosomal dominant limb-girdle muscular dystrophy. *Nat Genet* 1998; **18**: 365–8.

34. Betz RC, Schoser BG, Kasper D, et al. Mutations in CAV3 cause mechanical hyperirritability of skeletal muscle in rippling muscle disease. *Nat Genet* 2001; **28**: 218–19.

35. Aboumousa A, Hoogendijk J, Charlton R, et al. Caveolinopathy-new mutations and additional symptoms. *Neuromuscul Disord* 2008; **18**: 572–8.

36. Hayashi T, Arimura T, Ueda K, et al. Identification and functional analysis of a caveolin-3 mutation associated with familial hypertrophic cardiomyopathy. *Biochem Biophys Res Commun* 2004; **313**: 178–84.

37. Woodman SE, Sotgia F, Galbiati F, Minetti C, Lisanti MP. Caveolinopathies. Mutations in caveolin-3 cause four distinct autosomal dominant muscle diseases. *Neurology* 2004; **62**: 538–43.

38. Muller JS, Piko H, Schoser BGH, et al. Novel splice site mutation in the caveolin-3 gene leading to autosomal recessive limb-girdle muscular dystrophy. *Neuromusc Disord* 2006; **16**: 432–6.

39. Fanin M, Nascimbeni AC, Fulizio L, Angelini C. The frequency of limb-girdle muscular dystrophy 2A in northeastern Italy. *Neuromusc Disord* 2005; **15**: 218–24.

40. Richard I, Broux O, Allamand V, et al. Mutations in the proteolytic enzyme, calpain 3, cause limb-girdle muscular dystrophy type 2A. *Cell* 1995; **81**: 27–40.

41. Richard I, Roudaut C, Saenz A, et al. Calpainopathy—a survey of mutations and polymorphisms. *Am J Hum Genet* 1999; **64**: 1524–40.

42. Fanin M, Fulizio L, Nascimbeni AC, et al. Molecular diagnosis in LGMD2A: mutation analysis or protein testing? *Hum Mutat* 2004; **24**: 52–62.

43. Saenz A, Leturq F, Cobo AM, et al. LGMD2A: genotype-phenotype correlations based on a large mutational survey on the calpain 3 gene. *Brain* 2005; **128**: 732–42.

44. Piluso G, Politano L, Aurino S, et al. Extensive scanning of the calpain-3 gene broadens the spectrum of LGMD2A phenotypes. *J Med Genet* 2005; **42**: 686–93.

45. Pollitt C, Anderson LVB, Pogue R, Davison K, Pyle A, Bushby KMD. The phenotype of calpainopathy: diagnosis based on a multidisciplinary approach. *Neuromusc Disord* 2001; **11**: 287–96.

46. Bashir R, Britton S, Strachan T, et al. A gene related to *Caenorhabditis elegans* spermatogenesis factor *fer-1* is mutated in limb-girdle muscular dystrophy type 2B. *Nat Genet* 1998; **20**: 37–42.

47. Liu J, Aoki M, Illa I, et al. Dysferlin, a novel skeletal muscle gene, is mutated in Miyoshi myopathy and limb-girdle muscular dystrophy. *Nat Genet* 1998; **20**: 31–6.

48. Roberds SL, Leturq F, Allamand V, et al. Missense mutations in the adhalin gene linked to autosomal recessive muscular dystrophy. *Cell* 1994; **78**: 625–33.

49. Bonnemann CG, Modi R, Noguchi S, et al. Beta-sarcoglycan (A3b) mutations cause autosomal recessive muscular dystrophy with loss of the sarcoglycan complex. *Nat Genet* 1995; **11**: 266–73.

50. Noguchi S, McNally EM, Ben Othmane K, et al. Mutations in the dystrophin-associated protein gamma-sarcoglycan in chromosome 13 muscular dystrophy. *Science* 1995; **270**: 819–22.

51. Nigro V, Moreira ES, Piluso G, et al. Autosomal recessive limb-girdle muscular dystrophy, LGMD2F, is caused by a mutation in the delta-sarcoglycan gene. *Nat Genet* 1996; **14**: 195–8.

52. Ginjaar HB, van der Kooi A, Ceelie H, et al. Sarcoglycanopathies in Dutch patients with autosomal recessive limb-girdle muscular dystrophy. *J Neurol* 2000; **247**: 524–9.

53. Moreira ES, Wiltshire TJ, Faulkner G, et al. Limb-girdle muscular dystrophy type 2G is caused by mutations in the gene encoding the sarcomeric protein telethonin. *Nat Genet* 2000; **24**: 163–6.

54. Frosk P, Weiler T, Nylen E, et al. Limb-girdle muscular dystrophy type 2H associated with mutation in *TRIM32*, a putative E3-ubiquitin-ligase gene. *Am J Hum Genet* 2002; **70**: 663–72.

55. Brockington M, Yuva Y, Prandini P, et al. Mutations in the fukutin-related protein gene (FKRP) identify limb-girdle muscular dystrophy 2I as a milder allelic variant of congenital muscular dystrophy MDC1C. *Hum Mol Genet* 2001; **10**: 2851–59.

56. Poppe M, Cree L, Bourke J, et al. The phenotype of limb-girdle muscular dystrophy type 2I. *Neurology* 2003; **60**: 1246–51.

57. Brown SC, Torelli S, Brockington M, et al. Abnormalities in α-dystroglycan expression in MDC1C and LGMD2I muscular dystrophies. *Am J Pathol* 2004; **164**: 727–37.

58. Udd B, Vihola A, Sarparanta J, Richard I, Hackman P. Titinopathies and extension of the M-line phenotype beyond distal myopathy and LGMD2J. *Neurology* 2005; **64**: 636–42.

59. Ohlsson M, Hedberg C, Bradvik B, Lindberg C, Tajsharghi H, Danielsson O. Hereditary myopathy with early respiratory failure associated with a mutation in A-band titin. *Brain* 2012; **135**: 1682–94.

60. Pfeffer G, Barresi R, Wilson IJ, et al. Titin founder mutation is a common cause of myofibrillar myopathy with early respiratory failure. *J Neurol Neurosurg Psychiatry* 2013; doi: 10.1136/jnnp-2012-304728.

61. Bolduc V, Marlow G, Boycott KM, et al. Recessive mutations in the putative calcium-activated chloride channel Anoctamin 5 cause proximal LGMD2L and distal MMD3 muscular dystrophies. *Am J Hum Genet* 2010; **86**: 213–21.

62. Mahjneh I, Jaiswal J, Lamminen A, et al. A new distal myopathy with mutation in anoctamin 5. *Neuromusc Disord* 2010; **20**: 791–5.

63. Hilton-Jones D, Freebody J, Stein J. *Neuromuscular Disorders in the Adult: a Practical Manual.* Oxford: Oxford University Press, 2011.

64. Walter MC, Lochmuller H, Reilich P, et al. Creatine monohydrate in muscular dystrophies: a double-blind, placebo-controlled clinical study. *Neurology* 2000; **54**: 1848–50.

65. Angelini C, Fanin M, Menegazzo E, Freda MP, Duggan DJ, Hoffman EP. Homozygous α-sarcoglycan mutation in two siblings: one asymptomatic and one steroid-responsive mild limb-girdle muscular dystrophy patient. *Muscle Nerve* 1998; **21**: 769–75.

66. Walter MC, Reilich P, Theile S, et al. Treatment of dysferlinopathy with deflazacort: a double-blind, placebo-controlled clinical trial. *Orphanet J Rare Dis* 2013; **8**: 26.

CHAPTER 24

The congenital muscular dystrophies

Emma Clement and Heinz Jungbluth

Introduction

Congenital muscular dystrophies (CMDs) are a heterogeneous group of mainly autosomal recessive disorders associated with dystrophic changes on skeletal muscle biopsy. CMDs present at birth or within the first few months with muscular weakness, hypotonia, delayed motor milestones, and variable joint contractures. In addition, a proportion of affected individuals exhibit mental retardation, often associated with structural brain abnormalities [1,2].

CMDs usually arise as a result of mutations in genes that encode components of the muscle cells distinct from those affected in the congenital myopathies. Skeletal muscle is composed of individual myofibres bound by a plasma membrane (sarcolemma) and surrounded by a basement membrane comprising the outer reticular layer and the inner basal lamina. The outer reticular layer is fibrillar and contains collagen VI myofibrils, whereas the inner basal lamina comprises networks of non-fibrillar collagen VI and laminins linked by non-collagenous glycoproteins [3,4]. The basement membrane interacts with a network of other proteins including the dystrophin–glycoprotein complex (DGC) [5,6], a trans-membrane complex. Among other proteins, the DGC contains α-dystroglycan (ADG) and interacts with extracellular ligands including laminin. The nuclear envelope consists of an inner nuclear membrane (INM) and an outer nuclear membrane (ONM) separated by a perinuclear space. At the nuclear face of the INM lies the nuclear lamina, comprised largely of A-type and B-type lamins that form intermediate filaments providing structural and mechanical support to the nucleus [7,8]. Nesprin-1 is an integral part of the ONM and has a role in connecting the actin cytoskeleton to the nuclear lamins [9].

CMDs may be grouped according to those that occur as a result of abnormalities in external membrane, basal lamina, and extracellular matrix proteins and those CMDs resulting from abnormal glycosylation of ADG secondary to mutations in known/putative enzymes involved in this pathway. In addition, a specific form of CMD, rigid spine muscular dystrophy Type 1 (RSMD1), may result from mutations in *SEPN1*, a gene that encodes an endoplasmic reticulum protein and, more rarely, by mutations in nuclear envelope proteins [4,10]. The known genetic variants implicated in the CMDs are summarized in Table 24.1 [2,11,12] and the cellular location of the affected proteins is represented in Figure 24.1.

Whilst treatment is currently mainly supportive, identification of the molecular defects underlying specific CMDs offers the prospect of rational pharmacological therapies in the future.

Clinical features of the congenital muscular dystrophies

The muscular system is always affected in CMD, although the severity of symptoms and maximal motor achievement is very variable. The main musculoskeletal features are weakness, hypotonia, and muscle wasting (or, rarely, hypertrophy) but may also include torticollis, spinal rigidity, scoliosis, contractures, and congenital dislocation of the hips. In most forms, the weakness is usually relatively static with increasing disability more often the result of contractures and scoliosis [2].

Respiratory involvement may be a significant cause of morbidity if not managed proactively. Cardiac involvement in CMD is not usually a major feature, with a few exceptions: patients with congenital-onset Emery–Dreifuss muscular dystrophy Type 2 (EDMD2) are at risk of conduction defects [13] and dystroglycanopathy patients with *FKTN* and *FKRP* mutations may develop dilated cardiomyopathy or left ventricular systolic dysfunction [14–16]. Subclinical cardiac involvement is also thought to affect up to a third of patients with merosin-deficient congenital muscular dystrophy Type 1A (MDC1A) [17,18].

Structural and functional brain involvement is common in the CMDs. This may range from characteristic white matter changes, often seen in MDC1A, through to dramatic structural changes including agyria inevitably associated with profound mental retardation, as seen in Walker–Warburg syndrome (WWS). Seizures and learning difficulties are seen in a number of CMD subtypes, e.g. MDC1A. In others, such as Ullrich congenital muscular dystrophy (UCMD) and Bethlem myopathy (BM), intelligence and magnetic resonance imaging (MRI) of the brain is expected to be normal.

Eye involvement may be prominent in the more severe dystroglycanopathy phenotypes where structural abnormalities such as anterior chamber defects, retinal abnormalities, cataracts, and severe myopia are typical. In MDC1A, external ophthalmoplegia, pronounced on upward gaze, is a recognized feature and visual evoked responses are usually abnormal [19].

Specific CMDs are outlined in more detail in the rest of this chapter. For a clinical overview see Tables 24.2 and 24.3.

Table 24.1 Congenital muscular dystrophy variants with known gene defects

Functional classification	Protein	Gene	Gene ID*	Chromosomal location	Disease	OMIM number†
Structural protein of basement membrane, extracellular matrix or external membrane protein	Laminin α2	LAMA2	156225	6q2	MDC1A	607855
	Collagen VI	Col6A1	120220	21q2	UCMD	254090
		Col6A2	120240	21q2	BM	158810
		Col6A3	120250	2q3		
	Integrin α7	ITGA7	600536	12q	Integrin α7 deficiency	613204
	Integrin α9	ITGA9	603963	3p22	CMDH [124]	
Dystroglycanopathy	Protein-O-mannosyltransferase 1	POMT1	607423	9q34	MDDGA1 (WWS†)	236670
	Protein-O-mannosyltransferase 2	POMT2	607439	14q24	MDDGA2 (WWS†)	613150
	Protein-O-linked mannose beta 1,2-N-acetylglucosaminyltransferase	POMGNT1	606822	1p34	MDDGA3 (MEB†)	253280
	Fukutin	FKTN	607440	9q31	MDDGA4 (FCMD†)	253800
	Fukutin-related protein	FKRP	606596	19q13	MDDGB5 (MDC1C†)	606612
	Like-glycosyltransferase	LARGE	603590	22q12	MDDGB6 (MDC1D†)	608840
	Isoprenoid synthase domain containing	ISPD	614631	7p21	MDDGA7 (WWS†)	614643
	Glycosyltransferase-like domain-containing protein 2	GTDC2	614828	3p22	MDDGA8 (WWS†)	614830
	Transmembrane protein 5	TMEM5	605862	12q14	MDDGA10 (WWS†)	615041
	β-1,3-N-acetylglucosaminyltransferase 1	B3GNT1	605581	11q13	WWS† [89]	
	Dystroglycan-associated glycoprotein 1	DAG1	128239	3p21	MDDGC9	613818
Dystroglycanopathy– congenital disorder of glycosylation overlap	Dolichyl-phosphate mannosyltransferase polypeptide 3	DPM3	605951	1q22	CDG1o	612937
	Dolichyl-phosphate mannosyltransferase polypeptide 2	DPM2	603564	9q34	CDG1u	615042
	Dolichol kinase	DOLK	601746	9q34	CDG1m	610768
Endoplasmic reticulum protein	Selenoprotein N,1	SEPN1	606210	1p35-36	RSMD1§	602771
Phosphatidylcholine biosynthesis	Choline kinase beta	CHKB	612395	22q13	MDCMC	602541
Nuclear envelope protein	Lamin A/C	LMNA	150330	1q21	EDMD2¶	181350
	Nesprin	SYNE1	608441	6q25	CMD with adducted thumbs [121]	

MDC1A, congenital muscular dystrophy Type 1A; UCMD, Ullrich congenital muscular dystrophy; BM, Bethlem myopathy; WWS, Walker–Warburg syndrome; MEB, muscle–eye–brain disease, FCMD, Fukuyama congenital muscular dystrophy; MDC1C, merosin-deficient congenital muscular dystrophy Type 1C, MDC1D, merosin-deficient congenital muscular dystrophy Type 1D; CGD1o, congenital disorder of glycosylation Type 1o; CGD1u, congenital disorder of glycosylation Type 1u; CGD1m, congenital disorder of glycosylation type 1m; RSMD1, rigid spine muscular dystrophy; EDMD2, autosomal dominant Emery–Dreifuss muscular dystrophy.

*Entrez Gene Identifier from the NCBI database (<http://www.ncbi.nlm.nih.gov/>).

†Online Mendelian Inheritance in Man (<http://www.ncbi.nlm.nih.gov/OMIM>).

†Denotes original phenotype described in association with the gene; the dystroglycanopathies show considerable genetic heterogeneity and have recently been reclassified in OMIM as MDDG (muscular dystrophy–dystroglycanopathy) subtypes; however, the original phenotypic descriptions are still widely used.

§SEPN1 mutations may also be associated with other myopathy phenotypes.

¶LMNA mutations are associated with a number of other non-CMD phenotypes.

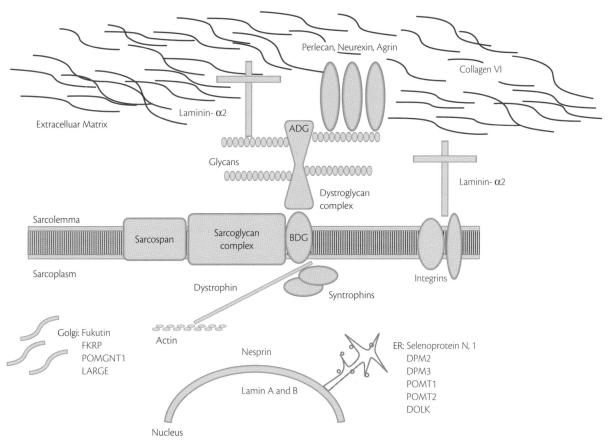

Fig. 24.1 Diagrammatic representation of the subcellular localization of congenital muscular dystrophy (CMD) proteins (where known) within skeletal muscle. Proteins highlighted in green are known to cause various forms of CMD. ER, endoplasmic reticulum; POMT1, protein-*O*-mannosyl transferase 1; POMT2, protein-*O*-mannosyl transferase 2; POMGNT1, protein-*O*-mannose 1,2-*N*-acetylglucosaminyltransferase 1; FKRP, fukutin-related protein; LARGE, like-glycosyltransferase; DPM3, dolichyl-phosphate mannosyltransferase polypeptide 3; DPM2, dolichyl-phosphate mannosyltransferase polypeptide 2; DOLK, dolichol kinase. The components of the core dystrophin–glycoprotein (dystroglycan) complex include the cytoplasmic proteins dystrophin and syntrophin (α and β), the transmembrane protein sarcospan, the glycoproteins dystroglycan (α, ADG; β, BDG) and sarcoglycan (α, β, γ, and δ).

Investigation, diagnosis, and differential diagnosis of the congenital muscular dystrophies

Patient history, examination, and baseline investigations

The baseline assessment for patients with CMD includes a detailed history and clinical examination. Features particularly relevant for CMD include age of onset, pattern of weakness and contractures, muscle wasting or hypertrophy, cardiorespiratory impairment, feeding difficulties, eye and brain involvement, and the presence of skin changes. A history of consanguinity should also be sought.

Serum creatine kinase (CK) determination is one of the most useful investigations, and the extent to which it is elevated may provide a clue to the specific diagnosis. In the dystroglycanopathies, CK is typically very high, sometimes up to 50 times the upper limit of normal, whilst in collagen VI myopathies and RSMD1 the CK is usually only mildly elevated or normal.

Skeletal muscle and skin biopsy

Skeletal muscle biopsy forms a key role in the diagnostic assessment of patients with CMD. Overtly dystrophic features, i.e. the

presence of necrotic and regenerating fibres, are supportive of the diagnosis but may be absent in some patients. There is no correlation between the extent of muscle biopsy changes and the severity of clinical disease. In addition, muscle involvement may be selective and change with disease progression, hence biopsy findings are dependent on the individual muscle sampled as well as the age of the patient at the time of biopsy. Immunochemical labelling, e.g. for laminin α2 in MDC1A [3], may provide a definitive diagnosis in some cases.

In patients where a muscle sample is not available, pathological analysis of a skin biopsy may be helpful. For example, in MDC1A laminin α2 may be reduced or absent in the epidermal–dermal junction [3]. Fibroblasts cultured from skin biopsy are of particular value in the investigation of collagen VI-related myopathies where fibroblasts may be used to extract RNA for protein expression studies or for analysis of collagen VI expression [20,21].

Molecular genetic testing

The gold standard diagnostic test in the investigation of CMD is the identification of a pathogenic genetic mutation. Screening of *SEPN1*, *FKRP*, and *LAMA2* is well established and the interpretation of results is usually uncomplicated. In other genes, in particular collagen VI, genetic investigations are more difficult to interpret

Table 24.2 Summary of clinical features seen in the main congenital muscular dystrophy (CMD) subtypes

CMD type	Brain malformation	Mental retardation	Ocular involvement	Weakness	Spine (rigidity/ weakness)	Contractures	Respiratory involvement	Cardiac involvement	Other features
MDC1A	+/++	+	+	+++	+++	++	+++	+	External ophthalmoplegia, feeding difficulties
UCMD	–	–	–	++/+++	+++	+++	+++	-	Distal laxity, CDH,skin changes
BM	–	–	–	+	–	+++	+	+	CDH, skin changes, long finger flexor contractures
WWS	+++	+++	+++	+++	++	–	+	+	Usually fatal within 12 months
MEB	++	++	++	++	+	–	+	+	
FCMD	++	++	++	++	+	–	++	++	Only common in Japanese population. Pseudohypertrophy
MDC1C	+	+	+	+++	+		++	++	Pseudohypertrophy
Congenital EDMD2	–	–	–	++	+	++	–	++	Cardiac conduction defects
RSMD1	–	–	–	+	+++	–	+++	+	Nasal voice, respiratory weakness disproportionate to muscle weakness

MDC1A, congenital muscular dystrophy Type 1A; UCMD, Ullrich congenital muscular dystrophy; BM, Bethlem myopathy; WWS, Walker–Warburg syndrome; MEB, muscle–eye–brain disease, FCMD, Fukuyama congenital muscular dystrophy; MDC1C, congenital muscular dystrophy Type 1C, EDMD2, autosomal dominant Emery–Dreifuss muscular dystrophy; RSMD1, rigid spine muscular dystrophy.

+, A rare or mild finding; ++, a common or moderate finding; +++, a prominent or severe finding; –, not a reported feature; CDH, congenital dislocation of the hip.

because of a large number of variations of uncertain significance. In such cases, alternative supportive evidence of pathogenicity is required and may include RNA studies and family segregation studies in conjunction with consistent pathological and clinical investigations.

Muscle and brain imaging

Muscle ultrasound used in the clinic setting may demonstrate increased echogenicity in muscles, indicative of muscle pathology. Muscle MRI, increasingly important in the investigation of muscle disorders, often shows a specific pattern of muscle involvement in the different subtypes of CMD and the congenital myopathies (Fig. 24.2) that may help direct molecular testing [22,23].

Several of the CMDs have associated brain abnormalities. These can have dramatic appearances on MRI brain scans and can be pathognomonic for a particular condition [24–26,27] (Fig. 24.3).

Electrophysiology

Electrophysiology does not play a major role in the assessment of the CMDs. However, in some variants, particularly MDC1A, abnormalities in keeping with peripheral nerve involvement may be observed on electrophysiological testing [19,28]. Rarely, electrophysiology may be required to investigate the possibility of a congenital myasthenic syndrome in cases with overlapping clinical features.

Differential diagnosis

CMDs shows considerable clinical and pathological overlap with the congenital myopathies and some of the congenital myasthenic syndromes and these disorders ought to be considered in the differential diagnosis [29]. Mutations in the *SEPN1* gene in particular have been associated with both myopathic and dystrophic manifestations [30]. Mutations in the skeletal muscle ryanodine receptor (*RYR1*) gene, one of the most common causes of congenital myopathy [31], may mimic both clinical and histopathological features of the CMDs at the most severe end of the spectrum [32].

Congenital muscular dystrophy variants

Merosin-deficient congenital muscular dystrophy Type 1A (MDC1A)

MDC1A (MIM #607855) was the earliest CMD pathologically defined due to a characteristic deficiency of merosin on skeletal muscle biopsy [33–35].

Laminins are situated in the cell basement membrane and act as barriers to cell penetration and infiltration. MDC1A is due to mutations in laminin α2 (*LAMA2*; MIM #156225), which encodes the laminin α2 chain that forms part of merosin (laminin 2). Merosin plays an essential role in maintaining integrity of the basement

Table 24.3 Summary of investigations and diagnostic features in the main congenital muscular dystrophy (CMD) subtypes

CMD type	Relative frequency in the UK*	Genes	Inheritance	CK (U L⁻¹)	Muscle biopsy	Muscle MRI	Brain MRI
MDC1A	~About 10%	LAMA2	AR	1000s	Absent/ reduced merosin	–	White matter change (100% > 6m), cerebellar hypoplasia (1/3), occipital agyria (minority)
UCMD	About 20% UCMD and BM combined	COL6A1 COL6A2 COL6A3	AR/AD	Normal/mild elevation	May show absent/reduced collagen VI	Diffuse involvement of thigh with relative sparing of anteromedial muscles	Normal
BM			AD	Normal	Collagen VI fibroblast studies may help	May be normal. Concentric muscle atrophy. 'Central shadow' in rectus	
WWS	All dystroglycanopathy phenotypes about 15%	POMT1 POMT2 POMGNT1 FKTN FKRP LARGE ISPD TMEM5 B3GNT1 DAG1 (DPM2, DPM3, DOLK)† >50% have no known mutation	AR	1000s	Reduced glycosylation ADG	–	Agyria or cobblestone lissencephaly, hydrocephalus, cerebellar abnormality brainstem abnormality
MEB							Pachygyria, polymicrogyria cerebellar abnormality including cysts, brainstem abnormality
FCMD							Pachygyria, polymicrogyria, cerebellar abnormality
MDC1C							Usually normal, subgroup with cerebellar cysts
Congenital ECMD2	<5%	LMNA	AD	100s–1000s	Not diagnostic	Calf: medial > lateral gastrocnemius. Thigh: vasti more affected	Normal
RSMD1	<5%	SEPN1	AR	Normal/mild elevation	Not diagnostic	Selective sartorius involvement	Normal

CK, creatine kinase; MDC1A, congenital muscular dystrophy Type 1A; UCMD, Ullrich congenital muscular dystrophy; BM, Bethlem myopathy; WWS, Walker–Warburg syndrome; MEB, muscle–eye–brain disease, FCMD, Fukuyama congenital muscular dystrophy; MDC1C, congenital muscular dystrophy Type 1C, EDMD2, autosomal dominant Emery–Dreifuss muscular dystrophy; RSMD1, rigid spine muscular dystrophy; ADG; α-dystroglycan.

*Fifty per cent of patients have all known genes excluded.

†Mutations in these genes give rise to phenotypes with overlap between the dystroglycanopathies and congenital disorders of glycosylation.

membrane during development and in adult life [36]. Most mutations in *LAMA2* result in a complete absence of laminin α2 protein, with a small minority causing a partial deficiency.

MDC1A with complete absence of merosin causes a severe predictable phenotype with CK levels typically exceeding 1000 U L⁻¹. It presents in the neonatal period or first few months of life with profound proximal and axial weakness, hypotonia, and delayed motor milestones. Affected individuals rarely acquire independent ambulation but most are able to sit unsupported; however, mobility is further compromised by the development of contractures and scoliosis. Most patients with complete absence of merosin will need ventilatory support and enteral feeding at some stage. Respiratory insufficiency, if left untreated, often leads to death in the first decade

of life. Other features include partial external ophthalmoplegia and cardiac abnormalities in the form of cardiomyopathy, hypokinesis, or subclinical cardiac involvement [17,18].

Intelligence is usually normal in MDC1A although some patients have mental retardation and seizures. MRI of the brain invariably reveals diffuse white matter changes after the age of 6 months [35,37,38], thought to be due to dysmyelination (see Fig. 24.3) and occasionally confused with hypoxic damage or primary white matter disease if the diagnosis of CMD has not already been established. Structural brain abnormalities may include hypoplasia of the cerebellum (up to a third) and occasionally neuronal migration abnormalities, usually of the occipital lobes [39]. MDC1A patients have a motor demyelinating neuropathy and reduced nerve conduction

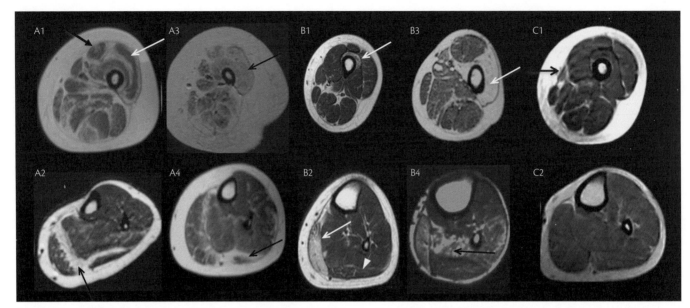

Fig. 24.2 Muscle MRI findings in patients with Bethlem myopathy (BM) and Ullrich congenital muscular dystrophy (UCMD) A), Emery–Dreifuss muscular dystrophy Type 2 (EDMD2) (B) and rigid spine muscular dystrophy Type 1 (RSMD1) (C). (A) Axial T_1-weighted images at thigh (A1, A3) and calf (A2, A4) level showing the gradient of muscle change from BM (A1, A2) to UCMD (A3, A4). Patients with BM have a typical peripheral involvement of the thigh muscles, especially of the vastus lateralis (A1, white arrow), and a 'central shadow' in the rectus (A1, black arrow). At calf level, there is obvious increased signal (thickening) of the fascia between gastrocnemius and soleus (arrow, A2). Patients with UCMD have a more diffuse involvement but sparing of the central portion of the thigh muscles (arrow, A3) and gastrocnemii (arrow, A4). (B) Axial T_1-weighted images at thigh (B1, B3) and calf (B2, B4) level in two patients with EDMD2. At the calf level the medial gastrocnemius (B2, white arrow) is more affected than the lateral gastrocnemius (B2, white arrowhead). There is variable soleus involvement (B4, arrow). At thigh level, the vasti are involved, limited to the intermedius in case B1 (arrow) and involving all vasti muscles in B3 (arrow). Patients with EDMD2 may have more diffuse thigh muscle involvement, especially in advanced disease. (C) Axial T_1-weighted images at thigh (C1) and calf (C2) level in a patient with RSMD1. Patients have a selective involvement of sartorius (arrow) with relative sparing of the other muscles.

velocities. In addition, visual and somatosensory evoked responses are usually abnormal [40].

Patients with partial merosin deficiency usually have a less severe phenotype, but there are notable exceptions to this rule [36,41–44].

Diagnosis is usually based on a suggestive combination of clinical features, muscle biopsy findings, and genetic studies. Muscle biopsies in MDC1A patients show a variable degree of fibre necrosis and regeneration, increased connective tissue, and inflammatory infiltrates. Immunocytochemically, the laminin α2 chain is deficient. ADG and integrin a7b1 show secondary reduction in labelling [45]. Absence of laminin α2 can be detected in skin biopsies where it may also be secondarily reduced in conditions such as the dystroglycanopathies [3].

Collagen-VI related disorders

The collagen VI- related disorders, UCMD (MIM #254090) and its milder allelic variant BM (MIM #158810), represent a significant proportion of diagnosed cases of CMD [46,47].

Collagen VI is an extracellular matrix protein composed of three chains— α1 and α2 encoded by *COL6A1* (MIM #120220) and

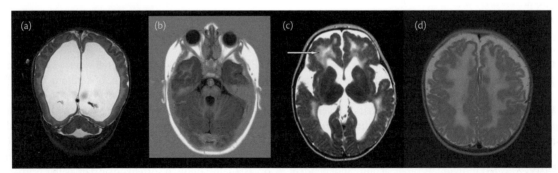

Fig. 24.3 Magnetic resonance imaging (MRI) brain changes in dystroglycanopathy patients (a–c). (a) Posterior inferior lissencephaly and dilated ventricles in a 4-week-old patient with Walker–Warburg syndrome. (b) T_1-weighted MRI brain scan of a 3-year-old patient with heterozygous *POMGNT1* mutations. Posterior cerebellar cysts are visible. Phenotypically this patient is at the milder end of the muscle-eye-brain disease (MEB) spectrum. (c) T_2-weighted MRI brain scan of an 8-month-old patient with typical MEB and heterozygous *POMGNT1* mutations. There is widespread bilateral polymicrogyria affecting predominantly the frontal and parietal lobes. White matter is reduced in volume with abnormally high signal intensity. Areas of lower signal intensity, mainly within the periventricular white matter (arrow), may represent heterotopic cells. (d) T_2 weighted MRI brain scan showing typical white matter changes seen in merosin-deficient congenital muscular dystrophy Type 1A.

COL6A2 (MIM #120240) and α3 encoded by the larger *COL6A3* (MIM #120250) [48–50]. The collagen chains undergo a complex assembly process, ultimately forming a microfibrillar network in the reticular layer of basement membranes [51,52]. Studies suggest that one of the main functions of collagen VI is in a structural role anchoring the basement membrane to the underlying connective tissue [53].

Both autosomal recessive and dominant mutations cause UCMD with approximately equal frequency [54,55]. It is characterized by neonatal onset, hypotonia, proximal muscle weakness, and contractures with distal joint laxity. Presenting features may also include congenital dislocation of the hip, torticollis, and kyphosis. Motor achievement is variable; some patients achieve independent ambulation but this is typically lost by the early teenage years. Functional motor ability is further compromised by the development of contractures, scoliosis, and spinal rigidity. Respiratory insufficiency requiring ventilatory support is almost invariable by the mid teenage years but cardiac abnormality is not a feature. Intelligence is normal. The development of characteristic skin changes including hyperkeratosis and abnormal scarring may facilitate the diagnosis [56]. CK is usually normal or mildly increased [21,46,55,57,58]. Muscle MRI changes are characteristic and include diffuse involvement of the thigh muscles with relative sparing of the anteromedial muscles (see Fig. 24.2) [59].

BM, usually an autosomal dominant entity, is a much milder disorder. It is a slowly progressive proximal myopathy with development of contractures of the wrists, elbows, ankles, and long finger flexors. Although the phenotype is milder than that of UCMD, BM patients may present in the first years of life, usually with hypotonia, torticollis, or congenital dislocation of the hip. Rarely, patients may develop respiratory insufficiency in later life [60,61]. Skin changes may be similar to those seen in UCMD. CK is normal or only mildly elevated [55]. Typical changes on muscle MRI include concentric muscle atrophy with peripheral involvement most evident in the vasti and gastrocnemii. There is often a characteristic 'central shadow' in the rectus femoris which may facilitate diagnosis (see Fig. 24.2) [59,62]. Patients may display an 'intermediate' phenotype, suggesting that BM and UCMD represent either end of a spectrum of collagen VI-related disorders [2].

Mutations in all three collagen VI genes cause BM and UCMD. The complex structure of collagen VI, the numerous polymorphisms in the three genes, and the high number of splice site mutations make mutation detection a lengthy task. RNA sequencing has become a commonly adopted strategy to overcome some of these obstacles [63]. Although there is often a positive family history in individuals with BM, *de novo* dominant *COL6* mutations are common.

Skeletal muscle biopsy in UCMD and BM may be dystrophic or myopathic. In BM, collagen VI immunohistochemistry is usually normal and therefore not of diagnostic use [58,64,65]. In UCMD, complete or partial depletion of collagen VI may be observed and hence facilitate a diagnosis. The analysis of fibroblasts derived from skin biopsies is a sensitive test of collagen VI abnormalities and has been used in diagnostic settings [20,21,51].

Dystroglycanopathies

The dystroglycanopathies are a heterogeneous group of autosomal recessive disorders characterized by hypoglycosylation of ADG on skeletal muscle biopsy. They include CMD variants with structural changes affecting the brain and eyes [Fukuyama CMD (FCMD; MIM #253800), muscle-eye-brain disease (MEB; MIM #253280),

WWS (MIM #236670)], as well as relatively milder forms, characterized by subtle or absent brain involvement and ranging in severity from CMD (MDC1C, MIM #606612; MDC1D, MIM #608840) to later-onset limb-girdle muscular dystrophy (LGMD) forms (LGMD2I, MIM #607155; LGMD2K, MIM #609308; LGMD2L, MIM #611307; and LGMD2M, MIM #611588) [2,66–69].

In an attempt to escape the pitfalls of eponymous syndromes in this group a new Online Mendelian Inheritance in Man (OMIM) classification has emerged, containing three broadly defined dystroglycanopathy groups. At the severe end of the spectrum lies muscular dystrophy–dystroglycanopathy A (MDDGA) defined as CMD with brain and eye abnormality, progressing to MDDGB defined as CMD with/without mental retardation, through to the milder end of the spectrum, MDDGC, defined as limb-girdle muscular dystrophy. These are further subdivided according to the gene involved. Whether or not this system will supersede the names given to the various conditions historically remains to be seen but it does provide a useful framework when considering this complex group of disorders [70].

Mutations in several genes give rise to dystroglycanopathy phenotypes. These include protein-*O*-mannosyl transferase 1 (*POMT1*; MIM #607423), protein-*O*-mannosyl transferase 2 (*POMT2*; MIM #607439), protein-*O*-mannose 1,2-*N*-acetylglucosaminyltransferase 1 (*POMGNT1*; MIM #606822), fukutin (*FKTN*; MIM #607440), fukutin-related protein (*FKRP*; MIM #606596), like-glycosyltransferase (*LARGE*; MIM #603590), isoprenoid synthase domain containing (*ISPD*; MIM #614631), glycosyltransferase-like domain-containing protein 2 (*GTDC2*; MIM #614828), transmembrane protein 5 (*TMEM5*; MIM #605862), β-1 ,3-*N*-acetylglucosaminyltransferase 1 (*B3GNT1*; MIM #605581), and dystroglycan associated glycoprotein 1 (*DAG1*; MIM #128239) [71–80]. Mutations in three further genes—dolichyl-phosphate mannosyltransferase polypeptide 3 (*DPM3*; MIM #605951), dolichyl-phosphate mannosyltransferase polypeptide 2 (*DPM2*; MIM #603564), and dolichol kinase (*DOLK*; MIM #601746) [81,82]—have been reported in conditions with features overlapping those of the dystroglycanopathies and congenital disorders of glycosylation [69].

The DGC is present along the sarcolemma of skeletal muscle fibres and contains a number of cytoplasmic, transmembrane, and extracellular matrix proteins (see Fig. 24.1) [83]. Central to the DGC are ADG and β dystroglycan (BDG), formed by post-translational cleavage of the dystroglycan peptide. The main function of the DGC in skeletal muscle is to confer structural stability to the sarcolemma during contraction and relaxation, acting as a 'shock absorber' protecting skeletal muscle from damage [84]. In the dystroglycanopathies, the common pathological feature is the finding of hypoglycosylation of ADG on skeletal muscle biopsy. The formation of the major *O*-linked mannose glycan on ADG involves the action of specific enzymes (glycosyltransferases) that add monosaccharides in a stepwise manner, a process that affects protein conformation and function [4,85]. Mutations in *DAG1*, encoding, the dystroglycan precursor protein, have been reported in a single case [80]. The remaining genes implicated in this group are putative or proven enzymes involved in the *O*-mannosylation of ADG [2]: POMT1 forms a complex with POMT2 that catalyses the first step in the assembly of the *O*-mannosyl glycan [76], whereas POMGNT1 is the second enzyme in the *O*-mannosylation process (Fig. 24.4). Mutations in these three genes interrupt the *O*-mannosylation pathway, resulting in hypoglycosylation of ADG. The precise function of FKTN, FKRP, LARGE, B3GNT1, GTDC2,

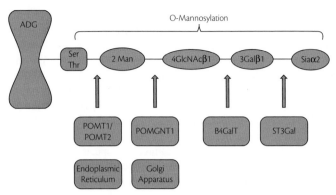

Fig. 24.4 Diagrammatic representation of the O-mannose-linked glycan attached to α-dystroglycan (ADG). Sugar residues are added in sequential order to the ADG backbone by the catalytic activity of glycosyltransferases. POMT1 and POMT2 act in the endoplasmic reticulum and catalyse the first step, the addition of mannose [80]. POMGNT1 catalyses the second step in the Golgi apparatus, the linkage of a N-acetylglucosamine residue to the mannose [73]. The functions of FKTN, FKRP, and LARGE have yet to be fully characterized.

TMEM5, and ISPD [78,86] in facilitating the glycosylation of ADG has yet to be elucidated [73,76,78,79,87–89].

Skeletal muscle biopsy in patients with dystroglycanopathies is usually dystrophic with a large proportion of fibres expressing neonatal myosin. A reduction in ADG on immunohistochemistry is apparent with normal expression of BDG [4]. Other features include a secondary reduction in labelling of laminin α2, although this is never absent as often seen in MDC1A [72]. In order to investigate the specific involvement of POMGNT1, POMT1, and POMT2, enzymatic activity can be studied in muscle biopsy samples, fibroblasts or Epstein–Barr virus-transformed lymphoblasts [87,90,91].

Dystroglycanopathy phenotypes

The dystroglycanopathies are a heterogeneous group of disorders with often uncertain boundaries; mutations in one gene may cause several phenotypes and some phenotypes may be caused by mutations in a number of different genes. Over 50% of dystroglycanopathy patients have no mutation in the known genes [92] and further heterogeneity is expected. However, several key phenotypes have been well described and are summarized in this section.

Walker–Warburg syndrome (MIM #236670)

This is a severe form of CMD with onset prenatally or at birth. Patients have structural brain abnormalities including complete agyria or severe 'cobblestone' lissencephaly, marked hydrocephalus, severe cerebellar involvement, and complete or partial absence of the corpus callosum. Eye abnormalities include congenital cataracts, microphthalmia, and buphthalmos. Motor development is minimal or absent and death before 1 year of age is usual [93].

The first gene identified in patients with WWS was POMT1, found to be mutated in 20% of a WWS patient cohort [74]. Mutations in POMT2, FKRP, FKTN, ISPD, GTDC2, B3GNT1, and TMEM5 were subsequently identified in WWS patients and, together with POMT1, are thought to account for more than a a third of patients with WWS [74,76,78,79,89,94–96].

Muscle–eye–brain disease (MIM #253280)

MEB is a CMD with brain abnormality less pronounced than that seen in WWS, originally reported in a Finnish population. MRI brain findings include cortical abnormalities including pachygyria and polymicrogyria, cerebellar abnormalities including hypoplasia, dysplasia, and cysts, and brainstem abnormalities. Structural eye involvement is a feature and may include congenital glaucoma, progressive myopia, retinal atrophy, and juvenile cataracts. Rarely, individuals may acquire the ability to walk, although this is delayed. Significant learning difficulties are expected, although patients occasionally manage to learn a few spoken words [93].

The first gene mutations were identified in POMGNT1 [73,97] with subsequent studies finding mutations also in FKRP and POMT2 [73,98,99].

Fukuyama congenital muscular dystrophy (MIM #253800)

FCMD is the second most frequent form of muscular dystrophy in Japan after Duchenne muscular dystrophy, due to the presence of a FKTN founder mutation within this population. Reports of the disease outside Japan are rare [100]. Affected children have generalized muscle weakness with marked motor delay. Pseudohypertrophy of the tongue, calves, and quadriceps muscles is common. Structural brain involvement includes cobblestone lissencephaly, white matter abnormalities, midbrain hypoplasia, and cerebellar abnormalities including polymicrogyria and cysts [26]. Mental retardation and seizures are common and respiratory failure in the mid-to-late teens is an invariable complication [71,101].

FCMD is due to mutations in FKTN with a common founder retrotransposal insertion found in more than 80% of FCMD chromosomes [71,102].

Congenital muscular dystrophy Type 1C (MDC1C; MIM #606612):

Mutations in FKRP are found in patients with MDC1C, a CMD characterized by pronounced muscle involvement with sparing of functional brain abnormality in most, but not all, cases [72]. Patients typically present in the first few months of life with hypotonia and weakness and do not acquire independent ambulation. Weakness is not particularly progressive but disability is compounded by the development of scoliosis and respiratory decline, usually necessitating non-invasive ventilation, in the second decade. Dilated cardiomyopathy is also a finding in some [72,99,103]. Limb-girdle muscular dystrophy Type 2I (LGMD2I; MIM #607155) is a milder condition allelic to MDC1C with variable severity [104,105].

Other dystroglycanopathy phenotypes

Other less common dystroglycanopathy phenotypes include congenital muscular dystrophy Type 1B (MDC1B; MIM #604801) linked to 1q42 [106], congenital muscular dystrophy Type 1D (MDC1D; MIM #608840) reported in a patient with mutations in the LARGE gene [75] and limb-girdle muscular dystrophy Type 2K (LGMD2K; MIM #609308), a condition found in the Turkish population, resulting from a founder mutation in POMT1 [67,107].

Congenital disorders of glycosylation

These include DPM3-related congenital disorder of glycosylation (CDG1O; MIM #612937), DPM2-related congenital disorder of glycosylation (CDG1u; MIM #615042), and DOLK-related congenital disorder of glycosylation (CDG1m; MIM #610768).

In 2009 Lefeber et al. [69] reported a patient presenting with mild muscular dystrophy, dilated cardiomyopathy, and stroke-like episodes with no associated brain or eye involvement. ADG immunoreactivity was reduced on skeletal muscle biopsy, consistent with a dystroglycanopathy, but transferrin isoelectric focusing studies in blood also revealed an abnormal transferrin profile, suggesting a congenital disorder of glycosylation. Mutation analysis subsequently revealed a homozygous mutation in *DPM3*, encoding one of three subunits in the Dol-P-Man synthase complex, a structure required for *N*-glycosylation, *C*-mannosylation, *O*-mannosylation, and glycosylphosphatidylinositol anchor formation, and a mutation would be expected to affect all four processes. It is speculated that *O*-mannosylation is more sensitive to the reduced binding capacity of DPM3 resulting from the reported mutation and consequently produces a phenotype that overlaps with that seen in dystroglycanopathy. Mutations in *DPM2*, another subunit of the Dol-P-Man synthase complex, were subsequently identified in siblings with CMD, severe mental retardation, microcephaly, myoclonic epilepsy, and cerebellar hypoplasia [82,108]. In 2011, Lefeber et al. [81] reported cases of CMD with cardiomyopathy, raised CK, and hypoglycosylation of ADG. Mutations in *DOLK* were found, a gene known to be mutated in patients with CDG1m. Prior to these reports, CDGs and dystroglycanopathies, although both disorders of glycosylation, were regarded as two separate disease entities.

Rigid spine muscular dystrophy

Mutations in selenoprotein N,1 (*SEPN1*; MIM #606210) give rise to four pathological phenotypes: rigid spine muscular dystrophy (RSMD1; MIM #602771), desmin-related myopathy with Mallory body-like inclusions (MB-DRM; MIM #602771), multiminicore disease (MmD, MIM #602771), and congenital fibre-type disproportion (CFTD MIM #255310). All are autosomal recessive conditions, and although RSMD1 is typically the only one considered a CMD they show considerable phenotypic overlap [30,109–112].

SEPN1 is a membrane bound glycoprotein, and whilst its specific function is unknown it is thought to have a role in early development and in protecting cells from oxidative stress damage [113,114]. Mutations in *SEPN1* have been found throughout the coding region, although homozygosity may be found even in individuals from non-consanguineous backgrounds due to the presence of founder mutations in European populations [30,109–112].

RSMD1 is characterized by early onset hypotonia and marked spinal rigidity. Weakness is classically axial, with head drop a finding in some. Facial and bulbar muscle weakness is frequently seen and palatal weakness with a nasal sounding voice is common. Patients often have a thin habitus. Respiratory involvement is prominent and disproportionate to the muscle weakness, which is often well preserved, with many patients remaining ambulant into adult life. Assisted nocturnal ventilation is usually required in childhood or early adolescence. Structural or functional brain involvement is not a feature of RSMD1. CK is usually normal or only mildly elevated [115,111,112,116,117]. Muscle MRI findings are characteristic, with prominent involvement of the sartorius and to a lesser degree adductors and biceps femoris (Fig. 24.2) [22].

The pathological changes in skeletal muscle biopsy of RSMD1 patients are not diagnostic. Muscle histology may show non-specific myopathic features, multiminicores or congenital fibre-type disproportion [117].

Congenital muscular dystrophies caused by mutations in nuclear envelope proteins

Mutations in the genes encoding the nuclear envelope proteins lamin A/C and nesprin-1 account for a relatively small number of reported cases of CMD. Lamins are structural proteins and have a function in determining nuclear shape and protecting the nuclear envelope from mechanical stress [118,119].

Autosomal dominant Emery–Dreifuss muscular dystrophy (EDMD2; MIM #181350) is one of a number of disorders caused by mutations in lamin A/C (*LMNA*; MIM #150330) [120] and whilst not usually viewed as a CMD, severe congenital cases have been reported. In these cases, onset of weakness may be prenatal with contractures evident at birth and early cardiorespiratory complications [13]. CK is normal or moderately elevated (two to twenty times the upper limit of normal). *LMNA* mutations have also been found in infants with a predominantly inflammatory myopathic appearance on muscle biopsy who later develop contractures and cardiac involvement [121].

Skeletal muscle biopsy is not diagnostic and shows non-specific myopathic or dystrophic changes. A predominance of Type 1 fibres may be present and structural changes such as cores may also be seen [3]. Electron microscopy may reveal specific alterations in nuclear architecture, including aggregation of chromatin. Immunostaining for lamins in EDMD2 muscle biopsies shows no detectable difference from normal controls, due to a functioning normal allele [122–124].

The distribution and type of *LMNA* mutations found in EDMD2 is variable with a large proportion of *de novo* events. Clinical heterogeneity may exist even between patients with the same mutation, suggesting that disease-modifying factors may be important in the pathogenesis of this group of conditions [120,125–129].

Mutations in *SYNE-1*, which encodes nesprin-1, give rise to a rare CMD variant with adducted thumbs, cerebellar hypoplasia, and cataracts [130].

Congenital muscular dystrophy due to integrin mutations

CMD due to integrin α7 deficiency (MIM #613204) is a rare form of CMD associated with mental retardation and mildly raised CK. It is due to mutations in the gene encoding integrin α7 (*ITGA7*; MIM #600536). Immunostaining of the skeletal muscle biopsy shows myopathic features with absent integrin α7 subunit and normal expression of laminin α2 [131,132].

Mutations in integrin α9 have been reported in a French-Canadian cohort with CMD and features overlapping those of the collagen VI disorders. In particular they had distal joint laxity, contractures, hypotonia, and a slowly progressive myopathy with mild to moderate respiratory impairment. Intelligence was usually normal and CK was normal or only mildly elevated [133,134].

Congenital muscular dystrophy caused by phosphatidylcholine biosynthesis abnormality

In a recent report from Japan, a defect in the gene encoding choline kinase beta (*CHKB*) has been identified in a group of patients with megaconial type CMD characterized by early onset muscle wasting, mental retardation, and enlarged mitochondria seen at the periphery of muscle fibres [135]. CHKB catalyses the first step in a biosynthetic pathway for phosphatidylcholine, a phospholipid prevalent in eukaryotes. This finding further expands the range of molecular pathologies known to give rise to CMD.

Treatment and potential therapeutic interventions

To date management of the CMDs has been mainly supportive. Interventions such as the introduction of non-invasive ventilation in subtypes with respiratory insufficiency have significantly improved life expectancy. Maximizing nutrition by ensuring appropriate caloric intake and gastrostomy insertion where indicated have also been important [117,136,137]. Other therapies, including physiotherapy and surgery for scoliosis and other orthopaedic complications, have also improved quality of life [138,139]. Standards of care for the CMDs have been recently summarized in a comprehensive consensus statement [140].

It has only been in recent years, with the improved knowledge and understanding of the molecular and genetic basis for this group of conditions, that a shift in direction towards trying to treat the underlying biochemical defects rather than physical symptoms has been possible. Several, largely disease-specific strategies, are currently being investigated. In the dystroglycanopathies research has focused on finding methods to enhance the glycosylation of ADG [141,142]. In the collagen VI-related disorders and MDC1A therapeutic strategies include searching for pharmacological agents capable of altering the pathological end point of myofibre apoptosis [143–148]. In RSMD1, research has shown the pathological importance of oxidative stress damage in patients with *SEPN1* mutations. Therapeutic agents that ameliorate this process, including *N*-acetylcysteine are currently being evaluated [114,149].

Conclusions and outlook

The term CMD encompasses a complex and heterogeneous group of disorders. Despite the progress made in understanding the molecular basis of CMD, approximately 50% of cases fulfilling the clinical and pathological diagnostic criteria for CMD remain without genetic diagnosis. This is probably due to the limitations of current mutation detection methods for known CMD genes and also that fact that there undoubtedly remain a number of CMD genes that have yet to be discovered. It is hoped, however, that the next decade will herald a turning point in CMD molecular diagnostics with the advent of technology including next-generation sequencing and collaborative neuromuscular disease screening projects.

Whilst much has been learnt over the last decade, further work is needed to refine the pathogenic mechanisms underlying these disorders in order to assist in the ultimate goal of achieving successful therapeutic intervention or cures for these devastating conditions.

Acknowledgements

The authors would like to acknowledge Professor Francesco Muntoni (Dubowitz Neuromuscular Centre, Institute of Child Health, London, UK) for providing MRI brain images and Professor Eugenio Mercuri (Institute of Neurology, Catholic University, Rome, Italy) for providing the MRI muscle images.

References

1. Mostacciuolo ML, Miorin M, Martinello F, Angelini C, Perini P, Trevisan CP. Genetic epidemiology of congenital muscular dystrophy in a sample from north-east Italy. *Hum Genet* 1996; **97**: 277–9.

2. Muntoni F, Voit T. The congenital muscular dystrophies in 2004: a century of exciting progress. *Neuromuscul Disord* 2004; **14**: 635–49.

3. Dubowitz V, Sewry CA. *Muscle Biopsy a Practical Approach*, 3rd edn. Philadelphia, PA: Saunders, 2007.

4. Jimenez-Mallebrera C, Brown SC, Sewry CA, Muntoni F. Congenital muscular dystrophy: molecular and cellular aspects. *Cell Mol Life Sci* 2005; **2**: 809–23.

5. Sanes JR. The basement membrane/basal lamina of skeletal muscle. *J Biol Chem* 2003; **278**: 12601–4.

6. Michele DE, Campbell KP. Dystrophin–glycoprotein complex: post-translational processing and dystroglycan function. *J Biol Chem* 2003; **278**: 15457–60.

7. Gerace L, Blum A, Blobel G. Immunocytochemical localization of the major polypeptides of the nuclear pore complex-lamina fraction. Interphase and mitotic distribution. *J Cell Biol* 1978; **79**: 546–66.

8. Burke B, Stewart CL. Life at the edge: the nuclear envelope and human disease. *Nat Rev Mol Cell Biol* 2002; **3**: 575–85.

9. Crisp M, Liu Q, Roux K, et al. Coupling of the nucleus and cytoplasm: role of the LINC complex. *J Cell Biol* 2006; **172**: 41–53.

10. Mercuri E, Poppe M, Quinlivan R, et al. Extreme variability of phenotype in patients with an identical missense mutation in the lamin A/C gene: from congenital onset with severe phenotype to milder classic Emery–Dreifuss variant. *Arch Neurol* 2004; **61**: 690–4.

11. Mahjneh I, Bushby K, Anderson L, et al. Merosin-positive congenital muscular dystrophy: a large inbred family. *Neuropediatrics* 1999; **30**: 22–8.

12. Muntoni F, Taylor J, Sewry CA, Naom I, Dubowitz V. An early onset muscular dystrophy with diaphragmatic involvement, early respiratory failure and secondary alpha2 laminin deficiency unlinked to the LAMA2 locus on 6q22. *Eur J Paediatr Neurol* 1998; **2**: 19–26.

13. Quijano-Roy S, Mbieleu B, Bonnemann CG, et al. *De novo* LMNA mutations cause a new form of congenital muscular dystrophy. *Ann Neurol* 2008; **64**: 177–86.

14. D'Amico A, Petrini S, Parisi F, et al. Heart transplantation in a child with LGMD2I presenting as isolated dilated cardiomyopathy. *Neuromuscul Disord* 2008; **18**: 153–5.

15. Murakami T, Hayashi YK, Noguchi S, et al. Fukutin gene mutations cause dilated cardiomyopathy with minimal muscle weakness. *Ann Neurol* 2006; **60**: 597–602.

16. Finsterer J, Ramaciotti C, Wang CH, et al. Cardiac findings in congenital muscular dystrophies. *Pediatrics* [review] 2010; **126**: 538–45.

17. Geranmayeh F, Clement E, Feng LH, et al. Genotype-phenotype correlation in a large population of muscular dystrophy patients with LAMA2 mutations. *Neuromuscul Disord* 2010; **20**: 241–50.

18. Jones KJ, Morgan G, Johnston H, et al. The expanding phenotype of laminin alpha2 chain (merosin) abnormalities: case series and review. *J Med Genet* 2001; **38**: 649–57.

19. Mercuri E, Muntoni F, Berardinelli A, et al. Somatosensory and visual evoked potentials in congenital muscular dystrophy: correlation with MRI changes and muscle merosin status. *Neuropediatrics* 1995; **26**: 3–7.

20. Jimenez-Mallebrera C, Maioli MA, Kim J, et al. A comparative analysis of collagen VI production in muscle, skin and fibroblasts from 14 Ullrich congenital muscular dystrophy patients with dominant and recessive COL6A mutations. *Neuromuscul Disord* 2006; **16**: 571–82.

21. Mercuri E, Yuva Y, Brown SC, et al. Collagen VI involvement in Ullrich syndrome: a clinical, genetic, and immunohistochemical study. *Neurology* 2002; **58**: 1354–9.

22. Mercuri E, Clements E, Offiah A, et al. Muscle magnetic resonance imaging involvement in muscular dystrophies with rigidity of the spine. *Ann Neurol* 2010; **67**: 201–8.

23. Astrea G, Schessl J, Clement E, et al. Muscle MRI in FHL1-linked reducing body myopathy. *Neuromuscul Disord* 2009; **19**: 689–91.

24. Quijano-Roy S, Marti-Carrera I, Makri S, et al. Brain MRI abnormalities in muscular dystrophy due to FKRP mutations. *Brain Dev* 2006; **28**: 232–42.

25. Philpot J, Cowan F, Pennock J, et al. Merosin-deficient muscular dystrophy: the spectrum of brain involvement on magnetic resonance imaging. *Neuromuscul Disord.* 1999; **9**: 81–5.

26. Clement E, Mercuri E, Godfrey C, et al. Brain involvement in muscular dystrophies with defective dystroglycan glycosylation. *Ann Neurol* 2008; **64**: 573–82.

27. Longman C, Mercuri E, Cowan F, et al. Antenatal and postnatal brain magnetic resonance imaging in muscle-eye-brain disease. *Arch Neurol* 2004; **61**: 1301–6.

28. Shorer Z, Philpot J, Muntoni F, Sewry C, Dubowitz V. Demyelinating peripheral neuropathy in merosin-deficient congenital muscular dystrophy. *J Child Neurol* 1995; **10**: 472–5.

29. Klein A, Clement E, Mercuri E, Muntoni F. Differential diagnosis of congenital muscular dystrophies. *Eur J Paediatr Neurol* 2008; **12**: 371–7.

30. Ferreiro A, Quijano-Roy S, Pichereau C, et al. Mutations of the selenoprotein N gene, which is implicated in rigid spine muscular dystrophy, cause the classical phenotype of multiminicore disease: reassessing the nosology of early-onset myopathies. *Am J Hum Genet* 2002; **71**: 739–49.

31. Jungbluth H, Sewry CA, Muntoni F. Core myopathies. *Semin Pediatr Neurol* 2011; **18**: 239–49.

32. Romero NB, Monnier N, Viollet L, et al. Dominant and recessive central core disease associated with RYR1 mutations and fetal akinesia. *Brain* 2003; **126**: 2341–9.

33. Hillaire D, Leclerc A, Faure S, et al. Localization of merosin-negative congenital muscular dystrophy to chromosome 6q2 by homozygosity mapping. *Hum Mol Genet* 1994; **3**: 1657–61.

34. Helbling-Leclerc A, Zhang X, Topaloglu H, et al. Mutations in the laminin alpha 2-chain gene (LAMA2) cause merosin-deficient congenital muscular dystrophy. *Nat Genet* 1995; **11**: 216–18.

35. Tome FM, Evangelista T, Leclerc A, et al. Congenital muscular dystrophy with merosin deficiency. *C R Acad Sci III* 1994; **317**: 351–7.

36. Hayashi YK, Tezak Z, Momoi T, et al. Massive muscle cell degeneration in the early stage of merosin-deficient congenital muscular dystrophy. *Neuromuscul Disord* 2001; **11**: 350–9.

37. Philpot J, Sewry C, Pennock J, Dubowitz V. Clinical phenotype in congenital muscular dystrophy: correlation with expression of merosin in skeletal muscle. *Neuromuscul Disord* 1995; **5**: 301–5.

38. Vainzof M, Marie SK, Reed UC, et al. Deficiency of merosin (laminin M or alpha 2) in congenital muscular dystrophy associated with cerebral white matter alterations. *Neuropediatrics* 1995; **26**: 293–7.

39. Dubowitz DJ, Tyszka JM, Sewry CA, Moats RA, Scadeng M, Dubowitz V. High resolution magnetic resonance imaging of the brain in the dy/dy mouse with merosin-deficient congenital muscular dystrophy. *Neuromuscul Disord* 2000; **10**: 292–8.

40. Matsumura K, Yamada H, Saito F, Sunada Y, Shimizu T. Peripheral nerve involvement in merosin-deficient congenital muscular dystrophy and dy mouse. *Neuromuscul Disord* 1997; **7**: 7–12.

41. Talts JF, Timpl R. Mutation of a basic sequence in the laminin alpha2LG3 module leads to a lack of proteolytic processing and has different effects on beta1 integrin-mediated cell adhesion and alpha-dystroglycan binding. *FEBS Lett* 1999; **458**: 319–23.

42. Nissinen M, Helbling-Leclerc A, Zhang X, et al. Substitution of a conserved cysteine-996 in a cysteine-rich motif of the laminin alpha2-chain in congenital muscular dystrophy with partial deficiency of the protein. *Am J Hum Genet* 1996; **58**: 1177–84.

43. Guicheney P, Vignier N, Zhang X, et al. PCR based mutation screening of the laminin alpha2 chain gene (LAMA2): application to prenatal diagnosis and search for founder effects in congenital muscular dystrophy. *J Med Genet* 1998; **35**: 211–17.

44. Pegoraro E, Marks H, Garcia CA, et al. Laminin alpha2 muscular dystrophy: genotype/phenotype studies of 22 patients. *Neurology* 1998; **51**: 101–10.

45. Muntoni F, Guicheney P. 85th ENMC International Workshop on Congenital Muscular Dystrophy. 6th International CMD Workshop. 1st Workshop of the Myo-Cluster Project 'GENRE'. 27–28th October 2000, Naarden, The Netherlands. *Neuromuscul Disord* 2002; **12**: 69–78.

46. Ullrich O. Kongenitale, atonisch-sklerotische Muskeldystrophie. *Monatsschr Kinderheilkd* 1930; **47**: 502–10.

47. Camacho Vanegas O, Bertini E, Zhang RZ, et al. Ullrich scleroatonic muscular dystrophy is caused by recessive mutations in collagen type VI. *Proc Natl Acad Sci USA* 2001; **98**: 7516–21.

48. Hessle H, Engvall E. Type VI collagen. Studies on its localization, structure, and biosynthetic form with monoclonal antibodies. *J Biol Chem* 1984; **259**: 3955–61.

49. von der Mark H, Aumailley M, Wick G, Fleischmajer R, Timpl R. Immunochemistry, genuine size and tissue localization of collagen VI. *Eur J Biochem* 1984; **142**: 493–502.

50. Bruns RR. Beaded filaments and long-spacing fibrils: relation to type VI collagen. *J Ultrastruct Res* 1984; **89**: 136–45.

51. Zhang RZ, Sabatelli P, Pan TC, et al. Effects on collagen VI mRNA stability and microfibrillar assembly of three COL6A2 mutations in two families with Ullrich congenital muscular dystrophy. *J Biol Chem* 2002; **277**: 43557–64.

52. Engvall E, Hessle H, Klier G. Molecular assembly, secretion, and matrix deposition of type VI collagen. *J Cell Biol* 1986; **102**: 703–10.

53. Kuo HJ, Maslen CL, Keene DR, Glanville RW. Type VI collagen anchors endothelial basement membranes by interacting with type IV collagen. *J Biol Chem* 1997; **272**: 26522–9.

54. Baker NL, Morgelin M, Peat R, et al. Dominant collagen VI mutations are a common cause of Ullrich congenital muscular dystrophy. *Hum Mol Genet* 2005; **14**: 279–93.

55. Lampe AK, Bushby KM. Collagen VI related muscle disorders. *J Med Genet* 2005; **42**: 673–85.

56. Nadeau A, Muntoni F. Skin changes in Ullrich congenital muscular dystrophy [case report]. *Neuromuscul Disord* 2008; **18**: 982.

57. Voit T. Congenital muscular dystrophies: 1997 update. *Brain Dev* 1998; **20**: 65–74.

58. Muntoni F, Bertini E, Bonnemann C, et al. 98th ENMC International Workshop on Congenital Muscular Dystrophy (CMD), 7th Workshop of the International Consortium on CMD, 2nd Workshop of the MYO CLUSTER project GENRE. 26–28th October, 2001, Naarden, The Netherlands. *Neuromuscul Disord* 2002; **12**: 889–96.

59. Mercuri E, Lampe A, Allsop J, et al. Muscle MRI in Ullrich congenital muscular dystrophy and Bethlem myopathy. *Neuromuscul Disord* 2005; **15**: 303–10.

60. Pepe G, Bertini E, Bonaldo P, et al. Bethlem myopathy (BETHLEM) and Ullrich scleroatonic muscular dystrophy: 100th ENMC international workshop, 23–24 November 2001, Naarden, The Netherlands. *Neuromuscul Disord* 2002; **12**: 984–93.

61. Haq RU, Speer MC, Chu ML, Tandan R. Respiratory muscle involvement in Bethlem myopathy. *Neurology* 1999; **52**: 174–6.

62. Mercuri E, Cini C, Counsell S, et al. Muscle MRI findings in a three-generation family affected by Bethlem myopathy. *Eur J Paediatr Neurol* 2002; **6**: 309–14.

63. Lampe AK, Dunn DM, von Niederhausern AC, et al. Automated genomic sequence analysis of the three collagen VI genes: applications to Ullrich congenital muscular dystrophy and Bethlem myopathy. *J Med Genet* 2005; **42**: 108–20.

64. Pepe G, de Visser M, Bertini E, et al. Bethlem myopathy (BETHLEM) 86th ENMC international workshop, 10–11 November 2000, Naarden, The Netherlands. *Neuromuscul Disord* 2002; **12**: 296–305.

65. Higuchi I, Suehara M, Iwaki H, Nakagawa M, Arimura K, Osame M. Collagen VI deficiency in Ullrich's disease. *Ann Neurol* 2001; **49**: 544.

66. Muntoni F, Brockington M, Torelli S, Brown SC. Defective glycosylation in congenital muscular dystrophies. *Curr Opin Neurol* 2004; **17**: 205–9.

67. Balci B, Uyanik G, Dincer P, et al. An autosomal recessive limb girdle muscular dystrophy (LGMD2) with mild mental retardation is allelic to Walker–Warburg syndrome (WWS) caused by a mutation in the POMT1 gene. *Neuromuscul Disord* 2005; **15**: 271–5.

68. Godfrey C, Escolar D, Brockington M, et al. Fukutin gene mutations in steroid-responsive limb girdle muscular dystrophy. *Ann Neurol* 2006; **60**: 603–10.

69. Lefeber DJ, Schonberger J, Morava E, et al. Deficiency of Dol-P-Man synthase subunit DPM3 bridges the congenital disorders of glycosylation with the dystroglycanopathies. *Am J Hum Genet* 2009; **85**: 76–86.

70. Godfrey C, Foley AR, Clement E, Muntoni F. Dystroglycanopathies: coming into focus. *Curr Opin Genet Dev* 2011; **21**: 278–85.

71. Kobayashi K, Nakahori Y, Miyake M, et al. An ancient retrotransposal insertion causes Fukuyama-type congenital muscular dystrophy. *Nature* 1998; **394**: 388–92.

72. Brockington M, Blake DJ, Prandini P, et al. Mutations in the fukutin-related protein gene (FKRP) cause a form of congenital muscular dystrophy with secondary laminin alpha2 deficiency and abnormal glycosylation of alpha-dystroglycan. *Am J Hum Genet* 2001; **69**: 1198–209.

73. Yoshida A, Kobayashi K, Manya H, et al. Muscular dystrophy and neuronal migration disorder caused by mutations in a glycosyltransferase, POMGnT1. *Dev Cell* 2001; **1**: 717–24.

74. Beltran-Valero de Bernabe D, Currier S, Steinbrecher A, et al. Mutations in the O-mannosyltransferase gene POMT1 give rise to the severe neuronal migration disorder Walker–Warburg syndrome. *Am J Hum Genet* 2002; **71**: 1033–43.

75. Longman C, Brockington M, Torelli S, et al. Mutations in the human LARGE gene cause MDC1D, a novel form of congenital muscular dystrophy with severe mental retardation and abnormal glycosylation of alpha-dystroglycan. *Hum Mol Genet* 2003; **12**: 2853–61.

76. van Reeuwijk J, Janssen M, van den Elzen C, et al. POMT2 mutations cause alpha-dystroglycan hypoglycosylation and Walker–Warburg syndrome. *J Med Genet* 2005; **42**: 907–12.

77. Willer T, Lee H, Lommel M, et al. ISPD loss-of-function mutations disrupt dystroglycan O-mannosylation and cause Walker–Warburg syndrome. *Nat Genet* 2012; **44**: 575–80.

78. Manzini MC, Tambunan DE, Hill RS, et al. Exome sequencing and functional validation in zebrafish identify GTDC2 mutations as a cause of Walker–Warburg syndrome. *Am J Hum Genet* 2012; **91**: 541–7.

79. Vuillaumier-Barrot S, Bouchet-Seraphin C, Chelbi M, et al. Identification of mutations in TMEM5 and ISPD as a cause of severe cobblestone lissencephaly. *Am J Hum Genet* 2012; **91**: 1135–43.

80. Hara Y, Balci-Hayta B, Yoshida-Moriguchi T, et al. A dystroglycan mutation associated with limb-girdle muscular dystrophy. *N Engl J Med* 2011; **364**: 939–46.

81. Lefeber DJ, de Brouwer AP, Morava E, et al. Autosomal recessive dilated cardiomyopathy due to DOLK mutations results from abnormal dystroglycan O-mannosylation. *PLoS Genet* 2011; **7**: e1002427.

82. Barone R, Aiello C, Race V, et al. DPM2-CDG: a muscular dystrophy-dystroglycanopathy syndrome with severe epilepsy. *Ann Neurol* 2012; **72**: 550–8.

83. Ervasti JM, Campbell KP. Membrane organization of the dystrophin-glycoprotein complex. *Cell* 1991; **66**: 1121–31.

84. Petrof BJ, Shrager JB, Stedman HH, Kelly AM, Sweeney HL. Dystrophin protects the sarcolemma from stresses developed during muscle contraction. *Proc Natl Acad Sci USA* 1993; **90**: 3710–14.

85. Chiba A, Matsumura K, Yamada H, et al. Structures of sialylated O-linked oligosaccharides of bovine peripheral nerve alpha-dystroglycan. The role of a novel O-mannosyl-type oligosaccharide in the binding of alpha-dystroglycan with laminin. *J Biol Chem* 1997; **272**: 2156–62.

86. Cirak S, Foley AR, Herrmann R, et al. ISPD gene mutations are a common cause of congenital and limb-girdle muscular dystrophies. *Brain* 2013; **136**: 269–81.

87. Manya H, Chiba A, Yoshida A, et al. Demonstration of mammalian protein O-mannosyltransferase activity: coexpression of POMT1 and POMT2 required for enzymatic activity. *Proc Natl Acad Sci USA* 2004; **101**: 500–5.

88. Willer T, Amselgruber W, Deutzmann R, Strahl S. Characterization of POMT2, a novel member of the PMT protein O-mannosyltransferase family specifically localized to the acrosome of mammalian spermatids. *Glycobiology* 2002; **12**: 771–83.

89. Buysse K, Riemersma M, Powell G, et al. Missense mutations in beta-1,3-N-acetylglucosaminyltransferase 1 (B3GNT1) cause Walker–Warburg syndrome. *Hum Mol Genet* 2013; **22**: 1746–54.

90. Zhang W, Vajsar J, Cao P, et al. Enzymatic diagnostic test for muscle-eye–brain type congenital muscular dystrophy using commercially available reagents. *Clin Biochem* 2003; **36**: 339–44.

91. Vajsar J, Zhang W, Dobyns WB, et al. Carriers and patients with muscle–eye–brain disease can be rapidly diagnosed by enzymatic analysis of fibroblasts and lymphoblasts. *Neuromuscul Disord* 2006; **16**: 132–6.

92. Godfrey C, Clement E, Mein R, et al. Refining genotype phenotype correlations in muscular dystrophies with defective glycosylation of dystroglycan. *Brain* 2007; **130**: 2725–35.

93. Cormand B, Pihko H, Bayes M, et al. Clinical and genetic distinction between Walker–Warburg syndrome and muscle–eye–brain disease. *Neurology* 2001; **56**: 1059–69.

94. Beltran-Valero de Bernabe D, Voit T, Longman C, et al. Mutations in the FKRP gene can cause muscle–eye–brain disease and Walker–Warburg syndrome. *J Med Genet*. 2004; **41**(5): e61.

95. de Bernabe DB, van Bokhoven H, van Beusekom E, et al. A homozygous nonsense mutation in the fukutin gene causes a Walker–Warburg syndrome phenotype. *J Med Genet* 2003; **40**: 845–8.

96. Roscioli T, Kamsteeg EJ, Buysse K, et al. Mutations in ISPD cause Walker–Warburg syndrome and defective glycosylation of alpha-dystroglycan. *Nat Genet* 2012; **44**: 581–5.

97. Cormand B, Avela K, Pihko H, et al. Assignment of the muscle-eye-brain disease gene to 1p32-p34 by linkage analysis and homozygosity mapping. *Am J Hum Genet* 1999; **64**: 126–35.

98. Mercuri E, D'Amico A, Tessa A, et al. POMT2 mutation in a patient with 'MEB-like' phenotype. *Neuromuscul Disord* 2006; **16**: 446–8.

99. Topaloglu H, Brockington M, Yuva Y, et al. FKRP gene mutations cause congenital muscular dystrophy, mental retardation, and cerebellar cysts. *Neurology* 2003; **60**: 988–92.

100. Fukuyama Y KM, Haruna H. A peculiar form of congenital progressive muscular dystrophy: report of fifteen cases. *Paediat Univ Tokyo* 1960; **4**: 5–8.

101. Toda T, Kobayashi K, Kondo-Iida E, Sasaki J, Nakamura Y. The Fukuyama congenital muscular dystrophy story. *Neuromuscul Disord* 2000; **10**: 153–9.

102. Toda T, Segawa M, Nomura Y, et al. Localization of a gene for Fukuyama type congenital muscular dystrophy to chromosome 9q31–33. *Nat Genet* 1993; **5**: 283–6.

103. Mercuri E, Sewry CA, Brown SC, et al. Congenital muscular dystrophy with secondary merosin deficiency and normal brain MRI: a novel entity? *Neuropediatrics* 2000; **31**: 186–9.

104. Brockington M, Yuva Y, Prandini P, et al. Mutations in the fukutin-related protein gene (FKRP) identify limb girdle muscular dystrophy 2I as a milder allelic variant of congenital muscular dystrophy MDC1C. *Hum Mol Genet* 2001; **10**: 2851–9.

105. Mercuri E, Brockington M, Straub V, et al. Phenotypic spectrum associated with mutations in the fukutin-related protein gene. *Ann Neurol* 2003; **53**: 537–42.

106. Brockington M, Sewry CA, Herrmann R, et al. Assignment of a form of congenital muscular dystrophy with secondary merosin deficiency to chromosome 1q42. *Am J Hum Genet* 2000; **66**: 428–35.

107. Dincer P, Balci B, Yuva Y, et al. A novel form of recessive limb girdle muscular dystrophy with mental retardation and abnormal expression of alpha-dystroglycan. *Neuromuscul Disord* 2003; **13**: 771–8.

108. Messina S, Tortorella G, Concolino D, et al. Congenital muscular dystrophy with defective alpha-dystroglycan, cerebellar hypoplasia, and epilepsy. *Neurology* 2009; **73**: 1599–601.

109. Clarke NF, Kidson W, Quijano-Roy S, et al. SEPN1: associated with congenital fiber-type disproportion and insulin resistance. *Ann Neurol* 2006; **59**: 546–52.

110. Ferreiro A, Ceuterick-de Groote C, Marks JJ, et al. Desmin-related myopathy with Mallory body-like inclusions is caused by mutations of the selenoprotein N gene. *Ann Neurol* 2004; **55**: 676–86.

111. Moghadaszadeh B, Petit N, Jaillard C, et al. Mutations in SEPN1 cause congenital muscular dystrophy with spinal rigidity and restrictive respiratory syndrome. *Nat Genet* 2001; **29**: 17–18.

112. Flanigan KM, Kerr L, Bromberg MB, et al. Congenital muscular dystrophy with rigid spine syndrome: a clinical, pathological, radiological, and genetic study. *Ann Neurol* 2000; **47**: 152–61.

113. Petit N, Lescure A, Rederstorff M, et al. Selenoprotein N: an endoplasmic reticulum glycoprotein with an early developmental expression pattern. *Hum Mol Genet* 2003; **12**: 1045–53.

114. Arbogast S, Beuvin M, Fraysse B, Zhou H, Muntoni F, Ferreiro A. Oxidative stress in SEPN1-related myopathy: from pathophysiology to treatment. *Ann Neurol* 2009; **65**: 677–86.

115. Dubowitz V. Rigid spine syndrome: a muscle syndrome in search of a name. *Proc R Soc Med* 1973; **66**: 219–20.

116. D'Amico A, Haliloglu G, Richard P, et al. Two patients with 'Dropped head syndrome' due to mutations in LMNA or SEPN1 genes. *Neuromuscul Disord* 2005; **15**: 521–4.

117. Schara U, Kress W, Bonnemann CG, et al. The phenotype and long-term follow-up in 11 patients with juvenile selenoprotein N1-related myopathy. *Eur J Paediatr Neurol* 2008; **12**: 224–30.

118. Fisher DZ, Chaudhary N, Blobel G. cDNA sequencing of nuclear lamins A and C reveals primary and secondary structural homology to intermediate filament proteins. *Proc Natl Acad Sci USA* 1986; **83**: 6450–4.

119. Dahl KN, Kahn SM, Wilson KL, Discher DE. The nuclear envelope lamina network has elasticity and a compressibility limit suggestive of a molecular shock absorber. *J Cell Sci* 2004; **117**: 4779–86.

120. Bonne G, Di Barletta MR, Varnous S, et al. Mutations in the gene encoding lamin A/C cause autosomal dominant Emery–Dreifuss muscular dystrophy. *Nat Genet* 1999; **21**: 285–8.

121. Komaki H, Hayashi YK, Tsuburaya R, et al. Inflammatory changes in infantile-onset LMNA-associated myopathy. *Neuromuscul Disord* 2011; **21**: 563–8.

122. Fidzianska A, Toniolo D, Hausmanowa-Petrusewicz I. Ultrastructural abnormality of sarcolemmal nuclei in Emery–Dreifuss muscular dystrophy (EDMD). *J Neurol Sci* 1998; **159**: 88–93.

123. Sewry CA, Brown SC, Mercuri E, et al. Skeletal muscle pathology in autosomal dominant Emery–Dreifuss muscular dystrophy with lamin A/C mutations. *Neuropathol Appl Neurobiol* 2001; **27**: 281–90.

124. Fidzianska A, Hausmanowa-Petrusewicz I. Architectural abnormalities in muscle nuclei. Ultrastructural differences between X-linked and autosomal dominant forms of EDMD. *J Neurol Sci* 2003; **210**: 47–51.

125. Brown SC, Piercy RJ, Muntoni F, Sewry CA. Investigating the pathology of Emery–Dreifuss muscular dystrophy. *Biochem Soc Trans* 2008; **36**: 1335–8.

126. Bonne G, Yaou RB, Beroud C, et al. 108th ENMC International Workshop, 3rd Workshop of the MYO-CLUSTER project: EUROMEN, 7th International Emery-Dreifuss Muscular Dystrophy (EDMD) Workshop, 13–15 September 2002, Naarden, The Netherlands. *Neuromuscul Disord* 2003; **13**: 508–15.

127. Bonne G, Mercuri E, Muchir A, et al. Clinical and molecular genetic spectrum of autosomal dominant Emery–Dreifuss muscular dystrophy due to mutations of the lamin A/C gene. *Ann Neurol* 2000; **48**: 170–80.

128. Vytopil M, Benedetti S, Ricci E, et al. Mutation analysis of the lamin A/C gene (LMNA) among patients with different cardiomuscular phenotypes. *J Med Genet* 2003; **40**(12): e132.

129. Krimm I, Ostlund C, Gilquin B, et al. The Ig-like structure of the C-terminal domain of lamin A/C, mutated in muscular dystrophies, cardiomyopathy, and partial lipodystrophy. *Structure* 2002; **10**: 811–23.

130. Voit T, Cirak S, Abraham S, et al. Congenital muscular dystrophy with adducted thumbs, mental retardation, cerebellar hypoplasia and cataracts is caused by mutation of Enaptin (Nesprin-1): The third nuclear enveloplathy with muscular dystrophy. *Neuromuscul Disord* 2007; **17**: 833–4.

131. Hayashi YK, Chou FL, Engvall E, et al. Mutations in the integrin alpha7 gene cause congenital myopathy. *Nat Genet* 1998; **19**: 94–7.

132. Vachon PH, Xu H, Liu L, et al. Integrins (alpha7beta1) in muscle function and survival. Disrupted expression in merosin-deficient congenital muscular dystrophy. *J Clin Invest* 1997; **100**: 1870–81.

133. Tetreault M, Thiffault I, Loisel L, et al. Mutations in the Integrin responsible for a congenital muscular dystrophy with hyperlaxity and their impact on normal cellular adhesion [abstract]. Presented at the 59th Annual Meeting of The American Society of Human Genetics, Honolulu, Hawaii, 20–24 October 2009.

134. Tetreault M, Duquette A, Thiffault I, et al. A new form of congenital muscular dystrophy with joint hyperlaxity maps to 3p23–21. *Brain* 2006; **129**: 2077–84.

135. Mitsuhashi S, Ohkuma A, Talim B, et al. A congenital muscular dystrophy with mitochondrial structural abnormalities caused by defective de novo phosphatidylcholine biosynthesis. *Am J Hum Genet* 2011; **88**: 845–51.

136. Nadeau A, Kinali M, Main M, et al. Natural history of Ullrich congenital muscular dystrophy. *Neurology* 2009; **73**: 25–31.

137. Ramelli GP, Aloysius A, King C, Davis T, Muntoni F. Gastrostomy placement in paediatric patients with neuromuscular disorders: indications and outcome. *Dev Med Child Neurol* 2007; **49**: 367–71.

138. Merlini L, Bernardi P. Therapy of collagen VI-related myopathies (Bethlem and Ullrich). *Neurotherapeutics* 2008; **5**: 613–18.

139. Takaso M, Nakazawa T, Imura T, et al. Surgical correction of spinal deformity in patients with congenital muscular dystrophy. *J Orthop Sci* 2010; **15**: 493–501.

140. Wang CH, Bonnemann CG, Rutkowski A, et al. Consensus statement on standard of care for congenital muscular dystrophies. *J Child Neurol* 2010; **25**: 1559–81.

141. Barresi R, Michele DE, Kanagawa M, et al. LARGE can functionally bypass alpha-dystroglycan glycosylation defects in distinct congenital muscular dystrophies. *Nat Med* 2004; **10**: 696–703.

142. Xia B, Martin PT. Modulation of agrin binding and activity by the CT and related carbohydrate antigens. *Mol Cell Neurosci* 2002; **19**: 539–51.

143. Merlini L, Angelin A, Tiepolo T, et al. Cyclosporin A corrects mitochondrial dysfunction and muscle apoptosis in patients with collagen VI myopathies. *Proc Natl Acad Sci USA* 2008; **105**: 5225–9.

144. Tiepolo T, Angelin A, Palma E, et al. The cyclophilin inhibitor Debio 025 normalizes mitochondrial function, muscle apoptosis and ultrastructural defects in Col6a1−/− myopathic mice. *Br J Pharmacol* 2009; **157**: 1045–52.

145. Irwin WA, Bergamin N, Sabatelli P, et al. Mitochondrial dysfunction and apoptosis in myopathic mice with collagen VI deficiency. *Nat Genet* 2003; **35**: 367–71.

146. Dominov JA, Kravetz AJ, Ardelt M, Kostek CA, Beermann ML, Miller JB. Muscle-specific BCL2 expression ameliorates muscle disease in laminin {alpha}2-deficient, but not in dystrophin-deficient, mice. *Hum Mol Genet* 2005; **14**: 1029–40.

147. Erb M, Meinen S, Barzaghi P, et al. Omigapil ameliorates the pathology of muscle dystrophy caused by laminin-alpha2 deficiency. *J Pharmacol Exp Ther* 2009; **331**: 787–95.

148. Girgenrath M, Beermann ML, Vishnudas VK, Homma S, Miller JB. Pathology is alleviated by doxycycline in a laminin-alpha2-null model of congenital muscular dystrophy. *Ann Neurol* 2009; **65**: 47–56.

149. Collins J, Bonnemann CG. Congenital muscular dystrophies: toward molecular therapeutic interventions. *Curr Neurol Neurosci Rep* 2010; **10**: 83–91.

CHAPTER 25

The myotonic dystrophies

Chris Turner and David Hilton-Jones

Introduction

The myotonic dystrophies Type 1 and Type 2 (DM1 and DM2) are progressive multisystem autosomal dominant disorders with several clinical and molecular genetic features in common. DM1 is the most common form of adult-onset muscular dystrophy, whereas DM2 is less common and is associated with a milder phenotype. Both are typical examples of unstable nucleotide repeat expansion disorders.

The molecular basis of DM1 and DM2

The mutation in DM1 is an expansion of an unstable trinucleotide (CTG) repeat sequence in an untranslated, but transcribed, portion of the 3' untranslated region (UTR) of the myotonic dystrophy protein kinase (*DMPK*) gene. There is little evidence that the mutant *DMPK* allele causes haploinsufficiency by a reduction in normal *DMPK* allele mRNA/protein levels or function. The *DMPK* mutation may alter the expression of adjacent genes [1], in particular *DMWD* and *SIX5* (Fig. 25.1). However, there is increasing evidence that the transcribed *DMPK* mRNA is directly toxic and results in abnormal splicing of other mRNA transcripts, such as the muscle chloride ion channel, *CLCN1*, resulting in myotonia [2]. Abnormal mRNA splicing may occur by the accumulation of splicing factors within ribonuclear accumulations of mutant *DMPK* or by mutant *DMPK* affecting splicing factors within the nucleus independent of the ribonuclear inclusions [3].

DM2 is also an autosomal dominant disorder, caused by a mutation in the *ZNF9* gene on chromosome 3q21. As in DM1, the mutation lies in an untranslated part of the gene. The first intron in ZNF9 contains a complex repeat motif $(TG)_n(TCTG)_n(CCTG)_n$. Expansion of the CCTG repeat causes DM2 [4]. A similar molecular mechanism of widespread cellular abnormalities of mRNA splicing has also been proposed for DM2. Figure 25.1 summarizes the molecular mechanisms of DM1 and DM2.

Myotonic dystrophy Type 1

Epidemiology

DM1 has a prevalence of between 3 and 15 per 100 000 [6]. Founder effects may have increased the prevalence in specific regions, such as Quebec, where the incidence rises to 1 in 500 [7].

Genetics

The *DMPK* gene codes for a myosin kinase expressed in skeletal muscle—'myotonin protein kinase' (Fig. 25.2). The gene is located on chromosome 19q13.3 [8]. An expansion of an unstable trinucleotide (CTG) repeat sequence in an untranslated, but transcribed, portion of the 3′UTR causes DM1. Normal individuals have between 5 and 37 CTG repeats. Patients with between 38 and 49 CTG repeats (the 'premutation allele') are asymptomatic but are at risk of having children with larger repeats caused by intergenerational repeat expansion due to anticipation [9]. These patients are rarely seen in everyday clinical practice. Fully penetrant alleles occur with repeats greater than CTG_{50}. Polymerase chain reaction (PCR) analysis is used to detect repeat lengths of less than 100 and Southern blot analysis to detect larger expansions. Allele sizes were established by the Second International Myotonic Dystrophy Consortium (IDMC) in 1999 [10]. Predictive testing in asymptomatic relatives as well as antenatal and preimplantation diagnosis can be performed.

DM1 demonstrates genetic 'anticipation'—increasing disease severity and decreasing age of onset in successive generations. However, the situation in DM1 is more complex. The molecular basis of anticipation is that the repeat expansion is unstable in meiosis and the child inherits a larger expansion than is present somatically in the parent. The inheritance of a very large expansion leads to 'congenital' DM1. This is not just of earlier onset than in the parent but, as noted in the section Congenital DM1, is associated with very specific clinical features, including substantial learning difficulties and cognitive problems, which are not a major early feature in 'adult' DM1. Conversely, in most cases the early onset is not associated with particularly severe weakness and myotonia is not an early feature [11,12]. A child with congenital DM1 almost always inherits the expanded mutant *DMPK* allele from its mother, in contrast to other triplet repeat disorders where anticipation tends to occur through the paternal lineage, e.g. Huntington disease. Paternal inheritance of congenital DM1 has been described, but is extremely rare [13]. It is postulated that in DM1 very large CTG expansions are toxic to developing sperm, or negatively select against sperm, whereas oocytes are unaffected by the large expansion. Congenital DM1 occurs when a mother with a moderate sized expansion passes on a very large expansion to the fetus (see Fig. 25.3). For smaller parental expansions, the increase in size of the expansion on transmission tends to be greater when the father is the transmitting parent (see Fig. 25.4), but this rarely leads to congenital DM1 [14,15]. The pattern and severity of anticipation are therefore dependent on the size of the repeat and the sex of the parent transmitting the mutation—all of which greatly complicates genetic counselling—added to which there is only a broad correlation between expansion size in leucocyte DNA with clinical pattern and severity.

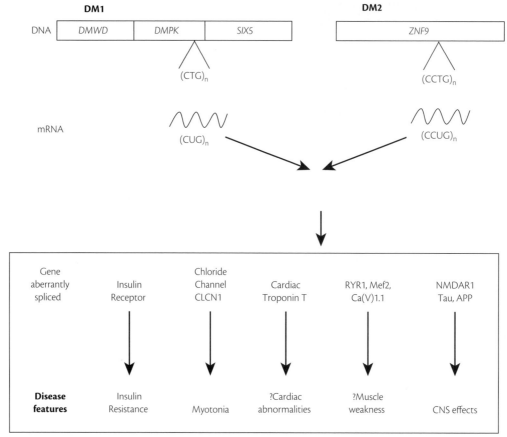

Fig. 25.1 Summary of the molecular pathogenesis of myotonic dystrophy Type 1 (DM1) and ype 2 (DM2), a 'spliceopathy'. Adapted from Gatchel JR, Zoghbi HY (2005). Diseases of unstable repeat expansion: mechanisms and common principles. *Nat Rev Genet.* **6**(10):743–55. Mef 2, myocyte enhancer factor; CLCN1, chloride channel, voltage-sensitive 1; Ca(V)1.1, calcium channel, voltage-dependent, L type, alpha 1S subunit; APP, amyloid precursor protein; RYR1, ryanodine receptor 1; NMDAR1, N-methyl-D-aspartate receptor subunit 1.

Genotype–phenotype correlations

There is a moderate correlation between longer CTG repeat expansions and an earlier age of onset and more severe disease. Diagnostic testing is only ever undertaken from leucocyte DNA. CTG repeat size in leucocytes correlates more significantly with age of onset and disease severity below 400 CTG repeats

[16]. One explanation for the poor correlation of phenotype with repeat size above 400 is that the *DMPK* CTG trinucleotide repeat length is unstable in individuals with DM1, which leads to somatic mosaicism for the size of the CTG expansion [17]. The repeat size is often stable in some postnatal tissues, e.g. leucocytes, but not in others, e.g. skeletal and cardiac muscle. Thus, the

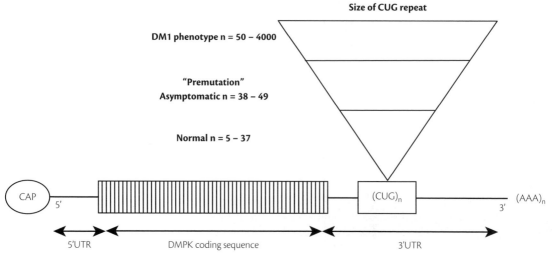

Fig. 25.2 *DMPK* mRNA with relationship between CUG repeat size and phenotype. UTR, untranslated region.

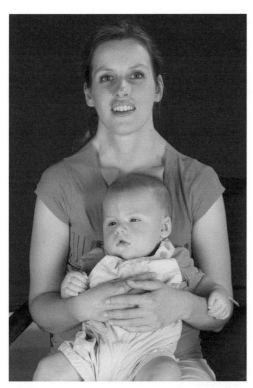

Fig. 25.3 This woman has adult-onset classical myotonic dystrophy Type 1 with a 'medium' expansion (200–700 CTG repeats) in the *DMPK* gene. Her son has congenital myotonic dystrophy Type 1 and has a 'large' expansion (>700 CTG repeats). Note that her son has a 'tent-like' mouth due to facial myopathy.

diagnostic test result does not correlate with expansion size in affected tissues and organs. Somatic instability occurs in mitotic and post-mitotic tissues, suggesting it is caused by changes in DNA repair mechanisms. The variation in disease severity between organs, within an individual, may partly be related to the level of somatic mosaicism.

Investigations

The diagnosis can only be confirmed by DNA analysis and this is the only diagnostic test required when the disease is suspected clinically. Although electromyography (EMG) shows highly characteristic features (myotonic discharges and myopathic changes), and was used as a diagnostic tool before DNA analysis became available, it is no longer required for diagnosis. However, in some patients not initially suspected of having DM1, the first clue may come from EMG findings when investigating somebody for a presumed myopathy or isolated myotonia.

Clinical features

Patients with DM1 can be divided into five main subtypes based on their clinical presentation (Table 25.1).

Congenital DM1

Congenital DM1 is not simply a severe, early form of 'classical' DM1, but a specific clinical phenotype with distinct clinical features. Congenital DM1 often presents before birth as polyhydramnios and reduced fetal movements. After delivery, the main features are generalized weakness, hypotonia, and respiratory failure. Affected infants have an inverted V-shaped (also termed 'tented' or 'fish-shaped') upper lip, which is characteristic of facial weakness originating *in utero* and makes suckling difficult. Mortality from respiratory failure is high. Failure to thrive, club feet, and feeding difficulties are common problems, but surviving infants experience gradual improvement in motor function and learn to walk, swallow, and independently ventilate. Cognitive and motor milestones are delayed and all patients with congenital DM1 develop learning difficulties which require special needs schooling and they rarely achieve independent living. Cerebral atrophy and ventricular enlargement are often present at birth [20,21]. Faecal soiling can be a problem. A progressive myopathy and the other features seen in the classical form of DM1 develop later, although this does not start until early adulthood and progresses slowly [22]. Congenitally affected patients typically die from cardiorespiratory complications in their third or fourth decade.

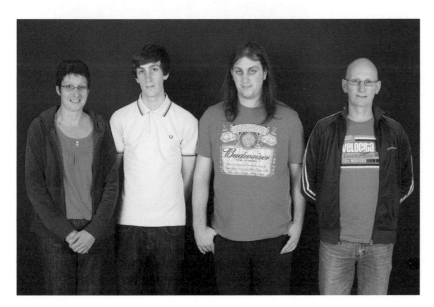

Fig. 25.4 The 51 year old father of this family (on the right) has very mild myotonic dystrophy associated with a 'very small' expansion (50–100 CTG repeats), early cataracts at the age of 50, and mild muscle aches. He was tested for DM1 when his eldest son (second from the right) was diagnosed with early adult-onset DM1 at the age of 21 associated with a 'medium' expansion (200–700 CTG repeats). The father's younger son (second from the left) has also been confirmed to have a medium expansion at the age of 19 and is less severely clinically affected than his elder brother. Their mother (on the left) is unaffected.

Table 25.1 A summary of clinical findings, phenotype, and CTG repeat length in myotonic dystrophy Type 1

Phenotype	Clinical signs	CTG repeat size	Age of onset (years)	Age of death (years)
Premutation	None	38–49	N/A	N/A
Mild/late-onset	Cataracts, mild myotonia	50–100	20–70	Normal life span
Classical	Weakness, myotonia, cataracts, conduction defects	50–1000	10–30	48-60
Childhood	Psychosocial problems, low IQ with classic features	Approx. 800	1–10	N/A
Congenital	Infantile hypotonia, respiratory failure, learning disabilities. Later classical features	>1000	Birth	45*

N/A, not applicable.

*Does not include neonatal deaths.

Adapted from [10], [18], and [19].

Childhood-onset DM1

The diagnosis of childhood DM1 is often missed initially due to the lack of specific physical neurological problems and apparently negative family history [6]. In contrast to congenital DM1, the sex of the transmitting parent is not relevant. Facial weakness is common, but without the characteristic 'tented' upper-lip appearance of the congenital form. Dysarthria and hand muscle myotonia may be prominent features with delayed motor development. Low intelligence and other psychosocial problems are often the principal management problem [23]. There is increasing evidence of early cardiac conduction abnormalities, and from the age of 10 annual electrocardiograms (ECGs) and consideration of electrophysiological studies should be a part of routine management.

'Classical' adult-onset DM1

Muscle

Muscle can be affected by the dystrophic process, causing weakness, and by a defect in muscle membrane excitability, causing myotonia. Head, neck, and distal limb muscles show a highly characteristic pattern of involvement. Facial weakness with ptosis, combined with atrophy of temporalis, causes the typical facial appearance (added to by premature hair loss, particularly in males). Neck flexion weakness (rarely neck extension weakness causing a "dropped head") is an early feature. In the upper limbs the long finger flexors are the earliest affected. This subsequently causes profound difficulties with hand grip and performing dexterous tasks. In the lower limbs, foot drop, associated with weakness in ankle dorsiflexion, is common. Muscle weakness progresses slowly over several years but substantial proximal weakness is only a late feature. An axonal peripheral neuropathy may add to the weakness [24].

Myotonia most commonly symptomatically affects handgrip but can also affect the face, jaw, tongue, and swallowing. Myotonia may improve with repeated contractions, and this is called the 'warm-up phenomenon' [25]. The warm-up phenomenon can also improve speech production [26]. The most sensitive way of detecting myotonia is by percussion of the thenar eminence with a tendon hammer, showing exaggerated contraction and delayed relaxation— 'percussion myotonia'. Maintained contraction of the eyes or hands— 'eye closure' and 'handgrip' myotonia—are less commonly elicited than percussion myotonia. Myotonia can also affect other muscles including the tongue (see Fig. 25.5). The severity of myotonia can vary throughout the day and is more marked in the cold.

Ocular

Posterior subcapsular cataracts develop in most patients at some time in their illness. Some patients develop cataracts at an early age and then prominent muscle symptoms later in life. A history of early onset cataracts in a parent of patients with adulthood-onset DM1 suggests that they may be the transmitting parent, but cataracts are so common in the general population that mistaken conclusions are common—specific diagnosis requires DNA analysis, following appropriate genetic counselling.

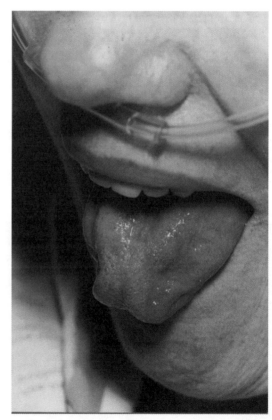

Fig. 25.5 This woman was diagnosed with DM1 at the age of 65 when she developed difficulties swallowing and handgrip myotonia and was admitted to hospital with a chest infection. She had cataracts removed at the age of 31 but had minimal muscle symptoms throughout most of her life. The photograph demonstrates tongue myotonia. She has subsequently required a permanent pacemaker for conduction block and has chronic atrial fibrillation.

Cardiac

Conduction disturbances and tachyarrhythmias are common in DM1 and contribute significantly to the morbidity and mortality of the disease [27–29]. The cardiac histopathology demonstrates fibrosis, particularly of the conducting system and sinoatrial node, myocyte hypertrophy, and fatty infiltration [30]. In one 10-year follow-up study [19], there was a 7.3 times greater mortality in DM1 than the general population, with a mean age of death at 53 years. There was a positive correlation between age of onset and age at death. Approximately 30% of the deaths were due to cardiac complications and 40% were due to respiratory complications. The cardiac abnormalities included sudden unexpected death, presumed to be due to a malignant arrhythmia, progressive LV dysfunction, and ischaemic heart disease, although there is no conclusive evidence of early atherosclerosis in DM1. The common ECG changes were prolonged PR interval (40%), a wide QRS (25%), sustained and paroxysmal AF (25%) as well as monomorphic and polymorphic ventricular tachycardia (VT) and ventricular fibrillation (VF). A study investigating sudden death in patients with DM1 found that a severe abnormality on the ECG (defined as a prolonged PR and/or QRS, second/third-degree heart block, or a non-sinus rhythm) or a diagnosis of an atrial tachyarrhythmia predicted sudden death [31]. Over a 5.7-year follow-up, 7% of patients experienced sudden death and 8% died from respiratory failure. In contrast to cardiac arrhythmias, cardiomyopathy is rarely a significant feature.

Central nervous system

Specific cognitive and intellectual deficits are frequent in adult DM1, but substantially milder and less of a clinical issue than in those with congenital and childhood DM1. The intelligence of patients with classical DM1 may be incorrectly assumed to be reduced because of the facial expression, speech disturbance, and apathy. Age-related cognitive decline has been reported in adults [32–35] but in clinical practice any such changes are much less striking than the physical progression of the disorder. DM1 patients have been found to have avoidant, obsessive–compulsive, paranoid, and aggressive personality features [36–38]. Deficits in recognition of facial emotion similar to patients with schizophrenia suggest a possible similar pathophysiology [39]. A broad range of neuropsychological defects in frontal, parietal, and temporal lobe functions have been described [38,40,41], although frontal lobe involvement predominates. White matter lesions are seen on MRI and can affect the anterior temporal lobes [40–42]. A reduction of the global grey matter, especially in the frontal and parietal lobes, and a reduction in bilateral hippocampal volumes was correlated specifically to both a clinical severity score and episodic memory deficits [40]. Patients rarely develop dementia in the typical sense of the meaning, and the cognitive phenotype remains complex and relatively uncharacterized despite it having a significant impact on the function and quality of life of the patient and relatives.

Neurons in the limbic system and/or brainstem contain tau-associated neurofibrillary tangles (NFTs) in DM1 and DM2, suggesting a common neuropathological process and a possible link with the central nervous system features of DM1, including apathy and sleepiness [43,44]. A unique abnormal pattern of tau isoform expression in DM1 and transgenic mice has been described. This consists of reduced exon 2/3-containing isoforms, hyperphosphorylated tau, and a predominance of shorter tau isoforms including exon 10 only or no additional exons [45,46].

Gastrointestinal (GI) tract

Prospective studies of GI symptoms in DM1 patients have found that abdominal pain (55%), dysphagia (45%), emesis (35%), chronic or episodic diarrhoea (33%), coughing while eating (33%), and anal incontinence (30%) are common symptoms [47,48]. Aspiration pneumonia is commonly due to the potent combination of poor cough, secondary to ventilatory muscle weakness, and dysphagia. This results in significant morbidity and mortality from pneumonia. The commonest GI symptom complex is similar to irritable bowel syndrome. The burden for patients of GI-related symptoms has generally been under-recognized [47,48]. Cholecystitis and gallstones are common, and cholecystectomy has a high morbidity due to postoperative respiratory complications (see the section Respiratory failure and excessive daytime sleepiness). Liver function tests are often elevated for unknown reasons [49].

Endocrinopathy

Endocrine abnormalities include disturbances of the thyroid, pancreas, hypothalamus, and gonads. Testicular atrophy, with atrophy of the seminiferous tubules, leads to infertility in males. Infertility may occur in otherwise asymptomatic patients [50]. In females, habitual abortion and menstrual irregularities are common. Although diabetes mellitus is probably no more common in DM1 than in the general population, a glucose tolerance test is often associated with abnormally high glucose levels, particularly at 3 h into the test, suggesting insulin insensitivity. An associated overproduction of insulin is due to insulin resistance secondary to abnormal splicing of the insulin receptor mRNA to a more insulin-insensitive isoform [51–53].

Skin

Patients commonly develop early frontal balding which is clinically more apparent in men than women. Pilomatrixomata and epitheliomas can occur, especially on the scalp, and can be confused with sebaceous cysts [54,55].

Respiratory failure and excessive daytime sleepiness

Excessive daytime sleepiness (EDS) and respiratory failure (RF) are very common in DM1. EDS and RF tend to occur independently of one another [56] and often significantly reduce quality of life. RF, usually in the context of aspiration pneumonia, is the commonest cause of early mortality in DM1 [19]. RF is caused by respiratory muscle (especially diaphragmatic) weakness, which can manifest as a poor cough and reduced vital capacity [57]. General anaesthesia often precipitates RF in patients who were previously clinically stable.

Patients have an abnormal central ventilatory response without the usual hyperpnoea produced by an increasing concentration of carbon dioxide. This is associated with an abnormal sensitivity to barbiturates, morphine, and other drugs that depress the ventilatory drive contributing to postoperative respiratory complications. General anaesthesia is associated with significant complications in DM1, which are usually respiratory. A 10% risk of postoperative complications due to general anaesthesia including prolonged respiratory depression from anaesthetic agents and postoperative pneumonia, especially following cholecystectomy, highlights the need for careful perioperative management of patients with DM [58].

EDS is present to varying degrees in at least 39% of patients with DM1 [59,60] and can have a major effect on quality of life for the patient and their family. Although it must be excluded, EDS is not often due to nocturnal hypoventilation or obstructive or central sleep apnoeas, and appears to originate from central nervous system dysfunction. Post-mortem studies of DM patients demonstrate reduced serotonergic neurons in the dorsal raphe and superior central nuclei [61–63]. The occurrence of sleep-onset rapid eye movement in patients also suggests a process with features similar to narcolepsy [64].

Psychiatry

Anxiety and depression are common and quality of life can be seriously impaired [65]. Patients often have apathy which may be confused with significant depression [59]. An inverse correlation between mood and fatigue and the degree of white matter involvement has been described [42,66]. If depressed mood was a consequence of neurodegeneration, a continuous worsening of depression would be expected as DM1 progresses, but that is not evident. The inverse correlation of white matter lesions with depression suggest that depression is a reactive adjustment disorder in the earlier stages of the disease when patients are more aware of their progressive disabilities.

Pregnancy

Women with DM1 are at risk of complications during pregnancy including an increased rate of spontaneous abortion, prolonged labour, retained placenta, and postpartum haemorrhage [67,68]. Anaesthesia, such as for Caesarean section, presents the respiratory and cardiac challenges discussed in Respiratory failure and excessive daytime sleepiness. However, most women can expect to have a normal vaginal delivery and the greatest obstetric/neonatal issues are seen when a congenitally affected child is born.

Mild/late-onset DM1

A study of 102 DM1 patients with between 50 and 200 CTG repeats found that most patients with between 50 and 99 repeats were asymptomatic, apart from 38% who had cataracts [69]. Myotonia, weakness, and EDS were far more common in patients with between 100 and 200 CTG repeats. Some patients with between 50 and 100 CTG repeats can nevertheless develop severe DM1, and some patients with between 300 and 500 CTG repeats can be asymptomatic for many years. This highlights the relatively poor correlation between CTG expansion size in leucocytes and clinical severity.

Myotonic dystrophy Type 2 (DM2)

DM2 was previously termed proximal myotonic myopathy (PROMM) and shares many of the multisystemic features of DM1 [70–73]. DM2 is important in the differential diagnosis of a limb-girdle myopathy. The repeat expansion for DM2 is much larger than for DM1, ranging from 75 to over 11 000 repeats. Unlike DM1, the size of the repeated DNA expansion does not correlate with the age of onset or disease severity in DM2 and obvious anticipation does not occur. A congenital form of DM2 has not been reported.

Clinical features of DM2

DM2 is a multisystem disorder characterized by myotonia (90%) and muscle weakness (82%). The onset of DM2 is typically in the third decade, but often much later, with the most common presenting symptom being muscle weakness, although myotonia during the first decade has been reported [72,73]. DM2 patients commonly have prominent muscle pain, stiffness, and fatigue in comparison to DM1 (Table 25.2), although muscle pain may be underestimated in DM1. The weakness typically affects proximal muscles, including the neck, elbow extension, and hip flexors in comparison to early DM1 which initially tends to affect the face, neck, and distal, rather than proximal, limb muscles [73]. DM2 patients less commonly require walking aids than in DM1, though they experience increasing difficulties climbing stairs as the disease progresses. Cardiac conduction defects [19%], posterior subcapsular cataracts, and endocrine changes including insulin insensitivity and testicular failure are common. Cognitive manifestations in DM2 are less severe than in DM1. Table 25.2 compares the main features of DM1 and DM2.

Table 25.2 Comparative features of myotonic dystrophy Type 1 (DM1) and Type 2 (DM2)

Feature	DM1	DM2
Epidemiology	Widespread	Regionally selective
Age of onset	Any	Adulthood
Anticipation	Yes	No/mild
Congenital form	Yes	No
Muscle		
Weak face/neck/swallow	Common	Uncommon
Weak limbs—proximal	Late	Early
Weak limbs—distal	Early	Late
Myotonia	Mild to moderate	Mild to moderate
Myalgia	Mild to moderate	Mild to severe
Systemic		
Cataracts	Very common/early	Common
Frontal balding	Very common	Uncommon
Cardiac arrhythmias	Very common/early	Common/late
Respiratory failure	Very common/late	Uncommon/late
Cognitive disorder	Common/mild to severe	Uncommon/mild
Gonadal failure	Common	Uncommon
Excessive daytime sleepiness	Very common and early	Common and late
Hyperhidrosis	Mild	Mild to severe
Laboratory		
Hyperinsulinaemia	Common/mild	Common/moderate
Electromyography: myotonia	Very common	Common
Chromosome	19q13.3	3q21
Gene	DMPK	ZNF9
Mutation type	CTG repeat	CCTG repeat
Repeat size	50–4000	Mean in 1000s

Adapted from Washington University Neuromuscular Disease Center website: <http://neuromuscular.wustl.edu/>.

Management

There is currently no cure for myotonic dystrophy. Cardiorespiratory disorders are responsible for 70% of mortality in DM1 and there is good evidence that active monitoring and timely intervention significantly reduce morbidity and mortality.

Muscle weakness

An initial pilot study suggested that dehydroepiandrosterone (DHEA) may improve myotonia and muscle strength in DM1 [74]. A multicentre randomized double-blind placebo-controlled trial found no evidence that 12-week treatment with replacement or pharmacologic doses of DHEA improved muscle power [75]. Mecasermin rinfabate (SomatoKine/iPLEX) is a combination of recombinant insulin-like growth factor 1 (IGF-1) and its binding protein, BP-3 (rhIGF-1/rhIGFBP-3). An open label trial of rhIGF-1/rhIGFBP-3 in DM1 found that treatment was associated with increased lean body mass and improvement in metabolism but not increased muscle strength or function [76]. A recent Cochrane review of creatine treatment in all muscle diseases came out in favour of creatine in the treatment of 'dystrophies'. The assessment included six trials of 'dystrophies' including two of DM1 and one of DM2 as well as three of dystrophinopathies. The first DM1 trial demonstrated a tendency to benefit [77] and the other trial demonstrated slight harm [78], with an overall non-significant effect of $Z = 0.66$ and $P = 0.51$. A small but significant benefit (an 8.8% increase in MVC) of creatine was found in patients with DM2 [79]. Routine use of any of these agents in DM1 or DM2 cannot be recommended on current evidence. A randomized trial compared the effect of strength training versus no training in 36 patients with DM1. There were no significant differences between training and non-training groups for the primary or secondary outcome measures [80]. However, moderate-intensity strength training appears not to cause harm in DM1, and despite the lack of evidence of benefit from this one study we strongly recommend that all patients undertake regular exercise which we believe is likely to help with muscle strength and fitness, general cardiovascular fitness, and weight control.

Myotonia

Many drugs have been given for the treatment of myotonia and have been the subject of a Cochrane review [81]. One small cross-over study, with a washout period, demonstrated a significant effect of clomipramine in myotonic dystrophy. The studies were all too small to enable meta-analysis to be performed. In practice, for most patients, hand weakness is more disabling than myotonia, and in our experience few patients note any useful benefit from anti-myotonia drugs. An exception is a small number of young patients with otherwise minimal symptoms, in whom myotonia, with little or no weakness, is a dominant problem, and for whom treatment of the myotonia may significantly improve hand function and quality of life. There are theoretical concerns about the potential cardiac side effects of the anti-myotonia drugs, noting the propensity for cardiac arrhythmia in the myotonic dystrophies. However, mexiletine at doses up to 200 mg three times a day has been found to be effective, safe (including with respect to the heart), and well tolerated as an anti-myotonia treatment [82].

Cardiac arrhythmias

We recommend yearly ECG, with a low threshold for cardiology referral if there is marked prolongation of the PR interval or QRS complex, any form of conduction block, or if the patient develops cardiac symptoms. A significant bradyarrhythmia can be treated with insertion of a permanent pacemaker. Eighteen per cent of patients with a normal 24-h Holter monitor have inducible VT in the absence of symptoms on electrophysiological studies (EPS) [83]. It is not certain how many of these patients develop dangerous arrhythmias and would benefit from insertion of an implantable cardioverter defibrillator (ICD). A recent study described the potential benefits on mortality of an 'invasive' versus a 'non-invasive' strategy for cardiac monitoring in DM1 [84]. An invasive strategy, consisting of electrophysiological cardiac studies, was associated with a higher rate of 9-year survival than a non-invasive strategy.

Physical activity precipitates arrhythmia, and therefore exercise testing with ECG is sometimes recommended in young patients with DM1 before intensive sports are undertaken [85].

There is no doubt that we still do not have enough knowledge to determine the optimal timing of cardiac interventions, and it is an area ripe for further study.

Respiratory

Regular screening for incipient respiratory failure is an important part of the management of DM1 patients. This should include annual assessment of vital capacity and overnight sleep oximetry (which can be done on a domiciliary basis) if the vital capacity is markedly reduced (<1.5 L) or, more importantly, if there are any symptoms suggestive of nocturnal hypoventilation or disturbed sleep (e.g. waking with headache/grogginess, EDS, observed apnoeas). If there is objective evidence of sleep apnoea, patients should be offered non-invasive ventilation (NIV). Even when nocturnal hypoventilation has been confirmed, many patients do not tolerate nocturnal NIV for reasons that have not been fully elucidated.

Excessive daytime sleepiness

Considerable experience indicates that most patients with EDS do not have clinically significant sleep apnoea and even those patients that do have sleep apnoea may have persisting EDS when apnoea is treated. In our experience EDS responds extremely well to the psychostimulant drug modafinil in a majority of affected patients, although the literature is contradictory. Three cross-over studies [86–88] and one open-label study [89] found benefit. A Cochrane review of psychostimulants in DM1 found the current level of evidence 'inconclusive' and suggested that further trials were needed [90]. Such trials are unlikely to happen due to the cost of detailed sleep studies, the relatively small number of patients affected, necessitating the complexity of multicentre studies, and the limited market interest for the pharmaceutical industry. Recent patient-centred observations provide strong support for a trial of modafinil in appropriately assessed patients [91]. We would therefore recommend modafinil at 200 mg in the morning, increased after 2 weeks to 200 mg in the morning and at lunchtime if there was no response at the lower dose. If there is still no clear benefit then the drug should be stopped. Theoretical risks of cardiac and psychiatric side effects have not been borne out in clinical trials or from extensive personal experience in DM1, or for other disorders such as narcolepsy. Severe, potentially fatal, skin eruptions have been reported rarely. Headache and GI upset tend to be the commonest side effects limiting usage.

Gastrointestinal

Dysphagia is common, but many patients will not complain of problems with swallowing even when there is significant aspiration on videofluoroscopy. Aspiration combined with respiratory muscle weakness contributes to the high morbidity and mortality associated with pneumonia. Simple approaches to management include cutting food into smaller pieces, avoiding problematic foods, adding thickeners to liquids, drinking whilst eating, and speech therapy advice. A few patients, after detailed investigation including videofluoroscopy and barium swallow, require intervention such as oesophageal balloon dilatation, cricopharyngeal myotomy, and, rarely, percutaneous endoscopic gastrostomy.

Cholestyramine improves diarrhoea, incontinence, and pain in many patients, possibly by preventing large-bowel osmotic diarrhoea due to failure of absorption of bile salts in the terminal ileum. Norfloxacin or other quinolones may be effective when cholestyramine fails by treating bacterial overgrowth, and erythromycin or domperidone may help improve gastric emptying by compensating for reduced motilin levels in DM1 [47,48].

Cataracts

Cataract formation occurs early in DM1 and visual impairment can significantly worsen balance which is already impaired by power loss. Patients should be aware of the need for early reporting of worsening vision so that a prompt referral for potential cataract surgery can be made.

Endocrine

The incidence of overt diabetes is probably no greater in DM1 than the general population despite laboratory evidence of impaired glucose tolerance.

Therapy services

Physiotherapy may help with the management of foot drop and gait by using ankle–foot orthoses and programmed exercises, and also with the treatment of respiratory failure and the encouragement of exercise. Occupational therapy (OT) may help hand function, but wrist splints are poorly tolerated by patients. The most important role of OT is with respect to home adaptations and the assessment of safety. Speech and language therapy is often helpful in assessing the degree of aspiration and for discussing treatment options for dysphagia and aspiration. A clinical nurse specialist with a specific interest in muscle disease often acts as a link with the main hospital and provides consistency in monitoring the patient. Social workers are vital for housing and social support.

Patient care and organizations

Patient-held care cards have been implemented in many centres and may improve compliance with monitoring the disease. In one study, 79% of cardholders had a recommended ECG within the last year compared with 3.5% of non-cardholders. In the UK the main charitable organizations are the Myotonic Dystrophy Support Group (MDSG) (<http://www.myotonicdystrophysupportgroup.org/>) and the Muscular Dystrophy Campaign (MDC) (<http://www.muscular-dystrophy.org/>). These organizations provide a significant support network for patients and carers as well as funding for research and treatment.

Gene therapy

The recent advances in our understanding of the underlying molecular mechanisms involved in myotonic dystrophy have generated new approaches for more specific and effective treatments for DM1 and DM2. The development of targeted molecular treatments, especially antisense therapy, has achieved success *in vitro* and in animal models, although the translation of this to human trials has understandably lagged behind. Some contributions to these achievements will be discussed.

One of the first studies of specific targeting of mutant DMPK described the hammerhead ribozyme (a form of post-transcriptional silencing distinct from antisense therapy)-mediated destruction of ribonuclear inclusions in myotonic dystrophy myoblasts and was associated with a preferential reduction in mutant DMPK mRNA [92].

Another study has demonstrated the reversal of abnormalities in DM1 myoblasts by preferential reduction of mutant DMPK using a retroviral vector to produce a 149-bp antisense RNA complementary to 13 CUG repeats and to the 110 bp region following the CUG repeat sequence in DMPK 3′ UTR [93].

The reversal of RNA missplicing and myotonia after overexpression of the splicing factor, MBNL1, in a mouse model of DM1 supports the role of MBNL1 in the pathogenesis of DM1. Overexpression of MBNL1 *in vivo* was achieved by injection of recombinant adeno-associated viral vector into skeletal muscle of the transgenic mice. This study was one of the first to demonstrate an improvement in phenotype after the onset of symptoms and pathology in an animal [94].

Mahadevan et al. [95] developed a conditional transgenic mouse model of DM1 by overexpression of a normal DMPK 3′UTR. This recapitulated the clinical and pathological features of DM1 in the absence of RNA inclusions but with increased CUG-BP1 levels, as described in DM1 tissues. By silencing the transgene, the phenotype dramatically improved, suggesting that the molecular deficits in DM1 can be reversed, although whether this can occur after decades of exposure to mutant DMPK in humans, in comparison to weeks in transgenic mice, remains unsubstantiated.

Altered splicing of the muscle-specific chloride channel 1 (ClC-1) has been shown to cause the myotonic phenotype of DM1, and this has recently been shown to be reversible in mouse models using morpholino (a small molecule to alter gene expression) antisense oligonucleotide to modify splicing of ClC-1 mRNA [96].

The reduction in ribonuclear foci and mRNA splicing defects has been shown using antisense oligonucleotides and small molecules *in vitro* and in animal models of DM1 [97,98]. This may occur by the complete elimination of expanded $(CUG)_n$ RNA transcripts or by the prevention of detrimental protein binding to thermodynamically stable $(CUG)_n$ hairpin structures. These developments offer new hope to patients with myotonic dystrophy, although obstacles such as toxicity and tissue-specific availability need to be overcome before small molecule and antisense treatments can be introduced into clinical practice [99].

Conclusions

DM1 is the commonest cause of muscular dystrophy. There is currently no cure, but effective management is likely to significantly reduce morbidity and mortality in patients who have perhaps in the past not received as much clinical attention as warranted. The enormous advances in the understanding of the molecular pathogenesis of DM1 and DM2 have resulted in the description of a novel disease mechanism potentially involved in several myoneurodegenerative disorders. These diseases have been called the 'spliceopathies' and are mediated by a primary disorder of RNA rather than proteins. This has heralded the use of gene therapy, which has already produced significant disease-modifying effects *in vitro* and in animal models. The dawn of gene therapy for DM1 and DM2 appears to be very close, and the near future is an exciting time for clinicians and patients alike.

References

1. Thornton CA, Wymer JP, Simmons Z, McClain C, Moxley RT 3rd. Expansion of the myotonic dystrophy CTG repeat reduces expression of the flanking DMAHP gene. *Nat Genet* 1997; **16**: 407–9.

2. Mankodi A, Takahashi MP, Jiang H, et al. Expanded CUG repeats trigger aberrant splicing of ClC-1 chloride channel pre-mRNA and hyperexcitability of skeletal muscle in myotonic dystrophy. *Mol Cell* 2002; **10**: 35–44.

3. Machuca-Tzili L, Brook D, Hilton-Jones D. Clinical and molecular aspects of the myotonic dystrophies: a review. *Muscle Nerve* 2005; **32**: 1–18.

4. Liquori CL, Ricker K, Moseley ML, et al. Myotonic dystrophy type 2 caused by a CCTG expansion in intron 1 of ZNF9. *Science* 2001; **293**: 864–7.

5. Gatchel JR, Zoghbi HY. Diseases of unstable repeat expansion: mechanisms and common principles. *Nat Rev Genet* 2005; **6**: 743–55.

6. Harper PS, Van Engelen B, Eymard B, Wilcox DE (ed). *Myotonic Dystrophy: Present Management, Future Therapy*. Oxford; Oxford University Press, 2004.

7. Yotova V, Labuda D, Zietkiewicz E, et al. Anatomy of a founder effect: myotonic dystrophy in Northeastern Quebec. *Hum Genet* 2005; **117**: 177–87.

8. Brook JD, McCurrach ME, Harley HG, et al. Molecular basis of myotonic dystrophy: expansion of a trinucleotide (CTG) repeat at the 3-prime end of a transcript encoding a protein kinase family member. *Cell* 1992; **68**: 799–808.

9. Martorell L, Monckton DG, Sanchez A, Lopez De Munain A, Baiget M. Frequency and stability of the myotonic dystrophy type 1 premutation. *Neurology* 2001; **56**: 328–35.

10. International Myotonic Dystrophy Consortium. New nomenclature and DNA testing guidelines for myotonic dystrophy type 1 (DM1). *Neurology* 2000; **54**: 1218–21.

11. De Temmerman N, Sermon K, Seneca S. Intergenerational instability of the expanded CTG repeat in the DMPK gene: studies in human gametes and preimplantation embryos. *Am J Hum Genet* 2004; **75**: 325–9.

12. Rakocevic-Stojanovic V, Savic D, et al. Intergenerational changes of CTG repeat depending on the sex of the transmitting parent in myotonic dystrophy type 1. *Eur J Neurol* 2005; **12**: 236–7.

13. Zeesman S, Carson N, Whelan DT. Paternal transmission of the congenital form of myotonic dystrophy type 1: a new case and review of the literature. *Am J Med Genet* 2002; **107**: 222–6.

14. Brunner HG, Bruggenwirth HT, Nillesen W, et al. Influence of sex of the transmitting parent as well as of parental allele size on the CTG expansion in myotonic dystrophy (DM). *Am J Hum Genet* 1993; **53**: 1016–23.

15. De Die-Smulders CE, Smeets HJ, Loots W, et al. Paternal transmission of congenital myotonic dystrophy. *J Med Genet* 1997; **34**: 930–3.

16. Hamshere MG, Harley H, Harper P, Brook JD, Brookfield JFY. Myotonic dystrophy: the correlation of (CTG) repeat length in leucocytes with age at onset is significant only for patients with small expansions. *J Med Genet* 1999; **36**: 59–61.

17. Lavedan C, Hofmann-Radvanyi H, Shelbourne P. Myotonic dystrophy: size- and sex-dependent dynamics of CTG meiotic instability, and somatic mosaicism. *Am J Hum Genet* 1993; **52**: 875–83.

18. De Die-Smulders CE, Howeler CJ, Thijs C, et al. Age and causes of death in adult-onset myotonic dystrophy. *Brain* 1998; **121**: 1557–63.

19. Mathieu J, Allard P, Potvin L, Prevost C, Begin P. A 10-year study of mortality in a cohort of patients with myotonic dystrophy. *Neurology* 1999; **52**: 1658–62.

20. Spranger M, Spranger S, Tischendorf M, Meinck HM, Cremer M. Myotonic dystrophy. The role of large triplet repeat length in the development of mental retardation. *Arch Neurol* 1997; **54**: 251–4.

21. Ashizawa T. Myotonic dystrophy as a brain disorder. [editorial; comment]. *Arch Neurol* 1998; **55**: 291–3.

22. Joseph JT, Richards CS, Anthony DC, Upton M, Perez-Atayde AR, Greenstein P Congenital myotonic dystrophy pathology and somatic mosaicism. *Neurology* 1997; **49**: 1457–60.

23. Steyaert J, Umans S, Willekens D, et al. A study of the cognitive and psychological profile in 16 children with congenital or juvenile myotonic dystrophy. *Clin Genet* 1997; **52**: 135–41.

24. Krishnan AV, Kiernan MC. Axonal function and activity-dependent excitability changes in myotonic dystrophy. *Muscle Nerve* 2006; **33**: 627–36.

25. Logigian EL, Blood CL, Dilek N, et al. Quantitative analysis of the "warm-up" phenomenon in myotonic dystrophy type 1. *Muscle Nerve* 2005; **32**: 35–42.

26. de Swart BJ, van Engelen BG, van de Kerkhof JP, Maassen BA. Myotonia and flaccid dysarthria in patients with adult onset myotonic dystrophy. *J Neurol Neurosurg Psychiatry* 2004; **75**: 1480–2.

27. Bassez G, Lazarus A, Desguerre I, et al. Severe cardiac arrhythmias in young patients with myotonic dystrophy type 1. *Neurology* 2004; **63**: 1939–41.

28. Chebel S, Ben Hamda K, Boughammoura A, Frih Ayed M, Ben Farhat MH. [Cardiac involvement in Steinert's myotonic dystrophy]. *Rev Neurol (Paris)* 2005; **161**: 932–9.

29. Dello Russo A, Pelargonio G, Parisi Q. Widespread electroanatomic alterations of right cardiac chambers in patients with myotonic dystrophy type 1. *J Cardiovasc Electrophysiol* 2006; **17**: 34–40.

30. Phillips MF, Harper PS. Cardiac disease in myotonic dystrophy. *Cardiovasc Res* 1997; **33**: 13–22.

31. Groh WJ, Groh MR, Saha C. Electrocardiographic abnormalities and sudden death in myotonic dystrophy type 1. *N Engl J Med* 2008; **358**: 2688–97.

32. Turnpenny P, Clark C, Kelly K. Intelligence quotient profile in myotonic dystrophy, intergenerational deficit, and correlation with CTG amplification. *J Med Genet* 1994; **31**: 300–5.

33. Modoni A, Silvestri G, Pomponi MG, et al. Characterization of the pattern of cognitive impairment in myotonic dystrophy type 1. *Arch Neurol* 2004; **61**: 1943–7.

34. Gaul C, Schmidt T, Windisch G, et al. Subtle cognitive dysfunction in adult onset myotonic dystrophy type 1 (DM1) and type 2 (DM2). *Neurology* 2006; **67**: 350–2.

35. Winblad S, Lindberg C, Hansen S. Cognitive deficits and CTG repeat expansion size in classical myotonic dystrophy type 1 (DM1). *Behav Brain Func* 2006; **2**: 16.

36. Delaporte C. Personality patterns in patients with myotonic dystrophy. *Arch Neurol* 1998; **55**: 635–40.

37. Winblad S, Lindberg C, Hansen S. Temperament and character in patients with classical myotonic dystrophy type 1 (DM-1). *Neuromuscul Disord* 2005; **15**: 287–92.

38. Sistiaga A, Urreta I, Jodar M, et al. Cognitive/personality pattern and triplet expansion size in adult myotonic dystrophy type 1 (DM1): CTG repeats, cognition and personality in DM1. *Psychol Med* 2010; **40**: 487–95.

39. Winblad S, Hellström P, Lindberg C, Hansen S. Facial emotion recognition in myotonic dystrophy type 1 correlates with CTG repeat expansion. *J Neurol Neurosurg Psychiatry* 2006; **77**: 219–23.

40. Weber YG, Roebling R, Kassubek J, et al. Comparative analysis of brain structure, metabolism, and cognition in myotonic dystrophy 1 and 2. *Neurology* 2010; **74**: 1108–17.

41. Romeo V, Pegoraro E, Ferrati C, et al. Brain involvement in myotonic dystrophies: neuroimaging and neuropsychological comparative study in DM1 and DM2. *J Neurol* 2010; **257**: 1246–55.

42. Minnerop M, Weber B, Schoene-Bake JC, et al. The brain in myotonic dystrophy 1 and 2: evidence for a predominant white matter disease. *Brain* 2011; **134**: 3530–46.

43. Maurage CA, Udd B, Ruchoux MM, et al. Similar brain tau pathology in DM2/PROMM and DM1/Steinert disease. *Neurology* 2005; **65**: 1636–8.

44. Oyamada R, Hayashi M, Katoh Y, et al. Neurofibrillary tangles and deposition of oxidative products in the brain in cases of myotonic dystrophy. *Neuropathology* 2006; **26**: 107–14.

45. Sergeant N, Sablonnière B, Schraen-Maschke S, et al. Dysregulation of human brain microtubule-associated tau mRNA maturation in myotonic dystrophy type 1. *Hum Mol Genet* 2001; **10**; 2143–55.

46. Seznec H, Agbulut O, Sergeant N. Mice transgenic for the human myotonic dystrophy region with expanded CTG repeats display muscular and brain abnormalities. *Hum Mol Genet* 2001; **10**; 2717–26.

47. Ronnblom A, Forsberg H, Danielsson A. Gastrointestinal symptoms in myotonic dystrophy. *Scand J Gastroenterol* 1996; **31**: 654–7.

48. Ronnblom A, Andersson S, Hellstrom PM, Danielsson A. Gastric emptying in myotonic dystrophy. *Eur J Clin Invest* 2002; **32**: 570–4.

49. Heatwole CR, Miller J, Martens B, Moxley RT, III. Laboratory abnormalities in ambulatory patients with myotonic dystrophy type 1. *Arch Neurol* 2006; **63**: 1149–53.

50. Garcia de Andoin N, Echeverria J, et al. A neonatal form of Steinert's myotonic dystrophy in twins after in vitro fertilization. *Fertil Steril* 2005; **84**: 756.

51. Barbosa J, Nuttall FQ, Kennedy W, Goetz F. Plasma insulin in patients with myotonic dystrophy and their relatives. *Medicine* 1974; **53**: 307.

52. Jakase S, Okita N, Sakuma H, et al. Endocrinological abnormalities in myotonic dystrophy: consecutive studies of eight tolerance tests in 26 patients. *Tohoku J Exp Med* 1987; **153**: 355–74.

53. Savkur RS, Philips AV, Cooper TA. Aberrant regulation of insulin receptor alternative splicing is associated with insulin resistance in myotonic dystrophy. *Nat Genet* 2001; **29**: 40–7.

54. Geh JL, Moss AL. Multiple pilomatrixomata and myotonic dystrophy: a familial association. *Br J Plast Surg* 1999; **52**: 143–5.

55. Cigliano B, Baltogiannis N, De Marco M, et al. Pilomatricoma in childhood: a retrospective study from three European paediatric centres. *Eur J Pediatr* 2005; **164**: 673–7.

56. Hanostia P, Frenz D. Hypersomonia associated with alveolar hypoventilation in myotonic dystrophy. *Neurology* 1981; **31**: 1336–7.

57. Bogaard JM, van der Meché FG, Hendriks I, Ververs, C. Pulmonary function and resting breathing pattern in myotonic dystrophy. *Lung* 1992; **170**: 143–53.

58. Mathieu J, Allard P, Gobeil G, et al. Anesthetic and surgical complications in 219 cases of myotonic dystrophy. *Neurology* 1997; **49**: 1646–50.

59. Rubinsztein JS, Rubinsztein DC, Goodburn S, Holland AJ. Apathy and hypersomnia are common features of myotonic dystrophy. *J Neurol Neurosurg Psychiatry* 1998; **64**: 510–15.

60. Hilton Jones D, Damian MS, Meola G. Somnolence and its management. In: Harper PS, Van Engelen B, Eymard B, Wilcox DE (ed) *Myotonic Dystrophy; Present Management, Future Therapy*, pp. 135–49. Oxford: Oxford University Press, 2004.

61. Ono S, Takahashi K, Jinnai K, et al. Loss of serotonin-containing neurons in the raphe of patients with myotonic dystrophy: a quantitative immunohistochemical study and relation to hypersomnia. *Neurology* 1998; **50**: 535–8.

62. Giubilei F, Antonini G, Bastianello S, et al. Excessive daytime sleepiness in myotonic dystrophy. *J Neurol Sci* 1999; **164**: 60–3.

63. van der Werf S, Kalkman J, Bleijenberg G et al. The relation between daytime sleepiness, fatigue,and reduced motivation in patients with adult onset myotonic dystrophy. *J Neurol Neurosurg Psychiatry* 2003; **74**: 138–9.

64. Gibbs JW, Ciafaloni E, Radtke RA. Excessive daytime somnolence and increased rapid eye movement pressure in myotonic dystrophy. *Sleep* 2002; **25**: 672–5.

65. Antonini G, Soscia F, Giubilei F, et al. Health related quality of life in myotonic dystrophy type 1 and its relationship with cognitive and emotional functioning. *J Rehabil Med* 2006; **38**: 181–5.

66. Winblad S, Jensen C, Mansson JE, Samuelsson L, Lindberg C. Depression in myotonic dystrophy type 1: clinical and neuronal correlates. *Behav Brain Funct* 2010; **6**: 25.

67. Sarnat HB, O'Connor T, Byrne PA. Clinical effects of myotonic dystrophy on pregnancy and the neonate. *Arch Neurol* 1976; **33**: 459–65.

68. Webb D, Muir I, Faulkner J, Johnson G. Myotonia dystrophica: obstetric complications. *Am J Obstet Gynecol* 1978; **132**: 265–70.

69. Arsenault ME, Prevost C, Lescault A, Laberge C, Puymirat J, Mathieu J. Clinical characteristics of myotonic dystrophy type 1 patients with small CTG expansions. *Neurology* 2006; **66**: 1248–50.

70. Meola G, Sansone V, Radice S, Skradski S, Ptacek L. A family with an unusual myotonic and myopathic phenotype and no CTG expansion (proximal myotonic myopathy syndrome): a challenge for future molecular studies. *Neuromuscul Disord* 1996; **6**: 143–50.

71. Udd B, Krahe R, Wallgren-Pettersson C, Falck B, Kalimo H. Proximal myotonic dystrophy--a family with autosomal dominant muscular dystrophy, cataracts, hearing loss and hypogonadism: heterogeneity of proximal myotonic syndromes? *Neuromuscul Disord* 1997; **7**: 217–28.

72. Day JW, Roelofs R, Leroy B, Pech I, Benzow K, Ranum LP. Clinical and genetic characteristics of a five-generation family with a novel form of myotonic dystrophy (DM2). *Neuromuscul Disord* 1999; **9**: 19–27.

73. Day JW, Ricker K, Jacobsen JF, et al. Myotonic dystrophy type 2: molecular, diagnostic and clinical spectrum. *Neurology* 2003; **60**: 657–64.

74. Sugino M, Ohsawa N, Ito T, et al. A pilot study of dehydroepiandrosterone sulfate in myotonic dystrophy. *Neurology* 1998; **51**: 586–9.

75. Pénisson-Besnier I, Devillers M, Porcher R, et al. Dehydroepiandrosterone for myotonic dystrophy type 1. *Neurology* 2008; **71**: 407–12.

76. Heatwole CR, Eichinger KJ, Friedman DI, et al. Open-label trial of recombinant human insulin-like growth factor 1/recombinant human insulin-like growth factor binding protein 3 in myotonic dystrophy type 1. *Arch Neurol* 2011; **68**: 37–44.

77. Walter MC, Reilich P, Lochmüller H, et al. Creatine monohydrate in myotonic dystrophy: a double-blind, placebo-controlled clinical study. *J Neurol* 2002; **249**: 1717–22.

78. Tarnopolsky M, Mahoney D, Thompson T, Naylor H, Doherty TJ. Creatine monohydrate supplementation does not increase muscle strength, lean body mass, or muscle phosphocreatine in patients with myotonic dystrophy type 1. *Muscle Nerve* 2004; **29**: 51–8.

79. Schneider-Gold C, Beck M, Wessig C, et al. Creatine monohydrate in DM2/PROMM: a double-blind placebo-controlled clinical study. Proximal myotonic myopathy. *Neurology* 2003; **60**: 500–2.

80. Lindeman E, Leffers P, Spaans F, et al. Strength training in patients with myotonic dystrophy and hereditary motor and sensory neuropathy: a randomized clinical trial. *Arch Phys Med Rehabil.* 1995; **76**: 612–20.

81. Trip J, Drost GG, van Engelen BGM, Faber CG. Drug treatment for myotonia. *Cochrane Database Syst Rev* 2007; issue 4, art. no.: CD004762.

82. Logigian EL, Martens WB, Moxley RT, 4th, et al. Mexiletine is an effective antimyotonia treatment in myotonic dystrophy type 1. *Neurology* 2010; **74**: 1441–8.

83. Lazarus A, Varin J, Ounnoughene Z, et al. Relationships among electrophysiological findings and clinical status, heart function, and extent of DNA mutation in myotonic dystrophy. *Circulation* 1999; **99**: 1041–6.

84. Wahbi K, Meune C, Porcher R, et al. Electrophysiological study with prophylactic pacing and survival in adults with myotonic dystrophy and conduction system disease. *J Am Med Assoc* 2012; **307**: 1292–301.

85. van Engelen B, Eymard B, Wilcox D. Workshop report: 123rd ENMC International Workshop: Management and Therapy in Myotonic Dystrophy, 6–8 February 2004, Naarden, The Netherlands. *Neuromuscul Disord* 2005; **15**: 389–94.

86. MacDonald JR, Hill JD, Tarnopolsky MA. Modafinil reduces excessive somnolence and enhances mood in patients with myotonic dystrophy. *Neurology* 2002; **59**: 1876–80.

87. Talbot K, Stradling J, Crosby J, Hilton-Jones D. Reduction in excess daytime sleepiness by modafinil in patients with myotonic dystrophy. *Neuromuscul Disord* 2003; **13**: 357–64.

88. Wintzen AR, Lammers GJ, van Dijk JG. Does modafinil enhance activity of patients with myotonic dystrophy? A double-blind placebo-controlled crossover study. *J Neurol* 2007; **254**: 26–8.

89. Damian MS, Gerlach A, Schmidt F, Lehmann E, Reichmann H. Modafinil for excessive daytime sleepiness in myotonic dystrophy. *Neurology* 2001; **56**: 794–6.

90. Annane D, Moore DH, Barnes PRJ, Miller RG. Psychostimulants for hypersomnia (excessive daytime sleepiness) in myotonic dystrophy. *Cochrane Database Syst Rev* 2006; Issue 3, art. no.: CD003218.

91. Hilton-Jones D, Bowler M, Lochmüeller H, et al. Modafinil for excessive daytime sleepiness in myotonic dystrophy type 1—the patients' perspective. *Neuromuscul Disord* 2012; **22**: 597–603.

92. Langlois M, Sook Lee N, Rossi J, Puymirat J. Hammerhead ribozyme-mediated destruction of nuclear foci in myotonic dystrophy myoblasts. *Molec Ther* 1999; **7**: 670–80.

93. Furling D, Doucet G, Langlois M-A, et al. Viral vector producing antisense RNA restores myotonic dystrophy myoblast functions. *Gene Ther* 2003; **10**: 795–802.

94. Kanadia RN, Shin J, Yuan Y, et al. Reversal of RNA missplicing and myotonia after muscleblind overexpression in a mouse poly(CUG) model for myotonic dystrophy. *Proc Natl Acad Sci USA* 2006; **103**: 11748–53.

95. Mahadevan MS, Yadava R, Yu Q, et al. Reversible model of RNA toxicity and cardiac conduction defects in myotonic dystrophy. *Nat Genet* 2006; **38**: 1066–70.

96. Wheeler TM, Lueck JD, Swanson MS, et al. Correction of ClC-1 splicing eliminates chloride channelopathy and myotonia in mouse models of myotonic dystrophy. *J Clin Invest* 2007; **117**: 3952–7.

97. Warf MB, Nakamori M, Matthys CM, Thornton CA, Berglund JA. Pentamidine reverses the splicing defects associated with myotonic dystrophy. *Proc Natl Acad Sci USA* 2009; **106**: 18551–6.

98. Mulders SA, van den Broek WJ, Wheeler TM, et al. Triplet-repeat oligonucleotide-mediated reversal of RNA toxicity in myotonic dystrophy. *Proc Natl Acad Sci USA* **106**: 13915–20.

99. Mulders SA, van Engelen BG, Wieringa B, Wansink DG. Molecular therapy in myotonic dystrophy: focus on RNA gain-of-function. *Neurology* 2010; **74**: 1108–17.

CHAPTER 26

Facioscapulohumeral muscular dystrophy

Elly L. van der Kooi, Silvere van der Maarel, and Baziel G.M. van Engelen

Clinical features

First clinical descriptions

It was probably Cruveilhier, in 1852, who first described post-mortem findings of a patient affected by facioscapulohumeral muscular dystrophy (FSHD). The brain, spinal cord, and peripheral nerves were unaffected [1,2]. Presumably this was an unexpected finding, as progressive muscle diseases were believed to have neurogenic causes. It was not until 1868 that the concept of primary muscle disorders was set out by Duchenne [3]. In his works concerning the differential diagnosis of the condition now carrying his name he described a facioscapulohumeral syndrome, most likely representing FSHD [3]. In 1884, the observations of Landouzy and Dejerine on 'la myopathie atrophique progressive: myopathie héréditaire débutant, dans l'enfance, par la face, sans alteration du système nerveux' were presented [4]. Their early reports actually describe all key elements of the disease which they named as a facioscapulohumeral type of progressive myopathy, only lacking an emphasis on the characteristic asymmetry in muscle involvement [4–6].

Pattern of muscle involvement

The median age of onset of FSHD is thought to be around 17 years with a wide range, varying at the most extreme from infancy to the seventh decade [1]. In general *de novo* cases report an earlier mean age of onset, whereas females may have a later age of onset [1,7,8]. FSHD is usually considered to be a slowly progressive disorder. However, the rate of progression can be highly variable: there may be periods of apparent clinical arrest with little or no deterioration in the patient's functioning, but also short periods of rapid progression. The well-known clinical variability of the disease concerns above all the rate and extent of the progression. The pattern in which muscles become clinically affected is rather uniform and recognizable [4–6,9]. The following description of the course of muscle involvement is based on previous descriptions by Padberg and by Rogers [1,9,10].

One of the main characteristics of FSHD is the early and often asymmetrical involvement of the facial muscles. Facial weakness is not necessarily present, and it often goes unrecognized. The most obviously affected facial muscles are the orbicularis oculi and oris. Weakness of the orbicularis oculi may lead to incomplete eye closure, which may cause Bell's phenomenon, exposure keratitis, and corneal scarring (Fig. 26.1).

When viewed from the side, the lips can have a pouting appearance. Involvement of the orbicularis oris and surrounding muscles causes difficulties in pursing the lips, whistling, sucking, or blowing (Fig. 26.2), and articulation difficulties.

Over 80% of patients notice shoulder-girdle weakness as the first symptom of the disease. Limited anteflexion and abduction due to weakness of the scapulofixators causes difficulties in handling objects above shoulder height, e.g. in combing the hair. On attempted anteflexion of the arms one can see a characteristic high rise of the winged scapula due to relative preservation of the deltoid muscle (Fig. 26.3). There is distinct involvement of the pectoralis muscles as well. Atrophy of the clavicular head of the pectoralis major produces a typical, almost horizontal, axillary fold. The weakness is often asymmetrical with a disputed and unexplained preference for involvement of the right side. Approximately 30% of all familial cases never progress beyond shoulder weakness.

In the majority of patients the weakness spreads to the upper arm affecting the triceps, followed by the biceps and brachioradialis [11,12]. Patients start having difficulties raising objects to their mouth. The atrophy in the upper arms may become very apparent, resulting in so-called Popeye arms, because of the relative sparing of the lower arm muscles.

At the same stage most patients develop foot extensor weakness. In moderate cases the front of the foot drops to the floor after heel strike, which is often better heard than seen, and prevents the striding leg from swinging through. In more severe cases toe strike may precede heel strike, which has a profound effect on gait. It results in a steppage gait and may lead to tripping or falling. Very occasionally, foot drop may be the presenting symptom.

The abdominal muscles are affected, but at this stage protuberance of the abdomen often goes unnoticed. A positive Beevor sign is often present. Lumbar lordosis may increase because of the combined weakness of abdominal, gluteal, and erector spinae muscles (Fig. 26.4).

In about one-fifth of cases with progression beyond shoulder-girdle involvement, weakness of the pelvic girdle and upper legs precedes that of the lower leg. Pelvic-girdle weakness gives a waddling gait and difficulties in rising from a chair or climbing stairs.

In severely affected patients wrist extensors become weak and patients start using wrist flexion to flex their elbows. Wrist flexion

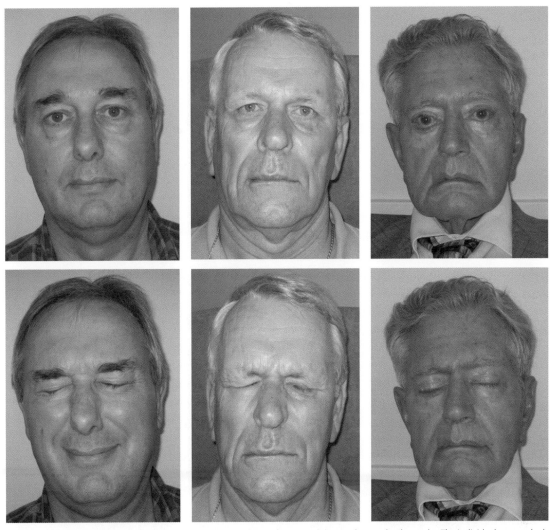

Fig. 26.1 Examples of several degrees of (asymmetrical) involvement of the face in facioscapulohumeral muscular dystrophy. The individuals were asked to: look neutral (top row) and close their eyes (bottom row).

functionally reduces grip strength. Finally, weakness of finger extensors and neck extensors (a dropped head) is occasionally seen.

Differential diagnosis

Despite the characteristic clinical presentation of FSHD, the combination of facial weakness and scapular winging can be seen in other myopathies, e.g. acid maltase deficiency, congenital myopathies, Davidenkow syndrome, inclusion body myositis/myopathy, limb-girdle muscular dystrophies, mitochondrial myopathies, neuralgic amyotrophy, polymyositis, proximal myotonic myopathy, scapuloperoneal muscular dystrophy, and scapuloperoneal spinal muscular atrophy [13].

Genetics, pathology, and physiology

Genetics and epigenetics

In the majority of cases, FSHD shows an autosomal dominant pattern of inheritance caused by contraction of the D4Z4 macrosatellite repeat in the subtelomeric region of chromosome 4q (FSHD1) [14]. Normal alleles contain between 11 and 100 D4Z4 repeat units

ordered head-to-tail, while in patients with FSHD1 one of the 4q chromosomes carries an array of one to ten D4Z4 units [15]. Contraction of the D4Z4 repeat in FSHD is associated with reduced levels of repressive chromatin markers: while D4Z4 is normally highly DNA methylated, D4Z4 at the disease allele is hypomethylated in FSHD. Similarly, there is a decrease of the repressive modification histone 3 lysine 9 trimethylation at D4Z4 in FSHD with secondary losses of other heterochromatic proteins [16–18].

In the subtelomeric region of chromosome 10q, a highly homologous repeat array structure has been found, but contractions of this repeat are generally non-pathogenic. D4Z4 repeat contractions need to occur on a specific genetic background, a so-called permissive chromosome, to be pathogenic [19–21]. Each D4Z4 repeat contains an open reading frame that encodes for the *DUX4* retrogene. In the absence of a polyadenylation (polyA) signal, transcripts from this retrogene are generally not stable. Recent data have demonstrated that permissive chromosomes 4, such as 4A161, contain an additional *DUX4* exon located immediately distal to the most telomeric D4Z4 unit which provides the transcript with a polyA signal [21–23]. This polyA signal enables the stabilization of the

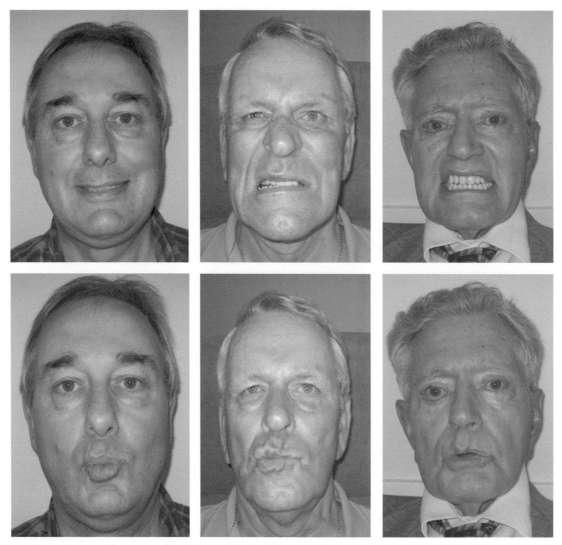

Fig. 26.2 Examples of several degrees of (asymmetrical) involvement of the face in facioscapulohumeral muscular dystrophy. The individuals were asked to: show their teeth (top row) and purse their lips (bottom row).

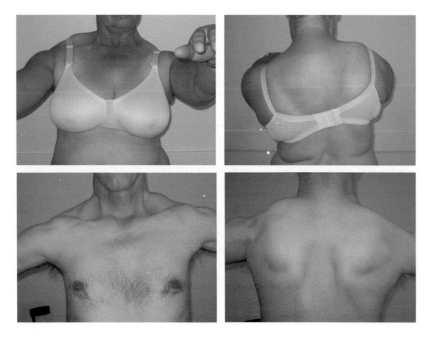

Fig. 26.3 Examples of shoulder-girdle and upper arm involvement. The person in the top row was asked to elevate her arms. The person in the bottom row was asked to abduct his arms.

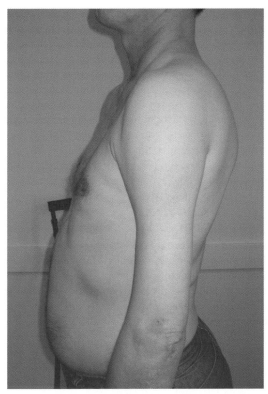

Fig. 26.4 Example of protrusion of the abdomen, increased lumbar lordosis, and atrophy of the upper arms.

DUX4 transcript emanating from the distal D4Z4 unit in skeletal muscle of FSHD1 patients, creating bursts of *DUX4* protein expression in sporadic myonuclei [23].

In accordance with genetic and epigenetic data supporting a pathogenic role for *DUX4* in FSHD, overexpression models show that somatic *DUX4* expression is toxic [24–27]. Although the exact pathophysiological role of *DUX4* is still under investigation, *DUX4* protein expression seems to cause cell death in a variety of cell types, with skeletal muscle being highly sensitive.

Genetic and prenatal counselling [13,28]

FSHD is inherited in an autosomal dominant manner with a previously reported penetrance of over 95% by the age of 20. However, in our experience and in a current Dutch genotype–phenotype study, penetrance appears to be about 80% with a wide range in the age of onset (unpublished). Approximately 70–90% of individuals have inherited the disease-causing deletion from a parent; and approximately 10–30% as the result of a *de novo* deletion. Offspring of an affected individual have a 50% chance of inheriting the deletion. There is no reliable correlation between genotype and phenotype, and there is large intrafamilial variability. However, the presence of only a small number of residual repeats, i.e. allele sizes of 10–19 kb, reliably predicts severe or infantile-onset FSHD.

Prenatal testing is possible if a D4Z4 contraction mutation has been identified in the family. Diagnosis on DNA isolated from chorionic villi is preferred over amniocentesis, because amniocentesis tests takes several weeks to complete. Preimplantation genetic diagnosis (PGD) is still difficult due to technical constraints.

Fertility, pregnancy, and delivery

There are no reports or data on (decreased) fertility. There is one German (from 1997) and one American (from 2006) case series on pregnancy and delivery in women with FSHD [29–31]. Altogether, outcome of 131 pregnancies in 49 women was generally favourable. There was no indication of increased risk of miscarriage, preterm labour, or perinatal death. However, there were higher rates of low birth weight and total operative deliveries. Worsening of weakness and pain occurred in about 25% of the pregnancies—generally not resolving after delivery.

The European Neuromuscular Centre (ENMC) recommends that pregnant women be followed by high-risk obstetricians and are delivered in a centre with comprehensive perinatal care. Additionally, pregnant women with reduced lung function should have serial monitoring of forced vital capacity (FVC) during their pregnancy [13].

Genotype and phenotype

What determines the severity and characteristic asymmetric pattern of FSHD is at least as important as the question of which gene causes it. An association between the residual D4Z4 fragment size, the age of onset, and disease severity has been observed in groups of patients from different ethnic backgrounds [32–35]. Smaller residual D4Z4 fragments are associated with an earlier age of onset and more severe forms of disease. However, there is large variability in disease expression within patients sharing the same residual D4Z4 fragment size, both interfamilial and intrafamilial [1,36]. So it is not possible to predict the likely severity of disease expression and rate of progression in individual patients based on the residual fragment size alone. Recent studies indicate that the degree of DNA methylation of the D4Z4 allele may also in part determine disease severity [17,37]. A comparative study of gene expression profiles in asymptomatic carriers and related affected patients identified differentially expressed genes that might contribute to the disease presentation and severity [38].

In FSHD there are rather consistent findings regarding gender differences in disease expression: females are more likely to be asymptomatic, to have a later onset, and a slower progression [1,8]. After the menopause disease progression appears to accelerate. Also, in mosaic patients with only a proportion of affected cells, males are more frequently symptomatic than females, and they require lower percentages of mutated cells (peripheral blood lymphocytes) to become clinically manifest [39]. It has been suggested that female sex hormones might have a mild protective effect on disease progression.

In 5% of patients with FSHD, no D4Z4 repeat contraction on chromosome 4q35 is observed [40]. Such patients, nowadays called patients with FSHD2, show loss of DNA methylation and heterochromatin markers at the D4Z4 repeat that are similar to patients with D4Z4 contractions. FSHD2 is no different in its clinical presentation, except for a (possible) absence of gender differences in disease severity and a higher incidence (67%) of sporadic cases. In FSHD2 disease severity is not influenced by D4Z4 repeat size and only slightly influenced by the degree of hypomethylation [40].

Muscle pathology and physiology

Neither muscle biopsy nor electrophysiological studies are indicated in the diagnostic assessment of suspected FSHD

(DNA testing is the first investigation), but such studies have been performed historically and may be undertaken in a patient presenting with muscle symptoms in whom the diagnosis of FSHD is not initially considered.

Muscle biopsy studies

Muscle histology in FSHD shows no disease-specific abnormalities. However, the presence of lobulated fibres, small angular fibres, and inflammatory infiltrates in combination with dystrophic features form a pattern suggestive of FSHD [9]. Dystrophic features include fibre necrosis and regeneration, increased variation in fibre size, increased numbers of internal nuclei, fibrosis, and fat replacement [41]. Occasionally the mononuclear cellular infiltrates may be large, falsely suggesting myositis [42]. The overall findings on electron microscopy, immunochemistry, and immunoblotting are generally consistent with a primary myopathic process, and do not demonstrate any consistent disease-specific findings [43]. Freeze fracture and electron microscopy studies suggest that the organization of the sarcolemma and its relationship to the underlying contractile apparatus is altered [44].

Myoblast studies

In recent myoblast studies FSHD myoblasts displayed a rather characteristic necrotic phenotype (swollen and vacuolated) [45]. A developmental stage-specific susceptibility to oxidative stress was hypothesized. An analysis of comparative gene expression profiles revealed consistent down-regulation of a set of transcripts involved in oxidative stress in FSHD myoblasts [46,47]. FSHD myoblasts showed a reduced replicative capacity and a morphological appearance resembling senescence in normal myoblasts [45]. However, more recent studies reported normal growth and regeneration ability of myoblasts and mesangioblasts from unaffected muscles of patients [48–51].

Electrophysiological studies

Overall findings on electromyography are generally consistent with a myopathic process, and do not demonstrate any disease-specific findings [1]. Occasionally, spontaneous activity is found [52]. Infrequently, neurogenic features may be present.

Interventions and intervention studies

Therapeutic interventions

In 1980 Dubowitz reviewed the results of therapeutic drug trials in muscular dystrophies [53]. Most of these studies grouped patients with different muscular dystrophies together, often including as many as one to ten FSHD patients. Dubowitz came across many claims for cures based on uncontrolled trials or anecdotal comments. Generally, the initial positive study was of poor quality and was followed by a well-controlled study proving the drug to be of no value. The following agents appeared not to be effective: vitamins B_6 and E, folic acid, anabolic steroids, corticosteroids, digitoxin, and a mixture of nucleotides. Dubowitz made a plea for reliable controlled and blinded studies in uniform groups of patients with durations of at least 2 years and more systematic and comprehensive assessments of muscle function.

However, effective therapeutic treatments are still lacking in FSHD and the majority of other muscular dystrophies. The following agents have been, or are currently being, tested in clinical intervention studies: the corticosteroid prednisone (one open-label pilot study; no significant changes on muscle strength or mass), the β2-adrenergic agonist albuterol or salbutamol (one open-label pilot study, three randomized, placebo-controlled trials; not effective or at best a temporary, very moderate gain in muscle strength and mass), creatine monohydrate (one uncontrolled trial; negative for participating FSHD patients), the calcium antagonist diltiazem (one open-label pilot study; no significant changes in muscle strength, function, or mass), the myostatin neutralizing antibody MYO-029 (one randomized, placebo-controlled safety trial; no significant improvement of muscle strength or function), and folic acid combined with methionine (one open-label pilot study; no effect on D4Z4 hypomethylation) [54–64]. Muscle stem cell therapy has also been put forward as a potential therapeutic strategy [48–51,65].

Other interventions

The absence of effective therapeutic treatment makes interventions aimed at the preservation of muscle function and the patient's functional capabilities of major importance. Possible interventions include surgical and non-surgical interventions for scapular winging and foot drop, exercise, physiotherapy, and more comprehensive rehabilitation programmes.

Scapular winging [65,66]

Different non-surgical and surgical interventions have been used to achieve better scapular stability: bracing, muscle transfer techniques, scapulodesis, and scapulopexy.

Bracing with orthotic devices such as figure-of-eight braces is often poorly tolerated and lacks sufficient force to fix the scapula to a degree needed for a meaningful improvement of shoulder function. Sometimes these braces are used for short periods of time to ease intractable shoulder pain due to laxity of the shoulder joint.

Muscle transfer techniques are inappropriate in progressive muscular dystrophies, as the dystrophic process will continue, eventually affecting the transferred muscle itself. In scapulodesis the scapula is fixed to the thoracic wall with screws, wires or plates with or without a bone graft to produce a solid fusion. In scapulopexy, fascial or synthetic slings are used to improve scapular fixation. There are no randomized controlled trials of scapular fixation in FSHD or other muscular dystrophies. A recently updated systematic review of all available non-randomized case reports and case series comprised one FSHD patient with an orthosis, six with scapulopexy, and 65 with mostly bilateral scapulodesis [66]. Operative interventions appeared to produce significant benefits regarding shoulder abduction, elevation, and functional use of the arm. However, these benefits need to be balanced against postoperative immobilization, the need for physiotherapy, and intra-operative and postoperative complications. Most stable results, but also most complications, were reached after scapulodesis. However, the limited published data on the other techniques preclude a fair comparison.

The ENMC recommends that patients considering surgery should have reasonable residual upper arm strength and should weigh the potential benefits against the possible complications of the procedure. The potential gain in range of motion from surgical fixation can be tested at the bedside by manual fixation of the scapula [13].

Foot drop [67]

Weakness of the ankle dorsiflexors and subsequent contracture of the ankle joint and Achilles tendon frequently cause 'floppy' foot drop. Foot drop can have a profound effect on gait and may lead to tripping or falling. The most frequently used interventions are orthopaedic shoes and custom moulded ankle–foot orthoses (AFOs). Floor reaction ankle–foot orthoses (FRAFO) or sometimes modern knee–ankle–foot orthoses (KAFO) are recommended for patients who have foot drop combined with weakness of the knee extensors [65]. Other suggested interventions are tendon transfers, surgery to fixate the ankle, and physiotherapy (including strengthening exercises and functional electrical stimulation) [67]. However, 1 year of strengthening exercise did not significantly affect the strength of the ankle dorsiflexors [57].

Exercise, physiotherapy, and rehabilitation programmes

A randomized controlled trial with 1 year of moderate-intensity strength training versus no training in 65 patients showed only a very limited positive effect on muscle strength, and no harmful effects [57,68–70]. A 12-week low-intensity aerobic exercise programme in eight patients appeared to improve their aerobic capacity without signs of muscle damage [71]. Five months of neuromuscular electrical stimulation strength training in nine patients increased muscle strength [72]. There is no specific literature or study known to us on the effects of physiotherapeutic interventions or more comprehensive rehabilitation programmes [70].

Based on this limited evidence we tell our patients that 'normal' participation in sports and work appears not to harm their muscles, but there is insufficient evidence to say that it offers benefit or for general prescription of exercise programmes. Any training should be done under the supervision of a specialized therapist who can monitor side effects and prevent injuries [68].

There is a high prevalence of falls in FSHD patients and a distinct relationship between their muscle weakness and instability [73]. In a questionnaire, 30% of patients reported falling at least once a month. Injuries occurred in almost 70% of these patients. Patients who fall tend to do this mainly at home and show instability while climbing stairs, rising from chairs, and standing with their eyes closed. Strategies for preventing falls should focus on home adaptations and these situations [73].

The ENMC recommends an initial rehabilitation consultation for all patients with functional limitations, and follow-up depending on the ongoing needs of the individual [13].

Associated clinical features and their management

The characteristic pattern of weakness and wasting of the skeletal muscles is the most prominent feature of FSHD. Nevertheless, there are other clinical features, associated complaints, and conditions [1,9]. Some of these features are clearly related to the dystrophic process; for others the causative relation with the pathogenetic mechanism of FSHD remains unclear. Some of these symptoms and conditions have only recently been recognized as relevant symptoms in FSHD, i.e. pain, fatigue, dysphagia, and respiratory insufficiency. Others have been known about and debated for some decades now, and have been studied more extensively, e.g. hearing loss, vascular retinopathy, and cardiac involvement. Knowledge of these associated features is important for medical management and so that patients can be given proper information.

Pain

In FSHD pain is rarely mentioned as an important clinical feature. However, in two questionnaire-based surveys 50–75% of patients indicated its presence [74,75]. In two subsequent studies about 80% of patients reported chronic persistent or periodic pains of mostly moderate intensity; multifocal, but most frequent of the neck, shoulder, lower back, and legs [69,76]. Remarkably, in the Dutch study [69] pain intensity ranged from mild to moderate, and in the American one [76] from moderate to severe. The role of biopsychosocial factors on chronic pain and its impact on quality of life in patients has been studied [77–79]. Considering its high frequency, it is surprising how little attention pain and its treatment has received. First-line analgesics are used by 11–46% of patients [69,74–76]. Dutch patients noticed only limited benefits from first-line analgesics, unlike most French patients who reported a clear beneficial effect [74,75]. In an American study of FSHD and myotonic dystrophy Type 1 patients together reported the greatest pain relief from using marijuana, followed by opioids, nerve blocks, massage, and chiropractic manipulation [76]. Further research on pain in FSHD should probably also take intercultural differences into account.

The ENMC recommends dealing with pain using standard approaches to the management of chronic pain such as, where appropriate, physical therapy and pain medications [13].

Fatigue

Until recently, fatigue was not considered an important feature of FSHD—yet, in a strength training and albuterol trial 34% of patients appeared to be severely fatigued [69]. In a subsequent questionnaire-based survey 61% of patients were considered to be severely fatigued [80]. The severity of the fatigue experienced was associated with the severity of functional impairments. Fatigue and its consequences in patients with neuromuscular disorders, including FSHD, is just starting to receive more attention [81,82]. At the moment there is no treatment available. A study on the effect of aerobic exercise training and cognitive behavioural therapy on chronic fatigue in neuromuscular disorders, including FSHD, is being conducted [83]. At present, the ENMC recommends energy conservation strategies and aerobic training, if necessary.

Hearing loss

Clinically significant hearing loss appears to be a prominent feature of infantile-onset FSHD. Audiological evaluation is advised in these patients as hearing aids may be necessary [9]. Recent audiometric studies did not find any significant difference in the prevalence of hearing impairment in adult-onset patients compared with the normal population [84,85]. So, screening in adult-onset patients without hearing problems is not necessary.

Vascular retinopathy

In 50–75% of patients subclinical vascular retinopathy can be detected by fluorescein angiography [86,87]. In less than 1% of these patients it will eventually lead to symptomatic exudative retinopathy (Coat syndrome) which can result in significant visual loss [86]. Timely photocoagulation may preserve sight, although not always [88]. Nowadays, the ENMC recommends that all patients with FSHD be referred to an ophthalmologist for dilated indirect ophthalmoscopy. If no significant retinal vascular disease is detected in adult patients, no further follow-up is warranted unless the patients develop visual symptoms. In early onset disease, where the incidence of Coat syndrome is more common, yearly follow-up with indirect ophthalmoscopy is recommended until the child is deemed mature enough to report visual symptoms [13].

Scoliosis/bent spine

Mild kyphoscoliosis and increased lumbar lordosis is seen in 30% of patients. In severely affected, wheelchair-dependent patients with an early onset kyphoscoliosis, the spinal deformity may eventually compromise respiratory function [1,9,89]. The management of spinal deformities is as recommended for patients with idiopathic adolescent scoliosis [90].

In recent years, patients with a predominant or isolated bent spine syndrome or captocormia due to severe involvement of the paraspinal muscles and hamstrings with relative sparing of the other muscles have been described [91,92].

Dysphagia

Involvement of the lingual and pharyngeal muscles was long considered to be an exclusion criterion for FSHD [93]. However, dysphagia and tongue atrophy have been reported in severely affected early onset patients [94,95]. In a survey on pulmonary function in 87 patients, ten reported problems with swallowing [94]. Ancillary studies in these patients indicated mild to moderate oropharyngeal dysfunction and relatively small tongue volumes. Dysphagia was associated with more severe muscle disease and pronounced weakness of the facial muscles. In FSHD, dysphagia seldom leads to aspiration. We refer patients with swallowing difficulties to a speech therapist. Special attention should be paid to patients with respiratory insufficiency and swallowing problems, because of a higher risk of aspiration [94]. A speech therapist might also be of help when patients have articulation problems due to orofacial weakness.

Ankle and other contractures

Ankle contractures occur in approximately 10% of patients. Occasionally, elbow and hip contractures are found. As the contractures are usually mild, they seldom warrant active treatment. Limited and dated experiences with techniques for elongating the Achilles tendon were negative [1].

Pectus excavatum

Pectus excavatum is present in approximately 5% of patients [1,9]. It can lead to cosmetic complaints. Combined with spinal deformities it might further compromise respiratory function [89]. Whether surgical correction will clinically improve respiratory function is not known.

Cardiac involvement

Cardiac involvement in FSHD has been debated for decades, but the current opinion is that symptomatic cardiac disease is rare. De Visser et al. [96] found no electrocardiographic or echocardiographic abnormalities, and no rhythm disturbances in 31 familial patients studied. More recent studies showed some evidence for cardiac abnormality in about 5–12% of patients, usually rhythm disturbances [97,98]. In addition, minor electrocardiographic abnormalities are reported in up to 60% of patients, and these are most likely of little clinical significance [97,99]. There is no special need for cardiac screening or surveillance [13].

Respiratory insufficiency/sleep-disordered breathing

The pulmonary function in a large group of ambulant and wheelchair-dependent patients was studied using facial mask-adjusted devices because of the orofacial weakness [100,101]. Ambulatory patients had a nearly normal FVC, but their maximal respiratory pressures tended to be 80% of predicted. Wheelchair-dependent patients with an early onset of disease, especially those with a kyphoscoliosis, showed restricted pulmonary function, i.e. mean FVC just above 60% and maximal respiratory pressures around 45% of predicted.

Nocturnal hypoventilation is known to be an early manifestation of respiratory insufficiency in patients with neuromuscular disease [102]. In general, patients with a FVC over 60% are at low risk of nocturnal hypoventilation; patients with a FVC of less than 40% have a significant risk [103]. Although respiratory insufficiency in FSHD is rare, approximately 1% of patients require (nocturnal) ventilatory support [89]. Severe muscle weakness, wheelchair dependency, and kyphoscoliosis appear to be risk factors for respiratory failure. Pectus excavatum might be an additional risk factor.

Current ENMC recommendations are to routinely screen patients with moderate to severe FSHD, i.e. those with proximal lower extremity weakness, for symptoms of hypoventilation. Supine and sitting FVC is recommended for any patient with FSHD prior to any surgical procedure requiring general anaesthesia or conscious sedation. FVC measurements should be performed with a full facial mask rather than a mouthpiece to avoid falsely low values from leakage of air due to weakness of lip closure [13,101]. Even in the absence of symptoms of nocturnal hypoventilation, yearly FVC is recommended for patients who are wheelchair bound, have pelvic-girdle weakness, superimposed pulmonary disease, moderate to severe kyphoscoliosis, lumbar hyperlordosis, or chest wall deformities such as pectus excavatum [13,89]. When symptoms of nocturnal hypoventilation are present, or FVC drops below 50% or maximum inspiratory pressure (MIP) below 30% of predicted, further analysis is needed and non-invasive ventilatory support considered [13,89,101]. Our patients on (nocturnal) ventilatory support all reported improved quality of life.

Currently, attention is being called to the high percentage, probably up to 50%, of patients, having an impaired sleep quality and sleep-disordered breathing, in particular obstructive apnoeas and rapid eye movement (REM)-related oxygen desaturations. Screening for sleep-disordered breathing should possibly be included in the clinical assessment of FSHD [104–106].

Keratitis

Occasionally incomplete lid closure leads to serious exposure keratitis and corneal scarring despite treatment with emollient eye drops and ointments, taping, or patches [107]. Gold-weight implants in the upper eyelid and reconstructive surgery of the lower lid can be considered to relieve discomfort and prevent severe keratopathy [108].

Mental retardation

Mental retardation and occasionally epilepsy are features seen in patients at the most extreme end of the FSHD spectrum: severe, early onset, mostly sporadic cases with small residual repeat sizes, i.e. a residual D4Z4 fragment size of one to three repeats [107,109].

These patients are likely to have hearing impairment and vascular retinopathy as well. Mental retardation and epilepsy have been frequently observed in Japanese infantile patients, and may reflect a population-dependent effect of the disease [107,109].

References

1. Padberg GW. *Facioscapulohumeral Disease* [thesis]. Leiden University, Leiden, 1982.

2. Cruveilhier J. Mémoire sur la paralysie musculaire atrophique. *Bull l'Acad Méd* 1982–1983; **18**: 490–502, 546–83.

3. Duchenne GBA. Recherches sur la paralysie musculaire pseudohypertrophique, ou paralysie myo-sclérosique. *Arch Gén Méd* 1868; **11**: 5–25, 179–209, 305–21, 421–43, 552–88.

4. Landouzy L, Dejerine J. De la myopathie atrophique progressive: myopathie héréditaire débutant, dans l'enfance, par la face, sans alteration du système nerveux. *C R Acad Sci (Paris)* 1884; **98**: 53–5.

5. Landouzy L. Note sur deux cas d'atrophie musculaire progressive de l'enfance. *Mem Soc Biol* 1874; 103–21.

6. Landouzy L, Dejerine J. De la myopathie atrophique progressive: myopathie sans neuropathie debutant d'ordinaire dans l'enfance par la face. *Rev Med (Paris)* 1885; **5**: 254–366.

7. Jardine PE, Koch MC, Lunt PW, et al. De novo facioscapulohumeral muscular dystrophy defined by DNA probe p13E-11 (D4F104S1). *Arch Dis Child* 1994; **71**: 221–7.

8. Zatz M, Marie SK, Cerqueira A, Vainzof M, Pavanello RC, Passos-Bueno MR. The facioscapulohumeral muscular dystrophy (FSHD1) gene affects males more severely and more frequently than females. *Am J Med Genet* 1998; **77**: 155–61.

9. Padberg GW. Facioscapulohumeral muscular dystrophy: a clinician's experience. In: Upadhyaya M, Cooper DN (ed) *Facioscapulohumeral Muscular Dystrophy. Clinical Medicine and Molecular Biology*, pp. 41–53. London and New York; Garland Science/BIOS Scientific Publishers, 2004.

10. Rogers MT. Facioscapulohumeral muscular dystrophy: historical background and literature review. In: Upadhyaya M, Cooper DN (ed) *Facioscapulohumeral Muscular Dystrophy. Clinical Medicine and Molecular Biology*, pp. 17–39. London and New York: Garland Science/BIOS Scientific Publishers, 2004.

11. Tyler FH, Stephens FE. Studies in disorders of muscle. II. Clinical manifestations and inheritance of facioscapulohumeral dystrophy in a large family. *Ann Int Med* 1950; **32**: 640–60.

12. Flanigan KM, Coffeen CM, Sexton L, Stauffer D, Brunner S, Leppert MF. Genetic characterization of a large, historically significant Utah kindred with facioscapulohumeral dystrophy. *Neuromuscul Disord* 2001; **11**: 525–9.

13. Tawil R, van der Maarel S, Padberg GW, van Engelen BG. 171st ENMC International Workshop: Standards of Care and Management of Facioscapulohumeral Muscular Dystrophy. *Neuromuscul Disord* 2010; **20**: 471–5.

14. Wijmenga C, Hewitt JE, Sandkuijl LA, et al. Chromosome 4q DNA rearrangements associated with facioscapulohumeral muscular dystrophy. *Nat Genet* 1992; **2**: 26–30.

15. van Deutekom JC, Bakker E, Lemmers RJ, et al. Evidence for subtelomeric exchange of 3.3 kb tandemly repeated units between chromosomes 4q35 and 10q26: implications for genetic counselling and etiology of FSHD1. *Hum Mol Genet* 1996; **5**: 1997–2003.

16. de Greef JC, Frants RR, van der Maarel SM. Epigenetic mechanisms of facioscapulohumeral muscular dystrophy. *Mutat Res* 2008; **647**: 94–102.

17. van Overveld PGM, Lemmers RJFL, Sandkuijl LA, et al. Hypomethylation of D4Z4 in 4q-linked and non-4q-linked facioscapulohumeral muscular dystrophy. *Nat Genet* 2003; **35**: 315–17.

18. Zeng W, de Greef JC, Chien R, et al. Specific loss of histone H3 lysine 9 trimethylation and HP1gamma/cohesin binding at D4Z4 repeats is associated with facioscapulohumeral dystrophy (FSHD). *PLoS Genet* 2009; **5**: e1000559.

19. Lemmers RJ, de Kievit P, Sandkuijl L, et al. Padberg GW, van Ommen GJ, Frants RR, van der Maarel SM. Facioscapulohumeral muscular dystrophy is uniquely associated with one of the two variants of the 4q subtelomere. *Nat Genet* 2002; **32**: 235–6.

20. Lemmers RJ, Wohlgemuth M, van der Gaag KJ, et al. Specific sequence variations within the 4q35 region are associated with facioscapulohumeral muscular dystrophy. *Am J Hum Genet* 2007; **81**: 884–94.

21. Lemmers RJ, van der Vliet PJ, Klooster R, et al. A unifying genetic model for facioscapulohumeral muscular dystrophy. *Science* 2010; **329**: 1650–3.

22. Dixit M, Ansseau E, Tassin A, et al. DUX4, a candidate gene of facioscapulohumeral muscular dystrophy, encodes a transcriptional activator of PITX1. *Proc Natl Acad Sci USA* 2007; **104**: 18157–62.

23. Snider L, Geng LN, Lemmers RJ, et al. Facioscapulohumeral dystrophy: incomplete suppression of a retrotransposed gene. *PLoS Genet* 2010; **6**: e1001181.

24. Bosnakovski D, Xu Z, Gang EJ, et al. An isogenetic myoblast expression screen identifies DUX4-mediated FSHD-associated molecular pathologies. *EMBO J* 2008; **27**: 2766–79.

25. Bosnakovski D, Daughters RS, Xu Z, Slack JM, Kyba M. Biphasic myopathic phenotype of mouse DUX, an ORF within conserved FSHD-related repeats. *PLoS One* 2009; **4**: e7003.

26. Kowaljow V, Marcowycz A, Ansseau E, et al. The DUX4 gene at the FSHD1A locus encodes a pro-apoptotic protein. *Neuromuscul Disord* 2007; **17**: 611–23.

27. Wuebbles RD, Long SW, Hanel ML, Jones PL. Testing the effects of FSHD candidate gene expression in vertebrate muscle development. *Int J Clin Exp Pathol* 2010; **3**: 386–400.

28. Lemmers RJLF, Miller DG, van der Maarel SM. Facioscapulohumeral muscular dystrophy. In: Pagon RA, Adam MP, Bird TD, et al. (ed) *GeneReviews*™ [Internet]. Seattle, WA: University of Washington, Seattle, March 8 1999 [updated 21 June 2012]. Available from: <http://www.ncbi.nlm.nih.gov/books/NBK1443/>.

29. Rudnik-Schöneborn S, Glauner B, Röhrig D, Zerres K. Obstetric aspects in women with facioscapulohumeral muscular dystrophy, limb-girdle muscular dystrophy, and congenital myopathies. *Arch Neurol* 1997; **54**: 888–94.

30. Ciafaloni E, Pressman EK, Loi AM, et al. Pregnancy and birth outcomes in women with facioscapulohumeral muscular dystrophy. *Neurology* 2006; **67**: 1887–9.

31. Argov Z, de Visser M. What we do not know about pregnancy in hereditary neuromuscular disorders. *Neuromuscul Disord* 2009; **19**: 675–9.

32. Lunt PW, Jardine PE, Koch MC, et al. Correlation between fragment size at D4F104S1 and age at onset or at wheelchair use, with a possible generational effect, accounts for much phenotypic variation in 4q35-facioscapulohumeral muscular dystrophy (FSHD). *Hum Mol Genet* 1995; **4**: 951–8.

33. Zatz M, Marie SK, Passos-Bueno MR, et al. High proportion of new mutations and possible anticipation in Brazilian facioscapulohumeral muscular dystrophy families. *Am J Hum Genet* 1995; **56**: 99–105.

34. Tawil R, Forrester J, Griggs RC, et al. Evidence for anticipation and association of deletion size with severity in facioscapulohumeral muscular dystrophy. The FSH-DY Group. *Ann Neurol* 1996; **39**: 744–8.

35. Hsu YD, Kao MC, Shyu WC, et al. Application of chromosome 4q35-qter marker (pFR-1) for DNA rearrangement of facioscapulohumeral muscular dystrophy patients in Taiwan. *J Neurol Sci* 1997; **149**: 73–9.

36. Ricci E, Galluzzi G, Deidda G, et al. Progress in the molecular diagnosis of facioscapulohumeral muscular dystrophy and correlation between the number of KpnI repeats at the 4q35 locus and clinical phenotype. *Ann Neurol* 1999; **45**: 751–7.

37. van Overveld PGM, Enthoven L, Ricci E, et al. Variable hypomethylation of D4Z4 in facioscapulohumeral muscular dystrophy. *Ann Neurol* 2005; **58**: 569–76.

38. Arashiro P, Eisenberg I, Kho AT, et al. Transcriptional regulation differs in affected facioscapulohumeral muscular dystrophy patients compared to asymptomatic related carriers. *Proc Natl Acad Sci USA* 2009; **106**: 6220–5.

39. van der Maarel SM, Deidda G, Lemmers RJ, et al. De novo facioscapulohumeral muscular dystrophy: frequent somatic mosaicism, sex-dependent phenotype, and the role of mitotic transchromosomal repeat interaction between chromosomes 4 and 10. *Am J Hum Genet* 2000; **66**: 26–35.

40. de Greef JC, Lemmers RJ, Camaño P, et al. Clinical features of facioscapulohumeral muscular dystrophy 2. *Neurology* 2010; **75**:1548–54.

41. Brooke MH. *A Clinician's View of Neuromuscular Diseases.* Baltimore, MD: Williams & Wilkins, 1986.

42. Arahata K, Ishihara T, Fukunaga H, et al. Inflammatory response in facioscapulohumeral dystrophy (FSHD): immunocytochemical and genetic analysis. *Muscle Nerve* 1995; **2**: S56–S66.

43. Rogers MT, Sewry AS, Upadhyahya M. Histological, immunocytochemical, molecular and ultrastructural characteristics of FSHD muscle. In: Upadhyaya M, Cooper DN (ed) *Facioscapulohumeral Muscular Dystrophy. Clinical Medicine and Molecular Biology*, pp. 277–98. London and New York: Garland Science/BIOS Scientific Publishers, 2004.

44. Reed P, Porter NC, Strong J, et al. Sarcolemmal reorganization in FSHD. In: Upadhyaya M, Cooper DN (ed) *Facioscapulohumeral Muscular Dystrophy. Clinical Medicine and Molecular Biology*, pp. 341–51. London and New York: Garland Science/BIOS Scientific Publishers, 2004.

45. Figlewicz DA, Barrett K, Haefele Leskovar A, et al. FSHD myoblasts: in vitro studies. In: Upadhyaya M, Cooper DN (ed) *Facioscapulohumeral Muscular Dystrophy. Clinical Medicine and Molecular Biology*, pp. 277–98. London and New York: Garland Science/BIOS Scientific Publishers, 2004.

46. Winokur ST, Chen YW, Masny PS, et al. Expression profiling of FSHD muscle supports a defect in specific stages of myogenic differentiation. *Hum Mol Genet* 2003; **12**: 2895–907.

47. Winokur ST, Barrett K, Martin JH, et al. Facioscapulohumeral muscular dystrophy (FSHD) myoblasts demonstrate increased susceptibility to oxidative stress. *Neuromuscul Disord* 2003; **13**: 322–33.

48. Vilquin JT, Marolleau JP, Sacconi S, et al. Normal growth and regenerating ability of myoblasts from unaffected muscles of facioscapulohumeral muscular dystrophy patients. *Gene Ther* 2005; **12**: 1651–62.

49. Desnuelle C, Sacconi S, Marolleau JP, Larghero J, Vilquin JT. [The possible place of autologus cell therapy in facioscapulohumeral muscular dystrophy.] *Bull Acad Natl Med* 2005; **189**: 697–713, 713–14.

50. Morosetti R, Mirabella M, Gliubizzi C, et al. Isolation and characterization of mesoangioblasts from facioscapulohumeral muscular dystrophy muscle biopsies. *Stem Cells* 2007; **25**: 3173–82.

51. Morosetti R, Gidaro T, Broccolini A, et al. Mesoangioblasts from Facioscapulohumeral Muscular Dystrophy display in vivo a variable myogenic ability predictable by their in vitro behavior. *Cell Transplant* 2011; **20**: 1299–313.

52. Munsat TL, Piper D, Cancilla P, Mednick J. Inflammatory myopathy with facioscapulohumeral distribution. *Neurology* 1972; **22**: 335–47.

53. Dubowitz V, Heckmatt J. Management of muscular dystrophy:\ pharmacological and physical aspects. *Br Med Bull* 1980; **36**: 139–44.

54. Tawil R, McDermott MP, Pandya S, et al. A pilot trial of prednisone in facioscapulohumeral muscular dystrophy. FSH-DY Group. *Neurology* 1997; **48**: 46–9.

55. Kissel JT, McDermott MP, Natarajan R, et al. Pilot trial of albuterol in facioscapulohumeral muscular dystrophy. FSH-DY Group. *Neurology* 1998; **50**: 1402–6.

56. Kissel JT, McDermott MP, Mendell JR, et al. Randomized, double-blind, placebo-controlled trial of albuterol in facioscapulohumeral muscular dystrophy. FSH-DY Group. *Neurology* 2001; **57**: 1434–40.

57. van der Kooi EL, Vogels OJ, van Asseldonk RJ, et al. Strength training and albuterol in facioscapulohumeral muscular dystrophy. *Neurology* 2004; **63**: 702–8.

58. Payan CA, Hogrel JY, Hammouda EH, et al. Periodic salbutamol in facioscapulohumeral muscular dystrophy: a randomized controlled trial. *Arch Phys Med Rehabil* 2009; **90**: 1094–101.

59. Matsumura T, Yokoe M, Nakamori M, et al. [A clinical trial of creatine monohydrate in muscular dystrophy patients]. *Rinsho Shinkeigaku* 2004; **44**: 661–6.

60. Walter MC, Lochmuller H, Reilich P, et al. Creatine monohydrate in muscular dystrophies: a double-blind, placebo-controlled clinical study. *Neurology* 2000; **54**: 1848–50.

61. Rose MR, Tawil R. Drug treatment for facioscapulohumeral muscular dystrophy. *Cochrane Database Syst Rev* 2004; **2**: CD002276.

62. Elsheikh BH, Bollman E, Peruggia M, King W, Galloway G, Kissel JT. Pilot trial of diltiazem in facioscapulohumeral muscular dystrophy. *Neurology* 2007; **68**: 1428–9.

63. Wagner KR, Fleckenstein JL, Amato AA, et al. A phase I/II trial of MYO-029 in adult subjects with muscular dystrophy. *Ann Neurol* 2008; **63**: 561–71.

64. van der Kooi EL, de Greef JC, Wohlgemuth M, et al. No effect of folic acid and methionine supplementation on D4Z4 methylation in patients with facioscapulohumeral muscular dystrophy. *Neuromuscul Disord* 2006; **16**: 766–9.

65. Tawil R. Facioscapulohumeral muscular dystrophy. *Neurotherapeutics* 2008; **5**: 601–6.

66. Orrell RW, Copeland S, Rose MR. Scapular fixation in muscular dystrophy. *Cochrane Database Syst Rev* 2010; **1**: CD003278.

67. Sackley C, Disler PB, Turner-Stokes L, Wade DT, Brittle N, Hoppitt T. Rehabilitation interventions for foot drop in neuromuscular disease. *Cochrane Database Syst Rev* 2009; **3**: CD003908.

68. van der Kooi EL, Lindeman E, Riphagen I. Strength training and aerobic exercise training for muscle disease. *Cochrane Database Syst Rev* 2005; **1**: CD003907.

69. van der Kooi EL, Kalkman JS, Lindeman E, et al. Effects of training and albuterol on pain and fatigue in facioscapulohumeral muscular dystrophy. *J Neurol* 2007; **254**: 931–40.

70. Voet NB, van der Kooi EL, Riphagen II, Lindeman E, van Engelen BG, Geurts ACh. Strength training and aerobic exercise training for muscle disease. *Cochrane Database Syst Rev* 2010; **1**: CD003907.

71. Olsen DB, Orngreen MC, Vissing J. Aerobic training improves exercise performance in facioscapulohumeral muscular dystrophy. *Neurology* 2005; **64**: 1064–6.

72. Colson SS, Benchortane M, Tanant V, et al. Neuromuscular electrical stimulation training: a safe and effective treatment for facioscapulohumeral muscular dystrophy patients. *Arch Phys Med Rehabil* 2010; **91**: 697–702.

73. Horlings CG, Munneke M, Bickerstaffe A, et al. Epidemiology and pathophysiology of falls in facioscapulohumeral disease. *J Neurol Neurosurg Psychiatry* 2009; **80**: 1357–63.

74. Koetsier CP. [*Pain related to FSH dystrophy. An underestimated problem? Results of an inquiry in the Netherlands*]. Baarn: Dutch Public Fund for Neuromuscular Disorders (VSN), 1997.

75. Association Française contre les Myopathies (AFM). *Myoline Dystrophie Musculaire Facio-scapulo-humérale.* Evry: Association Française contre les Myopathies (AFM), 1998.

76. Jensen MP, Hoffman AJ, Stoelb BL, et al. Chronic pain in persons with myotonic dystrophy and facioscapulohumeral dystrophy. *Arch Phys Med Rehabil* 2008; **89**: 320–8.

77. Miró J, Raichle KA, Carter GT, et al. Impact of biopsychosocial factors on chronic pain in persons with myotonic and

facioscapulohumeral muscular dystrophy. *Am J Hosp Palliat Care* 2009; **26**: 308–19.

78. Padua L, Aprile I, Frusciante R, et al. Quality of life and pain in patients with facioscapulohumeral muscular dystrophy. *Muscle Nerve* 2009; **40**: 200–5.

79. Nieto R, Raichle KA, Jensen MP, Miró J. Changes in pain-related beliefs, coping, and catastrophizing predict changes in pain intensity, pain interference, and psychological functioning in individuals with myotonic muscular dystrophy and facioscapulohumeral dystrophy. *Clin J Pain* 2012; **12**: 47–54.

80. Kalkman JS, Schillings ML, van der Werf SP, et al. Experienced fatigue in facioscapulohumeral dystrophy, myotonic dystrophy, and HMSN-I. *J Neurol Neurosurg Psychiatry* 2005; **76**: 1406–9.

81. Kalkman JS, Schillings ML, Zwarts MJ, van Engelen BG, Bleijenberg G. The development of a model of fatigue in neuromuscular disorders: a longitudinal study. *J Psychosom Res* 2007; **62**: 571–9.

82. Kalkman JS, Zwarts MJ, Schillings ML, van Engelen BG, Bleijenberg G. Different types of fatigue in patients with facioscapulohumeral dystrophy, myotonic dystrophy and HMSN-I. Experienced fatigue and physiological fatigue. *Neurol Sci* 2008; **29**: S238–S240.

83. Voet NB, Bleijenberg G, Padberg GW, van Engelen BG, Geurts AC. Effect of aerobic exercise training and cognitive behavioural therapy on reduction of chronic fatigue in patients with facioscapulohumeral dystrophy: protocol of the FACTS-2-FSHD trial. *BMC Neurol* 2010; **10**: 56.

84. Rogers MT, Zhao F, Harper PS, Stephens D. Absence of hearing impairment in adult onset facioscapulohumeral muscular dystrophy. *Neuromuscul Disord* 2002; **12**: 358–65.

85. Trevisan CP, Pastorello E, Ermani M, et al. Facioscapulohumeral muscular dystrophy: a multicenter study on hearing function. *Audiol Neurootol* 2008; **13**: 1–6.

86. Padberg GW, Brouwer OF, de Keizer RJ, et al. On the significance of retinal vascular disease and hearing loss in facioscapulohumeral muscular dystrophy. *Muscle Nerve* 1995; **2**: S73–S80.

87. Fitzsimons RB, Gurwin EB, Bird AC. Retinal vascular abnormalities in facioscapulohumeral muscular dystrophy. A general association with genetic and therapeutic implications. *Brain* 1987; **110**: 631–48.

88. Fitzsimons RB. Facioscapulohumeral muscular dystrophy. *Curr Opin Neurol* 1999; **12**: 501–11.

89. Wohlgemuth M, van der Kooi EL, van Kesteren RG, van der Maarel SM, Padberg GW. Ventilatory support in facioscapulohumeral muscular dystrophy. *Neurology* 2004; **63**: 176–8.

90. Birch JG. Orthopedic management of neuromuscular disorders in children. *Semin Pediatr Neurol* 1998; **5**: 78–91.

91. Kottlors M, Kress W, Meng G, Glocker FX. Facioscapulohumeral muscular dystrophy presenting with isolated axial myopathy and bent spine syndrome. *Muscle Nerve* 2010; **42**: 273–5.

92. Jordan B, Eger K, Koesling S, Zierz S. Camptocormia phenotype of FSHD: a clinical and MRI study on six patients. *J Neurol* 2011; **258**: 866–73.

93. Padberg GW, Lunt PW, Koch M, Fardeau M. Facioscapulohumeral muscular dystrophy. In: Emery AEH (ed) *Diagnostic Criteria for Neuromuscular Disorders*, pp. 9–15. Baarn: European Neuromuscular Center, 1997.

94. Wohlgemuth M, de Swart BJM, Kalf JG, Joosten FBM, van der Vliet AM, Padberg GW. Dysphagia in facioscapulohumeral muscular dystrophy. *Neurology* 2006; **66**: 1926–8.

95. Yamanaka G, Goto K, Hayashi YK, Miyajima T, Hoshika A, Arahata K. Clinical and genetical features of Japanese early onset facioscapulohumeral muscular dystrophy. *No To Hattatsu* 2002; **34**: 318–24.

96. de Visser M, de Voogt WG, la Riviere GV. The heart in Becker muscular dystrophy, facioscapulohumeral dystrophy, and Bethlem myopathy. *Muscle Nerve* 1992; **15**: 591–6.

97. Laforet P, de Toma C, Eymard B, et al. Cardiac involvement in genetically confirmed facioscapulohumeral muscular dystrophy. *Neurology* 1998; **51**: 1454–6.

98. Trevisan CP, Pastorello E, Armani M, et al. Facioscapulohumeral muscular dystrophy and occurrence of heart arrhythmia. *Eur Neurol* 2006; **56**: 1–5.

99. Stevenson WG, Perloff JK, Weiss JN, Anderson TL. Facioscapulohumeral muscular dystrophy: evidence for selective, genetic electrophysiologic cardiac involvement. *J Am Coll Cardiol* 1990; **15**: 292–9.

100. Wohlgemuth M, van der Kooi EL, Hendriks JC, Padberg GW, Folgering HT. Face mask spirometry and respiratory pressures in normal subjects. *Eur Respir J* 2003; **22**: 1001–6.

101. Wohlgemuth M, van der Kooi EL, Hendriks JC, Folgering HTh, van der Maarel SM, Padberg, GW. Respiratory function in facioscapulohumeral muscular dystrophy. Unpublished manuscript.

102. Perrin C, Unterborn JN, Ambrosio CD, Hill NS. Pulmonary complications of chronic neuromuscular diseases and their management. *Muscle Nerve* 2004; **29**: 5–27.

103. Wallgreb-Pettersson C, Bushby K, Mellies U, Simonds A. 117th ENMC Workshop: ventilatory support in congenital neuromuscular disorders-congenital myopathies, congenital muscular dystrophies, congenital myotonic dystrophy and SMA (II); 4–6 April 2003, Naarden, The Netherlands. *Neuromuscul Disord* 2004; **14**, 56–69.

104. Della Marca G, Frusciante R, Vollono C, et al. Sleep quality in Facioscapulohumeral muscular dystrophy. *J Neurol Sci* 2007; **263**: 49–53.

105. Della Marca G, Frusciante R, Dittoni S, et al. Sleep disordered breathing in facioscapulohumeral muscular dystrophy. *J Neurol Sci* 2009; **285**: 54–8.

106. Della Marca G, Pantanali F, Frusciante R, et al. Cephalometric findings in facioscapulohumeral muscular dystrophy patients with obstructive sleep apneas. *Sleep Breath* 2011; **15**: 99–106.

107. Padberg GW, Frants RR, Brouwer OF, Wijmenga C, Bakker E, Sandkuijl LA. Facioscapulohumeral muscular dystrophy in the Dutch population. *Muscle Nerve* 1995; **2**: S81–S84.

108. Sansone V, Boynton J, Palenski C. Use of gold weights to correct lagophthalmos in neuromuscular disease. *Neurology* 1997; **48**: 1500–3.

109. Funakoshi M, Goto K, Arahata K. Epilepsy and mental retardation in a subset of early onset 4q35-facioscapulohumeral muscular dystrophy. *Neurology* 1998; **50**: 1791–4.

CHAPTER 27

Distal and myofibrillar myopathies

Bjarne Udd

Introduction

The distal and myofibrillar myopathies are two heterogeneous groups of inherited or sporadic primary and progressive muscle disorders. Distal myopathy is a clinical concept characterized by predominant distal muscle weakness and atrophy in the hands, forearms, lower legs, or feet. Myofibrillar myopathy is a muscle pathology concept characterized by findings consisting of dark and hyaline cytoplasmic changes on trichrome stain, abnormal protein aggregations, disintegrated myofibrillar structures, and rimmed vacuoles. In this chapter a clinical and differential diagnostic approach is emphasized and some novel forms of distal myopathy are described.

Distal myopathy with myofibrillar pathology

The first known distal myopathies with myofibrillar pathology were desminopathy [1] and αB-crystallinopathy [2], and later myotilinopathy [3] and zaspopathy, as with Markesbery–Griggs late-onset distal myopathy [4]. In fact, the first family reported to have autosomal dominant distal myopathy [5] later proved to have desminopathy [6]. In filaminopathy the current situation is complex as the first missense mutations described in the rod and C-terminal domains caused a myofibrillar myopathy with both proximal and distal clinical involvement of muscles [7,8]. However, later identified missense mutations in the N-terminal actin-binding domain (ABD) [9] and a recently identified nonsense mutation in the 3′ end cause a distal myopathy without myofibrillar pathology [10].

General aspects of myofibrillar myopathy

Besides the frequent distal clinical presentation, many myofibrillar myopathies are associated with cardiomyopathy and some with respiratory failure [11–13]. Desmin was the first of the accumulating proteins to be studied, and thus the term 'desmin-related myopathies' was applied in the past [14]. The three major structural abnormalities in light as well as electron microscopy are: non-hyaline lesions consisting of foci of myofibrillar destruction, hyaline lesions composed of compacted and degraded myofibrillar elements (cytoplasmic or spheroid bodies), and rimmed vacuolar degeneration. The non-hyaline lesions appear dark green with the modified Gomori trichrome stain. These lesions contain desmin, dystrophin, neural cell adhesion molecule, gelsolin, and β-amyloid precursor protein but do not contain myosin, actin, or α-actinin [15–18]. The hyaline lesions are cytoplasmic inclusions, usually eosinophilic with the haematoxylin and eosin (H&E) stain and dark blue or purple-red with the modified Gomori trichrome stain. These lesions react with antibodies against dystrophin, gelsolin, β-amyloid precursor protein, titin, nebulin, actin, myosin, and α-actinin. Myotilin and αB-crystallin have proved to be very sensitive markers of protein accumulation [15–18]. A focal increase in desmin, however, is a non-specific finding—it can be seen in many neuromuscular diseases, including spinal muscular atrophy, congenital myotonic dystrophy, myotubular myopathy, and nemaline myopathy, as well as diffusely in regenerating muscle fibres of any aetiology. Besides desmin, αB-crystallin, myotilin, ZASP, and filamin-C, mutations in BAG3, FHL1, and SEPN1 have also been associated with myofibrillar pathology without a distal phenotype [18–20].

Distal and proximal phenotypes

For some disorders, mutations in the same gene may cause either a proximal or a distal phenotype, such as limb-girdle muscular dystrophy (LGMD) 2B or Miyoshi myopathy in dysferlinopathy [21], LGMD2L or calf distal myopathy in anoctaminopathy [22], and LGMD1A or very late-onset distal myopathy in myotilinopathy [23,24]. Nonaka distal myopathy with rimmed vacuoles, hereditary inclusion body myopathy, and quadriceps-sparing myopathy are all caused by mutations in GNE (UDP-N-acetylglucosamine 2-epimerase/N-acetylmannosamine kinase) and consequently are now considered to be the same disease, namely GNE myopathy [25]. Thus, future classifications of distal and myofibrillar myopathies may be based on the gene/protein mutation or affected molecular pathway rather than on the distribution of clinical or pathological findings. However, a classification based on age at onset and mode of inheritance is useful for the clinician and facilitates further diagnostic procedures (Table 27.1), especially when combined with the pattern of muscle involvement on MRI.

Late adult-onset autosomal dominant distal myopathies

Welander distal myopathy (WDM)

WDM is an autosomal dominant disease most prevalent in the Scandinavian populations in Sweden and Finland. Patients usually develop their first symptoms in the distal upper extremities in the fifth decade, typically with weakness of the finger and wrist extensors, more marked in the index finger (Fig. 27.1). Wasting of thenar and intrinsic hand muscles appears several years after the onset of weakness [26]. Some patients have onset of weakness as late as in

Table 27.1 Classification of genetically defined distal and myofibrillar myopathies

Type	Description	Inheritance	Locus/gene	Age of onset (years)	Early symptoms	CK	Pathology
Distal myopathies							
Welander myopathy	Welander 1951 [26]	AD	2p13/TIA1	>40	Hands, finger extensors	1–3×	Dystrophic, rimmed vacuoles
Tibial muscular dystrophy (Udd myopathy)	Udd 1993 [33]	AD	2q31/titin	>35	Anterior lower leg	1–4×	Dystrophic, rimmed vacuoles in tibial anterior muscle
Vocal cord and pharyngeal distal myopathy (VCPDM)	Feit 1998 [46]	AD	5q31/MATR3	40–60	Anterior lower leg, dysphonia	1–4×	Dystrophic, rimmed vacuoles
VCP-mutated distal myopathy	Palmio 2011 [49]	AD	9p13.3/VCP	>30	Anterior lower leg	1–3×	Rimmed vacuolar, ring fibers
Distal ABD-flaminopathy	Duff 2011 [9]	AD	7q32/FLNC	>20	Calf muscle weakness, grip weakness	1–4×	Non-specific myopathic
C-terminal distal filaminopathy	Guergueltcheva 2011 [10]	AD	7q32/FLNC	>20	Finger weakness	1–3×	Non-specific myopathic
Nonaka myopathy	Nonaka 1981 [58]	AR	9p1–q1/GNE	15–30	Anterior lower leg	3–4×	Dystrophic, prominent rimmed vacuoles
Miyoshi myopathy	Miyoshi 1986 [77]	AR	2p13/Dysferlin	15–30	Posterior lower leg, calf	20–150×	Dystrophic, dysferlin defect
Distal anoctaminopathy	Bolduc 2010 [92]	AR	11p14 /ANO5	18–35	Posterior lower leg, calf	20–150×	Scattered necrotic fibers
Laing myopathy (MPD1)	Laing 1995 [94]	AD	14q/beta myosin (MYH7)	3–25	Anterior lower leg	1–3×	Mild to moderate dystrophic
Distal nebulin myopathy	Wallgren-Pettersson 2007 [107]	AR	2q21/Nebulin	1–20	Anterior lower leg	1–3×	Myopathic, group atrophy, no rods on lightmicroscopy
KLHL9-mutated distal myopathy	Cirak 2010 [109]	AD	3p22/KLHL9	3–10	Anterior lower leg	1–4×	Myopathic
Distal myofibrillar myopathies							
Distal zaspopathy	Markesbery and Griggs 1974 [41]	AD	10q22/ZASP	40–50	Clinically anterior but posterior lower leg on muscle imaging	1–4×	Dystrophic, rimmed and non-rimmed vacuoles, desmin–myotilin aggregates
Distal desminopathy	Milhorat and Wolf 1943 [5]	AD	2q35/Desmin	> 15	Distal and proximal weakness, cardiomyopathy	1–4×	Dystrophic, rimmed vacuoles, desmin bodies
Distal αB-crystallinopathy	Reichlich 2010 [51]	AD	11q/αB-crystallin	> 50	Distal leg and hands, cardiomyopathy	1–2.5×	Rimmed vacuoles, desmin aggregates
Distal myotilinopathy	Penisson-Besnier 1998 [24]	AD	5q31/Myotilin	50–60	Posterior more than anterior distal leg	1–3×	Dystrophic, rimmed and non-rimmed vacuoles, myotilin aggregates
Other myofibrillar myopathies							
Myofibrillar filaminopathy	Vorgerd 2005 [7]	AD	7q32/FLNC	30–60	Axial, proximal and distal	1–4×	Myofibrillar myopathy vacuoles, protein aggregates
BAG3 myofibrillar myopathy	Selcen 2009 [20]	AD	10q25/BAG3	2–4	Toe walk, axial, general weakness	2–3×	

AD, autosomal dominant; AR, autosomal recessive.

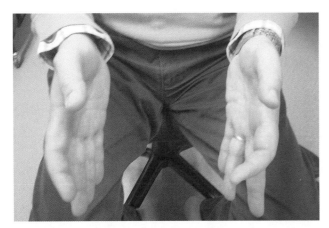

Fig. 27.1 Index finger extension weakness and mild thenar muscle atrophy in a 65-year-old male patient with Welander distal myopathy.

their seventies, and onset before age 30 years is unusual. Disease progression includes finger and wrist flexor weakness and gradual extension to the lower extremities, with weakness predominantly in toe and ankle extensors. Proximal weakness is uncommon even in senescence [26]. Tendon reflexes are preserved except for a loss of ankle reflexes later in the disease course. Patients may complain of a cold sensation in their hands but clinical sensory examination is usually normal. The progression of the disease is slow and most patients retain their activities except for manual skills and they have normal life span [26]. Cardiomyopathy has not been observed. Rare homozygous patients have a more severe disease with earlier age at onset, proximal muscle weakness, and loss of ambulance [27].

Laboratory findings

The serum creatine kinase (CK) level is normal or slightly elevated. Electromyography (EMG) shows small, brief motor unit potentials, early recruitment, and some fibrillations and complex repetitive discharges. Nerve conduction studies are normal, but on quantitative sensory testing mild deficits in vibration and temperature have been described. Mild abnormalities have also been reported in sural nerve biopsies suggesting a subclinical length-dependent, predominantly sensory small-fibre neuropathy [28]. Muscle biopsy findings largely depend on which muscle was obtained. The more affected muscle shows dystrophic features with variability in fibre size, increase in connective and fat tissue, central nuclei, and split fibres but rarely fibre necrosis. Rimmed vacuoles are frequent and 15- to 18-nm cytoplasmic and nuclear filaments have been reported [28]. The lack of inflammatory infiltrates helps to distinguish WDM from inclusion body myositis. Magnetic resonance imaging (MRI) provides additional information for diagnosis and the selection of the best muscle site for biopsy. Fatty degenerative changes are present early in posterior calf muscles without causing subjective weakness [29]. In some patients the disease starts in the lower legs and in these patients there is more marked involvement of anterior compartment muscles.

Molecular genetics

WDM was first linked to chromosome 2p13 in 1999 [30]. All currently known families have an identical haplotype on the chromosomal locus indicating a Nordic founder mutation [31]. The causative gene, *TIA1*, was recently identified [32].

When to think of Welander distal myopathy?

In a patient over the age of 40–45 years complaining of difficulties in fully extending their fingers without sensory defects.

Tibial muscular dystrophy (TMD, Udd myopathy)

TMD is characterized by the onset of ankle dorsiflexion weakness after the age of 35 years. Atrophy of the anterior compartment lower leg muscles becomes visible later (Fig. 27.2). Symptoms may start asymmetrically, progression is slow, and walking with minor aids is usually preserved into the 90th decade. A useful sign on clinical examination is the sparing of short toe extensor muscles (extensor digitorum brevis) as a distinction from neurogenic peroneal paresis. Upper limb and hand muscles are rarely affected [33], although phenotypic variations occur even with an identical mutation in 9% of patients [34]. Prevalence of the autosomal dominant disease is very high in Finland, calculated at 20 per 100 000 based on number of new diagnoses every year. TMD has been identified in Sweden, Norway, Germany, and Canada occurring in descendants of Finnish immigrants, and increasing numbers of TMD families without Finnish ancestry have been identified in France, Belgium, Spain, Italy, Portugal, and Switzerland [35].

Laboratory findings

Serum CK is normal or mildly elevated. EMG is myopathic with low-amplitude, short-duration motor unit potentials on moderate activity, frequent fibrillation potentials, and occasional high-frequency and complex repetitive discharges in the affected tibialis anterior muscle [33]. Polyphasic potentials may be recorded in clinically unaffected muscles [33]. Muscle MRI imaging is a very useful diagnostic tool, showing selective fatty degeneration first in the anterior tibial muscles and later in the long toe extensor and hamstring muscles (Fig. 27.3). Focal lesions may occur in soleus and medial gastrocnemius muscles [34].

Muscle biopsy findings depend on which muscle is obtained. In the target tibialis anterior muscle findings include variation in fibre size, thin atrophic fibres, central nuclei, structural changes within the fibres, endomysial fibrosis, and rimmed vacuoles, but with fatty replacement in end-stage muscle. Fibre necrosis is rare and both major fibre types are equally involved in the pathological process [33]. Many rimmed vacuoles are acid phosphatase positive, while others are ubiquitin positive and, with rare exceptions, they are not

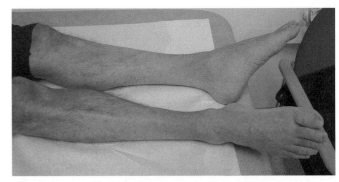

Fig. 27.2 The lower legs of a 53-year-old male patient with tibial muscular dystrophy (Udd myopathy) showing wasting of tibialis anterior muscles with prominence of the ventral edge of the tibial bone and mild foot drop.

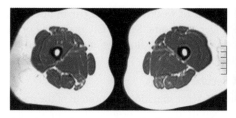 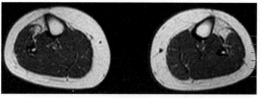

Fig. 27.3 Muscle T_1-weighted magnetic resonance imaging findings in a 62-year-old female patient with tibial muscular dystrophy (Udd myopathy) showing on the thigh level (left) early fatty degenerative change in the semimembranosus muscles and on the lower legs (right) complete replacement in tibialis anterior on both sides and long toe extensors on the left leg with early change in the long toe extensor muscles on the right leg.

lined by sarcolemmal membrane proteins. Congo red stains and immunohistochemistry for β-amyloid and amyloid precursor protein usually remain negative, in contrast to inclusion body myositis [36]. On electron microscopy the sarcomeric structure is preserved overall with dispersed autophagic vesicles, myeloid figures, and debris material without a surrounding membrane correlating to the rimmed vacuolar changes [36].

Molecular genetics

Mutations in the C-terminus of the huge sarcomeric protein titin, encoded by the *TTN* gene on chromosome 2q31, are responsible for TMD. In Finland one common founder mutation (FINmaj), a complex 11-bp insertion–deletion mutation changing four amino acids without frameshift, is present in all TMD patients [37]. Since the original gene discovery seven other mutations, both missense and nonsense, in the last or second to last exon of *TTN* have been identified in TMD patients in different European populations: three different mutations in France, one Belgian–French, one Iberian, one Italian, and one Swiss mutation [35]. In new, unrelated TMD patients, the mutations responsible can be identified by sequencing the last titin exons. Molecular genetics also confirmed homozygosity of the FINmaj titin mutation in rare patients presenting with a different phenotype: childhood-onset severe LGMD [37]. Since this specific phenotype is clearly recessive despite the parents having TMD, it was denominated LGMD2J [37].

Molecular pathology

Titin constitutes the third filament system of the sarcomere and is the third most abundant muscle protein after myosin and actin. Titin extends from the Z-disc to the M-line and binds a large number of ligands including calpain3 in the titin I-band and in its C-terminus in the M-line [37]. Homozygous LGMD2J patients show severe secondary calpain3 deficiency [38]. Mutant titin is incorporated in the sarcomere, as shown by immunohistochemistry with N-terminal antibodies in homozygous muscle. However, C-terminal antibodies show loss of epitopes over the three last domains indicating disruptive changes leading to mislocation of the ligands obscurin and obscurin-like protein [39]. M-line titin contains motifs for signalling, and a catalytic kinase domain with several interacting signalling molecules [40].

Zaspopathy (Markesbery–Griggs distal myopathy)

Late-onset ankle weakness, of both plantar and dorsal flexion, usually begins after the age of 40 years [41]. With disease progression finger and wrist extensors may be affected, and very late in life proximal weakness may also occur. Exceptionally there is rapid progression with loss of ambulation after 15 or 20 years of disease

and complete incapacity after 30 years. One patient in the first described family had cardiomyopathy with heart block requiring a pacemaker [41]. Facial, bulbar, and respiratory muscles are not affected [41]. This form of late-onset, dominantly inherited distal myopathy has been reported and identified in families of English, French, and German descent [4,15].

Laboratory findings

Serum CK levels can be normal or elevated three- to fourfold. EMG reveals small, brief-duration motor unit potentials with early recruitment in affected muscles [41]. Muscle imaging at first symptoms shows early changes in the posterior compartment, and later severe involvement of all lower leg muscles with moderate involvement of the proximal leg muscles [4]. Muscle biopsy shows prominent rimmed vacuoles together with non-rimmed vacuoles and dark structures in trichrome stain compatible with myofibrillar myopathy [41,42]. Immunohistochemical stains for desmin, myotilin, ZASP, and αB-crystallin reveal abnormal cytoplasmic aggregation in which there is also aberrant dystrophin expression [4].

Molecular genetics

There are two frequently recurring mutations in ZASP (Z-disc alternatively spliced PDZ-domain containing protein, encoded by the *LDB3* gene) associated with this type of distal myopathy [15]. The causative A165V mutation in the Markesbery–Griggs family was shown to be an ancient European founder mutation based on a relatively short common haplotype around the mutation in six unrelated families tested [4]. The other recurring ZASP mutation, A147T, causes an identical phenotype.

Distal myotilinopathy

Myotilinopathy was first associated with a dominant limb-girdle phenotype (LGMD1A). The late-onset distal phenotype was identified in patients classified histologically as having myofibrillar myopathy. Subsequent studies showed that myofibrillar myotilinopathy much more frequently presents with a distal phenotype than with LGMD [11,16]. In some families the first symptom was loss of ankle dorsiflexion between the ages of 50 and 60 years, followed by plantar flexion weakness [11,16]. In others weakness and atrophy of calf muscles was the first sign followed by a period of pain and cramps [43]. Involvement of upper limbs or proximal leg muscles was moderate or severe at later stages. Dysphonia or respiratory defect was not part of the distal phenotype [16,43].

Laboratory findings

Serum CK levels ranged from normal to twofold. EMG is myopathic with fibrillations and complex repetitive discharges. Computed tomography (CT) or MRI imaging show fatty degenerative changes in calf muscles and milder proximal leg muscle involvement

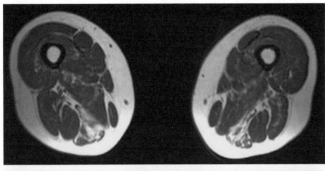
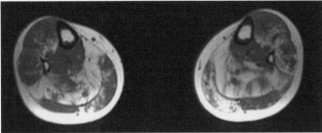

Fig. 27.4 Muscle T_1-weighted magnetic resonance imaging findings in a 58-year-old female patient with myotilinopathy showing on the thigh level (upper images) fatty degeneration in the semimembranosus muscles with minor diffuse changes in other thigh muscles, and on the lower legs (lower images) severe fatty degeneration in soleus on both sides with moderate changes in the medial gastrocnemii and anteriolateral compartment muscles slightly more on the left than on the right leg.

(Fig. 27.4) [16,44]. Muscle biopsy findings are frequent large non-rimmed vacuoles and focal cytoplasmic H&E-basophilic and trichrome dark material in both fibre types, consistent with myofibrillar myopathy. Other features included occasional rimmed vacuoles and fibre splitting [16]. Electron microscopy shows autophagic vacuoles and large zones of myofibrillar disorganization with characteristic filament bundles. An early change is widening of the dark material of the Z-disc [45]. Of the different proteins associated with myofibrillar myopathy, myotilin shows the highest degree of abnormal irregularly aggregated and mislocated protein [3,11,16].

Molecular genetics

Irrespective of clinical phenotype most reported mutations in myotilin are dominant missense mutations located within the serine rich second domain. Mutations outside the second domain have not been associated with the distal phenotype. Myotilin is an integral part of the sarcomeric Z-disc structure with many interactions, but the MYOT knock-out mouse shows normal muscle development. The previously described spheroid body myopathy also proved to be caused by myotilin mutation [17].

When to think of myotilinopathy?

In a patient over the age of 50 complaining of ankle weakness and tripping showing both dorsal and plantar flexion weakness of the feet.

Vocal cord and pharyngeal distal myopathy (VCPDM, MPD2)

This disease has so far been identified in only two families. It is characterized by late-onset distal upper and lower limb weakness together with symptoms of vocal cord and pharyngeal weakness.

The onset of weakness may occur in ankle and toe extensors or in finger extensors. Serum CK is normal or moderately elevated and muscle biopsy findings are dominated by rimmed vacuolar changes [46].

Molecular genetics

One missense mutation in a protein of the nuclear matrix, Matrin3, was reported in the original US family and in one Bulgarian family [47].

Valosin-containing protein (VCP)-mutated distal myopathy

Mutations in VCP were first identified in patients with multi-organ disease: rimmed vacuolar myopathy, Paget disease, and frontotemporal dementia (IBMPFD) [48]. The muscle phenotype usually shows a proximal or scapuloperoneal distribution [48], but VCP mutations may also cause a late-onset distal myopathy which is clinically indistinguishable from WDM or TMD [49]. In the reported distal family, Paget disease was not part of the disease and the myopathy was slowly progressive but remained distal. Rapidly progressive lethal frontotemporal dementia appeared very late, 20–25 years after the onset of muscle symptoms. CK levels were slightly elevated, muscle biopsy showed rimmed vacuolated fibres combined with ring fibres. Muscle MRI revealed fatty degeneration in the anterior compartment muscles of the lower legs [49].

αB-crystallin-mutated myofibrillar and distal myopathy

The first reports of myofibrillar myopathy combined with dilated cardiomyopathy and cataracts caused by mutations in *CRYAB* gene described the muscle phenotype as both distal and proximal [2]. Just a few rare families were reported. There have been later reports of two other phenotypes. One severe infantile early lethal form was described in Canadian aboriginals caused by a homozygous 1-bp deletion null mutation, g.60Cdel [50]. Another distinct late-onset distal myopathy, without respiratory dysfunction or significant cataracts, is caused by C-terminal *CRYAB* mutation [51]. Muscle biopsy showed rimmed vacuolar pathology without granulofilamentous inclusions on ultrastructure. Mutations in the C-terminal extension destabilize the protein and increase its tendency to self-aggregate, which is thought to be the major pathogenic mechanism in the adult forms.

Early adult-onset dominant distal and myofibrillar myopathies

Desminopathy

The first reported family with a distal phenotype, later confirmed to be a true myopathy, had desminopathy [1,5,6]. Characteristic clinical findings are early adult-onset distal leg weakness with signs of cardiomyopathy and/or respiratory failure frequently occurring as part of the disease spectrum. Cardiac involvement may also include atrioventricular conduction defect. The disease is usually rapidly progressive with proximal and generalized muscle weakness and wasting after a few years [52,53]. The variability of clinical presentation is shown by the fact that the classic scapuloperoneal syndrome of Kaeser, originally reported to be a neurogenic disease, was found to be caused by desmin mutation [54]. There are no epidemiological studies available, but more than 40 different mutations have been reported in many populations and the approximate prevalence could be about 1 per million [52].

Laboratory findings

CK levels are usually mildly or moderately elevated. EMG is myopathic, but can apparently be confusing in some patients reported as having neurogenic findings [54]. Muscle MRI shows more anterior and lateral than posterior compartment involvement. The pathological hallmark of desminopathy is increased cytoplasmic desmin aggregations on muscle biopsy together with general myofibrillar myopathy findings [6,11,19,53]. However, the pathological findings in desminopathy may not always be of a highly myofibrillar myopathy [54]. On electron microscopy the main features consist of granulofilamentous changes that are different from the filamentous bundles in myotilinopathy and zaspopathy [45].

Molecular genetics

Desmin is a muscle protein forming intermediate filaments with a Z-disc and subsarcolemmal location in skeletal, cardiac, and smooth muscle, where the filaments serve as a major scaffold structure linking the Z-discs to the plasma membrane. *DES* knockout mice develop normally and are fertile. Cells transfected with mutant desmin protein (L385P) show *DES*-positive aggregates, suggesting misfolding and reduced turnover of mutant desmin [55].

αB-crystallin is a molecular chaperone and is believed to interact with DES in the assembly of intermediary filaments.

Filaminopathies

There are three types of filaminopathy:

* distal ABD-filaminopathy
* proximodistal myofibrillar myopathy
* C-terminal nonsense mutated distal myopathy.

As indicated in the Introduction, mutations in muscle-specific filamin-C may cause a range of different dominant presentations, of which the N-terminal actin-binding domain (ABD)-filaminopathy [9] and the C-terminal nonsense mutated filaminopathy [10] show a clear distal phenotype with uncharacteristic pathology, whereas the rod domain and C-terminal Ig-like domain mutations cause later-onset generalized myopathy with a clearly myofibrillar pathology [7,8].

ABD-filaminopathy

In ABD-filaminopathy weakness of handgrip in the early twenties marks the onset, followed by thenar atrophy and calf weakness in the forties. The progression is very slow and most patients retain walking capacity despite late proximal limb weakness [9,56].

Laboratory features

CK levels are normal or mildly elevated. EMG is myopathic and muscle biopsy findings are non-specific, without any rimmed vacuoles or pathology of the myofibrillar myopathy type being present.

Molecular genetics

Filamins are actin-binding cytoskeletal proteins. The muscle-specific isoform filamin-C is localized at the periphery of the Z-discs in direct interaction with myotilin. Filamin-C also binds sarcolemmal proteins and is cleaved by calpain3 [7]. In the case of distal ABD-filaminopathy, so far identified only in a few families, the mutations are located in the N-terminal ABD [9].

Myofibrillar filaminopathies

The myofibrillar filaminopathies have a later adult onset in the thirties or forties with more proximal than distal lower and upper limb weakness. The slow progression includes paravertebral muscles with scapular winging and, in some, the respiratory muscles and loss of ambulance [7,8,57].

Laboratory features

CK levels are normal or up to tenfold elevated. EMG is myopathic and muscle biopsy findings clearly show myofibrillar pathology with abundant accumulations of Z-disc and other proteins. The rimmed vacuolar pathology is less marked [7,8,57].

Molecular genetics

In the cases of myofibrillar filaminopathy seen so far three different mutations have been identified—p.W2710X as a founder mutation in Germany in the 24th Ig-like repeat and two complex in frame deletion and deletion–insertion mutations in the seventh Ig-like repeat: p.V930_T933del and p.K899_V904/V899_C900 del/ins [9].

C-terminal nonsense mutated distal filaminopathy

The C-terminal nonsense mutated distal filaminopathy is clinically more similar to distal ABD-filaminopathy with onset of finger weakness from the age 20 causing later severe atrophy of the hand muscles. The lower leg weakness is slightly different in that these patients also have involvement of anterior lower leg muscle in contrast to patients with distal ABD filaminopathy. There is slow progression to proximal limb weakness but no cardiac or respiratory involvement [10].

Laboratory features

CK levels are normal to slightly elevated. MRI clearly shows involvement of both the posterior and anterior compartments of the lower leg muscles. EMG is myopathic and muscle biopsy findings are non-specific, without any rimmed vacuoles or pathology of the myofibrillar myopathy type, in line with ABD-distal filaminopathy [10].

Molecular genetics

This type of C-terminal nonsense mutated distal filaminopathy has been identified in Bulgarian families with an identical c.5160delC mutation in exon 30, resulting in a frameshift and a premature stop codon p.F1720LfsX63 [10].

Early adult-onset autosomal recessive distal myopathies

GNE myopathy (distal myopathy with rimmed vacuoles, Nonaka distal myopathy)

GNE-myopathy was first described in Japanese patients and subsequently the disease has been reported in many other populations. The first symptoms usually become apparent in the late second or the third decade, and later onset has occasionally been reported [58–60]. Weakness starts in the ankle dorsiflexor and toe extensor muscles, causing foot drop and a steppage gait. Mild distal upper-extremity weakness may also be present. Later on, patients develop proximal weakness, although the quadriceps muscles remain relatively spared. Disease progression including neck flexors makes most patients lose their ability to walk some 10 to 15 years after disease onset [58–60]. Cranial muscles are not involved. Cardiomyopathy is not part of the disease but cardiac arrhythmia and pacemaker implant have been reported.

Laboratory findings

The serum CK level is slightly or moderately elevated. EMG is myopathic with small, brief motor unit potentials and fibrillation potentials [58–60]. Morphological findings on muscle biopsy are dominated by prominent rimmed vacuolar changes, also evident in less weak proximal muscles. The vacuolar regions have increased acid phosphatase activity and also contain increased ubiquitinated material. Electron microscopy reveals 15- to 18-nm filamentous inclusions in the nucleus and cytoplasm, in addition to the autophagic vacuoles [61–63].

Molecular genetics and epidemiology

Patients in the Middle East first reported as having quadriceps-sparing myopathy, later termed hereditary inclusion body myopathy (HIBM), proved to have the same disease as the Japanese Nonaka distal myopathy patients, currently together termed GNE myopathy. The prevalence is more than 1 per million in the populations with founder mutations. HIBM was first, and Nonaka myopathy later, linked to chromosome 9p12–13 [64–66]. The gene responsible was later identified in patients with HIBM, and subsequently confirmed in Nonaka myopathy [67–69]. Patients in Jewish families from Middle Eastern countries were homozygous for a missense mutation (M712T) in the kinase domain of GNE [66]. In Japanese patients one mutation is a more frequent founder mutation, V572L [68,69], and families of different ethnic origin (Asian Indian, North American, and Caribbean) were heterozygous for distinct missense mutations in the kinase and epimerase domains of GNE [67].

GNE is a bifunctional enzyme that catalyses the first two steps in the biosynthesis of N-acetylneuraminic acid or sialic acid and has been shown to be the rate-limiting enzyme in the sialic acid biosynthetic pathway. Sialic acid modification of glycoproteins and glycolipids expressed at the cell surface is crucial for their function in many biological processes, including cell adhesion and signal transduction [70]. Hyposialylation of proteins in affected muscles has been proposed as the molecular pathomechanism in Nonaka myopathy [71,72], but has not been confirmed by others [73].

Therapy

The phenotype of a mouse model of GNE myopathy with rimmed vacuolar myopathology was ameliorated with direct substitution of the sialic acid prerequisites N-acetylneuraminic acid, N-acetylmannosamine, sialyllactose, and even with a synthetic derivative, thus forming the basis for human treatment trials [74]. Direct GNE-gene delivery has been performed in one single patient but the final outcome is not available [75].

Miyoshi distal myopathy

Miyoshi reported the first patients from Japan in the 1970s [76,77]. The same disease was later identified in many different populations with an overall prevalence estimated at around 1 per million [78–82]. Onset of the disease is usually between the ages of 15 and 25 years with the first symptoms relating to the calf muscles, either as exercise discomfort or weakness in ankle plantar flexion; the weakness affects climbing stairs because of reduced push-off. Calf muscles become atrophic, and ankle reflexes are lost. Later, anterior and lateral compartment muscles become involved [76,77]. With progression of the disease, proximal muscles in the legs and arms become weaker, and after 20 years of the disease course the two phenotypes of dysferlinopathy, Miyoshi myopathy and LGMD2B, are no longer distinct [83]. About one-third of patients will be confined to a wheelchair within 10 years of onset of symptoms. Onset in the anterior rather than posterior compartment, and more rapid progression of the disease, has also been reported [84].

Laboratory findings

In contrast to dominant distal myopathies CK levels are highly increased, ranging from 20 to 150 times the upper limit of normal. Elevated CK levels may even be detected before the onset of symptoms or abnormal signs. EMG findings are myopathic with small, brief motor unit potentials and early recruitment with spontaneous activity in calf muscles [76,77]. Severely atrophic gastrocnemius muscles may show long-duration polyphasic motor unit potentials with reduced recruitment. Muscle pathology in severely affected gastrocnemius muscle biopsy shows 'end-stage' pathology. The major finding in less severely affected muscle is scattered fibre necrosis with macrophages and occasional infiltrates without rimmed vacuolar or myofibrillar changes [82]. After identification of the genetic defect and development of antibodies, the diagnosis of Miyoshi myopathy can now be confirmed by an absence of immunohistochemical dysferlin label on the sarcolemma or by semiquantitative Western blotting [81,82].

Molecular genetics

Mutation of the dysferlin gene (DYSF) in patients with Miyoshi myopathy was the first to be identified as a cause in any distal myopathy [85,86]. Interestingly, identical mutations may cause Miyoshi myopathy, LGMD2B, or distal myopathy with clinical onset in anterior tibial muscles, even in the same family [87]. The reason for the difference in phenotype at disease onset is not known. Dysferlin is not homologous to other known mammalian proteins. It is expressed in many tissues, including heart, skeletal muscle, kidney, stomach, liver, spleen, lung, uterus, and, to a lesser extent, brain and spinal cord. Dysferlin is localized mainly to the plasma membrane in muscle, interacting with caveolin-3, but does not interact with dystrophin, sarcoglycans, or dystroglycans [88,89]. The presence of C2 domains in dysferlin suggests that it may play an important role in signalling pathways. C2 domains are believed to bind calcium and thereby trigger signal transduction and membrane trafficking events. Indeed, structural abnormalities of the sarcolemma, including subsarcolemmal vacuoles and papillary projections, have been reported in patients with Miyoshi myopathy [90]. Further studies on dysferlin indicate essential functions in the membrane repair mechanisms [91].

Distal anoctaminopathy

Anoctaminopathy is a recessive disease but may present with various clinical phenotypes from relatively severe limb-girdle ones to more or less asymptomatic hyperCKaemia. One phenotype is early adult-onset distal myopathy with asymmetric calf involvement. First symptoms may be exercise-induced pain in the calf muscles, and even occasionally hypertrophy, which turns into weakness and atrophy within a few years later [22,92,93]. Similar to dysferlinopathy, patients have very high CK levels, up to 100 times the upper limit of normal. EMG shows myopathic changes but may be normal if the medial gastrocnemius muscle is not examined. Muscle biopsy shows just a scattered few necrotic fibres and later

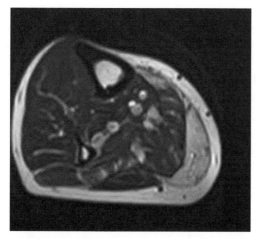
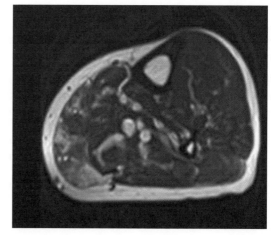

Fig. 27.5 Muscle T_2-weighted magnetic resonance imaging findings in a 32-year-old female patient with distal anoctaminopathy showing fatty replacement of the right medial gastrocnemius muscle and early degenerative change in medial gastrocnemius on the right leg and both soleus muscles.

non-specific dystrophic myopathology. Muscle MRI is useful for demonstrating the fatty degenerative changes in the calf muscles (Fig. 27.5). The evolution is remarkably slow despite the high CK levels, and patients remain ambulant until old age [22,92,93].

Molecular genetics and epidemiology

ANO5/TMEM16E codes for a putative cytoplasmic calcium-activated chloride channel protein anoctamin-5, but the exact role of this protein in muscle is not known. Anoctaminopathy seems to be one of the most common causes of muscular dystrophy with mutations spread all over the gene [22,92]. Diagnosis is currently made by molecular genetic sequencing techniques as protein diagnostics in muscle are not available yet.

Early onset distal myopathies

Laing distal myopathy (LDM, MPD1)

The disease is inherited as an autosomal dominant trait but many patients are sporadic cases because of frequent *de novo* mutations [94]. Usually the first symptoms of ankle dorsiflexion weakness appear in childhood, but may remain undiagnosed because of minimal impact on activities in mild cases. Juvenile or early adult onset is not unusual, and even late onset has been reported [95–98]. Weakness in ankle dorsiflexors, toe extensors, and neck flexor muscles is prominent. Finger extensors and shoulder muscles are affected later. The disease does not shorten the life span and most patients remain ambulant. Cardiomyopathy may be associated with LDM but is rare [99,100]. No exact epidemiological data are available and the disease is still under-diagnosed. Based on several different mutations occurring even in smaller populations such as the Finnish, Norwegian, and Valencian, LDM should be present in all populations [99–104].

Laboratory findings

Serum CK level is normal or mildly elevated. EMG is myopathic and shows short, brief myopathic potentials, but has occasionally been interpreted as neurogenic because of loss of motor units in the anterior tibial muscle [95–100]. MRI shows consistent fatty degeneration of tibialis anterior and, depending on disease duration, variably in other anterior compartment muscles and to a lesser extent in calf muscles (Fig. 27.6). Muscle biopsy findings are most

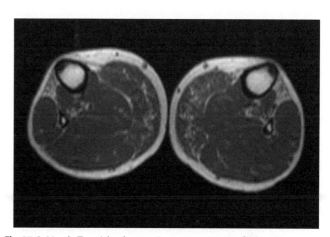

Fig. 27.6 Muscle T_1-weighted magnetic resonance imaging findings in a 32-year-old male patient with Laing distal myopathy showing fatty degenerative atrophy in tibialis anterior and long toe extensors on both sides combined with compensatory hypertrophic bulging of the lateral peroneal muscle into the anterior compartment and early fatty degenerative change in hypertrophic medial gastrocnemius muscles on both sides.

consistent with congenital fibre type disproportion, showing small and moderately atrophic Type 1 fibres. Core structures are common and rimmed vacuoles infrequent [95–100].

Molecular genetics

In 1995 LDM became the first distal myopathy disease to be linked to a certain chromosomal locus, 14q11 [94]. The responsible gene, *MYH7*, encodes slow beta myosin heavy chain protein, which is the main myosin isoform in Type 1 slow muscle fibres and in cardiac muscle fibres [95,96]. Most mutations so far identified in LDM are located in the tail region of the MYH7 molecule between the positions 1500 and 1800, but with exceptions [98–104]. Mutations in more N-terminal parts, the head and neck regions or even the rod domain of MYH7, give rise to cardiomyopathy [105], and mutations in the ultimate C-terminus are known causes of hyaline body myopathy [106].

Distal nebulin myopathy

In contrast to Laing distal myopathy this is an autosomal recessive disease. The first symptoms, ankle dorsiflexion weakness, are observed in early childhood. Later in adolescence finger and hand extensors and neck flexors may be moderately involved [107]. The overall progression is mild with some proximal weakness in the sixties and retained ambulation.

Laboratory findings

Muscle MRI shows selective fatty degeneration in the anterior tibial muscles, EMG is myopathic, and CK is normal or mildly elevated. Muscle biopsy findings are different compared with other distal myopathies and may show grouped atrophic fibres, easily misinterpreted as neurogenic change. Nemaline rods are not observed on light microscopy, although small numbers of rods associated with Z-discs can be discerned on electron microscopy in some but not all patients [107].

Molecular genetics

Recessive mutations in nebulin are known causes of autosomal recessive nemaline myopathy. In the first set of patients identified with this new clinical distal phenotype the mutations were missense on both alleles in contrast to patients with common nemaline myopathy who carry more disruptive mutations on at least one allele [107]. These less severe missense mutations may also be the reason for the different pathology and absence of nemaline rods on light microscopy. In line with this concept, three patients with a distal myopathy without generalized weakness have been reported with more disrupting nebulin mutations and with nemaline rods in the muscle biopsy on light microscopy [108].

KLHL9-mutated distal myopathy

This autosomal dominant disease has been reported in one German family. Muscle weakness starts in early childhood with weakness of ankle dorsiflexion. Later patients also have atrophy of intrinsic hand muscles together with moderate proximal limb weakness [109]. EMG is myopathic and muscle biopsy shows non-specific myopathic changes without rimmed vacuoles. CK levels are mildly to moderately elevated [109]. One missense mutation reported was identified in the *KLHL9* gene which encodes a kelch-like homologue protein implicated in turnover degradation pathways [109].

Distal caveolinopathy

Mutations in the caveolin-3 gene cause dominant disorders of various clinical forms (caveolinopathies) including LGMD1C, hyper-CKaemia, rippling muscle disease, and distal myopathy [110,111]. One sporadic patient had atrophy and moderate weakness of small muscles in the hands and feet at the age of 12 years. CK levels were elevated, EMG showed myopathic potentials in hand muscles, and muscle biopsy from a proximal muscle showed non-specific myopathy. Loss of immunoreactivity for caveolin-3 antibodies is a diagnostic hallmark of most caveolinopathies. In the reported patient, Western blot showed absent caveolin-3. Molecular genetics revealed a known missense mutation [110].

BAG3-mutated myofibrillar myopathy

This autosomal dominant disease has so far been described in only a few patients. Myofibrillar myopathies usually show adult onset and slow progression. However, BAG3 mutations cause onset in childhood, rapid progression, and have a poor prognosis with respiratory and cardiac involvement. Proximal weakness, rigid spine, and Achilles tendon contractures are features of the muscle phenotype.

One mutation, p.Pro209Leu, is more common and seems to reoccur independently as a *de novo* mutation, although other mutations have been reported [111,112].

Distal myopathy with unknown molecular cause

Juvenile-onset sporadic/recessive oculopharyngodistal myopathy has been described in a several reports and certainly represents at least one distinct entity. This is also true for adult-onset dominant oculopharyngeal distal myopathy, even if the molecular genetics is not settled [114–119]. Recently a large number of both recessive and dominant families from Turkey were reported [120].

A number of distal myopathies have been reported in single families and shown to be distinct from any of the other known entities by phenotype or molecular genetic linkage at the time of study:

- distal myopathy with thenar atrophy and sarcoplasmic bodies [121]
- distal neuromyopathy with pes cavus (MIM #601846) [122]
- autosomal dominant distal myopathy in a Polish–American family [123]
- adult-onset dominant distal myopathy MPD3 (MIM #610099) [124,125]
- late-onset recessive calf distal myopathy [126].

Distal muscle phenotype in other myopathies (Table 27.2)

Besides all the previously detailed distinct disorders many other myopathies may present with clinical distal muscle weakness and wasting, and these occasionally need to be considered in differential diagnosis [127–131]. Facioscapulohumeral dystrophy can have onset in the lower legs without overt weakness in the upper regions [132,133]. Dynaminopathy shows distal weakness in the limbs, although facial weakness is always an important diagnostic feature [134]. Similarly, in myotonic dystrophy Type 1 the muscle phenotype is distal but at the stage of distal weakness other features of the disease are usually apparent and will direct the diagnostic efforts.

Conclusion

Molecular definition has considerably increased awareness of distal and myofibrillar myopathies and continues to identify new entities. The gold standard for diagnosis is thus molecular genetic definition

Table 27.2 Distal weakness and/or atrophy as the presenting finding in other myopathies

1. Facioscapulohumeral dystrophy
2. Dynamin2 mutated centronuclear myopathy
3. Myotonic dystrophy Type 1
4. Telethoninopathy
5. Branching and debranching glycogenoses
6. Nemaline myopathy
7. Sporadic inclusion body myositis

of the disease. For a diagnosis of myofibrillar myopathy the histopathological findings in muscle biopsy are required and sufficient. However, even with a histopathological diagnosis, the further identification of the underlying gene defect is advised in the myofibrillar myopathies because of the great differences in prognosis that have a direct impact on management. Histopathology in the differentiation of other distal myopathies is currently restricted to dysferlinopathy and caveolinopathy using immunohistochemistry or Western blotting. Muscle imaging is an effective tool for directing the further molecular genetic diagnostics towards a limited number of diseases [135].

Treatment is in most diseases limited to providing correct management based on exact diagnosis, physiotherapy, and rehabilitative efforts, including orthotic measures when applicable. However, as shown with the example of GNE myopathy, gene therapies and specific therapies based on understanding the molecular pathophysiology are on the move and will probably change the prognosis of these genetic diseases in the future.

References

1. Sjöberg G, Saavedra-Matiz CA, Rosen DR, et al. A missense mutation in the desmin rod domain is associated with autosomal dominant distal myopathy, and exerts a dominant negative effect on filament formation. *Hum Mol Genet* 1999; **8**: 2191–8.

2. Vicart P, Caron A, Guicheney P, et al. A missense mutation in the alphaB-crystallin chaperone gene causes a desmin-related myopathy. *Nat Genet* 1998; **20**: 92–5.

3. Penisson-Besnier I, Talvinen K, Dumez C, et al. Myotilinopathy in a family with late onset myopathy. *Neuromuscul Disord* 2006; **16**: 427–31.

4. Griggs R, Vihola A, Hackman P, et al. Zaspopathy in a large classic late onset distal myopathy family. *Brain* 2007; **130**: 1477–84.

5. Milhorat AT, Wolff HG. Studies in diseases of muscle: XIII. Progressive muscular dystrophy of atrophic distal type: report on a family: report of autopsy. *Arch Neurol Psychiatry* 1943; **49**: 655.

6. Horowitz S, Schmalbruch H. Autosomal dominant distal myopathy with desmin storage: a clinicopathologic and electrophysiologic study of a large kinship. *Muscle Nerve* 1994; **17**: 151–60.

7. Vorgerd M, van der Ven PF, Bruchertseifer V, et al. A mutation in the dimerization domain of filamin c causes a novel type of autosomal dominant myofibrillar myopathy. *Am J Hum Genet* 2005; **77**: 297–304.

8. Shatunov A, Olivé M, Odgerel Z, et al. In-frame deletion in the seventh immunoglobulin-like repeat of filamin C in a family with myofibrillar myopathy. *Eur J Hum Genet* 2009; **17**: 656–63.

9. Duff R, Tay V, Hackman P, et al. Mutations in the N-terminal actin-binding domain of filamin C cause a distal myopathy. *Am J Hum Genet* 2011; **88**: 729–40.

10. Guergueltcheva V, Peeters K, Baets J, et al. Distal myopathy with upper limb predominance caused by filamin C haploinsufficiency. *Neurology*, 2011; **77**: 2105–14.

11. Selcen D, Ohno K, Engel AG. Myofibrillar myopathy: clinical, morphological and genetic studies in 63 patients. *Brain* 2004; **127**: 439–51.

12. Amato A, Kagan-Hallet K, Jackson C, et al. The wide-spectrum of myofibrillar myopathy suggests a multifactorial etiology and pathogenesis. *Neurology* 1998; **51**: 1646–55.

13. Melberg A, Oldfors A, Blomstrom-Lundqvist C, et al. Autosomal dominant myofibrillar myopathy with arrhythmogenic right ventricular cardiomyopathy linked to chromosome 10q. *Ann Neurol* 1999; **46**: 684–92.

14. Goebel HH, Müller HD. Protein aggregate myopathies. *Semin Pediatr Neurol* 2006; **13**: 96–103.

15. Selcen D, Engel AG. Mutations in ZASP define a novel form of muscular dystrophy in humans. *Ann Neurol* 2005; **57**: 269–76.

16. Olive M, Goldfarb LG, Shatunov A, et al. Myotilinopathy: refining the clinical and myopathological phenotype. *Brain* 2005; **128**: 2315–26.

17. Foroud T, Pankratz N, Batchman AP, et al. A mutation in myotilin causes spheroid body myopathy. *Neurology* 2005; **65**: 1936–40.

18. Selcen D, Bromberg MB, Chin SS, Engel AG. Reducing bodies and myofibrillar myopathy features in FHL1 muscular dystrophy. *Neurology* 2011; **77**: 1951–9.

19. Olivé M, Odgerel Z, Martínez A, et al. Clinical and myopathological evaluation of early—and late-onset subtypes of myofibrillar myopathy. *Neuromuscul Disord* 2011; **21**: 533–42.

20. Selcen D, Muntoni F, Burton BK, et al. Mutation in BAG3 causes severe dominant childhood muscular dystrophy. *Ann Neurol* 2009; **65**: 83–9.

21. Illarioshkin S, Ivanova-Smolenskaya IA, Greenberg CR, et al. Identical dysferlin mutation in limb-girdle muscular dystrophy type 2B and distal myopathy. *Neurology* 2000; **55** 1931–3.

22. Penttilä S, Palmio J, Suominen T, et al. Eight new mutations and the expanding phenotype variability in muscular dystrophy caused by ANO5. *Neurology* 2012; **78**: 897–903.

23. Hauser S, Horrigan SK, Salmikangas P, et al. Myotilin is mutated in limb girdle muscular dystrophy 1A. *Hum Mol Genet* 2000; **9**: 2141–7.

24. Penisson-Besnier I, Dumez C, Chateau D, et al. Autosomal dominant late adult onset distal leg myopathy. *Neuromuscul Disord* 1998; **8**: 459–66.

25. Udd B. 165th ENMC International Workshop: Distal myopathies III. *Neuromuscul Disord* 2009; **19**: 429–38.

26. Welander L. Myopathia distalis tarda hereditaria. *Acta Med Scand* 1951; **141** (Suppl. 265): 1.

27. Welander L. Homozygous appearance of distal myopathy. *Acta Genet* 1957; **7**: 321–5.

28. Borg K, Ahlberg G, Borg J, et al. Welander's distal myopathy: clinical, neurophysiological and muscle biopsy observations in young and middle aged adults with early symptoms. *J Neurol Neurosurg Psychiatry* 1991; **54**: 494–8.

29. Åhlberg G, Jakobsson F, Fransson A, et al. Distribution of muscle degeneration in Welander distal myopathy—a magnetic resonance imaging and muscle biopsy study. *Neuromuscul Disord* 1994; **4**: 55–62.

30. Åhlberg G, von Tell D, Borg K, et al. Genetic linkage of Welander distal myopathy to chromosome 2p13. *Ann Neurol* 1999; **46**: 399–404.

31. von Tell D, Somer H, Udd B, et al. Welander distal myopathy outside the Swedish population: phenotype and genotype. *Neuromuscul Disord* 2002; **12**: 544–7.

32. Hackman P, Sarparanta J, Lehtinen S, et al. Welander distal myopathy is caused by a mutation in the RNA-binding protein TIA1. *Ann Neurol* 2013; **73**: 500–9.

33. Udd B, Partanen J, Halonen P, et al. Tibial muscular dystrophy. Late adult-onset distal myopathy in 66 Finnish patients. *Arch Neurol* 1993; **50**: 604–8.

34. Udd B, Vihola A, Sarparanta J, et al. Titinopathies and extension of the M-line mutation phenotype beyond distal myopathy and LGMD2J. *Neurology* 2005; **64**: 636–42.

35. Hackman P, Marchand S, Sarparanta J, et al. Truncating mutations in C-terminal titin may cause more severe tibial muscular dystrophy (TMD). *Neuromuscul Disord* 2008; **18**: 922–8.

36. Udd B, Haravuori H, Kalimo H, et al. Tibial muscular dystrophy—from clinical description to linkage on chromosome 2q31. *Neuromuscul Disord* 1998; **8**: 327–32.

37. Hackman P, Vihola A, Haravuori H, et al. Tibial muscular dystrophy is a titinopathy caused by mutations in TTN, the gene encoding the giant skeletal-muscle protein titin. *Am J Hum Genet* 2002; **71**: 492–500.

38. Haravuori H, Vihola A, Straub V, et al. Secondary calpain3 deficiency in 2q linked muscular dystrophy—titin is the candidate gene. *Neurology* 2001; **56**: 869–77.

39. Fukuzawa A, Lange S, Holt M, et al. Interactions with titin and myomesin target obscurin and its small homologue, obscurin-like 1, to

the sarcomeric M-band: implications for hereditary myopathies. *J Cell Sci* 2008; **121**: 1841–51.

40. Lange S, Xiang F, Yakovenko A, et al. The kinase domain of titin controls muscle gene expression and protein turnover. *Science* 2005; **308**: 1599–603.

41. Markesbery WR, Griggs RC, Leach RP, et al. Late onset hereditary distal—myopathy. *Neurology* 1974; **23**: 127–34.

42. Markesbery WR, Griggs RC, Herr B. Distal myopathy: electron microscopic and histochemical studies. *Neurology* 1997; **27**: 727–41.

43. Penisson-Besnier I, Dumez C, Chateau D, et al. Autosomal dominant late adult onset distal leg myopathy. *Neuromuscul Disord* 1998; **8**: 459–66.

44. Fischer D, Kley R, Strach K, et al. Distinct muscle imaging patterns in myofibrillar myopathies. *Neurology* 2008; **71**: 758–65.

45. Claeys K, Udd B, Stoltenburg G. Electron microscopy in myofibrillar myopathies reveals clues to the mutated gene. *Neuromuscul Disord* 2008; **18**: 656–66.

46. Feit H, Silbergleit A, Schneider LB, et al. Vocal cord and pharyngeal weakness with autosomal distal myopathy: clinical description and gene localization to chromosome 5q31. *Am J Hum Genet* 1998; **63**: 1732–44.

47. Senderek J, Garvey SM, Krieger M, et al. Autosomal-dominant distal myopathy associated with a recurrent missense mutation in the gene encoding the nuclear matrix protein, matrin 3. *Am J Hum Genet* 2009; **84**: 511–18.

48. Kimonis V, Mehta S, Fulchiero E, et al. Clinical studies in familial VCP myopathy associated with Paget disease of bone and frontotemporal dementia. *Am J Med Genet* 2008; **146A**: 745–57.

49. Palmio J, Sandell S, Suominen T, et al. Distinct distal myopathy phenotype caused by VCP gene mutation in a Finnish family. *Neuromuscul Disord* 2011; **21**: 551–5.

50. Del Bigio M, Chudley A, Sarnat H, Campbell C, Goobie S, Chodirker B, Selcen D. Infantile muscular dystrophy in Canadian aboriginals is an alpha-B-crystallinopathy. *Ann Neurol* 2011; **69**: 866–71.

51. Reichlich P, Schoser B, Schramm N, et al. The p.G154S mutation of the alpha-B crystallin gene (CRYAB) causes late-onset distal myopathy. *Neuromuscul Disord* 2010; **20**: 255–9.

52. van Spaendonck-Zwarts K, van Hessem L, Jongbloed J, et al. Desmin-related myopathy. *Clin Genet* 2011; **80**: 354–66.

53. Dalakas M, Park KY, Semino-Mora C, et al. Desmin myopathy, a skeletal myopathy with cardiomyopathy caused by mutations in the desmin gene. *N Engl J Med* 2000; **342**: 770–80.

54. Walter MC, Reilich P, Huebner A, et al. Scapuloperoneal syndrome type Kaeser and a wide phenotypic spectrum of adult-onset, dominant myopathies are associated with the desmin mutation R350P. *Brain* 2007 **130**: 1485–96.

55. Sugawara M, Kato K, Komatsu M, et al. A novel de novo mutation in the desmin gene causes desmin myopathy with toxic aggregates. *Neurology* 2000; **55**: 986–90.

56. Williams DR, Reardon K, Roberts L, et al. A new dominant distal myopathy affecting posterior leg and anterior upper limb muscles. *Neurology* 2005; **64**: 1245–54.

57. Kley R, Hellenbroich Y, van der Ven P, et al. Clinical and morphological phenotype of the filamin myopathy: a study of 31 German patients. *Brain* 2007 **130**: 3250–64.

58. Nonaka I, Sunohara N, Ishiura S, et al. Familial distal myopathy with rimmed vacuole and lamellar (myeloid) body formation. *J Neurol Sci* 1981; **51**: 141–55.

59. Nonaka I, Sunohara N, Satoyoshi E, et al. Autosomal recessive distal muscular dystrophy: A comparative study with distal myopathy with rimmed vacuole formation. *Ann Neurol* 1985; **17**: 51–9.

60. Sunohara N, Nonaka I, Kamei N, et al. Distal myopathy with rimmed vacuole formation. a follow up study. *Brain* 1989; **112**: 65–83.

61. Murakami N, Ihara Y, Nonaka I, et al. Muscle fiber degeneration in distal myopathy with rimmed vacuoles. *Acta Neuropathol* 1995; **89**: 29–34.

62. Mizusawa H, Kurisaki H, Takatsu M, et al. Rimmed vacuolar distal myopathy: an ultrastructural study. *J Neurol* 1987; **234**: 137–47.

63. Kumamoto T, Ito T, Horinouchi H, et al. Increased lysosome-related proteins in the skeletal muscles of distal myopathy with rimmed vacuoles. *Muscle Nerve* 2000; **23**: 1686–93.

64. Mitrani-Rosenbaum S, Argov Z, Blumenfeld A, et al. Hereditary inclusion body myopathy maps to chromosome 9p1-q1. *Hum Mol Genet* 1996; **5**: 159–63.

65. Ikeuchi T, Asaka T, Saito M, et al. Gene locus for autosomal recessive distal myopathy with rimmed vacuoles maps to chromosome 9. *Ann Neurol* 1997; **41**: 432–7.

66. Mirabella M, Christodoulou K, Di Giovanni S, Ricci E, Tonali P, Servidei S. An Italian family with autosomal recessive quadriceps-sparing inclusion body myopathy (ARQS-IBM) linked to chromosome 9p1. *Neurolog Sci* 2000; **21**: 99–102.

67. Eisenberg I, Avidan N, Potikha T, et al. UDP-N-Acetylglucosamine 2-epimerase/N-Acetylemannosamine kinase is mutated in recessive hereditary inclusion body myopathy. *Nat Genet* 2001; **29**: 83–7.

68. Nishino I, Noguchi S, Murayama K, et al. Distal myopathy with rimmed vacuoles is allelic to hereditary inclusion body myopathy. *Neurology* 2002; **59**: 1689–93.

69. Kayashima T, Matsuo H, Satoh A, et al. Nonaka myopathy is caused by mutations in the UDP-N-acetylglucosamine-2-epimeras e/N-acetylmannosamine kinase gene (GNE). *J Hum Genet* 2002; **47**: 77–9.

70. Krause S, Aleo A, Hinderlich S, et al. GNE protein expression and subcellular distribution are unaltered in HIBM. *Neurology* 2007; **69**: 655–9.

71. Nishino I, Malicdan MC, Murayama K, et al. Molecular pathomechanism of distal myopathy with rimmed vacuoles. *Acta Myol* 2005; **24**: 80–3.

72. Gagiannis D, Orthmann A, Danssmann I, et al. Reduced sialylation status in UDP-N-acetylglucosamine-2-epimerase/N-acetylmannosamine kinase (GNE)-deficient mice. *Glycoconj J* 2007; **24**: 125–30.

73. Salama I, Hinderlich S, Shlomai Z, et al. No overall hyposialylation in hereditary inclusion body myopathy myoblasts carrying the homozygous M712T GNE mutation. *Biochem Biophys Res Commun* 2005; **328**: 221–6.

74. Malicdan M, Noguchi S, Tokutomi T, et al. Peracetylated N-acetylmannosamine, a synthetic sugar molecule, effectively rescues muscle phenotype and biochemical defects in a mouse model of sialic acid deficient myopathy. *J Biol Chem* 2012; **287**: 2689–705.

75. Nemunaitis G, Jay C, Maples P, et al. Hereditary inclusion body myopathy: single patient response to intravenous dosing of GNE gene lipoplex. *Hum Gene Ther* 2011; **22**: 1331–41.

76. Miyoshi K, Iwasa M, Kawai H, et al. Autosomal recessive distal muscular dystrophy: a new variety of distal muscular dystrophy predominantly seen in Japan. *Nippon Rinsho (Tokyo)* 1977; **35**: 3922.

77. Miyoshi K, Kawai H, Iwasa M, et al. Autosomal recessive distal muscular dystrophy as a new type of progressive muscular dystrophy: seventeen cases in eight families, including an autopsied case. *Brain* 1986; **109**: 31–54.

78. Argov Z, Sadeh M, Mazor K, et al. Muscular dystrophy due to dysferlin deficiency in Libyan Jews. Clinical and genetic features. *Brain* 2000; **123**: 1229–37.

79. Cupler EJ, Bohlega S, Hessler R, et al. Miyoshi myopathy in Saudi Arabia: clinical, electrophysiological, histopathological and radiological features. *Neuromuscul Disord* 1998; **8**: 321–6.

80. Eymard B, Laforet P, Tome FM, et al. Miyoshi distal myopathy: specific signs and incidence [in French]. *Rev Neurol* 2000; **156**: 161–8.

81. Barohn RJ, Sadeh M, Mazor K. Autosomal recessive distal dystrophy. *Neurology* 1991; **41**: 1365–9.

82. Gallardo E, Rojas-Garcia R, de Luna N, et al. Inflammation in dysferlin myopathy: immunohistochemical characterization of 13 patients. *Neurology* 2002; **57**: 2136–8.

83. Paradas C, Llauger J, Diaz-Manera J, et al. Redefining dysferlinopathy phenotypes based on clinical findings and muscle imaging studies. *Neurology* 2010; **75**: 316–23.

84. Illa I, Serrano-Munuera C, Gallardo E, et al. Distal anterior compartment myopathy: a dysferlin mutation causing a new muscular dystrophy phenotype. *Ann Neurol* 2001; **49**: 130–4.

85. Bejaoui K, Hirabayashi K, Hentati F, et al. Linkage of Miyoshi myopathy (distal autosomal recessive muscular dystrophy) to chromosome 2p12–14. *Neurology* 1995; **45**: 494–8.

86. Liu J, Aoki M, Illa I, et al. Dysferlin, a novel skeletal muscle gene, is mutated in Miyoshi myopathy and limb girdle muscular dystrophy. *Nat Genet* 1998; **20**: 31–40.

87. Illarioshkin S, Ivanova-Smolenskaja I, Tanaka H, et al. Clinical and molecular analysis of large family with three distinct phenotypes of progressive muscular dystrophy. *Brain* 1996; **119**: 1895–909.

88. Matsuda C, Aoki M, Hayashi YK, et al. Dysferlin is a surface membrane-associated protein that is absent in Miyoshi myopathy. *Neurology* 1999; **53**: 1119–22.

89. Matsuda C, Hayashi YK, Ogawa M, et al. The sarcolemmal proteins dysferlin and caveolin-3 interact in skeletal muscle. *Hum Mol Genet* 2001; **17**: 1761–6.

90. Selcen D, Stilling G, Engel A. The earliest pathologic alterations in dysferlinopathy. *Neurology* 2001; **56**: 1472–81.

91. Bansal D, Campbell KP. Dysferlin and the plasma membrane repair in muscular dystrophy. *Trends Cell Biol* 2004; **14**: 206–13.

92. Bolduc V, Marlow G, Boycott KM, et al. Recessive mutations in the putative calcium-activated chloride channel anoctamin 5 cause proximal LGMD2L and distal MMD3 muscular dystrophies. *Am J Hum Genet* 2010; **86**: 213–21.

93. Bouquet F, Cossée M, Béhin A, et al. Miyoshi-like distal myopathy with mutations in anoctamin 5 gene. *Rev Neurol (Paris)* 2012; **168**: 135–41.

94. Laing N, Laing BA, Meredith C, et al. Autosomal dominant distal myopathy: linkage to chromosome 14. *Am J Hum Gen* 1995; **56**: 422–7.

95. Mastaglia FL, Phillips BA, Cala LA et al. Early onset chromosome 14-linked distal myopathy (Laing). *Neuromuscul Disord* 2002; **12**: 350–7.

96. Meredith C, Herrmann R, Parry C, et al. Mutations in the slow skeletal muscle fiber myosin heavy chain gene (MYH7) cause Laing early-onset distal myopathy (MPD1). *Am J Hum Genet* 2004; **75**: 703–8.

97. Meredith C. Distal myopathy. *Thesis*. University of Western Australia, Perth, 2001.

98. Auer Grumbach M, John E, Wallefeld W, et al. A novel slow-skeletal myosin (MYH7) mutation in a large Austrian family presenting as late onset distal myopathy. *Neuromuscul Disord* 2007; **17**: 883.

99. Hedera P, Petty EM, Bui MR, et al. The second kindred with autosomal dominant distal myopathy linked to chromosome 14q: genetic and clinical analysis. *Arch Neurol* 2003; **60**: 1321–5.

100. Muelas N, Hackman P, Luque H, et al. MYH7 gene tail mutation causing myopathic profiles beyond Laing distal myopathy. *Neurology* 2010; **75**: 732–41.

101. Zimprich F, Djamshidian A, Hainfellner JA, et al. An autosomal dominant early adult-onset distal muscular dystrophy. *Muscle Nerve* 2000; **23**: 1876–9.

102. Voit T, Kutz P, Leube B, et al. Autosomal dominant distal myopathy: further evidence of a chromosome 14 locus. *Neuromuscul Disord* 2001; **11**: 11–19.

103. Lamont P, Udd B, Mastaglia FL, et al. Laing early onset distal myopathy: slow myosin defect with variable abnormalities on muscle biopsy. *J Neurol Neurosurg Psychiatry* 2006; **77**: 208–15.

104. Dubourg O, Maisonobe T, Behin A, et al. A novel MYH7 mutation occurring independently in French and Norwegian Laing distal myopathy families and de novo in one Finnish patient. *J Neurol* 2011; **258**: 1157–63.

105. Blair E, Redwood C, de Jesus Oliveira M, et al. Mutations of the light meromyosin domain of the beta-myosin heavy chain rod in hypertrophic cardiomyopathy. *Circ Res* 2002; **90**: 263–9.

106. Tajsharghi H, Thornell LE, Lindberg C, Lindvall B, Henriksson KG, Oldfors A. Myosin storage myopathy associated with a heterozygous missense mutation in MYH7. *Ann Neurol* 2003; **54**: 494–500.

107. Wallgren-Pettersson C, Lehtokari V-L, Kalimo H, et al. Distal myopathy caused by homozygous missense mutations in the nebulin gene. *Brain* 2007; **130**: 1465–76.

108. Lehtokari V, Pelin K, Herczegfalvi A, et al. Nemaline myopathy caused by mutations in the nebulin gene may present as a distal myopathy. *Neuromuscul Disord* 2011; **21**: 556–62.

109. Cirak S, v Deimling F, Sahdev S, et al. Kelch-like homologue 9 mutation is associated with an early onset autosomal dominant distal myopathy. *Brain* 2010; **133**: 2123–35.

110. Tateyama M, Aoki M, Nishino I, et al. Mutation in the caveolin-3 gene causes a peculiar form of distal myopathy. *Neurology* 2002; **58**: 323–5.

111. Sotgia F, Woodman SE, Bonuccelli G, et al. Phenotypic behavior of caveolin-3 R26Q, a mutant associated with hyperCKemia, distal myopathy, and rippling muscle disease. *Am J Physiol Cell Physiol* 2003; **285**: C1150–C1160.

112. Selcen D, Muntoni F, Burton BK, Pegoraro E, Sewry C, Bite AV, Engel AG. Mutation in BAG3 causes severe dominant childhood muscular dystrophy. *Ann Neurol* 2009; **65**: 83–9.

113. Lee H, Cherk S, Chan S, et al. BAG3-related myofibrillar myopathy in a Chinese family. *Clin Genet* 2012; **81**: 394–8.

114. Goto I, Kato H, Kase M, et al. Oculopharyngeal myopathy with distal and cardiomyopathy. *J Neurol Neurosurg Psychiatry* 1977; **40**: 600–7.

115. Satoyoshi E, Kinoshita M. Oculopharyngodistal myopathy: report of four families. *Arch Neurol* 1977; **34**: 89–92.

116. Scrimgeour E, Mastaglia F. Oculopharyngeal and distal myopathy. A case study from Papua New Guinea. *Am J Med Genet* 1984; **17**: 763–71.

117. Uyama E, Uchino M, Chateau D, et al. Autosomal recessive oculopharyngodistal myopathy in light of distal myopathy with rimmed vacuoles and oculopharyngeal muscular dystrophy. *Neuromuscul Disord* 1998; **8**: 119–25.

118. Witoonpanich R, Phankhian S, Sura T, et al. Oculopharyngodistal myopathy in a Thai family. *J Med Assoc Thai* 2004; **87**: 1518–21.

119. van der Sluijs BM, ter Laak HJ, Scheffer H, et al. Autosomal recessive oculopharyngodistal myopathy: a distinct phenotypical, histological, and genetic entity. *J Neurol Neurosurg Psychiatry* 2004; **75**: 1499–501.

120. Durmus H, Laval S, Deymeer F, et al. Oculopharyngeal distal myopathy is a distinct entity. *Neurology* 2011; **76**: 227–35.

121. Edström L, Thornell LE, Eriksson A. A new type of hereditary distal myopathy with characteristic sarcoplasmic bodies and intermediate (skeletin) filaments. *J Neurol Sci* 1980; **47**: 171–89.

122. Servidei S, Capon F, Spinazzola A, et al. A distinctive autosomal dominant vacuolar neuromyopathy linked to 19p13. *Neurology* 1999; **53**: 830–7.

123. Felice K, Meredith C, Binz N, et al. Autosomal dominant distal myopathy not linked to the known distal myopathy loci. *Neuromuscul Disord* 1999; **9**: 59–65.

124. Mahjneh I, Haravuori H, Paetau A, et al. A distinct phenotype of distal myopathy in a large Finnish family. *Neurology* 2003; **61**: 87–92.

125. Haravuori H, Siitonen HA, Mahjneh I, et al. Linkage to two separate loci in a family with a novel distal myopathy phenotype (MPD3). *Neuromuscul Disord* 2004 **14**: 183–7.

126. Linssen W, de Visser M, Notermans NC, et al. Genetic heterogeneity in Miyoshi type distal muscular dystrophy. *Neuromuscul Disord* 1998; **8**: 317–20.

127. Clemens PR, Yamamoto M, Engel AG. Adult phosphorylase b kinase deficiency. *Ann Neurol* 1990; **28**: 529–36.

128. DiMauro S, Hartwig GB, Hays A, et al. Debrancher deficiency: Neuromuscular disorder in five adults. *Ann Neurol* 1979; **5**: 422–31.

129. Moreira E, Vainzof M, Marie SK, et al. The seventh form of autosomal recessive limb-girdle muscular dystrophy is mapped to 17q11–12. *Am J Hum Genet* 1997; **61**: 151–9.

130. Moxley RT, Griggs RC, Markesbery WR, et al. Metabolic implications of distal atrophy: Carbohydrate metabolism in centronuclear myopathy. *J Neurol Sci* 1978; **39**: 247–60.

131. Vester U, Schubert M, Offner G, et al. Distal myopathy in nephropatic cystinosis. *Pediatr Nephrol* 2000; **14**: 36–8.

132. Van der Koi A, Visser MC, Rosenberg N, et al. Extension of the clinical range of facioscapulohumeral dystrophy: report of six cases. *J Neurol Neurosurg Psychiatry* 2000; **69**: 114–16.

133. Ricker K, Mertens HG. The differential diagnosis of the myogenic (facio) scapulo-peroneal syndrome. *Eur Neurol* 1968; **1**: 275–9.

134. Schessl J, Medne L, Hu Y, et al. MRI in DNM2-related centronuclear myopathy: evidence for highly selective muscle involvement. *Neuromuscul Disord* 2007; **17**: 28–32.

135. Udd B. Distal myopathies. *Neuromuscul Disord* 2012; **22**: 5–12.

CHAPTER 28

Congenital/ultrastructural myopathies

Gianina Ravenscroft, Nigel F. Clarke, and Nigel G. Laing

Introduction

The congenital myopathies are a broad group of disorders characterized by the presence of specific structural or ultrastructural abnormalities such as central cores, central nuclei, minicores, and nemaline bodies in the muscle biopsy. Almost all patients have generalized muscle weakness and hypotonia although rare hypertonic patients have been described. The various subtypes of congenital myopathy are defined by the predominance of a particular structural abnormality [1] (Table 28.1). The congenital myopathies share many clinical features, and cannot usually be distinguished from each another on clinical grounds alone (Table 28.2). In recent years, the genetic basis of many congenital myopathies has been clarified, but the muscle biopsy has remained central to the diagnosis of the congenital myopathies, excluding other conditions, and directing genetic testing. Low-cost diagnostic next-generation sequencing (NGS) of multiple disease genes is becoming widely available and it is possible that this will prompt a change in this paradigm.

The congenital myopathies account for a small proportion of patients with genetic muscle disease, in the vicinity of 2% of patients overall [2]. The incidence of the different congenital myopathies is not well characterized and rates may vary in different populations. The most common forms are thought to be multiminicore disease, central core disease, and nemaline myopathy with a point prevalence of around 2–4 patients per million for each subtype [2–4].

In this chapter, we will focus on the clinical and histological features of the main forms of congenital myopathy, discuss current

Table 28.1 Correlation between pathologies and disease genes in the congenital myopathies

Gene	Actin aggregates	Caps	Central cores	Central/internalised nuclei	CFTD	Cores and rods	Intranuclear rods	Multiminicores or atypical cores	Hyaline bodies	Nemaline bodies	Type 1 fibre uniformity	Zebra bodies
ACTA1	✓	✓			✓	✓	✓			✓		✓
BIN1				✓								
CFL2								✓		✓		
DNM2				✓								
KBTBD13						✓				✓		
KLHL40										✓		
KLHL41										✓		
MYH7								✓	✓			
MTM1				✓								
NEB						✓				✓		
RYR1			✓	✓	✓	✓		✓			✓	
SEPN1								✓				
TNNT1										✓		
TPM2		✓			✓					✓		
TPM3		✓			✓					✓		

Table 28.2 Clinical features associated with some of the specific subsets of the congenital myopathies

	RYR1 CCD	MTM1 MM	DNM2 CNM	BIN1 CNM	RYR1 MmD, CNM, and CFTD	SEPN1 MmD	MYH7 MSM	NEB NM	ACTA1 myopathies	TPM3 myopathies	TPM2 myopathies	KBTBD13 NM
Presentation												
Congenital onset	✓	✓✓✓	✓	✓✓	✓✓	✓	✓✓	✓✓	✓✓✓	✓✓	✓✓	–
Childhood onset	✓✓	(✓)	✓✓✓	✓✓	✓	✓✓✓	✓✓	✓✓	✓	✓✓	✓✓	✓✓
Adult onset	✓	(✓)	✓	✓	–	✓	✓	–	✓	✓	✓	✓
Weakness												
Axial	✓	✓✓	✓✓	–	✓✓✓	✓✓✓	✓✓	✓✓	✓✓	✓✓	✓✓	✓
Proximal limb	✓✓✓	✓✓	✓✓	✓✓	✓✓	✓✓	✓✓	✓	✓✓	✓✓	✓✓	✓✓
Distal limb		✓✓	✓✓	✓	✓	✓	✓✓	✓✓	✓✓	✓✓	✓✓	✓
Facial	✓	✓✓✓	✓✓	✓✓	✓✓	–	✓	✓✓	✓✓	✓	✓	–
Bulbar	✓	✓✓✓	✓✓	✓	✓✓	–	–	✓✓	✓✓	–	–	–
Eye movement	✓	✓✓✓	✓✓	✓✓	✓✓	–	–	–	–	–	–	–
Respiratory	✓	✓✓✓	✓✓	–	✓	✓✓✓	✓	✓✓	✓✓	✓✓	✓✓	–
Cardiac involvement	–			✓	–	–	✓✓	–	(✓)	–	✓	–
Malignant hyperthermia	✓✓✓	–	–		✓✓	–	–	–	–	–	–	–
Scoliosis	✓	✓	✓✓	–	✓✓	✓✓✓	✓	✓	✓✓	✓	✓	–
Congenital hip dislocation	✓✓✓	–	–		✓✓	–	–	–	(✓)	–	–	–

CCD, central core disease; MM, Myotubular myopathy; CNM, centronuclear myopathy; MmD, multiminicore disease; CFTD, congenital fibre–type disproportion; MSM, myosin storage myopathy; NM, nemaline myopathy.

✓✓✓, important diagnostic feature; ✓✓, common; ✓, occasional; (✓), rare.

Approach to diagnosis

Clinical examination and several common tests play an important role in the diagnosis of congenital myopathies. The first task for the clinician is to determine whether a congenital myopathy is likely (in which case a muscle biopsy will contribute important information) and to exclude other neuromuscular disorders that are best diagnosed using other tests. The most important neuromuscular conditions to exclude when considering a diagnosis of a congenital myopathy are congenital myotonic dystrophy, congenital muscular dystrophies, congenital myasthenic syndromes, and mitochondrial myopathies.

There are several clinical features that are common to most congenital myopathies. If weakness is severe there is usually early onset generalized muscle weakness and hypotonia that is evident at birth; however, if weakness is mild, patients may not present until infancy or early childhood. When there is moderate or marked generalized weakness the following features are common: difficulty feeding, reduced muscle bulk, a long face, high-arched palate, pronounced facial weakness, and absent or hypoactive tendon reflexes (Fig. 28.1). Ophthalmoplegia, prominent axial muscle weakness, spinal rigidity, and early respiratory muscle involvement occur in a range of congenital myopathies. The clinical course is usually stable or only slowly progressive. Vignette 1 provides an example of the common clinical features and complications that can be associated with moderate weakness. Clinical features that are *uncommon* in congenital myopathies are raised plasma creatine kinase (more than three times normal), cardiac involvement, rapidly progressive weakness, prominence of joint contractures (other than Achilles tendon), intellectual disability, fluctuating weakness, and predominantly distal limb muscle involvement. Although they occasionally occur in specific forms of congenital myopathy, the presence of one or more of these features should prompt the clinician to consider other diagnoses. Nerve conduction tests are usually normal and electromyography may be normal or show myopathic changes.

The text at the top of the page reads: "approaches to diagnosis, and highlight the most important aspects of clinical care."

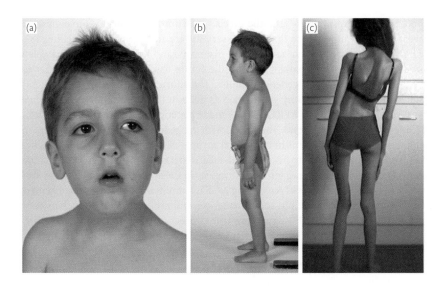

Fig. 28.1 Common clinical features of congenital myopathies. Two individuals with heterozygous mutations in *TPM3* aged 3 years (a, b), and 33 years (c). (a), (b) Note the myopathic face, mild ptosis, and hypotonic standing posture. (c) Generalized muscle atrophy is present in most congenital myopathies and scoliosis is common when there is moderate or severe generalized muscle weakness. Adapted with permission from Figure 2 in Clarke NF et al., *Ann Neurol* 2008; **63**: 329–37.

The long-term prognosis is an important issue for both clinicians and families with genetic myopathies. In general, patients with congenital myopathies have good long-term outcomes since weakness usually remains relatively stable, unless there is severe congenital weakness. In children with severe congenital weakness, establishing an early genetic diagnosis is often helpful. Patients with severe nemaline myopathy, *DNM2*-related centronuclear myopathy (CNM), and *RYR1*-related myopathies may improve with supportive care after 1 or 2 months, while the long-term prognosis is usually poor for boys with X-linked myotubular myopathy.

Involvement of the respiratory muscles is common in many forms of congenital myopathy, and fully ambulant patients may present in respiratory failure, especially those with *SEPN1* and *TPM3* mutations. Untreated nocturnal hypoventilation can lead to right-heart failure or sudden death, but non-invasive nocturnal ventilation is almost always effective if patients can tolerate it. For this reason, careful monitoring of respiratory function with lung function tests and/or sleep studies is important in all undiagnosed patients. Dysphagia is a common cause of failure to thrive and aspiration pneumonia in all congenital myopathies with moderate to

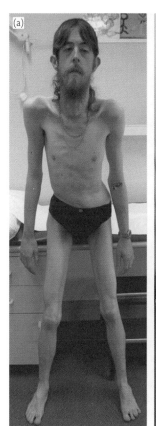
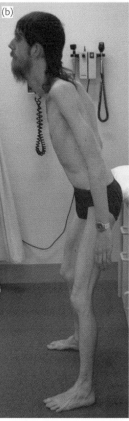
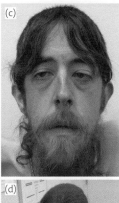
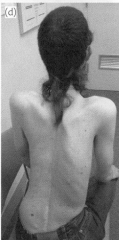

Vignette 1 This patient had moderate stable generalized muscle weakness from birth and his forced vital lung capacity was 50% of predicted in teenage years. He has ophthalmoplegia, ptosis, long myopathy face (C), scoliosis (D; post-fixation), and a histological diagnosis of congenital fibre-type disproportion (CFTD). Creatine kinase levels were normal. RYR1 was the likely genetic cause since involvement of the eye muscle is not reported in the other known causes of CFTD. Muscle magnetic resonance imaging would be likely to give further useful diagnostic information but spinal rods were a contraindication here. Regular respiratory function tests and/or sleep studies are recommended. All patients with possible or suspected *RYR1* mutations require precautions against malignant hyperthermia for all general anaesthetic procedures. This patient has compound heterozygous mutations in *RYR1*. Adapted from Figure 1 in Clarke NF et al., *Hum Mut* 2010; **31**: E1544–E1550.

severe muscle weakness. Gastrostomy tube feeding is an effective treatment. Scoliosis commonly arises in patients with severe weakness and is particularly associated with mutations in *SEPN1* and *RYR1*. Timely surgical fixation results in a good outcome for most patients.

In the last 20 years, the genetic basis of many congenital myopathies has been clarified, allowing a molecular diagnosis to be established in a large proportion of patients (see Table 28.1). Congenital myopathies may have autosomal dominant (AD), autosomal recessive (AR), or X-linked inheritance. They also may arise from *de novo* mutations [5]. There is considerable genetic heterogeneity within several forms of congenital myopathy, with mutations in multiple genes causing the same pathology. For example, there are nine characterized genetic causes of nemaline myopathy (NEM1-8 and KLHL41). In addition, mutations in one particular gene can cause multiple pathologies (see Table 28.1). Thus, even though the muscle biopsy provides important clues, it often remains a challenge to predict the causative gene, and several genes may be analysed before a molecular diagnosis is made. Currently, some patients with typical clinical and histological features of a congenital myopathy remain without a genetic diagnosis, even in the best diagnostic centres, because it is likely that many congenital myopathy genes remain uncharacterized.

Challenges in establishing a genetic diagnosis

For patients with all forms of genetic myopathy, it is becoming increasingly important to determine the specific gene that is responsible, and the precise mutation. This clarifies the pattern of inheritance that is necessary for accurate genetic counselling, is a prerequisite for prenatal diagnosis, and helps the clinician to plan optimal patient care. In the future it will be essential in order to prescribe genetic therapies. The enormous size of several congenital myopathy genes, such as nebulin (*NEB*) [6] and the ryanodine receptor (*RYR1*) [7] has made genetic testing expensive and difficult to access. This, along with the genetic heterogeneity inherent in many forms of congenital myopathy, and the fact that many genes have still to be identified, means that many patients currently lack a molecular diagnosis. Advances in the ability to sequence many disease genes at once using NGS is simplifying many aspects of genetic diagnosis, but some challenges will probably remain, such as confidently distinguishing true disease-causing mutations from rare, harmless sequence changes (genetic polymorphisms).

Nemaline myopathies

The cardinal feature of NEMs is the presence of electron-dense nemaline bodies or rods within the skeletal muscle (Fig. 28.2a,d). These rods are usually present in the sarcoplasm, but may be in the nuclei alone (intranuclear rod myopathy) or both. There are nine known NEM genes, with more to be identified [8]. The established causes of NEM in approximate descending order of incidence are *NEB, ACTA1, KLHL40, TPM2, TPM3, CFL2,* and *TNNT1*. The incidences of *KBTBD13*- and *KLHL41*-related NEM appear similar to the *TPM2* and *TPM3* genes, but this requires further study. Magnetic resonance imaging (MRI) of muscle appears to be less helpful in distinguishing between genetic causes in NEM than in other congenital myopathies, but experience is limited.

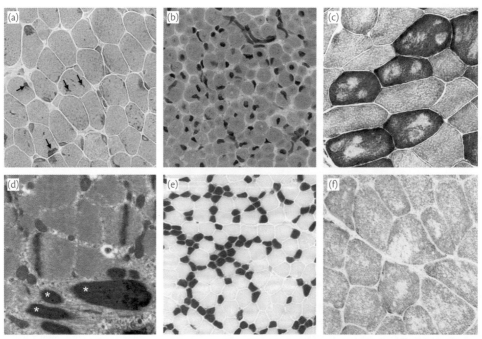

Fig. 28.2 The main histological features of common congenital myopathies. (a), (d) Nemaline myopathy. Intensely staining inclusions (arrows) on the Gomori trichrome stain (a) represent clumps of nemaline bodies, which appear as electron-dense rods (*) on electron microscopy (d). (b) *MTM1*-related centronuclear myopathy. There are numerous internalized nuclei, many of which occupy central positions, on haematoxylin and eosin staining. (c) Central core disease (CCD). Nicotinamide adenine dinucleotide tetrazolium reductase (NADH-TR) staining shows large cores limited to Type 1 (dark) fibres. Many CCD muscle biopsies also show complete Type 1 fibre predominance, not present here. (e) Congenital fibre-type disproportion due to a heterozygous mutation in *TPM3*. An ATPase 4.3 stain shows marked consistent smallness of Type 1 (dark staining) fibres compared with Type 2 (pale) fibres. (f) Succinate dehydrogenase stain showing multiminicores in most fibres. (See also figure in colour plate section)

NEM1 (MIM #609284) due to *TPM3* mutations

The first genetic cause of NEM to be identified was the *TPM3* gene, which encodes α-tropomyosin$_{slow}$ (MIM #191030) [9]. *TPM3* is a relatively uncommon cause of NEM with either AD or AR inheritance and is associated with a wide range of disease severity. Two large dominant families with disease onset in childhood or adulthood have been reported [9,10] and severe [11] or intermediate [12] neonatal-onset NEM due to homozygous recessive mutations have also been reported. A strong clue to the diagnosis of *TPM3*-related NEM is that nemaline bodies are only present in Type 1 (slow twitch) muscle fibres, since α-tropomyosin$_{slow}$ protein is not expressed in fast muscle fibres.

Recent reports suggest that the majority of patients with *TPM3* mutations do not have nemaline bodies and that congenital fibre-type disproportion (CFTD) is the most frequent histopathological pattern [13,14]. Respiratory muscle weakness is commonly associated with dominant *TPM3* mutations, and even though most patients remain ambulant until old age almost all will require nocturnal ventilatory support at some stage during adulthood, some from early childhood [13]. An 8 year old boy with CFTD due to a de novo mutation in TPM3 is shown in video 28.2.

NEM2 (MIM #256030) due to *NEB* mutations

Linkage mapping and positional cloning of seven families with AR typical NEM identified nebulin (*NEB*; MIM #161650) as the most common cause of NEM, responsible for around 50% of families [15–17]. To date, all patients with NEM2 have had recessive disease. The most common pattern is for children to have moderate generalized weakness and hypotonia from birth, and for there to be prominent weakness of the bulbar, face, neck flexor, and respiratory muscles [18]. Some patients have severe disease, characterized by the absence of spontaneous movements or respiration at birth, congenital contractures, or fractures and many do not survive, although aggressive supportive care will enable some patients to wean from full-time ventilation after 1 or 2 months of life [19]. Dysphagia, nocturnal hypoventilation, and scoliosis are common complications in patients with moderate or severe weakness, and these respond well to clinical intervention. Recently, *NEB* mutations have been defined as a cause of NEM presenting clinically as a distal myopathy, and it is possible that this gene is responsible for a still wider spectrum of phenotypes [20]. *Nebulin* is one of the largest known proteins and the *NEB* gene is expensive to sequence using standard techniques. Historically, this has been a major barrier to patient diagnosis and research but this impasse should be solved when diagnostic laboratories adopt NGS techniques.

NEM3 (MIM #161800) due to *ACTA1* mutations

Mutations in the skeletal muscle α-actin gene (*ACTA1*; MIM #102610) account for about 20–25% of all NEM [21], but are found in more than 50% of the NEM patients with severe congenital weakness [22]. Most of the over 200 different *ACTA1* mutations cause dominant disease [5] (see also the *ACTA1* Locus Specific Database at <http://www.waimr.uwa.edu.au/research/lovd.html>) and many of these arise de novo in affected children. Around 10% of mutations abolish actin expression or are functional nulls, and result in severe AR disease. Some of these patients survive after birth due to persistent expression of cardiac α-actin in skeletal muscles beyond the foetal period [23]. Patients with the most severe *ACTA1*-related NEM will not establish independent respiration and most die in the neonatal period. Most of these children have de novo dominant *ACTA1* mutations, in which case the recurrence risk for further siblings is low but dependent on the level of gonadal mosaicism in the parent. Patients follow a stable clinical course and proactive management of dysphagia, respiratory infections, nocturnal hypoventilation, and scoliosis in those with moderate or severe weakness can have a major impact on the quality and length of life.

The extraocular muscles are almost always spared in *ACTA1*-related NEM, even in patients with profound weakness. This is probably due to abundant cardiac α-actin expression in these muscles [24,25]. This can be a useful diagnostic clue, since ophthalmoplegia is a feature of several other severe forms of congenital myopathy. Recently three NEM patients with *ACTA1* mutations and with malformations of the central nervous system and skeleton, liver, and renal tract have been reported [26].

NEM4 (MIM #609285) due to *TPM2* mutations

Mutations in the gene that encodes β-tropomyosin (*TPM2*; MIM #190990) are an uncommon cause of dominant NEM and most families have had mild or moderate generalized weakness [27,28]. Regular cardiac assessments are advised in NEM4, as cardiomyopathy has been reported in one patient with *TPM2*-related cap myopathy [29].

NEM5—Amish type (MIM #605355) due to *TNNT1* mutations

NEM5 or AR Amish NEM is caused by a single founder mutation in the gene encoding slow muscle troponin T (*TNNT1*; MIM #191041) and had until recently only been reported in the Old-order Amish community [30]. All affected neonates presented with severe muscle weakness and generalized tremors at or soon after birth. In the first 2–3 months of life tremors typically subside but most children die in their second year of life from progressive generalized weakness, muscle atrophy, large joint contractures, pectus carinatum, and respiratory muscle weakness [30]. See Box 28.1 for NEM5 outside the Amish community.

NEM6 (MIM #609273) due to *KBTBD13* mutations

NEM6 is an AD disorder characterized by childhood onset of slowly progressive proximal muscle weakness, exercise intolerance, and a distinctive difficulty in moving quickly (slow movements). As a result, patients cannot run and may have difficulty preventing themselves from falling if they stumble. As well as having nemaline bodies, muscle biopsies often show cores and predominance of hypertrophic Type 1 (slow twitch) fibres, which is opposite to other characterized forms of NEM that usually have hypotrophic (small) Type 1 fibres. In five unrelated families (three of Dutch origin) [31,32], three missense mutations were identified in the kelch repeat and BTB/POZ domains containing protein 13 gene (*KBTBD13*; MIM #613727) [33]. The genetic basis of this form of NEM was therefore identified only recently and the full spectrum of phenotypes associated with mutations in *KBTBD13* may be broader than is currently appreciated. Some NEM patients with slow movements have normal *KBTBD13* gene sequencing, indicating that mutations in other genes can also cause this phenotype (unpublished observations).

NEM7 (MIM #610687) due to *CFL2* mutations

NEM7 is a rare form of NEM caused by AR mutations in the *CLF2* gene (MIM #601443), reported in only two families to date. The first reported family had congenital hypotonia, delayed motor milestones, and an inability to run [34]. Nemaline bodies, occasional minicores, concentric laminated bodies, and filamentous actin accumulations were present in the muscle biopsy. To date only one other family has been described with a *CFL2* mutation [35] and *CFL2* mutations were not present in over 100 undiagnosed NEM patients, suggesting that NEM7 accounts for less than 1% of affected families [34]. A lack of facial weakness or foot drop may be a diagnostic clue but clinical experience is very limited at present.

See Box 28.1 at the end of the chapter for information about NEM8 (MIM #615348) due to *KLHL40* mutations and *KLHL41*-related NEM, two further recently identified forms of NEM.

Core/minicore myopathies

The core myopathies collectively account for more congenital myopathy patients than any other group and encompass central core disease (CCD), multiminicore disease (MmD), and atypical core myopathies. The central abnormality in all core myopathies is the presence of 'cores', which are regions that lack staining on the standard oxidative stains succinate dehydrogenase (SDH), nicotinamide adenine dinucleotide tetrazolium reductase (NADH-TR), and cytochrome *c* oxidase (COX) (Fig. 28.2c,f). Cores are seen on electron microscopy as regions that lack mitochondria. Sarcomeric disorganization is also common in core lesions, particularly in minicores. Even though there is overlap between CCD and MmD, and some patients share features of both conditions, it has been useful to retain these as separate diagnoses because the patterns of inheritance, genetic causes, and severities differ between these disorders.

Central core disease (MIM #117000)

CCD was the first form of congenital myopathy to be recognized and has a distinctive histological pattern that makes diagnosis of most CCD patients straightforward. The hallmark abnormality on muscle cross-section is the presence of large cores (which may occupy eccentric positions) that typically have well-defined boundaries (Fig. 28.2.c) and extend the entire length of Type 1 myofibres. Complete Type 1 fibre predominance is very common. Most patients with CCD have mild or moderate, stable proximal limb-girdle weakness and remain ambulant into late adulthood. However, moderate intrafamilial variability in disease severity is common. Facial and eye movements are usually normal. Some CCD patients have severe weakness and develop similar health problems to MmD patients with severe weakness (see section on Multiminicore disease). Congenital hip dislocation is common, even in patients with mild weakness, and should be excluded in all infants with CCD. A mother and daughter with moderately severe AD CCD due to RYR1 are shown in video 28.1.

Over 90% of typical CCD is caused by mutations in the ryanodine receptor Type 1 gene (*RYR1*) [7,36]. Dominant mutations cluster in three hotspot regions of the gene but many mutations lie elsewhere. An AD family history or *de novo* dominant mutations

in a proband (more common in severely affected patients) are the most common patterns of inheritance, but occasional typical CCD patients have AR disease. The *RYR1* gene is large (106 exons) and therefore expensive to sequence. Splice-site mutations, which may be difficult to find or correctly classify, are relatively common. This, together with the polymorphic nature of the gene sequence in normal individuals and variable inheritance patterns, can complicate the interpretation of results. If there is any doubt, it is wise to seek the advice of an experienced testing laboratory or clinical genetics service. All patients with core disease who lack a genetic diagnosis and all patients with *RYR1* mutations require precautions against malignant hyperthermia (MH) during anaesthetic procedures due to a high risk of this condition unless, perhaps, an individual has had a negative *in vitro* MH contracture test.

Multiminicore disease (MIM #117000)

In MmD the cores are usually small, randomly scattered in myofibres, lack well-defined boundaries, and extend only a short distance longitudinally (Fig. 28.2f). Electron microscopy is worthwhile to confirm the diagnosis, and to distinguish between true minicores and artefacts of biopsy processing. The two main established causes of MmD are the *SEPN1* gene (MIM #606210), which encodes selenoprotein N, and *RYR1*. *SEPN1*-related myopathy follows an AR inheritance pattern and is associated with a relatively consistent clinical phenotype, which becomes easier to identify from late childhood. Head drop (due to neck extensor weakness) is a common sign in infancy. Children may be slow to walk but often have normal early motor milestones and may not present until mid or late childhood with mild generalized weakness. A rigid spine usually develops during childhood, and typically a scoliosis that requires surgical fixation arises during early adolescence. Most patients require nocturnal non-invasive ventilation from their early to mid teenage years. A small number of patients will present with respiratory failure in early childhood and the occasional patient may first present during adulthood. The vast majority of *SEPN1*-related myopathy patients remain ambulant into adulthood, and can work and lead independent lives, despite having significant respiratory muscle weakness [37]. Some patients have dystrophic changes on the muscle biopsy and can be diagnosed with rigid spine muscular dystrophy (MIM #602771). The history and clinical presentation are often more helpful in diagnosing *SEPN1*-related myopathy than the histology, and a typical history is outlined in Vignette 2. Patients with MmD due to *RYR1* mutations have a wide spectrum of disease severity, but are typically weaker than patients with CCD. Many have marked motor delay and some never walk. Facial weakness, ptosis, ophthalmoplegia, osteopenia, and scoliosis are common and respiratory failure can develop when there is severe generalized weakness.

Atypical core diseases

Some patients have additional histological features that are atypical for standard CCD or MmD, such as abundant internal nuclei, protein accumulations, prominent dystrophic features, or widespread sarcomeric disorganization, and these are often grouped together under the term 'atypical core myopathies'. The list of genes responsible for atypical core myopathies is broader than for CCD or MmD and includes *RYR1, SEPN1, ACTA1* [5], *TTN* [38], *DOK7* [39], and *MYH7* [40].

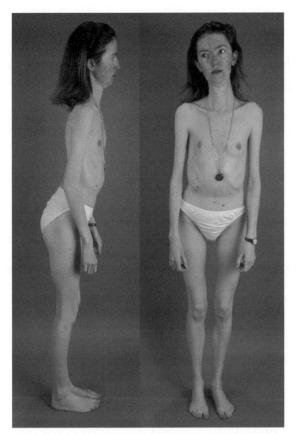

Vignette 2 This patient presented at the age of 1 year with truncal hypotonia and poor head control but had normal early motor milestones. She developed mild generalized weakness from mid childhood, required scoliosis fixation at the age of 14, and required nocturnal non-invasive ventilation from the age of 21. At the age of 30 her forced vital lung capacity was 25% of predicted and she remained ambulant. A muscle biopsy given at the age of 7 showed non-specific myopathy changes (mild Type 1 fibre smallness). This patient has a homozygous missense mutation in the *SEPN1* gene. Clinical features provide the most useful diagnostic clues in *SEPN1*-related myopathy. Muscle magnetic resonance imaging may also give useful diagnostic information. The prominence of scoliosis and respiratory muscle weakness (usually in the teenage years) in the context of preserved limb strength is typical of this condition. The absence of facial weakness, ptosis, or ophthalmoplegia and the relative severity of respiratory muscle weakness differentiate this presentation from myopathies due to *RYR1*. Close monitoring of respiratory function is essential in all patients suspected or confirmed to have *SEPN1*-related myopathies. Adapted from Figure 2 in Clarke NF et al., *Ann Neurol* 2006; **59**: 546–552.

Centronuclear and myotubular myopathies

The centronuclear myopathies are a group of congenital myopathies that were initially defined by the presence of abnormally high numbers of myofibres with nuclei organized in rows in the central portion of the myofibres [41] (Fig. 28.2b). The three established genetic causes of this classical CNM pattern are *DNM2*, *MTM1*, and *BIN1*. Recently, patients who have markedly increased numbers of internalized nuclei (which may not be geographically central) as the main histological abnormality, have also been referred to as having CNM [42]. Mutations in *RYR1*

account for a large proportion of patients with this phenotype. Early data suggest that mutations in *TTN* may be another important cause. Each of these forms of CNM differs in histopathological presentation, mode of inheritance, and clinical phenotype, although overlaps can make predicting the correct genetic cause difficult [41,43]. On average, *DNM2*-related CNM (AD) has a later onset and milder course than the X-linked form (*MTM1*), and the recessive forms (*BIN1*, *RYR1*) are intermediate with respect to severity. Many CNM patients remain without a genetic diagnosis after tests of the known genes, indicating that further genetic causes probably remain undiscovered [44]. Muscle MRI can provide useful information for prioritization of genetic testing, especially in children over the age of 5 years who do not require an anaesthetic.

Centronuclear myopathy 1 (MIM #160150) due to *DNM2* mutations

CNM due to mutations in *DNM2* most frequently follows AD (or *de novo* dominant) inheritance and is a common form of CNM [45]. Most patients present during infancy or early childhood (classical form) with weakness in the limb-girdle, trunk, and neck muscles. However, distal muscle involvement (ankle dorsiflexor weakness especially) can be prominent. Ptosis and limited eye movements frequently occur but the latter may not manifest at first presentation. The most severely affected individuals present at birth with respiratory insufficiency, generalized weakness, and dysphagia that often improves after several months. Mildly affected patients may only present in the third decade of life. Respiratory failure, scoliosis, difficulty walking, and dysphagia are common in late childhood in severely affected patients and may arise in patients with the classical phenotype during adulthood. A different range of dominant *DNM2* mutations cause Charcot–Marie–Tooth disease 1B [46]. The presence of radial sarcoplasmic strands in the muscle biopsy on NADH stains are a strong indication of *DNM2*-related CNM, but can occur in CNM due to *BIN1* (CNM2). Neuropathic changes, neutropenia, and cataracts are uncommon associations in *DNM2*-related CNM but may be clues to the diagnosis. MRI of the lower limb muscles can be a useful investigation to guide genetic testing in CNM, particularly in children over age 5 years who do not require a general anaesthetic, as different, relatively consistent, patterns of muscle involvement have been reported for patients with *DNM2* and *RYR1* mutations [47,48]. Muscle MRI appearances for the other forms of CNM have not yet been well characterized.

Centronuclear myopathy 2 (MIM #255200) due to *BIN1* mutations

AR mutations in *BIN1* are a rare cause of CNM, reported in fewer than ten families to date (*BIN1*; MIM #601248) [49–51]. CNM2 has many clinical features in common with moderate to severe *DNM2*-related CNM, such as facial weakness, ptosis, external ophthalmoplegia, and weakness of the chewing muscles. Proximal weakness is prominent; however, there may also be distal weakness and wasting of the lower limbs with foot abnormalities. Scoliosis is common, respiratory involvement may be severe [44,51], and *BIN1* is the only cause of CNM associated with cardiomyopathy

[44,50]. In addition, some CNM2 patients have a mild intellectual disability [50,51].

Myotubular myopathy (MIM #310400)

X-linked CNM due to mutations in the *MTM1* gene is, for historical reasons and because the clinical presentation and histological features are relatively distinct from other types of CNM, more often referred to as myotubular myopathy. Most affected males have severe, generalized weakness at birth, together with hypotonia, external ophthalmoplegia, and respiratory failure. Reduced foetal movements, polyhydramnios, and a family history of male neonatal death or miscarriages are common. Affected infants are often macrosomic (length greater than the 90th percentile). Most affected males die within the first few months of life from respiratory complications, but some patients with attenuated forms, or with intensive respiratory support, survive into late childhood and beyond.

Most female carriers of X-linked myotubular myopathy are asymptomatic, but a small percentage have mild muscle weakness or pronounced weakness due to skewed X-inactivation [52]. When there is only one affected male in a family, around 80–90% of mothers will carry the mutation as well. In 10–20% of families the mutation likely arises *de novo* in the affected boy, but maternal mosaicism cannot be excluded and families are advised to have genetic counselling. A presumptive diagnosis can be made rapidly in most males from the severe congenital presentation and the presence of numerous myofibres with central nuclei surrounded by a clear halo on haematoxylin and eosin (H&E) stain (that resemble foetal myotubes). The main differential diagnosis for this presentation is congenital myotonic dystrophy (DM1), which can have similar clinical and histological features. Genetic testing can reliably diagnose DM1 and is informative in most families with *MTM1* mutations. Mildly affected males and symptomatic females may be diagnosed late, as clinical and histological signs overlap other forms of CNM and the possibility of *MTM1* mutations may not be considered. The presence of necklace fibres appears to be a useful marker of *MTM1*-related CNM but these are occasionally seen in CNM due to *DNM2* and *RYR1* mutations (unpublished observations) [53,54].

Myopathy with prominent internal nuclei due to *RYR1* mutations

Some patients with *RYR1* mutations have markedly increased numbers of internalized nuclei as the main histological abnormality on muscle biopsy and are diagnosed with CNM if a broad definition for this condition is used [53,55,56]. *RYR1*-related CNM is best discriminated from other characterized forms of CNM based on the relative proportions of internalized nuclei that adopt central versus non-central positions. *RYR1*-related CNM most often follows AR inheritance, although patients with likely dominant mutations have been reported. The clinical course largely depends on the severity of weakness, and the range of clinical issues that can arise is the same as in *RYR1*-related MmD. Early reports suggest that *RYR1*-related CNM is relatively common.

Other rare forms of congenital myopathy

A number of rare congenital myopathies can be considered variants of NEM because they overlap in histological features or genetic cause. Actin accumulation myopathy is characterized by homogeneous protein inclusions comprising actin filaments (best appreciated on electron microscopy) that can occupy large areas in muscle fibres. In intranuclear rod myopathy, nemaline bodies are seen inside myonuclei, with or without coexisting cytoplasmic rods. For both myopathies, dominant mutations in *ACTA1* are the only known cause. Cap myopathy is characterized by subsarcolemmal accumulations of thin filament proteins that stain negative for myosin. The known genetic causes of cap myopathy in descending order of frequency are *TPM2*, *TPM3*, and *ACTA1* [29,57]. When both cores and rods are present in the muscle biopsy, the term core–rod myopathy is used. Established genetic causes of core–rod myopathy are *RYR1* [58], *ACTA1* [59], *NEB* [60], and *KBTBD13* [33].

Congenital fibre-type disproportion (CFTD) is sometimes regarded as a less robust diagnosis than other forms of congenital myopathy but it is useful in practice because the genetic basis can be identified in many patients [61]. The defining feature of CFTD is that Type 1 myofibres are consistently smaller than Type 2 (fast twitch) myofibres by at least 35% as the main histological abnormality on muscle biopsy (Fig. 28.2e). Patients should also have clinical features of a congenital myopathy. Over half of patients with this clinical–histological pattern have mutations in the following genes (listed in descending order of frequency): *TPM3*, *RYR1*, *ACTA1*, *TPM2*, and *MYH7* [62]. An 8 year old boy with CFTD due a de novo AD mutation in TPM3 is shown in video 28.2.

Future directions

The widespread introduction of high-throughput sequencing approaches into diagnostic laboratories [63–65] promises to greatly simplify molecular diagnosis of the congenital myopathies, especially for forms with many possible genetic causes like NEM and CNM or those that that involve large genes like *NEB* and *RYR1*. It is reasonable to expect that an affordable genetic diagnosis will be possible in most families in the near future.

There is a pressing need for effective treatments that improve strength and quality of life and reduce mortality in the congenital structural myopathies. There are anecdotal and empirical reports [66,67] and animal studies [68] that support the use of L-tyrosine in NEM in increasing function and, especially, in control of oral secretions in patients. Ongoing studies into the basis of muscle dysfunction and muscle weakness in various congenital myopathies are likely to eventually provide the most useful therapeutic targets.

The most recent developments in the genetic basis of the congenital myopathies are summarized in Box 28.1.

Box 28.1 Recent developments

An increase in the availability of genetic tests that use next-generation sequencing to screen panels of genes has led to several recent developments in understanding the genetic basis of the congenital myopathies [1].

Hypertonic congenital myopathy

Hypertonic nemaline myopathy has been associated with a particular mutation of *ACTA1* [2], while recessive null mutation of αB-crystallin (*CRYAB*) has been associated with myofibrillar myopathy with stiffness [3].

NEM

NEM5 (*TNNT1* NEM) has recently been reported outside the Amish community in a Dutch family and shown to be caused by different mutations to the founder mutation in the Amish [4]. NEM5 may well be present in other communities.

Two novel NEM genes

Two novel disease genes encoding skeletal muscle-specific BTB-Kelch proteins have been identified as causes of nemaline myopathy. Autosomal recessive mutations in *KLHL40* were found to be a relatively common cause of severe nemaline myopathy (NEM8; MIM #615318), with many cases presenting *in utero*. Congenital fractures and contractures were frequently observed in *KLHL40* patients, and may serve as a useful diagnostic clue to this disorder. Due to a founder effect of the p.G1u528Lys substitution in Japan, *KLHL40* mutation is the most frequent cause of severe nemaline myopathy in Japan [5]. Autosomal recessive mutations of *KLHL41* were subsequently identified as a less frequent cause of severe nemaline myopathy [6].

Core disease genes

RYR1

Autosomal recessive *RYR1* mutations are a relatively common cause of severe congenital myopathy (often with symptoms noted *in utero*) [7,8]. In many of these cases, the muscle biopsy shows a dystrophic pattern, without prominent myofibre degeneration, a pattern not typically associated with *RYR1* mutations in the past [8].

Multiminicore disease

In addition, classic multiminicore disease has recently been associated with a dominant mutation in slow skeletal beta cardiac myosin (*MYH7*) [9].

Centronuclear myopathy

Autosomal recessive *DNM2* mutations were reported in a single family presenting with a lethal congenital syndrome associated with akinesia, joint contractures, hypotonia, skeletal, and vascular abnormalities [10]. Autosomal recessive truncating *TTN* mutations have recently been described in patients presenting with a myopathy characterized by the presence of internal nuclei and/or core-like regions on muscle biopsy and also heart disease in some cases [11–13].

References

1. Bohm J, Vasli N, Malfatti E, et al. An integrated diagnosis strategy for congenital myopathies. *PLoS ONE* 2013; **8**: e67527.
2. Jain RK, Jayawant S, Squier W, et al. Nemaline myopathy with stiffness and hypertonia associated with an ACTA1 mutation. *Neurology* 2012; **78**: 1100–3.
3. Forrest KM, Al-Sarraj S, Sewry C, et al. Infantile onset myofibrillar myopathy due to recessive CRYAB mutations. *Neuromuscul Disord* 2011; **21**: 37–40.
4. Van der Pol LW, Leijenaar JF, Spliet WGM, et al. Nemaline myopathy caused by TNNT1 mutations in a Dutch pedigree. *Mol Genet Genom Med* 2013; published online 12 December, doi: 10.1002/mgg3.52
5. Ravenscroft G, Miyatake S, Lehtokari VL, et al. Mutations in KLHL40 are a frequent cause of severe autosomal-recessive nemaline myopathy. *Am J Hum Genet* 2013; **93**: 6–18.
6. Gupta VA, Ravenscroft G, Shaheen R, et al. Identification of KLHL41 mutations implicates BTB-kelch-mediated ubiquitination as an alternate pathway to myofibrillar disruption in nemaline myopathy. *Am J Hum Genet* 2013; **93**: 1108–17.
7. Amburgey K, Bailey A, Hwang JH, et al. Genotypephenotypecorrelations in recessive RYR1-related myopathies. *Orphanet J Rare Dis* 2013; **8**: 117.
8. Bharucha-Goebel DX, Santi M, Medne L, et al. Severe congenital RYR1-associated myopathy: the expanding clinicopathologic and genetic spectrum. *Neurology* 2013; **80**: 1584–9.
9. Cullup T, Lamont PJ, Cirak S, et al. Mutations in MYH7 cause multi-minicore disease (MmD) with variable cardiac involvement. *Neuromuscul Disord* 2012; **22**: 1096–104.
10. Koutsopoulos OS, Kretz C, Weller CM, et al. Dynamin 2 homozygous mutation in humans with a lethal congenital syndrome. *Eur J Hum Genet* 2013; **21**: 637–42.
11. Ceyhan-Birsoy O, Agrawal PB, Hidalgo C, et al. Recessive truncating titin gene, TTN, mutations presenting as centronuclear myopathy. *Neurology* 2013; **81**: 1205–14.
12. Chauveau C, Bonnemann CG, Julien C, et al. Recessive TTN truncating mutations define novel forms of core myopathy with heart disease. *Hum Mol Genet* 2013; published online 8 October, doi: 10.1093/hmg/ddt494
13. Palmio J, Evila A, Chapon F, et al. Hereditary myopathy with early respiratory failure:occurrence in various populations. *J Neurol Neurosurg Psychiatry* 2013; published online 19 April, doi: 10.1136/jnnp-2013-304965

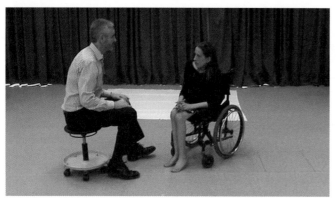

📹 **Video 28.1** Mother and daughter with moderately severe autosomal dominant central core disease due to a *RYR1* gene mutation.

References

1. Wallgren-Petterson C, Laing NG. Congenital Myopathies. In: Karpati G, Hilton-Jones D, Bushby K, Griggs RC (ed) *Disorders of Voluntary Muscle*, 8th edn, pp. 282–98. New York: Cambridge University Press, 2010.

2. Norwood FL, Harling C, Chinnery PF, Eagle M, Bushby K, Straub V. Prevalence of genetic muscle disease in northern England: in-depth analysis of a muscle clinic population. *Brain* 2009; **132**: 3175–86.

3. Amburgey K, McNamara N, Bennett LR, McCormick ME, Acsadi G, Dowling JJ. Prevalence of congenital myopathies in a representative pediatric united states population. *Ann Neurol* 2011; **70**: 662–5.

4. Maggi L, Scoto M, Cirak S, et al. Congenital myopathies—clinical features and frequency of individual subtypes diagnosed in a five-year perod: the UK experience. *Neuromuscul Disord* 2011; **21**: 691.

5. Laing NG, Dye DE, Wallgren-Pettersson C, et al. Mutations and polymorphisms of the skeletal muscle alpha-actin gene (ACTA1). *Hum Mutat* 2009; **30**: 1267–77.

6. Donner K, Sandbacka M, Lehtokari VL, Wallgren-Pettersson C, Pelin K. Complete genomic structure of the human nebulin gene and identification of alternatively spliced transcripts. *Eur J Hum Genet* 2004; **12**: 744–51.

7. Robinson R, Carpenter D, Shaw MA, Halsall J, Hopkins P. Mutations in RYR1 in malignant hyperthermia and central core disease. *Hum Mutat* 2006; **27**: 977–89.

8. Jeannet PY, Mittaz L, Dunand M, Lobrinus JA, Bonafe L, Kuntzer T. Autosomal dominant nemaline myopathy: a new phenotype unlinked to previously known genetic loci. *Neuromuscul Disord* 2007; **17**: 6–12.

9. Laing NG, Wilton SD, Akkari PA, et al. A mutation in the alpha tropomyosin gene TPM3 associated with autosomal dominant nemaline myopathy. *Nat Genet* 1995; **9**: 75–9.

10. Penisson-Besnier I, Monnier N, Toutain A, Dubas F, Laing N. A second pedigree with autosomal dominant nemaline myopathy caused by TPM3 mutation: a clinical and pathological study. *Neuromuscul Disord* 2007; **17**: 330–7.

11. Tan P, Briner J, Boltshauser E, et al. Homozygosity for a nonsense mutation in the alpha-tropomyosin slow gene TPM3 in a patient with severe infantile nemaline myopathy. *Neuromuscul Disord* 1999; **9**: 573–9.

12. Lehtokari VL, Pelin K, Donner K, et al. Identification of a founder mutation in TPM3 in nemaline myopathy patients of Turkish origin. *Eur J Hum Genet* 2008 **16**: 1055–61.

13. Clarke NF, Kolski H, Dye DE, et al. Mutations in TPM3 are a common cause of congenital fiber type disproportion. *Ann Neurol* 2008; **63**: 329–37.

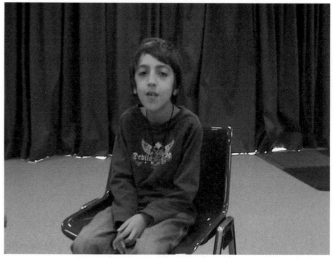

📹 **Video 28.2** Eight-year-old boy with congenital fibre type disproportion (CFTD) due to a *de novo* dominant mutation in *TPM3*.

14. Lawlor MW, Dechene ET, Roumm E, Geggel AS, Moghadaszadeh B, Beggs AH. Mutations of tropomyosin 3 (TPM3) are common and associated with type 1 myofiber hypotrophy in congenital fiber type disproportion. *Hum Mutat* 2010; **31**: 176–83.

15. Wallgren-Pettersson C, Avela K, Marchand S, et al. A gene for autosomal recessive nemaline myopathy assigned to chromosome 2q by linkage analysis. *Neuromuscul Disord* 1995; **5**: 441–3.

16. Pelin K, Hilpela P, Donner K, et al. Mutations in the nebulin gene associated with autosomal recessive nemaline myopathy. *Proc Natl Acad Sci USA* 1999; **96**: 2305–10.

17. Lehtokari VL, Pelin K, Sandbacka M, et al. Identification of 45 novel mutations in the nebulin gene associated with autosomal recessive nemaline myopathy. *Hum Mutat* 2006; **27**: 946–56.

18. Wallgren-Pettersson C, Pelin K, Hilpela P, et al. Clinical and genetic heterogeneity in autosomal recessive nemaline myopathy. *Neuromuscul Disord* 1999; **9**: 564–72.

19. Wallgren-Pettersson C, Donner K, Sewry C, et al. Mutations in the nebulin gene can cause severe congenital nemaline myopathy. *Neuromuscul Disord* 2002; **12**: 674–9.

20. Lehtokari VL, Pelin K, Herczegfalvi A, et al. Nemaline myopathy caused by mutations in the nebulin gene may present as a distal myopathy. *Neuromuscul Disord* 2011; **21**: 556–62.

21. Nowak KJ, Wattanasirichaigoon D, Goebel HH, et al. Mutations in the skeletal muscle alpha-actin gene in patients with actin myopathy and nemaline myopathy. *Nat Genet* 1999; **23**: 208–12.

22. Wallgren-Pettersson C, Pelin K, Nowak KJ, et al. Genotype-phenotype correlations in nemaline myopathy caused by mutations in the genes for nebulin and skeletal muscle alpha-actin. *Neuromuscul Disord* 2004; **14**: 461–70.

23. Nowak KJ, Sewry CA, Navarro C, et al. Nemaline myopathy caused by absence of alpha-skeletal muscle actin. *Ann Neurol* 2007; **61**: 175–84.

24. Ryan MM, Schnell C, Strickland CD, et al. Nemaline myopathy: a clinical study of 143 cases. *Ann Neurol* 2001; **50**: 312–20.

25. Ravenscroft G, Colley SM, Walker KR, et al. Expression of cardiac alpha-actin spares extraocular muscles in skeletal muscle alpha-actin diseases—quantification of striated alpha-actins by MRM-mass spectrometry. *Neuromuscul Disord* 2008; **18**: 953–8.

26. Saito Y, Komaki H, Hattori A, et al. Extramuscular manifestations in children with severe congenital myopathy due to ACTA1 gene mutations. *Neuromuscul Disord* 2011; **21**: 489–93.

27. Donner K, Ollikainen M, Ridanpaa M, et al. Mutations in the beta-tropomyosin (TPM2) gene—a rare cause of nemaline myopathy. *Neuromuscul Disord* 2002; **12**: 151–8.

28. Tajsharghi H, Ohlsson M, Lindberg C, Oldfors A. Congenital myopathy with nemaline rods and cap structures caused by a mutation in the beta-tropomyosin gene (TPM2). *Arch Neurol* 2007; **64**: 1334–8.

29. Clarke NF, Domazetovska A, Waddell L, Kornberg A, McLean C, North KN. Cap disease due to mutation of the beta-tropomyosin gene (TPM2). *Neuromuscul Disord* 2009; **19**: 348–51.

30. Johnston JJ, Kelley RI, Crawford TO, et al. A novel nemaline myopathy in the Amish caused by a mutation in troponin T1. *Am J Hum Genet* 2000; **67**: 814–21.

31. Gommans IM, Davis M, Saar K, et al. A locus on chromosome 15q for a dominantly inherited nemaline myopathy with core-like lesions. *Brain* 2003; **126**: 1545–51.

32. Olive M, Goldfarb LG, Lee HS, et al. Nemaline myopathy type 6: clinical and myopathological features. *Muscle Nerve* 2010; **42**: 901–7.

33. Sambuughin N, Yau KS, Olive M, et al. Dominant mutations in KBTBD13, a member of the BTB/kelch family, cause nemaline myopathy with cores. *Am J Hum Genet* 2010; **87**: 842–7.

34. Agrawal PB, Greenleaf RS, Tomczak KK, et al. Nemaline myopathy with minicores caused by mutation of the CFL2 gene encoding the skeletal muscle actin-binding protein, cofilin-2. *Am J Hum Genet* 2007; **80**: 162–7.

35. Ockeloen CM, Gilhuis HJ, Pfundt R, et al. Nemaline myopathy caused by a novel missense mutation in the CFL2 gene. *Neuromuscul Disord* 2011; **21**: 696.

36. Wu S, Ibarra MC, Malicdan MC, et al. Central core disease is due to RYR1 mutations in more than 90% of patients. *Brain* 2006; **129**: 1470–80.

37. Clarke NF, Kidson W, Quijano-Roy S, et al. SEPN1: associated with congenital fiber-type disproportion and insulin resistance. *Ann Neurol* 2006; **59**: 546–52.

38. Carmignac V, Salih MA, Quijano-Roy S, et al. C-terminal titin deletions cause a novel early-onset myopathy with fatal cardiomyopathy. *Ann Neurol* 2007; **61**: 340–51.

39. Kinali M, Beeson D, Pitt MC, et al. Congenital myasthenic syndromes in childhood: diagnostic and management challenges. *J Neuroimmunol* 2008; **201–202**: 6–12.

40. Muelas N, Hackman P, Luque H, et al. MYH7 gene tail mutation causing myopathic profiles beyond Laing distal myopathy. *Neurology* 2010; **75**: 732–41.

41. Romero NB. Centronuclear myopathies: a widening concept. *Neuromuscul Disord* 2010; **20**: 223–8.

42. Hanisch F, Muller T, Dietz A, et al. Phenotype variability and histopathological findings in centronuclear myopathy due to DNM2 mutations. *J Neurol* 2011; **258**: 1085–90.

43. Toussaint A, Cowling BS, Hnia K, et al. Defects in amphiphysin 2 (BIN1) and triads in several forms of centronuclear myopathies. *Acta Neuropathol* 2011; **121**: 253–66.

44. Jungbluth H, Wallgren-Pettersson C, Laporte J. Centronuclear (myotubular) myopathy. *Orphanet J Rare Dis* 2008; **3**: 26.

45. Bitoun M, Maugenre S, Jeannet PY, et al. Mutations in dynamin 2 cause dominant centronuclear myopathy. *Nat Genet* 2005; **37**: 1207–9.

46. Zuchner S, Noureddine M, Kennerson M, et al. Mutations in the pleckstrin homology domain of dynamin 2 cause dominant intermediate Charcot–Marie–Tooth disease. *Nat Genet* 2005; **37**: 289–94.

47. Schessl J, Medne L, Hu Y, et al. MRI in DNM2-related centronuclear myopathy: evidence for highly selective muscle involvement. *Neuromuscul Disord* 2007; **17**: 28–32.

48. Klein A, Jungbluth H, Clement E, et al. Muscle magnetic resonance imaging in congenital myopathies due to ryanodine receptor type 1 gene mutations. *Arch Neurol* 2011; **68**: 1171–9.

49. Nicot AS, Toussaint A, Tosch V, et al. Mutations in amphiphysin 2 (BIN1) disrupt interaction with dynamin 2 and cause autosomal recessive centronuclear myopathy. *Nat Genet* 2007; **39**: 1134–9.

50. Bohm J, Yis U, Ortac R, et al. Case report of intrafamilial variability in autosomal recessive centronuclear myopathy associated to a novel BIN1 stop mutation. *Orphanet J Rare Dis* 2010; **5**: 35.

51. Claeys KG, Maisonobe T, Bohm J, et al. Phenotype of a patient with recessive centronuclear myopathy and a novel BIN1 mutation. *Neurology* 2010; **74**: 519–21.

52. Schara U, Kress W, Tucke J, Mortier W. X-linked myotubular myopathy in a female infant caused by a new MTM1 gene mutation. *Neurology* 2003; **60**: 1363–5.

53. Wilmshurst JM, Lillis S, Zhou H, et al. RYR1 mutations are a common cause of congenital myopathies with central nuclei. *Ann Neurol* 2010; **68**: 717–26.

54. Bevilacqua JA, Bitoun M, Biancalana V, et al. 'Necklace' fibers, a new histological marker of late-onset MTM1-related centronuclear myopathy. *Acta Neuropathol* 2009; **117**: 283–91.

55. Jungbluth H, Zhou H, Sewry CA, et al. Centronuclear myopathy due to a de novo dominant mutation in the skeletal muscle ryanodine receptor (RYR1) gene. *Neuromuscul Disord* 2007; **17**: 338–45.

56. Bevilacqua JA, Monnier N, Bitoun M, et al. Recessive RYR1 mutations cause unusual congenital myopathy with prominent nuclear internalization and large areas of myofibrillar disorganization. *Neuropathol Appl Neurobiol* 2011; **37**: 271–84.

57. Ohlsson M, Quijano-Roy S, Darin N, et al. New morphologic and genetic findings in cap disease associated with beta-tropomyosin (TPM2) mutations. *Neurology* 2008; **71**: 1896–901.

58. Scacheri PC, Hoffman EP, Fratkin JD, et al. A novel ryanodine receptor gene mutation causing both cores and rods in congenital myopathy. *Neurology* 2000; **55**: 1689–96.

59. Kaindl AM, Ruschendorf F, Krause S, et al. Missense mutations of ACTA1 cause dominant congenital myopathy with cores. *J Med Genet* 2004; **41**: 842–8.

60. Romero NB, Lehtokari VL, Quijano-Roy S, et al. Core–rod myopathy caused by mutations in the nebulin gene. *Neurology* 2009; **73**: 1159–61.

61. Clarke NF. Congenital fibre type disproportion—a syndrome at the crossroads of the congenital myopathies. *Neuromuscul Disord* 2011; **21**: 252–3.

62. Clarke NF, Waddell LB, Cooper ST, et al. Recessive mutations in RYR1 are a common cause of congenital fiber type disproportion. *Hum Mutat* 2010; **31**: E1544–E1550.

63. Hoischen A, Gilissen C, Arts P, et al. Massively parallel sequencing of ataxia genes after array-based enrichment. *Hum Mutat* 2010; **31**: 494–9.

64. Simpson DA, Clark GR, Alexander S, Silvestri G, Willoughby CE. Molecular diagnosis for heterogeneous genetic diseases with targeted high-throughput DNA sequencing applied to retinitis pigmentosa. *J Med Genet* 2011; **48**: 145–51.

65. Walsh T, Lee MK, Casadei S, et al. Detection of inherited mutations for breast and ovarian cancer using genomic capture and massively parallel sequencing. *Proc Natl Acad Sci USA* 2010; **107**: 12629–33.

66. Kalita D. A new treatment for congenital nonprogressive nemaline myopathy. *J Orthomol Med* 1989; **4**: 70–4.

67. Ryan MM, Sy C, Rudge S, Ellaway C, et al. Dietary L-tyrosine supplementation in nemaline myopathy. *J Child Neurol* 2008; **23**: 609–13.

68. Nguyen MA, Joya JE, Kee AJ, et al. Hypertrophy and dietary tyrosine ameliorate the phenotypes of a mouse model of severe nemaline myopathy. *Brain* 2011; **134**: 3513–26.

CHAPTER 29

Metabolic myopathies

Mette C. Ørngreen and John Vissing

Introduction

Metabolic myopathies are hereditary muscle disorders caused by specific enzymatic defects of intermediary metabolism. The disorders are generally subdivided in two major groups affecting either carbohydrate metabolism (the glycogenoses also known as glycogen storage diseases) or lipid metabolism (Figs 29.1 and 29.2). The respiratory chain defects (mitochondrial myopathies) comprise a third group of metabolic myopathies, but these are classically described separately under mitochondrial disorders (see Chapter 30). In older children and adults, disorders of lipid and carbohydrate metabolism can share two common clinical presentations: (1) recurrent episodes of exercise intolerance, coupled with muscle contractures/stiffness and pain, which in severe cases result in breakdown of skeletal muscle fibre (rhabdomyolysis) and myoglobinuria; (2) static, often progressive, muscle weakness and atrophy. If symptomatic at birth or in infancy, these disorders typically present affecting multiple organs, involving episodes of hypoglycaemia, encephalopathy, and sudden death.

Exercise-related symptoms in patients with metabolic myopathies are caused by a mismatch between energy demand and supply [1]. The common symptoms of exertional fatigue, muscle contractures, and pain can make it difficult to pinpoint the exact defect based on clinical presentation. Furthermore, exercise-related symptoms are also common among the general population, which highlights the importance of being able to distinguish these disorders from the very common symptoms of myalgia and exercise intolerance in people without muscle disease. A further complicating factor in the diagnostic workup is that a number of non-metabolic myopathies may also present with a picture characteristic of the metabolic myopathies. Exercise-related muscle pain and even myoglobinuria are not rare in certain types of limb-girdle muscular dystrophy (Type 2I and sarcoglycanopathies) and Becker muscular dystrophy [2]. Exercise-related pain is also commonly found in other muscle diseases such as facioscapulohumeral muscular dystrophy, channelopathies, and thyroid gland diseases. Therefore it is important to have knowledge about the distinct clinical presentations of these patient groups to make the correct diagnosis.

In the differentiation between defects in fat and carbohydrate metabolism, it helps to interview the patient about when in exercise the symptoms occur (Fig. 29.3). At the start of exercise and during strenuous exercise energy production depends primarily on muscle glycogenolysis and glycolysis, and symptoms evoked by such exercise therefore suggest an underlying glycogenosis. During prolonged, low-intensity exercise, energy production depends primarily on oxidation of fatty acids, and symptoms provoked by such exercise would therefore point towards a disorder of lipid metabolism.

During dynamic exercise, such as walking, running, or cycling, energy comes from ATP generated through oxidative phosphorylation of muscle glycogen and free fatty acids (FFAs) [3,4]. The fraction of substrates oxidized depends on the intensity and duration of exercise:

1. At low intensity (<60% of maximal oxygen uptake, $V_{O_{2max}}$), energy primarily comes from the oxidation of fatty acids [3,4].

2. At moderate intensity (>60% and <75% of $V_{O_{2max}}$), ATP is regenerated by high-energy phosphates, followed by breakdown of muscle glycogen during the first 5 to 10 min of exercise [3,4]. As an indication of glycogen breakdown, lactate rises sharply in the first 10 min of exercise. During continued exercise, lactate levels drop as muscle triglycerides and blood-borne fuels are increasingly oxidized [5,6–8].

3. During high-intensity exercise (>75% of $V_{O_{2max}}$) oxidation of muscle carbohydrate is the major fuel source [4]. Carbohydrates from muscle and hepatic glycogenolysis and blood glucose are much more limited than energy reserves bound in fat, and can just support high-intensity exercise for approximately an hour [3,4].

4. During anaerobic exercise, ATP production primarily relies on anaerobic glycogenolysis, and the ADP phosphorylation by the creatine kinase and myoadenylate deaminase reactions [3]. Anaerobic glycolysis plays a smaller role in total energy production, and is usually only activated during anaerobic conditions such as sustained isometric contraction or high-intensity exercise >90% of $V_{O_{2max}}$ when blood flow and delivery of oxygen to exercising muscle are relatively insufficient [1].

Glycogenoses in skeletal muscle

In 1951, Brian McArdle demonstrated blocked lactate production in a patient performing ischaemic handgrip exercise [9]. He cleverly deduced that the patient had an enzymatic defect of muscle glycogenolysis, and some years later the defect was confirmed to be myophosphorylase deficiency [10,11]. Since then, approximately 14 other defects of glycogenolysis and glycolysis have been reported, the most recent one being phosphoglucomutase deficiency [glycogen storage disease (GSD) Type XIV] [12]. The glycogenoses are inherited as an autosomal recessive trait, except for phosphoglycerate kinase and phosphorylase b kinase deficiencies, which are X-linked recessive.

In the majority of glycogenoses affecting skeletal muscle, symptoms are dynamic and exercise-related, because the enzymatic defect limits energy supply initially during exercise when intact

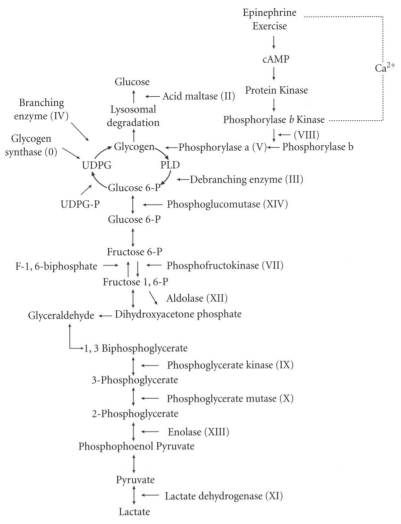

Fig. 29.1 The glycogenolytic pathway. Roman numerals refer to the muscle glycogenoses caused by the enzymes denoted: acid maltase (II), debrancher (III), brancher (IV), phosphorylase (V), phosphofructokinase (VII), phosphorylase b kinase (VIII), phosphoglycerate kinase (IX), phosphoglycerate mutase (X), lactate dehydrogenase (XI), aldolase (XII), enolase (XIII), phosphoglucomutase (XIV).

muscle glycogenolysis and glycolysis are essential for ATP production [13]. Most patients have lifelong exercise intolerance and typically have symptoms of muscle fatigue, pain, contractures, and episodes of myoglobinuria [13]. A smaller group of muscle glycogenoses present primarily with muscle weakness and wasting, and may resemble muscular dystrophies, although the two types of GSD may overlap in phenotype. In the rest of this section GSDs are described, based on their clinical presentation and divided into those with exercise-related dynamic symptoms and those with static symptoms of muscle wasting and weakness.

Glycogenoses with dynamic symptoms

McArdle disease

Patients with GSD V (McArdle disease) typically have a complete block in breakdown of muscle glycogen. Patients carry mutations in the myophosphorylase gene (*PYGM*) on chromosome 11 that encodes muscle glycogen phosphorylase [14]. The disease is autosomal recessively inherited and the most common mutation is the Arg50stop mutation [15]. This is the most common GSD with an estimated prevalence of 1 in 100 000.

Clinical features

Patients experience exercise intolerance, muscle fatigue, and exercise-induced muscle contractures and pain [16]. Eighty per cent have onset of these symptoms before the age of 10 [17]. Muscle cramps periodically lead to myoglobinuria in about two-thirds of cases, and a fraction of these patients have experienced acute renal failure [18]. Patients with McArdle disease have severely limited anaerobic and aerobic exercise capacity [16], and the maximal O_2 uptake is 35–50% of normal [13]. Patients with McArdle disease all develop a second-wind phenomenon after the first 5–8 min of exercise, which so far has only been observed in this condition. Most, but not all, patients can spontaneously report the second wind. In the first minutes of exercise, McArdle patients have an energy crisis due to the blocked muscle glycogenolysis and low availability of extramuscular fuels. This energy crisis results in tachycardia [140–150 beats min^{-1} (bpm)], but when extramuscular fuel supplies become more readily available for combustion after 6–8 min of exercise, a second wind kicks in with a spontaneous drop in heart rate of usually 30 bpm, and a great drop in perceived exertion [18].

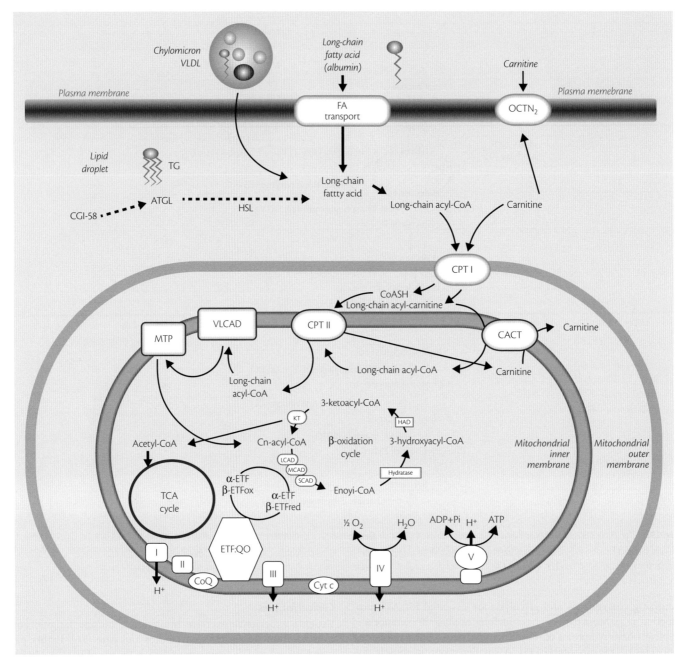

Fig. 29.2 The fatty acid oxidation pathway. ATGL, adipose triglyceride lipase; ATP, adenosine-5'-triphosphate; CACT, carnitine/acylcarnitine translocase; CGI-58, comparative gene identification-58; CoA, coenzyme A; CoASH, coenzyme A; CoQ, coenzyme Q; CPT I, carnitine palmitoyltransferase I; CPT II, carnitine palmitoyltransferase II; Cyt c, cytochrome c oxidase; ETF, electron transfer flavoprotein; ETF-QO, ETF coenzyme Q oxidoreductase; HAD, L-3-hydroxyacyl-CoA dehydrogenase; HSL, hormone-sensitive lipase; LCAD, long chain acyl-CoA dehydrogenase; MCAD, medium chain acyl-CoA dehydrogenase; MTP, mitochondrial trifunctional protein; OCTN2, sodium-dependent carnitine transporter; SCAD, short chain acyl-CoA dehydrogenase; TCA, tricarboxylic acid; VLCAD, very long chain acyl-CoA dehydrogenase; VLDL, very low-density lipoprotein; I, respiratory chain complex I; II, respiratory chain complex II; III, respiratory complex III; IV, respiratory complex IV; respiratory chain complex V.

A third of patients develop fixed weakness, primarily affecting the shoulder girdle, after the age of 40 [19].

Differential diagnosis

So far, the second-wind phenomenon is pathognomic for McArdle disease. Otherwise, the other glycogenoses are the most likely differential diagnoses. Creatine kinase (CK) levels are usually constantly elevated in McArdle disease and phosphofructokinase (PFK) deficiency (PFKD), but are normal between attacks in other muscle glycogenoses with dynamic symptoms.

Treatment

Oral sucrose supplementation and a carbohydrate-rich diet improves exercise tolerance in patients with McArdle disease [20–22]. Aerobic exercise training is also beneficial [23].

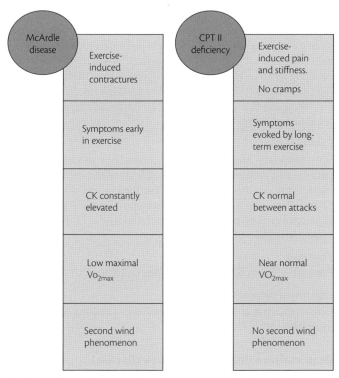

Fig. 29.3 Differences between glycogenoses represented by McArdle disease and fatty acid oxidation disorders represented by carnitine palmitoyl transferase II (CPT II) deficiency. CK, creatine kinase.

Phosphofructokinase deficiency (Tarui disease)

PFK is the rate-limiting enzyme of glycolysis, and catalyses the irreversible conversion of fructose-6-phosphate to fructose-1,6-biphosphate [24]. The muscle defect (GSD VII) is caused by mutations in the *PFKM* gene. The functional PFK molecule is a tetramer with various combinations of three subunits, the combination of which depends on tissue type: muscle (M4 subunits), liver (L4 subunits), and platelet (both M and L subunits) [25,26]. GSD VII shows autosomal recessive inheritance and patients have loss of PFK activity in skeletal muscle and also partial loss in the erythrocytes [27]. Fewer than 150 patients have been described in the world, and around 20 disease-causing mutations have been identified in *PFKM*.

Clinical features

Two phenotypes are described: (1) a very rare, severe, infantile form with hypotonia, limb weakness, progressive myopathy, and respiratory failure leading to early death, and (2) the adult-onset form with exercise intolerance, myopathy, and muscle contractures that can lead to myoglobinuria. Myoglobinuria and contractures are, however, less common than in McArdle disease. As in patients with McArdle disease, PFKD patients develop muscle weakness; however, the frequency is unknown. Haemolytic anaemia is a common finding.

Treatment

No dietary interventions have proven helpful. Experimentally, lipid and lactate infusions improve and glucose infusion worsens exercise tolerance [28].

Differential diagnosis

Symptoms are very similar to those in McArdle disease, but exercise intolerance is more severe, and there is no second wind in PFKD [29].

Phosphorylase b kinase deficiency

Phosphorylase b kinase (PHK) deficiency is a rare glycogen storage disease (GSD VIII) which impairs glycogen breakdown by decreasing the phosphorylation of glycogen phosphorylase from the inactive (b) to the active (a) form. Because of the mild phenotype, the condition may be underdiagnosed [30]. The functional PHK molecule is a polymer with four subunits, α, β, γ, and δ. Subunits α and β regulate phosphorylation, γ is the catalytic subunit, and δ is identical to calmodulin and confers Ca^{2+} sensitivity to the enzyme [16,31]. For the α and γ subunits, tissue-specific isoforms are known for muscle ($α_M$, $γ_M$), liver ($α_L$), and testis ($γ_T$) [32,33]. The inheritance is X-linked for the α subunit [33,34] and autosomal for the β, γ, and δ subunits [34].

Clinical features

Fewer than 10 patients with mutations in the gene encoding the X-linked muscle-specific α subunit (*PHKA1*) have been reported [30,35–38]. Since the biochemical defect of PHK deficiency affects the function of myophosphorylase, patients with PHK deficiency are expected to clinically mimic patients with McArdle disease, who have a primary defect of myophosphorylase. In agreement with this, the symptoms of exercise intolerance, myoglobinuria, and exercise-induced muscle contractures and pain reported in patients with PHK deficiency resemble those observed in McArdle disease, although they seem to be less severe [30]. Patients with PHK deficiency do not experience a second wind [30,39].

Differential diagnosis and diagnosis

Most patients with PHK deficiency are characterized by normal lactate production during ischaemic forearm exercise, but ammonia responses may be elevated, and lactate production may be impaired during dynamic, moderate-intensity exercise. Thus, the metabolic block is only partial. Diagnosis rests on demonstration of low PHK activity in muscle and demonstration of a relevant mutation in *PHKA1*.

Phosphoglycerate kinase deficiency

Phosphoglycerate kinase (PGK) deficiency was identified in 1981 [40]. The defect is an autosomal X-linked disorder caused by mutation in the *PGK* gene [41,42]. Unlike most other glycolytic enzymes, PGK exists in only one isoform (except in spermatogenic cells). However, heterogeneous phenotypes exist.

Clinical features

PGK deficiency may present with severe haemolytic anaemia, seizures and mental retardation, and myopathies with episodes of myoglobinuria. Only nine patients have been reported with the pure myopathic form, characterized by symptoms and signs of exercise intolerance, muscle contractures, and myoglobinuria [43–49]. With just one isoform of the enzyme, it is still not understood why the phenotype has such great variation.

Phosphoglycerate mutase deficiency

Phosphoglycerate mutase deficiency (GSD X) is caused by mutations in the muscle phosphoglycerate mutase (*PGAM2*) gene [50]. PGAM is a glycolytic enzyme converting 3-phosphoglycerate to 2-phosphoglycerate, present in muscle (M-isoform) and brain (B-isoform). The isoforms are mixed in most tissues, but the M-isoform predominates in sperm cells and skeletal and cardiac muscles [50].

Clinical features

Symptoms only develop in skeletal muscle and are exercise-induced contractures, muscle pain and myoglobinuria, and intolerance to strenuous exercise. A common histopathological finding is tubular aggregates. Both periodically and persistently elevated CK have been reported [51–53].

Lactate dehydrogenase deficiency

Lactate dehydrogenase deficiency (GSD XI) was first reported in 1980 and is caused by deficiency of the muscle isoform of lactate dehydrogenase A (LDHA) induced by mutations in the *LDHA* gene [54]. Lactate dehydrogenase catalyses the last step of the glycolytic pathway from pyruvate to lactate, an oxidoreduction reaction. Biochemically this defect results in impaired reoxidation of NADH. The increased level of NADH is partly reoxidized by the action of α-glycerophosphate dehydrogenase instead, which simultaneously drains triose phosphate from the glycolytic pathway, resulting in impaired ATP production and attacks of rhabdomyolysis [54].

Clinical features

Muscle symptoms with exercise-induced myoglobinuria and high plasma CK levels. Patients typically also present with intermittent erythematous skin rashes.

Phosphoglucomutase deficiency

Phosphoglucomutase deficiency (GSD XIV) is caused by mutation in the phosphoglucomutase 1 (*PGM1*) gene. Phosphoglucomutase catalyses the second step in glycogen degradation after the phosphorylation of glycogen, which is proximal in the glycolytic pathway, like the defect of myophosphorylase in patients with McArdle disease [12]. The defect has only recently been described, and so far in only one patient [12].

Clinical features

The patient suffered from myopathy characterized by exercise-induced intolerance with episodes of rhabdomyolysis, and normal elevation of lactate, but hyperammonaemia on a forearm exercise test.

Treatment

Intravenous glucose improves exercise capacity [55. These results indicates that patients also might benefit from oral glucose; however, this has not been tested [55].

Differential diagnosis

Of all glycogenoses, only patients with PGM1 deficiency and McArdle disease have been shown to benefit from intravenous glucose. An important difference between these two disorders is that the phosphoglucomutase-deficient patient has a normal oxidative capacity and production of lactate, demonstrating that the enzyme defect is partial.

Muscle β-enolase deficiency

Muscle β-enolase deficiency (GSD XIII) is caused by mutation in the gene encoding β-enolase (*ENO3*), which predominates in muscle. GSD XIII has only been described in one patient; a 47-year-old man affected with exercise intolerance, myalgias, and increased CK. Furthermore, lactate production was blocked during the ischaemic forearm exercise test [56].

Glycogenoses with static symptoms

Glycogen storage disease 0

GSD 0 can present as a skeletal and cardiac-muscle form (GSD 0b) caused by mutations in the *GYS1* gene on chromosome 19q13.3, and a hepatic form (GSD 0a) caused by mutations in the *GYS2* gene on chromosome 12p12.2 [57]. GSD 0b is caused by deficient activity of glycogen synthase 1 (GYS1), which impairs the transfer of the activated glucosyl moiety of UDP-glucose to a glycogen molecule, resulting in severely reduced levels of glycogen in skeletal and cardiac muscles [57]. Muscle GSD 0 was first described in 2007, and only three families (five patients) with the muscle form have been identified [58–60].

Clinical features

Symptoms are mainly static with muscle weakness; however, patients also present with exercise intolerance and cardiac involvement. Tonic–clonic seizures were described in two of the patients. One patient also suffered from syncope. Three of the patients developed cardiac arrest and died at the ages of 8, 11, and 12 years, respectively [58–60].

Treatment

Beta-receptor blockade for cardiac protection [58].

Differential diagnosis

GYS1 deficiency could be a common cause of sudden cardiac death in children [59].

Acid maltase deficiency (Pompe disease)

Acid maltase deficiency (GSD II, Pompe disease) is an autosomal recessive disorder caused by mutations in the *GAA* gene on chromosome 17q25.3 encoding acid α-1,4-glucosidase (acid maltase), which leads to the accumulation of glycogen in lysosomes of several tissue and cell types, particularly cardiac, skeletal, and smooth muscle cells. More than 200 different mutations have been reported, the most common is the c.-32-13T->G mutation, which accounts for up to 75% of mutated alleles in adult cases [61]. A phenotype–genotype correlation exits [61]. Pathogenesis may be related to: (1) large accumulation of glycogen in muscle, displacing cellular organelles, (2) abnormal lysosomal activity which promotes autophagy, or (3) effects on intermediary metabolism.

Clinical features

Three phenotypes are described:

1. Classic infantile onset of Pompe disease with progressive weakness, enlargement of the tongue, feeding difficulties, and heart, liver, and respiratory insufficiency with death before the age of 3, if untreated [62].

2. Non-classic, infantile-onset Pompe disease with a milder clinical course, presenting in the first years of life, primarily affecting respiratory skeletal muscle and proximal skeletal muscles. Unlike the infantile cases, cardiac involvement is very rare [63].

3. The most common form with adult onset, which resembles the juvenile form but with a milder phenotype. In a third of the adult cases, respiratory distress is the presenting symptom [61].

Infantile onset is a result of a structural mutation causing synthesis of a catalytically inactive (cross-reacting material positive) enzyme protein. Adult-onset cases typically have residual GAA activities of 10–30% of normal [64]. GAA activity can be easily assessed in blood, and should be the preferred first-line diagnostic tool for Pompe disease. In adult-onset cases, muscle biopsy is often non-informative.

Treatment

Enzyme replacement therapy with recombinant α-glucosidase (rGAA) has shown major benefit on survival and cardiomyopathy in infantile Pompe disease. In late-onset patients, enzyme replacement therapy is less effective and difficult to assess, because of the heterogeneous clinical features and slow progression of the disease. A randomized, double-blind study of the effect of rGAA in patients with the late-onset form has shown improvement in walking and stabilization of respiratory function [65]. Due to the adverse and heterogeneous symptoms, treatment calls for interdisciplinary cooperation between different health specialities.

Differential diagnosis

In contrast to many of the other GSDs with static symptoms, hypoglycaemia has not been observed in GSD II. Furthermore, there is no enzymatic defect of the cytoplasmic breakdown of glycogen in GSD II. Infantile cases may be mistaken for mitochondrial disorders, spinal muscular atrophy, and congenital myasthenia and myopathy. In late-onset cases, differential diagnoses are limb-girdle muscular dystrophy, branching and debranching enzyme deficiencies, rigid spine syndrome (rare), and unexplained hyperCKaemia and respiratory insufficiency.

Debrancher deficiency

GSD III, also known as debrancher deficiency or Cori–Forbes disease, is caused by deficient activity of glycogen debranching enzyme (GDE) due to mutations in the *AGL* gene on chromosome 1p21. More than 20 different mutations have been identified in this gene [66]. Debranching enzyme is required for complete hydrolysis of glycogen, and GSD III is associated with an accumulation of abnormal glycogen with short outer chains [24]. Debranching enzyme is a bifunctional enzyme (4-α-D-glucanotransferase activity and amylo-α-1,6-glucosidase activity), that catalyses two reactions necessary for debranching of glycogen [24]. Four subtypes are described:

1. Type IIIa (the most common) that affects enzymes in the liver and the skeletal and cardiac muscle.

2. Type IIIb (about 15% of patients) involves only the liver enzyme.

3. Type IIIc (rare) with a selective loss of only one of the two GDE activities affecting muscle.

4. Type IIId (rare) with loss of the transferase, affecting muscle and liver [66].

Clinical features

Dominant features during infancy and childhood are hepatomegaly, hypoglycaemia, hyperlipidaemia, and growth retardation. Hepatic symptoms usually resolve after puberty [67]. Muscle weakness and wasting typically show in the third decade. Weakness can be both proximal and distal. Electromyography (EMG) and muscle biopsy show myopathic changes, and with large glycogen deposits in muscle [68]. Cardiomyopathy often develops, and can be asymptomatic or symptomatic, leading to early death.

Treatment

Treatment of debrancher deficiency is symptomatic, with emphasis on avoiding fasting in infants to prevent hypoglycaemia. Furthermore, patients should follow the national vaccination programme, and should be offered immunization for influenza to prevent illness and the subsequent risk of developing hypoglycaemia

[68]. Beta blockers should be used with caution due to their potential to mask symptoms of hypoglycaemia [68].

Differential diagnosis

Differential diagnosis of GSD III is extensive due to the broad spectrum of symptoms. The most common alternative diagnosis is GSD Ia (not described in this chapter); however, GSD III has similarities with several other GSDs, disorders of fructose metabolism, gluconeogenoses, primary liver diseases, and other metabolic disorders. For more detailed information on the distinguishing features the work by Kishnani et al. [68] is recommended.

Brancher deficiency (Andersen disease)

GSD IV (brancher deficiency) is caused by mutation in the glycogen branching enzyme 1 (*GBE*) gene. GBE catalyses the last step in glycogen synthesis by transferring the chains of glucose molecules with α-1,4-linked glucosyl units to the α-1,6-glucosidic links found in glycogen [24,69]. GSD IV causes accumulation of an abnormal glycogen known as polyglucosans, made of long chains of glucose units, which only infrequently branch [69].

Clinical features

GSD IV is a clinically heterogeneous disorder, characterized by three neuromuscular phenotypes and two hepatic forms (not described here):

1. The congenital form is further divided into two subgroups. (a) A severe perinatal form presenting with fetal akinesia deformation sequence (FADS) with multiple congenital contractures (arthrogryopsis multiplex congenita), and hydrops fetalis leading to perinatal death. (b) A severe congenital myopathy form inconsistently associated with cardiomyopathy, often simulating Werding–Hoffman disease.

2. A juvenile phenotype with myopathy, exercise intolerance, and cardiomyopathy.

3. An adult form presenting with isolated myopathy or as a multisystemic disorder with dysfunction of the central and peripheral nervous systems [69].

Aldolase deficiency

GSD XII is caused by deficiency in aldolase A enzyme activity. Aldolase A is a tetramer, composed of four identical subunits encoded by a single gene located on chromosome 16 [70].

Clinical features

Only one patient has been described, a 4½-year-old boy with predominantly myopathic symptoms of proximal muscle weakness and premature muscle fatigue. He had several episodes of jaundice and anaemia within the first year of life. Furthermore, hepatomegaly and splenomegaly occurred during febrile illness [70].

Lipid metabolism disorders in skeletal muscle

A disorder of lipid metabolism in skeletal muscle was first reported in 1969. DiMauro and DiMauro [71] identified the first enzyme defect of fatty acid oxidation (FAO), carnitine palmitoyltransferase (CPT) II deficiency, in a patient suffering from exercise-induced recurrent episodes of muscle pain, myoglobinuria, and renal failure [71]. Since then, more than 15 defects of mitochondrial FAO have been identified, involving almost all enzymatic steps of the β-oxidation pathway. Eight of these defects affect skeletal muscle, and are described in this chapter. All the disorders have an autosomal recessive inheritance.

At rest, and during prolonged, low-intensity exercise, energy supply, especially in skeletal muscle, heart, and liver, primarily relies on FAO of FFAs derived mainly from triglycerides stored in adipose tissue, and to a lesser extent from intracellular triglyceride lipid droplets in muscle cells [4]. Short and medium chain fatty acids cross freely into the mitochondrial matrix for oxidation. Long chain fatty acids require binding to carnitine in order to cross the inner mitochondrial membrane [3]. FAO is dependent on acyl-CoA dehydrogenases to cleave the chains of fatty acids before oxidation can occur. Failure in one of these processes, transport into the mitochondria, or defects in intramitochondrial dehydrogenases result in a disorder of lipid metabolism [3].

Disorders of lipid metabolism affecting skeletal muscle are characterized by two phenotypes: an infantile, severe form often, presenting with hypoketotic hypoglycaemia and hepatomegaly, and sometimes cardiac involvement; and an adult form, which can be characterized by either dynamic or static symptoms:

1. Dynamic; acute, recurrent episodes of rhabdomyolysis induced by exercise, fasting or infections [72]. In contrast to glycogenoses with dynamic symptoms, disorders of FAO typically present with symptoms later in exercise (>10–15 min) [72].

2. Static; a chronic myopathy with weakness and atrophy, usually characterized by an abnormal accumulation of lipid in muscle fibres.

Lipid metabolism disorders with dynamic symptoms

Carnitine palmitoyltransferase I deficiency
The mitochondrial CPTs are required to transport long chain fatty acids from the cytoplasm into the mitochondria for β-oxidation [73,74]. CPT I resides in the outer mitochondrial membrane and CPT II in the inner mitochondrial membrane. Mutation in the *CPT1* gene causes severe episodes of hypoketotic hypoglycaemia occurring after fasting or illness with onset in infancy or early childhood, but without prominent muscle symptoms [73,74].

Carnitine palmitoyltransferase II deficiency
CPT II deficiency is one of the most common inborn errors of FAO [1], impairing the transport of long chain fatty acids into the mitochondrial matrix [75]. The most common mutation is p.Ser113Leu [76]. The muscular form of the disease is always associated with some residual functional CPT II activity, whereas mutations which abolish enzyme activity are associated with the lethal early onset form. The functional CPT II molecule is a tetramer, and some carriers of single *CPT2* gene mutations may become symptomatic during exercise, perhaps due to a negative dominant effect of aberrant units on the wild-type CPT II molecule [77].

Clinical features
Mutations in the *CPT2* gene can result in three phenotypes: (1) a rare lethal neonatal form with seizures, hypoketotic hypoglycaemia, and hepatomegaly; (2) a life-threatening infantile form with hepato-cardio-muscular involvement; and (3) a more prevalent adult myopathic form, which is the most common cause of rhabdomyolysis and myoglobinuria [71,78]. Disease severity generally correlates with residual CPT II enzyme activity [78,79]. Symptoms are provoked by fasting, prolonged exercise, anxiety, shivering with cold, and febrile episodes [7]. In approximately 20% of the cases, attacks may occur without any apparent cause.

Paraclinical findings
During attacks, serum CK increases (20- to 400-fold) and the urinary excretion of myoglobin is elevated (>200 ng ml^{-1}). CK levels are typically normal between attacks. Plasma acylcarnitine profiling can be suggestive of the diagnosis, showing slightly elevated long chain acylcarnitines (C_{16}, $C_{18:1}$, C_{18}) (Fig. 29.4).

Treatment
To avoid symptoms, patients are recommended to follow a carbohydrate-rich diet, consisting mainly of polysaccharides [80]; mono- and disaccharides have no beneficial effect [81].

Differential diagnosis
Patients with CPT II deficiency have paroxysmal myoglobinuria associated with pain and stiffness without cramps, in contrast to patients with glycogenoses who develop muscle contractures. Furthermore, unlike patients with glycogenoses, patients with CPT II deficiency do not have a second wind and do not show reduced tolerance to short-term, strenuous exercise (Fig. 29.3).

Very long chain acyl-CoA dehydrogenase (VLCAD) deficiency
VLCAD was identified in 1992 as a key enzyme in mitochondrial long chain fatty acid β-oxidation [82]. VLCAD degrades very long chain fatty acids from food and fats stored in the body. Mutations in the *VLCAD* gene lead to reduced levels of VLCAD. Adult patients have enough residual enzyme activity to maintain basal FAO, but the reduced enzyme concentration causes impaired FAO during exercise, when symptoms are evoked [83].

Clinical features
Mutations in the *VLCAD* gene may cause three phenotypes: (1) a fatal infantile form presenting with hypertrophic cardiomyopathy, hepatocellular disease, and hypoketotic hypoglycaemia; (2) a childhood onset form with Reye-like disease and hypoketotic hypoglycaemia; and (3) an adult-onset myopathic form characterized by muscle pain, rhabdomyolysis, and myoglobinuria after prolonged exercise or fasting [84,85]. The first myopathic cases of VLCAD deficiency were published in 1993 [85,86], and more than 100 patients have since been reported.

Paraclinical findings
Plasma acylcarnitine profiling reveals an elevation of $C_{14:1}$, $C_{14:2}$ (Fig. 29.4). The elevation of $C_{14:1}$, $C_{14:2}$ persists even after the patients have fully recovered. Serum CK increases markedly during attacks (20- to 200-fold).

Treatment
Clinical experience suggests that patients should avoid prolonged periods of fasting and follow a carbohydrate-rich and low-LCFA diet. Oral supplementation with medium chain triglycerides (MCTs) may not be beneficial in mildly affected patients [81].

Differential diagnosis
Myalgia is more severe and episodes of rhabdomyolysis more numerous than in CPT II deficiency, which is the primary differential diagnosis.

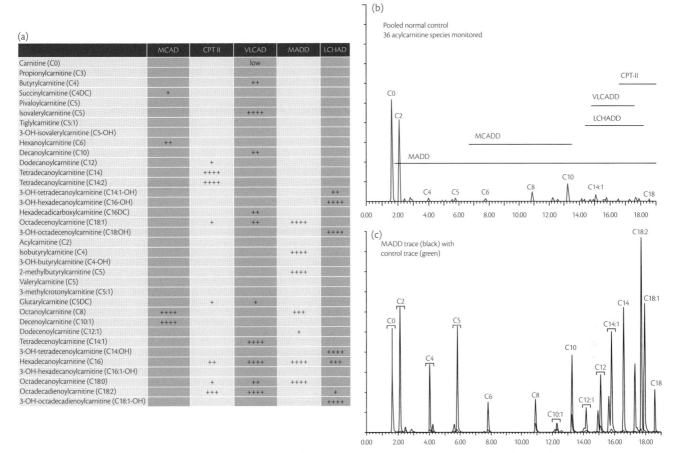

	MCAD	CPT II	VLCAD	MADD	LCHAD
Carnitine (C0)			low		
Propionylcarnitine (C3)					
Butyrylcarnitine (C4)			++		
Succinylcarnitine (C4DC)	+				
Pivaloylcarnitine (C5)					
Isovalerylcarnitine (C5)			++++		
Tiglylcarnitine (C5:1)					
3-OH-isovalerylcarnitine (C5-OH)					
Hexanoylcarnitine (C6)	++				
Decanoylcarnitine (C10)			++		
Dodecanoylcarnitine (C12)		+			
Tetradecanoylcarnitine (C14)		++++			
Tetradecanoylcarnitine (C14:2)		++++			
3-OH-tetradecanoylcarnitine (C14:1-OH)					++
3-OH-hexadecanoylcarnitine (C16-OH)					++++
Hexadecadicarboxylcarnitine (C16DC)			++		
Octadecenoylcarnitine (C18:1)		+	++	++++	
3-OH-octadecenoylcarnitine (C18:OH)					++++
Acylcarnitine (C2)					
Isobutyrylcarnitine (C4)				++++	
3-OH-butyrylcarnitine (C4-OH)					
2-methylbutyrylcarnitine (C5)				++++	
Valerylcarnitine (C5)					
3-methylcrotonylcarnitine (C5:1)					
Glutarylcarnitine (C5DC)		+	+		
Octanoylcarnitine (C8)	++++			+++	
Decenoylcarnitine (C10:1)	++++				
Dodecenoylcarnitine (C12:1)				+	
Tetradecenoylcarnitine (C14:1)			++++		
3-OH-tetradecenoylcarnitine (C14:OH)					++++
Hexadecanoylcarnitine (C16)		++	++++	+++	+++
3-OH-hexadecanoylcarnitine (C16:1-OH)					
Octadecanoylcarnitine (C18:0)		+	++	++++	
Octadecadienoylcarnitine (C18:2)		+++	++++		+
3-OH-octadecadienoylcarnitine (C18:1-OH)					++++

Fig. 29.4 (a) Diagnostic acylcarnitine patterns for the defects involving deficiencies of MAD (multiple acyl-CoA dehydrogenase), MCAD (medium chain acyl-CoA dehydrogenase), VLCAD (very long chain acyl-CoA dehydrogenase), LCHAD (long chain acyl-CoA dehydrogenase), CPT II (carnitine palmitoyl transferase II). More crosses indicate higher concentrations of acylcarnitines (b) Composite ion currents for 36 acylcarnitine species measured with tandem mass spectrometry in a patient with multiple acyl-CoA dehydrogenase deficiency (MADD) (black trace) and in a normal control pool (green trace). (c) Composite ion currents for 36 acylcarnitine species measured by tandem mass spectrometry in a normal control pool (green trace). Approximate elution ranges of diagnostic acylcarnitines for the myopathic fatty acid oxidation deficiencies are indicated with horizontal bars.

Acylcarnitine measurements and chromatograms were provided by courtesy by J. H. Olesen and the Metabolic Laboratory, Copenhagen University Hospital, Rigshospitalet, Denmark.

Medium chain acyl-CoA dehydrogenase (MCAD) deficiency

MCAD deficiency is the most common disorder of β-oxidation. It is an autosomal recessive disease caused by mutation in the *ACADM* gene with an incidence in northern Europe of 1 in 9000 to 1 in 10 000 [87]. The defect causes a defective breakdown of C_4 to C_{12} straight chain acyl-CoAs [88].

Clinical features

Two phenotypes are described:

1. A childhood form with episodes of encephalopathy due to accumulation of medium chain acyl-CoA intermediates inhibiting mitochondrial β-oxidation and inadequate ketone body synthesis, possibly complicated by hypoketotic hypoglycaemia as a late sign. Mortality is up to 25% [88].

2. An adolescent and adult form with broad phenotypic heterogeneity. Patients present acutely with organ involvement including neurological, muscular, hepatic, or cardiac symptoms [88].

Paraclinical findings

Patients with the adolescent and adult form present with metabolic decompensation, with metabolic acidosis, hyperammonaemia,

hyperlactacidaemia, and hypoglycaemia, and increased serum CK to 3000–4000 U L^{-1} [88]. The acylcarnitine profile shows increased (C_8, $C_{10:1}$) (Fig. 29.4).

Treatment

More than 10 years of screening has been shown to be beneficial in reducing the adverse events, including death. Avoidance of fasting periods and a high-carbohydrate diet are recommended [88].

Mitochondrial trifunctional protein (MTP) deficiency

Mitochondrial trifunctional protein (MTP) is a hetero-octamer composed of four α and four β subunits that catalyse the last three steps in the mitochondrial β-oxidation of (1) long chain 3-hydroxyacyl-CoA dehydrogenase (LCHAD); (2) long chain enoyl-CoA hydrates; and (3) long chain thiolase. MTP deficiency is caused by mutations in either the α subunit (*HADHA*) or the β subunit (*HADHB*) and is characterized by decreased activity of all three enzymes [89].

Classic trifunctional protein deficiency

Three clinical phenotypes are described: (1) a severe, lethal neonatal form; (2) infantile onset of a hepatic, Reye-like syndrome; and (3) a late-onset, adult myopathic form [90].

Long chain 3-hydroxy/acyl-CoA dehydrogenase (LCHAD) deficiency

Isolated LCHAD deficiency is often associated with the common α-subunit mutation Glu510Gln. This results in a mutant protein which confers a significantly reduced LCHAD activity; however, the activity of the two other enzymes in the MTP complex remains >60% of normal [89]. No apparent genotype–phenotype correlation has been observed, as patients homozygous for this mutation show widely different phenotypes [89]. LCHAD deficiency appears to be a relatively common β-oxidation defect (1 in 50 000 births in northern Europe).

Clinical features

In childhood, LCHAD deficiency is characterized by early onset cardiomyopathy, hypoglycaemia, neuropathy, and pigmentary retinopathy. Mortality is high (approximately 50%). However, patients who survive acute episodes of cardiomyopathy tend to resolve with dietary therapeutic measures [89].

Treatment

Avoidance of fasting periods and a diet high in carbohydrates and low in long chain fatty acids with oral MCT oil supplementation is recommended [91]. Cod liver oil extract high in docosahexaenoic acid (DHA) has shown positive effect upon visual function in patients with LCHAD deficiency [92] and on neuropathy in one patient with LCHAD deficiency [93].

Differential diagnosis

Progressive pigmentary retinopathy and peripheral neuropathy are not observed in any of the other β-oxidation defects. Acylcarntine profiling shows increase in ($C_{14\text{-OH}}$, $C_{14:1\text{-OH}}$, $C_{16\text{-OH}}$, $C_{16:1\text{-OH}}$, $C_{18\text{-OH}}$, $C_{18:1\text{-OH}}$) (Fig. 29.4).

Lipid metabolism disorders with static symptoms

Primary carnitine deficiency

Primary carnitine deficiency (PCD), also called carnitine transporter deficiency, is an autosomal recessive disorder caused by mutations in the *SLC22A5* gene. Several mutations have been reported. The mutations lead to absent sodium-dependent carnitine transporter (OCTN2) activity (premature stop codons) or variable, residual OCTN2 enzyme activity of carnitine transport. Carnitine is involved in the transport of long chain fatty acids from the cytoplasm to the mitochondrial matrix for β-oxidation. Defects of the carnitine transporter therefore result in the accumulation of long chain fatty acids and triglycerides, seen as lipid droplets. Disease frequency is 1 in 37 000 to 1 in 100 000 [94].

Clinical features

Three phenotypes are described: (1) an infantile form with hypotonia, Reye-like syndrome, and cardiomyopathy; (2) an isolated cardiomyopathy ranging from mild to lethal metabolic decompensation; and (3) a myopathic form ranging from asymptomatic to mild with muscle weakness. Some patients who have been asymptomatic for their whole life may be identified because of their affected children or siblings [95,96].

Paraclinical findings

Plasma free carnitine and acylcarnitine species are extremely low. Muscle pathology is characterized by the accumulation of lipid droplets.

Treatment

Patients respond very well to high-dose L-carnitine supplementation (100–400 mg kg^{-1} day^{-1}). Early treatment before irreversible organ damage has occurred may prevent the need for cardiac transplantation. Furthermore, hypoglycaemic episodes tend to disappear with age [94].

Multiple acyl-CoA dehydrogenase deficiency

Multiple acyl-CoA dehydrogenase deficiency (MADD), also known as glutaric aciduris Type II, is caused by defects in electron transfer flavoprotein (ETF) or ETF dehydrogenase (ETFDH), also called ETF-ubiquinone oxidoreductase. ETF transfers high-energy electrons from the mitochondrial matrix to the respiratory chain. ETFDH is located in the inner mitochondrial membrane and passes electrons to ubiquinone in the respiratory chain. Riboflavin (vitamin B$_2$) is the precursor of the coenzyme flavin adenine dinucleotide (FAD). Five flavin-containing enzymes play an essential role in energy metabolism in mitochondria. One is the flavin-linked EFT. Other enzymes involved are the acyl-CoA dehydrogenases (SCAD, MCAD, LCAD, VLCAD, and ACAD9), which are important in the first dehydrogenation reaction in β-oxidation [24] Therefore, MADD is characterized by impaired oxidation of fatty acids due to multiple deficiencies of SCAD, MCAD, LCAD, and VLCAD. Mutations in the *ETFA* and *ETFB* genes, encoding the α and β subunits of ETF, tend to cause neonatal forms. Mutation in the *ETFDH* gene causes the later-onset form [97].

Clinical features

The clinical phenotypes are heterogeneous and are classified as neonatal-onset forms with or without congenital anomalies, often resulting in early death. A milder late-onset form with proximal myopathy often presents with hepatomegaly, encephalopathy, episodic lethargy, vomiting, and hypoglycaemia, which can be lethal [97].

Paraclinical findings

Muscle pathology is characterized by the accumulation of lipid droplets. Plasma acylcarnitine profiling reveals elevated acylcarnitines (Fig. 29.4), especially medium and long chain species (C_4–C_{18}).

Treatment

Riboflavin supplementation (100–400 mg day^{-1}) improves clinical symptoms in some patients [98].

Neutral lipid storage disease/Chanarian–Dorfman syndrome

Neutral lipid storage disease is caused by mutations in the genes for CGI58 or PNPLA2. Mutations in the gene coding for CGI58 (*ABHD5*) are responsible for a paediatric disease, neutral lipid storage disease with ichthyosis (NLDSI), also called Chanarin–Dorfman syndrome [99–101]. Mutation in the pastatin-like phospholipase domain-containing protein 2 (*PNPLA2*) gene causes skeletal and cardiac muscle disease only [102]. PNPLA2 is also known as adipose triglyceride lipase (ATGL) or desnutrin. PNPLA2 specifically catalyses the first step in the hydrolysis of triacylglycerol (TAG), generating FFAs and diacylglycerol. This enzyme requires the activator protein CGI58 (a protein of the esterase/lipase/thioesterase subfamily) located on the surface of cytoplasmic lipid droplets. A defect in this pathway leads to intracellular accumulation of TAGs that affects energy metabolism [103].

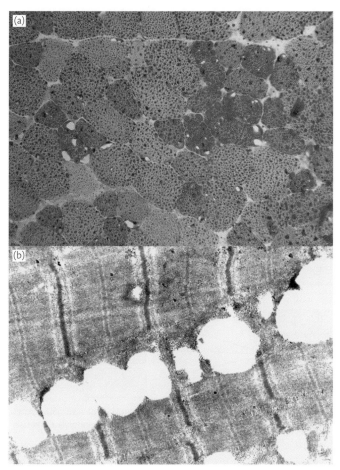

Fig. 29.5 Massive lipid accumulation is observed in skeletal muscle of a patient with neutral lipid storage disease myopathy (NLSDM) with optic oil red O (a) and electronic microscopy (b).

Reprinted from Neuromuscular Disorders, 20, Pascal Laforêt, Christine Vianey-Saban, Disorders of muscle lipid metabolism: Diagnostic and therapeutic challenges, 693–700, Copyright (2010), with permission from Elsevier. Histological and electron microscopy photos were provided by courtesy of Drs P. Laforêt[1], B. Eymard[1], and N. B. Romero[2] ([1]Centre de Référence de Pathologie Neuromusculaire Paris-Est, Groupe Hospitalier Pitié-Salpêtrière, Assistance Publique-Hôpitaux de Paris, Paris, France, [2]Département de Neurologie, Hôpitaux Universitaires, Strasbourg, France). (See also figure in colour plate section)

Clinical features

Patients may present initially with walking delay and exercise intolerance during childhood, but they generally exhibit a slowly progressive muscle weakness in the proximal and distal limb muscles starting between the second and third decades. Furthermore, some patients develop dilated cardiomyopathy leading to heart failure and severe arrhythmia.

Paraclinical findings

Muscle biopsy shows a massive lipidosis (Fig. 29.5), and neutral lipid storage diseases share the diagnostic hallmark of TAG-containing lipid vacuoles in leucocytes observed in peripheral blood smear, called the Jordan anomaly.

Paraclinical investigations

Glycogenoses

When it comes to glycogenoses, one of the most used diagnostic tests is the ischaemic forearm handgrip exercise test that evaluates muscle production of lactate and ammonia [104]. In recent years, the ischaemic model has been replaced by an aerobic forearm test that is equally as diagnostic as the ischaemic test but with much less discomfort to the patient and less chance of rhabdomyolysis [104]. In the glycogenoses with no residual enzyme, such as McArdle disease and PFK deficiency, the exercise-induced lactate response is absent due to the blocked glycogenolysis (in fact there is a small decrease in lactate due to the CK reaction), and ammonia production is increased more than fourfold as a result of a lack of energy from ATP (Figs 29.6 and 29.7) [104].

The exercise-induced lactate response is blunted or normal and ammonia production is increased in the partial enzymatic defects of muscle glycogenolysis/glycolysis such as deficiencies of PHK, PGM, LDH, PGK, PGAM, and debrancher deficiency (Figs 29.6 and 29.7).

Cycling exercise tests are only useful in patients with McArdle disease and PFK deficiency, in whom the cycling test can be used to distinguish between the two disorders: patients with McArdle disease and those with PFK deficiency have an absent lactate response to exercise, but only patients with McArdle disease develop a second wind, which has never been observed in PFK; also patients with McArdle disease benefit from oral glucose supplementation, whereas oral glucose worsens exercise capacity in patients with PFK deficiency [28].

^{31}P-magentic resonance spectroscopy (MRS) can be used to distinguish between McArdle disease, PFK deficiency, and the partial glycogenolytic defects: patients with McArdle disease have lack of muscle acidification and no accumulation of phosphomonoesters. Patients with PFK deficiency have a combined lack of acidification and phosphomonoesters are present. Patients with partial defects are characterized by normal acidification and the presence of phosphomonoesters. However, phosphorus MRS is expensive, time-consuming, and not readily available, and should not be considered a routine test in the evaluation of metabolic myopathies.

Lipid metabolism disorders in skeletal muscle

Plasma acylcarnitine profiling provides a quantitative evaluation of carnitine and individual acylcarnitine species. The test is cheap, provides rapid results, and should always be the first diagnostic test performed when a diagnosis of a lipid disorder is suspected (Fig. 29.6). Acylcarntine profiling is more informative after provocation with exercise or fasting (the most common procedure is to take a blood sample after an overnight fast), and can help to identify fatty acid oxidation defects such as VLCAD deficiency, where $C_{14:1}$ and $C_{14:2}$ are elevated, CPT II deficiency, where long chain acylcarnitines C_{16} and $C_{18:1}$ are (slightly) elevated, MCAD deficiency, where plasma levels of C_6, C_8, and $C_{10:1}$ are elevated, MTP and LCHAD deficiency, where 3-hydroxylated long chain acylcarnitines are elevated ($C_{14\text{-OH}}$, $C_{14:1\text{-OH}}$, $C_{16\text{-OH}}$, $C_{16:1\text{-OH}}$, $C_{18\text{-OH}}$, $C_{18:1\text{-OH}}$), and MADD where especially medium and long chain acylcarnitines are elevated (C_4–C_{18}) (Fig. 29.4). Acylcarnitine profiling is now used in the screening of several β-oxidation defects to identify and treat the neonatal forms before the onset of symptoms. Abnormal acylcarnitine profiles, although often highly suggestive of a specific disorder of lipid metabolism, should always be followed up by determination of specific enzyme activities in cultured fibroblasts, muscle tissue, or leucocytes, and/or confirmed by genetic testing if possible.

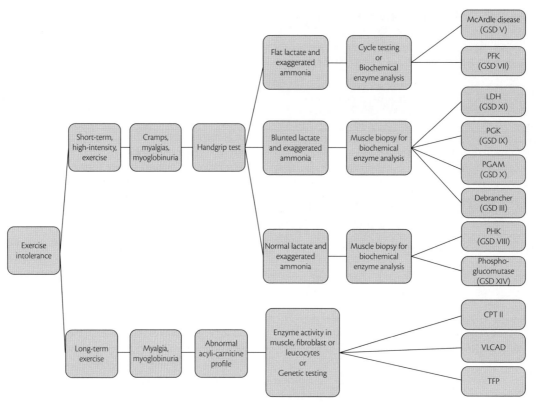

Fig. 29.6 Diagnostic flowchart for patients with exercise intolerance under suspicion of having a metabolic myopathy. CPT, carnitine palmitoyl transferase; GSD, glycogen storage disease; LDH, lactate dehydrogenase; PFK, phosphofructokinase; PGAM, phosphoglycerate mutase; PGK, phosphoglycerate kinase; PHK, phosphorylase b kinase; TFP, trifunctional protein deficiency; VLCAD, very long chain acyl-coenzyme A dehydrogenase.

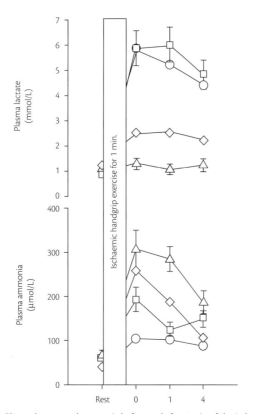

Fig. 29.7 Plasma lactate and ammonia before and after 1 min of the ischaemic forearm exercise test in seven patients with McArdle disease (Δ), one patient with phosphofructokinase deficiency (◊), one patient with phosphorylase b kinase deficiency (□), and nine healthy controls (○).

References

1. Haller RG, Lewis SF, Cook JD, Blomqvist CG. Myophosphorylase deficiency impairs muscle oxidative metabolism. *Ann Neurol* 1985; **17**: 196–9.
2. Sveen ML, Schwartz M, Vissing J. High prevalence and phenotype-genotype correlations of limb girdle muscular dystrophy type 2I in Denmark. *Ann Neurol* 2006; **59**: 808–15.
3. Romijn JA, Coyle EF, Sidossis LS, et al. Regulation of endogenous fat and carbohydrate metabolism in relation to exercise intensity and duration. *Am J Physiol* 1993; **265**: E380–E391.
4. van Loon LJ, Greenhaff PL, Constantin-Teodosiu D, Saris WH, Wagenmakers AJ. The effects of increasing exercise intensity on muscle fuel utilisation in humans. *J Physiol* 2001; **536**: 295–304.
5. Tein I. Metabolic myopathies. *Semin Pediatr Neurol* 1996; **3**: 59–98.
6. Felig P, Wahren J. Fuel homeostasis in exercise. *N Engl J Med* 1975; **293**: 1078–84.
7. Lithell H, Hellsing K, Lundqvist G, Malmberg P. Lipoprotein-lipase activity of human skeletal-muscle and adipose tissue after intensive physical exercise. *Acta Physiol Scand* 1979; **105**: 312–15.
8. Lithell H, Orlander J, Schele R, Sjodin B, Karlsson J. Changes in lipoprotein-lipase activity and lipid stores in human skeletal muscle with prolonged heavy exercise. *Acta Physiol Scand* 1979; **107**: 257–61.
9. McArdle B. Myopathy due to a defect in muscle glycogen breakdown. *Clin Sci* 1951; **10**: 13–33.
10. Mommaerts WF, Illingworth B, Pearson CM, Guillory RJ, Seraydarian K. A Functional disorder of muscle associated with the absence of phosphorylase. *Proc Natl Acad Sci USA* 1959; **45**: 791–7.
11. Schmid R, Mahler R. Chronic progressive myopathy with myoglobinuria: demonstration of a glycogenolytic defect in the muscle. *J Clin Invest* 1959; **38**: 2044–58.
12. Stojkovic T, Vissing J, Petit F, et al. Muscle glycogenosis due to phosphoglucomutase 1 deficiency. *N Engl J Med* 2009; **361**: 425–7.

13. Lewis SF, Haller RG. The pathophysiology of McArdle's disease: clues to regulation in exercise and fatigue. *J Appl Physiol* 1986; **61**: 391–401.

14. Burke J, Hwang P, Anderson L, Lebo R, Gorin F, Fletterick R. Intron/exon structure of the human gene for the muscle isozyme of glycogen phosphorylase. *Proteins* 1987; **2**: 177–87.

15. Bartram C, Edwards RH, Clague J, Beynon RJ. McArdle's disease: a nonsense mutation in exon 1 of the muscle glycogen phosphorylase gene explains some but not all cases. *Hum Mol Genet* 1993; **2**: 1291–3.

16. DiMauro S, Servidei S, Tsujino S, Disorders of carbohydrate metabolism: glycogen storage diseases. In: Rosenberg RN, Prusiner SB, Di Mauro S, Barchi RL (ed) *The Molecular and Genetic Basis of Neurological Disease*, 2nd edn, pp. 1067–97. Boston, MA: Butterworth-Heinemann, 1997.

17. Quinlivan R, Buckley J, James M, et al. McArdle disease: a clinical review. *J Neurol Neurosurg Psychiatry* 2010; **81**: 1182–8.

18. Pearson CM, Rimer DG, Mommaerts WF. A metabolic myopathy due to absence of muscle phosphorylase. *Am J Med* 1961; **30**: 502–17.

19. Nadaj-Pakleza AA, Vincitorio CM, Laforet P, et al. Permanent muscle weakness in McArdle disease. *Muscle Nerve* 2009; **40**: 350–7.

20. Andersen ST, Haller RG, Vissing J. Effect of oral sucrose shortly before exercise on work capacity in McArdle disease. *Arch Neurol* 2008; **65**: 786–9.

21. Andersen ST, Vissing J. Carbohydrate- and protein-rich diets in McArdle disease: effects on exercise capacity. *J Neurol Neurosurg Psychiatry* 2008; **79**: 1359–63.

22. Vissing J, Haller RG. The effect of oral sucrose on exercise tolerance in patients with McArdle's disease. *N Engl J Med* 2003; **349**: 2503–09.

23. Haller RG, Wyrick P, Taivassalo T, Vissing J. Aerobic conditioning: an effective therapy in McArdle's disease. *Ann Neurol* 2006; **59**: 922–8.

24. Harris RA, Devlin TM. *Textbook of Biochemistry with Clinical Correlations*. New York: Wiley-Liss, 1997.

25. Vora S, Corash L, Engel WK, Durham S, Seaman C, Piomelli S. The molecular mechanism of the inherited phosphofructokinase deficiency associated with hemolysis and myopathy. *Blood* 1980; **55**: 629–35.

26. Raben N, Sherman JB. Mutations in muscle phosphofructokinase gene. *Hum Mutat* 1995; **6**: 1–6.

27. Layzer RB, Rowland LP, Bank WJ. Physical and kinetic properties of human phosphofructokinase from skeletal muscle and erythrocytes. *J Biol Chem* 1969; **244**: 3823–31.

28. Haller RG, Lewis SF. Glucose-induced exertional fatigue in muscle phosphofructokinase deficiency. *N Engl J Med* 1991; **324**: 364–9.

29. Haller RG, Vissing J. No spontaneous second wind in muscle phosphofructokinase deficiency. *Neurology* 2004; **62**: 82–6.

30. Preisler N, Orngreen MC, Echaniz-Laguna A, et al. Muscle phosphorylase kinase deficiency: a neutral metabolic variant or a disease? *Neurology* 2012; **78**: 265–8.

31. Chen YT, Burchell A. Glycogen storage diseases. In: Scriver CR, Beaudet AL, Sly WS, Valle D (Vol. 1) *The Metabolic and Molecular Basis of Inherited Disease*, pp. 935–66. New York: McGraw Hill, 2007.

32. Calalb MB, Fox DT, Hanks SK. Molecular cloning and enzymatic analysis of the rat homolog of 'PhK-gamma T', an isoform of phosphorylase kinase catalytic subunit. *J Biol Chem* 1992; **267**: 1455–63.

33. Davidson JJ, Ozcelik T, Hamacher C, Willems PJ, Francke U, Kilimann MW. cDNA cloning of a liver isoform of the phosphorylase kinase alpha subunit and mapping of the gene to Xp22.2-p22.1, the region of human X-linked liver glycogenosis. *Proc Natl Acad Sci USA* 1992; **89**: 2096–100.

34. Francke U, Darras BT, Zander NF, Kilimann MW. Assignment of human genes for phosphorylase kinase subunits alpha (PHKA) to Xq12-q13 and beta (PHKB) to 16q12-q13. *Am J Hum Genet* 1989; **45**: 276–82.

35. Bruno C, Manfredi G, Andreu AL, et al. A splice junction mutation in the alpha(M) gene of phosphorylase kinase in a patient with myopathy. *Biochem Biophys Res Commun* 1998; **249**: 648–51.

36. Burwinkel B, Hu B, Schroers A, et al. Muscle glycogenosis with low phosphorylase kinase activity: mutations in PHKA1, PHKG1 or six other candidate genes explain only a minority of cases. *Eur J Hum Genet* 2003; **11**: 516–26.

37. Wehner M, Clemens PR, Engel AG, Kilimann MW. Human muscle glycogenosis due to phosphorylase kinase deficiency associated with a nonsense mutation in the muscle isoform of the alpha subunit. *Hum Mol Genet* 1994; **3**: 1983–7.

38. Wuyts W, Reyniers E, Ceuterick C, Storm K, de BT, Martin JJ. Myopathy and phosphorylase kinase deficiency caused by a mutation in the PHKA1 gene. *Am J Med Genet A* 2005; **133**: 82–4.

39. Orngreen MC, Schelhaas HJ, Jeppesen TD, et al. Is muscle glycogenolysis impaired in X-linked phosphorylase b kinase deficiency? *Neurology* 2008; **70**: 1876–82.

40. DiMauro S, Dalakas M, Miranda AF. Phosphoglycerate kinase deficiency: a new cause of recurrent myoglobinuria. *Trans Am Neurol Assoc* 1981; **106**: 202–5.

41. Yoshida A, Watanabe S, Chen SH, Giblet ER, Malcolm LA. Human phosphoglycerate kinase. II. Structure of a variant enzyme. *J Biol Chem* 1972; **247**: 446–9.

42. Yoshida A, Watanabe S. Human phosphoglycerate kinase. I. Crystallization and characterization of normal enzyme. *J Biol Chem* 1972; **247**: 440–5.

43. Rosa R, George C, Fardeau M, Calvin MC, Rapin M, Rosa J. A new case of phosphoglycerate kinase deficiency: PGK Creteil associated with rhabdomyolysis and lacking hemolytic anemia. *Blood* 1982; **60**: 84–91.

44. DiMauro S, Dalakas M, Miranda AF. Phosphoglycerate kinase deficiency: another cause of recurrent myoglobinuria. *Ann Neurol* 1983; **13**: 11–19.

45. Sugie H, Sugie Y, Nishida M, et al. Recurrent myoglobinuria in a child with mental retardation: phosphoglycerate kinase deficiency. *J Child Neurol* 1989; **4**: 95–9.

46. Ookawara T, Dave V, Willems P, et al. Retarded and aberrant splicings caused by single exon mutation in a phosphoglycerate kinase variant. *Arch Biochem Biophys* 1996; **327**: 35–40.

47. Hamano T, Mutoh T, Sugie H, Koga H, Kuriyama M. Phosphoglycerate kinase deficiency: an adult myopathic form with a novel mutation. *Neurology* 2000; **54**: 1188–90.

48. Spanu C, Oltean S. Familial phosphoglycerate kinase deficiency associated with rhabdomyolysis and acute renal failure: abnormality in mRNA splicing? *Nephrol Dialysis Transplant* 2003; **18**: 445–6.

49. Shirakawa K, Takahashi Y, Miyajima H. Intronic mutation in the PGK1 gene may cause recurrent myoglobinuria by aberrant splicing. *Neurology* 2006; **66**: 925–7.

50. Naini A, Toscano A, Musumeci O, Vissing J, Akman HO, DiMauro S. Muscle phosphoglycerate mutase deficiency revisited. *Arch Neurol* 2009; **66**: 394–8.

51. DiMauro S, Miranda AF, Khan S, Gitlin K, Friedman R. Human muscle phosphoglycerate mutase deficiency: newly discovered metabolic myopathy. *Science* 1981; **212**: 1277–9.

52. Bresolin N, Ro YI, Reyes M, Miranda AF, DiMauro S. Muscle phosphoglycerate mutase (PGAM) deficiency: a second case. *Neurology* 1983; **33**: 1049–53.

53. Tsujino S, Shanske S, Sakoda S, Fenichel G, DiMauro S. The molecular genetic basis of muscle phosphoglycerate mutase (PGAM) deficiency. *Am J Hum Genet* 1993; **52**: 472–7.

54. Kanno T, Sudo K, Takeuchi I, et al. Hereditary deficiency of lactate dehydrogenase M-subunit. *Clin Chim Acta* 1980; **108**: 267–76.

55. Preisler N, Orngreen MC, Laforet P, et al. No second wind phenomenon, but glucose improves exercise capacity in phosphoglucomutase deficiency. *Neuromuscul Disord* 2011; **21**: 738.

56. Comi GP, Fortunato F, Lucchiari S, et al. Beta-enolase deficiency, a new metabolic myopathy of distal glycolysis. *Ann Neurol* 2001; **50**: 202–7.

57. Shulman GI, Rothman DL, Jue T, Stein P, DeFronzo RA, Shulman RG. Quantitation of muscle glycogen synthesis in normal subjects and

subjects with non-insulin-dependent diabetes by 13C nuclear magnetic resonance spectroscopy. *N Engl J Med* 1990; **322**: 223–8.

58. Kollberg G, Tulinius M, Gilljam T, et al. Cardiomyopathy and exercise intolerance in muscle glycogen storage disease 0. *N Engl J Med* 2007; **357**: 1507–14.

59. Cameron JM, Levandovskiy V, MacKay N, et al. Identification of a novel mutation in GYS1 (muscle-specific glycogen synthase) resulting in sudden cardiac death, that is diagnosable from skin fibroblasts. *Mol Genet Metab* 2009; **98**: 378–82.

60. Sukigara S, Liang WC, Komaki H, et al. Muscle glycogen storage disease 0 presenting recurrent syncope with weakness and myalgia. *Neuromuscl Disord* 2012; **22**: 162–5.

61. Bembi B, Cerini E, Danesino C, et al. Diagnosis of glycogenosis type II. *Neurology* 2008; **71** (Suppl 2): S4–S11.

62. van den Hout HM, Hop W, van Diggelen OP, et al. The natural course of infantile Pompe's disease: 20 original cases compared with 133 cases from the literature. *Pediatrics* 2003; **112**: 332–40.

63. Slonim AE, Bulone L, Ritz S, Goldberg T, Chen A, Martiniuk F. Identification of two subtypes of infantile acid maltase deficiency. *J Pediatr* 2000; **137**: 283–5.

64. Beratis NG, LaBadie GU, Hirschhorn K. Characterization of the molecular defect in infantile and adult acid alpha-glucosidase deficiency fibroblasts. *J Clin Invest* 1978; **62**: 1264–74.

65. Angelini C, Semplicini C, Tonin P, et al. Progress in enzyme replacement therapy in glycogen storage disease type II. *Ther Adv Neurol Disord* 2009; **2**: 143–53.

66. Shen J, Bao Y, Liu HM, Lee P, Leonard JV, Chen YT. Mutations in exon 3 of the glycogen debranching enzyme gene are associated with glycogen storage disease type III that is differentially expressed in liver and muscle. *J Clin Invest* 1996; **98**: 352–7.

67. Coleman RA, Winter HS, Wolf B, Gilchrist JM, Chen YT. Glycogen storage disease type III (glycogen debranching enzyme deficiency): correlation of biochemical defects with myopathy and cardiomyopathy. *Ann Intern Med* 1992; **116**: 896–900.

68. Kishnani PS, Austin SL, Arn P, et al. Glycogen storage disease type III diagnosis and management guidelines. *Genet Med* 2010; **12**: 446–63.

69. Bruno C, Cassandrini D, Assereto S, Akman HO, Minetti C, Di Mauro S. Neuromuscular forms of glycogen branching enzyme deficiency. *Acta Myol* 2007; **26**: 75–8.

70. Kreuder J, Borkhardt A, Repp R, et al. Brief report: inherited metabolic myopathy and hemolysis due to a mutation in aldolase A. *N Engl J Med* 1996; **334**: 1100–4.

71. DiMauro S, DiMauro PM. Muscle carnitine palmityltransferase deficiency and myoglobinuria. *Science* 1973; **182**: 929–31.

72. Bruno C, Dimauro S. Lipid storage myopathies. *Curr Opin Neurol* 2008; **21**: 601–6.

73. Bonnefont JP, Djouadi F, Prip-Buus C, Gobin S, Munnich A, Bastin J. Carnitine palmitoyltransferases 1 and 2: biochemical, molecular and medical aspects. *Mol Aspects Med* 2004; **25**: 495–520.

74. Saudubray JM, Martin D, de Lonlay P, et al. Recognition and management of fatty acid oxidation defects: a series of 107 patients. *J Inherit Metab Dis* 1999; **22**: 488–502.

75. Bieber LL. Carnitine. *Annu Rev Biochem* 1988; **57**: 261–83.

76. Bonnefont JP, Demaugre F, Prip-Buus C, et al. Carnitine palmitoyltransferase deficiencies. *Mol Genet Metab* 1999; **68**: 424–40.

77. Orngreen MC, Duno M, Ejstrup R, et al. Fuel utilization in subjects with carnitine palmitoyltransferase 2 gene mutations. *Ann Neurol* 2005; **57**: 60–6.

78. Demaugre F, Bonnefont JP, Colonna M, Cepanec C, Leroux JP, Saudubray JM. Infantile form of carnitine palmitoyltransferase II deficiency with hepatomuscular symptoms and sudden death. Physiopathological approach to carnitine palmitoyltransferase II deficiencies. *J Clin Invest* 1991; **87**: 859–64.

79. Bonnefont JP, Taroni F, Cavadini P, et al. Molecular analysis of carnitine palmitoyltransferase II deficiency with hepatocardiomuscular expression. *Am J Hum Genet* 1996; **58**: 971–8.

80. Orngreen MC, Ejstrup R, Vissing J. Effect of diet on exercise tolerance in carnitine palmitoyltransferase II deficiency. *Neurology* 2003; **61**: 559–61.

81. Orngreen MC, Norgaard MG, van Engelen BG, Vistisen B, Vissing J. Effects of IV glucose and oral medium-chain triglyceride in patients with VLCAD deficiency. *Neurology* 2007; **69**: 313–15.

82. Izai K, Uchida Y, Orii T, Yamamoto S, Hashimoto T. Novel fatty acid beta-oxidation enzymes in rat liver mitochondria. I. Purification and properties of very-long-chain acyl-coenzyme A dehydrogenase. *J Biol Chem* 1992; **267**: 1027–33.

83. Orngreen MC, Norgaard MG, Sacchetti M, van Engelen BG, Vissing J. Fuel utilization in patients with very long-chain acyl-coa dehydrogenase deficiency. *Ann Neurol* 2004; **56**: 279–83.

84. Minetti C, Garavaglia B, Bado M, et al. Very-long-chain acyl-coenzyme A dehydrogenase deficiency in a child with recurrent myoglobinuria. *Neuromuscl Disord* 1998; **8**: 3–6.

85. Straussberg R, Harel L, Varsano I, Elpeleg ON, Shamir R, Amir J. Recurrent myoglobinuria as a presenting manifestation of very long chain acyl coenzyme A dehydrogenase deficiency. *Pediatrics* 1997; **99**: 894–6.

86. Aoyama T, Uchida Y, Kelley RI, et al. A novel disease with deficiency of mitochondrial very-long-chain acyl-CoA dehydrogenase. *Biochem Biophys Res Commun* 1993; **191**: 1369–72.

87. Grosse SD, Khoury MJ, Greene CL, Crider KS, Pollitt RJ. The epidemiology of medium chain acyl-CoA dehydrogenase deficiency: an update. *Genet Med* 2006; **8**: 205–12.

88. Schatz UA, Ensenauer R. The clinical manifestation of MCAD deficiency: challenges towards adulthood in the screened population. *J Inherit Metab Dis* 2010; **33**: 513–20.

89. Olpin SE, Clark S, Andresen BS, et al. Biochemical, clinical and molecular findings in LCHAD and general mitochondrial trifunctional protein deficiency. *J Inherit Metab Dis* 2005; **28**: 533–44.

90. Spiekerkoetter U, Sun B, Khuchua Z, Bennett MJ, Strauss AW. Molecular and phenotypic heterogeneity in mitochondrial trifunctional protein deficiency due to beta-subunit mutations. *Hum Mutat* 2003; **21**: 598–607.

91. Gillingham MB, Scott B, Elliott D, Harding CO. Metabolic control during exercise with and without medium-chain triglycerides (MCT) in children with long-chain 3-hydroxy acyl-CoA dehydrogenase (LCHAD) or trifunctional protein (TFP) deficiency. *Mol Genet Metab* 2006; **89**: 58–63.

92. Harding CO, Gillingham MB, van Calcar SC, Wolff JA, Verhoeve JN, Mills MD. Docosahexaenoic acid and retinal function in children with long-chain 3-hydroxyacyl-CoA dehydrogenase deficiency. *J Inherit Metab Dis* 1999; **22**: 276–80.

93. Tein I, Vajsar J, MacMillan L, Sherwood WG. Long-chain L-3-hydroxyacyl-coenzyme A dehydrogenase deficiency neuropathy: response to cod liver oil. *Neurology* 1999; **52**: 640–3.

94. Longo N, Amat di San Filippo C, Pasquali M. Disorders of carnitine transport and the carnitine cycle. *Am J Med Genet C* 2006; **142C**: 77–85.

95. Wang Y, Korman SH, Ye J, et al. Phenotype and genotype variation in primary carnitine deficiency. *Genet Med* 2001; **3**: 387–92.

96. El-Hattab AW, Li FY, Shen J, et al. Maternal systemic primary carnitine deficiency uncovered by newborn screening: clinical, biochemical, and molecular aspects. *Genet Med* 2010; **12**: 19–24.

97. Antozzi C, Garavaglia B, Mora M, et al. Late-onset riboflavin-responsive myopathy with combined multiple acyl coenzyme A dehydrogenase and respiratory chain deficiency. *Neurology* 1994; **44**: 2153–8.

98. DiDonato S, Taroni, F. *Disorders of Lipid Metabolism*. New York: McGraw-Hill, 2004.

99. Dorfman ML, Hershko C, Eisenberg S, Sagher F. Ichthyosiform dermatosis with systemic lipidosis. *Arch Dermatol* 1974; **110**: 261–6.

100. Chanarin I, Patel A, Slavin G, Wills EJ, Andrews TM, Stewart G. Neutral-lipid storage disease: a new disorder of lipid metabolism. *Br Med J* 1975; **1**(5957): 553–5.

101. Yamaguchi T, Osumi T. Chanarin-Dorfman syndrome: deficiency in CGI-58, a lipid droplet-bound coactivator of lipase. *Biochim Biophys Acta* 2009; **1791**: 519–23.

102. Fischer J, Lefevre C, Morava E, et al. The gene encoding adipose triglyceride lipase (PNPLA2) is mutated in neutral lipid storage disease with myopathy. *Nat Genet* 2007; **39**: 28–30.

103. Laforêt P, Ørngreen M, Preisler N, Andersen G, Vissing J. Muscle fat oxidation is blocked during exercise in neutral lipid storage disease. *Arch Neurol* 2012; **69**: 530–3.

104. Kazemi-Esfarjani P, Skomorowska E, Jensen TD, Haller RG, Vissing J. A nonischemic forearm exercise test for McArdle disease. *Ann Neurol* 2002; **52**: 153–9.

CHAPTER 30

Mitochondrial cytopathies

Gerald Pfeffer and Patrick F. Chinnery

Introduction

Mitochondrial cytopathies (also known as mitochondrial disorders or mitochondrial syndromes) are disorders resulting from primary dysfunction of the mitochondrial respiratory chain. Several important characteristics of mitochondria are important for understanding the pathogenesis of these disorders. Mitochondria are intracellular organelles which are present in all mammalian cells and are responsible for aerobic energy production. They contain their own genetic material, in the form of a circular 16.5-kbp genome, and there are multiple copies of this genome in each mitochondrion. This genome encodes for a critical part of the mitochondrion's separate replicative, transcriptional, and translational machinery, as well as for components of complexes I, III, IV, and V. However, the majority of proteins for mitochondrial function are encoded by the nuclear genome.

From these characteristics we can infer many of the clinical features of mitochondrial syndromes. These disorders can affect multiple organ systems, and tend to preferentially affect organs with higher energy requirements. They can occur due to mutations in mitochondrial DNA (mtDNA) or nuclear DNA (nDNA). Mutations in mtDNA can occur in a proportion of genomes (heteroplasmic) or in all genomes (homoplasmic). The extent to which a tissue is affected by such mutations may depend on the proportion of mutated genomes.

Numerous other diseases have mitochondrial dysfunction as a component of their pathogenesis, including common neurodegenerative [1], neurovascular [2], and traumatic neurological disorders. Other genetic conditions are caused by primary dysfunction of mitochondrial dynamics [3], resulting in secondary mtDNA abnormalities; these conditions are not generally considered in the same category as mitochondrial cytopathies, although clinical overlap in some of these conditions (such as progressive external ophthalmoplegia with multiple mtDNA deletions, which may occur with *OPA1* mutations) may render the disorders indistinguishable at the bedside.

This chapter will focus on the major clinical syndromes caused by primary dysfunction of the mitochondrial respiratory chain. The various other mitochondrial syndromes will be summarized in tabular format, with general principles discussed in the text.

General principles in mitochondrial cytopathies

Mitochondrial diseases are among the most common inherited neuromuscular diseases, and have an estimated prevalence in adults and children of 1 in 10 000 [4]. The carrier frequency of mtDNA mutations appears to be much higher, at only 1 in 200 [5]. The reason for the large discrepancy is the low heteroplasmy level in most carriers, the variable penetrance and expressivity of mtDNA disorders, and the difficulty in correctly identifying patients with mtDNA disease.

Clinical presentation

The most common disorder of mtDNA is Leber hereditary optic neuropathy (LHON), which has a restricted phenotype and clinically affects vision due to dysfunction of the retinal ganglion cells. Otherwise, as a general rule, patients with mitochondrial cytopathies have multisystem disease; the various types of organ dysfunction which can occur are summarized in Table 30.1. Some component of the central or peripheral nervous systems is nearly always affected because of the high energy requirements of these tissues. In particular, the ocular system is often affected, most frequently retinal pathology and/or the ocular muscles but also by disorders of the optic nerve and lens. It is also important to mention cardiac dysfunction because the complications are treatable and may be life-threatening if unidentified.

The various organ system dysfunctions can occur in any combination, although they often occur in constellations of symptoms or signs that form recognizable clinical syndromes. The clinical syndromes are summarized in Table 30.2. It is necessary to mention that the phenotypic variability in these disorders is extensive and overlap between syndromes is common—many patients may not fit into a single diagnostic category. The categorization of the various syndromes is difficult, again relating to phenotypic variability but also the broad variability within syndromes; nonetheless attempts at various categorizations are provided in Table 30.3. As mentioned, the most prevalent mitochondrial cytopathies in adults primarily involve neuro-ophthalmological features, and are LHON followed by progressive external ophthalmoplegia (PEO).

The classification of mitochondrial diseases is difficult because of the wide variety of overlapping clinical features in different patients with the same, or different, genetic mitochondrial diseases (see Table 30.1). To assist understanding, we have classified the disorders by clinical syndrome (Table 30.2), major disease categories (Table 30.3; note the overlap of the syndromes), and genetic aetiology (Table 30.4).

The example of PEO is particularly illustrative of the clinical heterogeneity of mitochondrial syndromes. PEO may occur as an isolated ocular myopathy (with ptosis and ophthalmoparesis) or in combination with any of the other features of mitochondrial dysfunction listed in Table 30.1. PEO also variably occurs as a

Table 30.1 Clinical features of mitochondrial cytopathies, by organ system, with common investigations and symptomatic therapies

Symptom	Investigation/abnormality	Treatment
Ocular		
Ophthalmoparesis		For diplopia: prism glasses or strabismus surgery
Ptosis		When visual fields obscured: frontalis slings or levator palpebrae resection.
Optic atrophy Pigmentary retinopathy		Referral for services as appropriate for level of visual disability; driving restrictions. Potential benefits from idebenone in LHON
Cataract		Surgical resection
Central neurological		
Ataxia		
Movement disorder		Symptomatic therapy
Spasticity		Symptomatic therapy
Seizures (generalized, focal, and/or myoclonic)	EEG (epileptiform abnormality)	Anticonvulsants (avoid VPA if possible)
Migraine		Analgesics and/or tryptans; prophylactic therapy when appropriate
Encephalopathy	MRI (nonspecific white matter or basal ganglia signal abnormalities). EEG (diffuse slowing)	Supportive therapy. Avoidance of precipitating factors or medications
Stroke-like episodes	MRI (high-signal T_2 abnormality not conforming to vascular territories, posterior-predominant)	L-arginine may be effective
Peripheral neurological		
Axonal polyneuropathy Sensory neuronopathy/ganglionopathy	EMG, nerve conduction studies	Symptomatic treatment and mobility aids
Sensorineural hearing loss	Audiography	Auditory aids, cochlear implantation
Autonomic dysfunction	Orthostatic vital signs. Clinical history for gastrointestinal dysmotility	Symptomatic treatment of orthostatic hypotension; dietary modification for gastrointestinal dysmotility
Musculoskeletal		
Skeletal myopathy (ocular > axial/proximal > distal > respiratory)	Pulmonary function testing and/or sleep studies for respiratory muscle weakness. CK normal or mildly elevated (or highly elevated in CoQ_{10} deficiency myopathy). EMG: myopathic changes	Mobility aids. Exercise therapy. CPAP/BiPAP for respiratory failure
Smooth muscle myopathy (dysphagia)	Oesophageal motility studies	Dietary modification
Cardiac		
Cardiomyopathy	Echocardiogram	ACE blockade
Conduction defects	Electrocardiogram, Holter monitor	Pacemaker, antiarrhythmics
Endocrine		
Diabetes mellitus	Fasting glucose, oral glucose tolerance test, HbA1c	Oral antihyperglycaemics, insulin
Hypothyroidism	TSH, T3, T4	Hormone replacement
Hypoparathyroidism	PTH, serum Ca	
Growth hormone deficiency	GH; GHRH-arginine test or insulin tolerance test	
Gonadal failure	LH, FSH	Hormone replacement in selected cases
Gastrointestinal		
Dysmotility: dysphagia, gastroparesis, diarrhoea, constipation, and/or pseudo-obstruction	Swallowing studies: cricopharyngeal achalasia or oesophageal dysmotility	Dietary modification, symptomatic therapy
Hepatic failure	Serum liver enzyme elevations, liver biopsy	

(continued)

Table 30.1 Continued

Symptom	Investigation/abnormality	Treatment
Neuropsychiatric		
Cognitive impairment	Mental status testing	Caregiver support, lifestyle modifications, assessment for driving and competency
Fatigue		
Depression	Psychiatric assessment	Antidepressants
Psychosis		Neuroleptics
Other		
Short stature		
Spontaneous abortion		

LHON, Leber hereditary optic neuropathy; VPA, valproic acid; MRI, magnetic resonance imaging EEG, electroencephalogram; EMG, electromyogram; CK, creatine kinase; CoQ$_{10}$, coenzyme Q10; CPAP, continuous positive airway pressure; BiPAP, bilevel positive airway pressure; ACE, angiotensin-converting enzyme; Hb, haemoglobin; TSH, thyroid-stimulating hormone; T3, triiodothyronine; T4, thyroxine; PTH, parathyroid hormone; GH, growth hormone; GHRH, growth hormone releasing hormone; LH, luteinizing hormone; FSH, follicle-stimulating hormone.

Table 30.2 Clinical syndromes of mitochondrial cytopathies. Note that the genetic aetiology is continuously changing. (This list is far from exhaustive.)

Syndrome	Clinical symptoms/signs	Age of onset	Genetics
Leber hereditary optic neuropathy (LHON)	Serial monocular visual loss	Adulthood	mtDNA point mutations (m.11778G>A, m.3460G>A, m.14484T>C)
Progressive external ophthalmoplegia (PEO)	Ptosis, ophthalmoparesis. Proximal myopathy often present. Various other clinical features variably present	Any age of onset. Typically more severe phenotype with younger onset.	mtDNA single deletions. mtDNA point mutations (including m.3243A>G, m.8344A>G). nDNA mutations (POLG1, POLG2, SLC25A4, C10orf2, RRM2B, TK2, and OPA1)
Kearns–Sayre syndrome (KSS)	PEO, ptosis, pigmentary retinopathy, cardiac conduction abnormality, ataxia, CSF elevated protein, diabetes mellitus, sensorineural hearing loss, myopathy	<20 years	mtDNA single deletions
Ataxia neuropathy syndromes (ANS): including MIRAS, SCAE, SANDO, MEMSA	SANDO: PEO, dysarthria, sensory neuropathy, cerebellar ataxia. Other ANS: Sensory axonal neuropathy with variable degrees of sensory and cerebellar ataxia. Epilepsy, dysarthria, or myopathy are present in some	Teens or adulthood	nDNA mutations (POLG, C10orf2, OPA1)
Mitochondrial neurogastrointestinal encephalopathy (MNGIE)	PEO, ptosis, GI dysmotility, proximal myopathy, axonal polyneuropathy, leucodystrophy	Childhood to early adulthood	nDNA mutations in TYMP; MNGIE-like syndromes may occur due to nDNA gene mutations with PEO
Mitochondrial encephalomyopathy with lactic acidosis and stroke-like episodes (MELAS)	Stroke-like episodes with encephalopathy, migraine, seizures. Variable presence of myopathy, cardiomyopathy, deafness, endocrinopathy, ataxia. A minority of patients have PEO	Typically <40 years of age but childhood more common	mtDNA point mutations (m.3243A>G in 80%, m.3256C>T, m.3271T>C, m.4332G>A, m.13513G>A, m.13514A>G)
Myoclonic epilepsy with ragged-red fibres (MERRF)	Stimulus sensitive myoclonus, generalized seizures, ataxia, cardiomyopathy. A minority of patients have PEO	Childhood	mtDNA point mutations (m.8344A>G most common; m.8356T>C, m.12147G>A)
Mitochondrial myopathy (isolated)	Axial/proximal myopathy. May have other features of mitochondrial disease (ataxia, polyneuropathy)	Any age of onset	mtDNA point mutations (multiple, including m.3243A>G; m.3302A>G, m.14709T>C). mtDNA single large scale deletions

(continued)

Table 30.2 Continued

Syndrome	Clinical symptoms/signs	Age of onset	Genetics
Mitochondrial DNA depletion syndrome	Diffuse myopathy, or encephalopathy, or hepatocerebral syndrome	Congenital or infantile presentation, with hypotonia, respiratory weakness, and death within a few years of birth. Infantile COX-deficiency myopathy occasionally reverses after first year of life	nDNA mutations (*DGUOK, TK2, C10orf2, POLG, RRM2B, SUCLA2, SUCLG1, MPV17*)
Infantile myopathy with COX deficiency	Diffuse myopathy, lactic acidosis, encephalopathy	Congenital/infantile onset. Fatal in first year, or reversible after first year in some patients	mtDNA mutation (m.14674T>C) in the reversible form
Neurogenic weakness with ataxia and retinitis pigmentosa (NARP)	Ataxia, pigmentary retinopathy, weakness	Childhood	*MTATP6* mutation (usually at m.8993)
Leigh syndrome	Encephalopathy precipitated by illness, brainstem and cerebellar dysfunction, neuropathy, cardiomyopathy	Infancy	Recessive or X-linked mutations in nDNA-encoded respiratory chain components, and less commonly mtDNA point mutations (usually *MTATP6*)
Alpers syndrome; childhood myocerebral hepatopathy syndrome (MCHS)	Seizures, developmental delay, hypotonia, hepatic failure	Infancy/childhood	Recessive mutations in *POLG*, or unknown for Alpers syndrome; for MCHS mutations in *POLG, c10orf2, MPV17, DGUOK*
Pearson syndrome	Sideroblastic anaemia, pancreatic failure	Infancy	Single large-scale mtDNA deletions
Maternally inherited diabetes and deafness	Type II diabetes. Sensorineural hearing loss	Adulthood	mtDNA point mutations (m.3243A>G, various other point mutations described in isolated reports)
Deafness sensorineural hearing loss	Sensorineural hearing loss	Childhood	mtDNA point mutations (m.1095T>C, m.1555A>G, m.7445A>G, and other mutations from isolated reports)
Mitochondrial cardiomyopathy	Cardiomyopathy (hypertrophic or dilated)	Infancy, childhood or adulthood	mtDNA point mutations (m.3243A>G, m.3260A>G, m.4300A>G, and various other mutations from isolated reports). nDNA mutations *COX15, SLC25A3*

mtDNA, mitochondrial DNA; nDNA, nuclear DNA; CSF, cerebrospinal fluid; MIRAS, mitochondrial recessive ataxia syndrome; SCAE, spinocerebellar ataxia with epilepsy; SANDO, sensory ataxia, neuropathy, dysarthria, ophthalmoplegia; MEMSA, myoclonic epilepsy, myopathy, sensory ataxia; GI, gastrointestinal; COX, cytochrome *c* oxidase.

component of other mitochondrial syndromes, such as Kearns–Sayre syndrome, mitochondrial encephalomyopathy with lactic acidosis and stroke-like episodes (MELAS), myoclonic epilepsy with ragged red fibres (MERRF), mitochondrial neurogastrointestinal encephalopathy (MNGIE), and in some of the ataxia–neuropathy syndromes (ANS) (namely sensory ataxia, neuropathy, dysarthria, ophthalmoplegia; SANDO). However, for the purposes of nomenclature, patients are given a diagnosis of PEO, or 'PEO-plus', if their clinical features do not meet criteria for another syndrome and their clinical presentation includes ocular myopathy.

Particular clinical syndromes will often suggest the genetic aetiology, although many of these syndromes have diverse genetic aetiologies and clinical features are unable to distinguish the various genetic causes. Here PEO is again illustrative of this point: identical clinical phenotypes may be caused by a broad repertoire of genetic defects, including single large-scale mtDNA deletions, numerous mtDNA point mutations, and a number of mutations in nuclear-encoded mitochondrial genes (*POLG1, POLG2, SLC25A4, C10orf2, RRM2B, TK2,* and *OPA1*). Similarly, defects in particular mitochondrial genes or specific mtDNA abnormalities are capable

of producing unrelated clinical phenotypes. Here the example of the m.3243A>G mutation is most illustrative. This mutation may cause maternally inherited diabetes and deafness, cardiomyopathy, PEO, isolated mitochondrial myopathy, or MELAS. *POLG* is also another example of this phenomenon, in which mutations at the same position can cause a relatively mild syndrome (PEO) or severe infantile-onset syndromes such as mtDNA depletion syndromes or myocerebrohepatopathy. Genetic defects which cause disparate clinical phenotypes, and their associated clinical syndromes, are summarized in Table 30.4. Determining the genetic aetiology is important for purposes of genetic counselling, since all modes of inheritance appear in mitochondrial cytopathies (maternal, dominant, recessive, and X-linked), and in the case of single large-scale mtDNA deletions, are only inherited in 4% of cases [6].

One problematic issue is determination of the pathogenicity of mtDNA variants because the mitochondrial genome is extensively polymorphic. As a result, a high burden of proof is required before a variant can be considered to be a mutation of proven pathogenicity. Criteria have been suggested for this purpose [7]: these include that the variant must not be a previously described polymorphism,

Table 30.3 Clinical disease categories of mitochondrial syndromes

Category	Syndromes
Neuro-ophthalmologic	Leber hereditary optic neuropathy (LHON)
	Progressive external ophthalmoplegia (PEO)
	Kearns–Sayre syndrome (KSS)
	Neurogenic weakness with ataxia and retinitis pigmentosa (NARP)
	Ataxia neuropathy syndromes (ANS) including MIRAS, SCAE, SANDO, MEMSA
	Myoclonic epilepsy with ragged-red fibres (MERRF)
	Mitochondrial encephalomyopathy with lactic acidosis and stroke-like episodes (MELAS)
	Mitochondrial neurogastrointestinal encephalopathy (MNGIE)
	Pearson syndrome
Presentation with ocular myopathy (or, progressive external ophthalmoplegia)	Progressive external ophthalmoplegia
	Kearns–Sayre syndrome
	MERRF
	MNGIE
	ANS (in about 50%)
	MELAS (minority)
Presentation with seizures and/or encephalopathy	MERRF
	MELAS
	Alpers syndrome
	NARP
	Leigh syndrome
	Infantile myopathy with COX deficiency
	Mitochondrial DNA depletion syndrome
	ANS
Mitochondrial myopathies	PEO
	KSS
	ANS including MIRAS, SCAE, SANDO, MEMSA
	MNGIE
	MELAS
	MERRF
	Mitochondrial myopathy (isolated)
	Mitochondrial DNA depletion syndrome
	Infantile myopathy with COX deficiency
Presentation with cardiomyopathy and/or cardiac conduction defects	Mitochondrial cardiomyopathy
	Maternally inherited diabetes and deafness
	MERRF
	MELAS
	PEO
	KSS

MIRAS, mitochondrial recessive ataxia syndrome; SCAE, spinocerebellar ataxia with epilepsy; SANDO, sensory ataxia, neuropathy, dysarthria, ophthalmoplegia; MEMSA, myoclonic epilepsy, myopathy, sensory ataxia; COX, cytochrome c oxidase.

Table 30.4 Genetic abnormalities causing multiple mitochondrial disease phenotypes

Mutation type	Gene and/or mutation	Clinical syndromes
mtDNA single large-scale deletion		Progressive external ophthalmoplegia (PEO)
		Kearns–Sayre syndrome
		Pearson syndrome
		Isolated mitochondrial myopathy
mtDNA point mutations	m.3243A>G	Mitochondrial encephalomyopathy with lactic acidosis and stroke-like episodes (MELAS)
		PEO
		Isolated mitochondrial myopathy
		Cardiomyopathy
		Maternally inherited diabetes and deafness
	MTATP6 (commonly m.8993T>C or m.8993T>G)	Neurogenic weakness with ataxia and retinitis pigmentosa (NARP)
		Leigh syndrome
		Adult-onset ataxia and/or spasticity
	m.8344A>G	Myoclonic epilepsy with ragged-red fibres (MERRF)
		PEO
nDNA mutations	POLG	PEO
		Alpers syndrome
		Childhood myocerebral hepatopathy syndrome
		mtDNA depletion syndrome
		Ataxia-neuropathy syndrome
		Hereditary sensorimotor neuropathy
		Familial parkinsonism
		MELAS-like syndrome
	C10orf2	PEO
		mtDNA depletion syndrome
		Ataxia-neuropathy syndrome
	RRM2B, TK2	PEO
		mtDNA depletion syndrome
mtDNA depletion	DGK, TK2, C10orf2, POLG, RRM2B	Myopathic syndrome (TK2, RRM2B)
		Encephalopathic syndrome (SUCLA2, SUCLG1)
		Hepatocerebral syndrome (DGUOK, MPV17, POLG, SUCLG1, C10orf2)

mtDNA, mitochondrial DNA.

the nucleotide must be conserved, the variant is (preferably) heteroplasmic, and affected tissues contain a higher mutation burden (ideally substantiated with single-fibre muscle studies). As a result a large number of variants that have been associated with mitochondrial disease phenotypes in isolated cases remain unproven. In the tables in this chapter we include proven mutations for the various syndromes, although this list is being updated over time as more evidence is collected. We suggest that readers consult <http://www.mitomap.org/>, a useful reference which provides updated information regarding confirmed and provisional mtDNA mutations, polymorphic variants of mtDNA, as well as a list of 'unpublished' mtDNA variants which may be of possible clinical significance. However, not all of the mutations described on this database are definitely pathogenic. An international initiative is currently under way to address this.

Clinical investigation

Diagnostic testing for mitochondrial disorders should be guided by the pattern of organ involvement. Genetic testing may be preferable as an initial investigation when a clear-cut clinical syndrome is present. Mutations in mtDNA are detectable in leucocyte DNA for LHON (homoplasmic mutations) as well as other mtDNA mutations such as common mutations for MERRF or MELAS syndromes. Mutations in nDNA, when present, are always detectable from leucocyte DNA. For the m.3243A>G mutation this can easily be detected in urine, and the mutation load may even provide prognostic information [8]. Elevations of plasma and urine thymidine are seen in MNGIE syndrome due to mutations in *TYMP*. However, where other mtDNA abnormalities are suspected analysis should be performed on DNA extracted from an affected tissue, which is usually skeletal muscle (the high replication rate of blood cells selects against pathogenic mtDNA abnormalities, therefore many mtDNA abnormalities are often not detectable in blood). Genetic testing for mtDNA includes long polymerase chain reaction (PCR) and/or Southern blot for large-scale rearrangements and targeted assays for common mtDNA point mutations, and mtDNA genome sequencing to uncover less common variants.

Muscle biopsy is therefore useful in order to provide DNA for the testing just described, although it also frequently provides important diagnostic information using histopathology and electron microscopy. Muscle biopsy is typically taken from a limb muscle, such as quadriceps femoris, or deltoid (although in PEO, studies have considered the diagnostic value of levator palpebrae and orbicularis oculi biopsy [9–12]). The testing should include a variety of histochemical functional assays, and be performed in a centre with experience in the diagnosis of mitochondrial disease. The major diagnostic feature is the presence of fibres deficient in cytochrome *c* oxidase (COX) activity, which represents poor activity of complex IV in the respiratory chain (and is encoded by both mtDNA and nDNA genes). However, COX-negative fibres accumulate with age, therefore there is an age-dependent threshold for the criteria for a mitochondrial disorder to be met (>2% for those under 50, and >5% for those above 50) [13]. COX-negative fibres are best identified by serially staining muscle for COX, followed by succinate dehydrogenase (SDH) which stains for complex II (and is encoded entirely by nuclear genes). The demonstration of COX-deficient, SDH-positive muscle fibres is thought to have the best sensitivity and specificity for mitochondrial disease, particularly in adults [14]. The subsarcolemmal accumulation of mitochondria is a classic feature of mitochondrial myopathy, and can be demonstrated by SDH histochemistry (so-called 'ragged blue fibres') or the Gomori trichrome stain (so-called 'ragged red fibres' or RRFs). Again, a low frequency of RRFs (<5%) can be seen in healthy aged individuals. However, the detection of RRFs in individuals younger than 50 years of age, or >5% RRFs at any age, is highly suggestive of mitochondrial myopathy. Clinical correlation

remains important because RRFs can be present at high levels in other muscle diseases such as sporadic inclusion body myositis or myotonic dystrophy (see Fig. 30.1).

The findings on muscle biopsy may provide guidance for appropriate genetic testing. As a general rule, a mosaic appearance of COX-negative fibres suggests a mtDNA mutation (due to the variable degrees of heteroplasmy between muscle cells), whereas uniformly decreased COX activity suggests a nDNA mutation (which would be equally present in all muscle cells). Other characteristic features include the presence of strongly SDH-positive blood vessels in patients with the m.3243A>G mutation [15].

Electron microscopy (EM) may also be performed on muscle specimens and may demonstrate enlarged pleiomorphic mitochondria and paracrystalline inclusions. At present EM is thought to provide minor criteria for the diagnosis of mitochondrial disease because the findings are often non-specific [16]. EM may provide additional diagnostic information in some patients with normal histochemistry [17], although this should be carefully interpreted in the context of genetic studies and the clinical picture. An important limitation of muscle biopsy is that histochemistry and/or EM may be normal even in the context of genetically proven mitochondrial syndromes [18], particularly early in the disease course or when the biochemical defect does not involve complex IV (COX).

Another test that can be done with muscle tissue is respiratory chain enzyme (RCE) analysis. This testing must be done either on fresh or snap-frozen muscle samples. RCE is technically difficult to perform, even in specialist laboratories [14,19,20], and the results should be interpreted in the context of the other investigations. Demonstrating a defect in RCEs is an important diagnostic step in patients with normal or near-normal muscle histochemistry, particularly children. In conditions such as Leigh syndrome, which is caused by a large array of nuclear gene defects, the demonstration of a specific RCE complex defect can guide the genetic investigations to confirm the diagnosis. However, RCE abnormalities can also occur early in the course of mtDNA depletion syndromes, and therefore the presence of a specific complex deficiency does not guarantee that a mutation in a specific complex assembly factor is present. It is important to note that complex V (ATP synthase) is rarely measured in diagnostic laboratories, but a defect of ATP synthase may be the only biochemical abnormality in some patients.

Diagnostic information can also be obtained from fibroblast cultures, established from a skin biopsy, which can be used for RCE analysis and with the DNA for genetic studies. However, this tissue has lower sensitivity than muscle because the RCE defect or molecular genetic defect may not be present in fibroblasts in all patients [21]. Liver biopsy is appropriate in selected situations with an important component of hepatic failure, providing there is no coagulopathy. In these situations the biopsy is helpful to exclude other disorders and is a tissue source for histological, EM, RCE, and DNA analysis.

Mitochondrial myopathy due to coenzyme Q10 (CoQ_{10}) biosynthetic defects is diagnosed by the demonstration of CoQ_{10} deficiency in muscle tissue, and may be supported by decreased levels in other tissues such as fibroblasts and white blood cells [20,22]. Plasma levels have a broad reference range and may be normal in this condition [20]. RCE analysis on muscle tissue may demonstrate the combination of either complex I and III deficiency or complex II and III deficiency, since these complexes are CoQ_{10}-dependent [23].

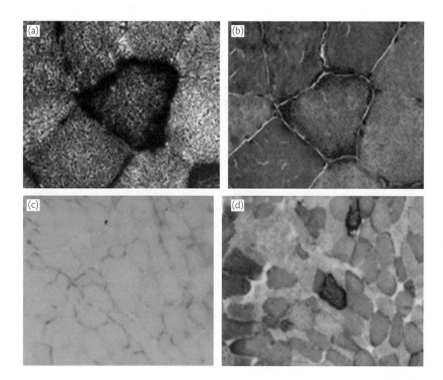

Fig. 30.1 (a) Succinate dehydrogenase (SDH) histochemistry and (b) Gomori trichrome histochemistry, both demonstrating subsarcolemmal accumulation of mitochondria in a 'ragged red fibre'. Cytochrome *c* oxidase (COX) histochemistry demonstrates diffusely COX-negative fibres in a nuclear gene defect (c) and serial COX/SDH assay reveals mosaic pattern of COX deficiency in a heteroplasmic mitochondrial DNA disorder (d).
Adapted from Chinnery PF, Betts J, Jaros E, Turnbull DM, DiMauro S, Perry R. Mitochondrial diseases. Chapter 8. *Greenfields Neuropathology*, 8th Edition, 2008. Editors: Love S, Louis DN, Ellison BW. pp. 601–642. With thanks to Prof Robert Taylor. (See also figure in colour plate section)

Non-invasive tests for mitochondrial disorders include exercise testing. There are numerous described protocols for testing using cycle ergometry or treadmill exercise [24]. The specificity [25,26] and sensitivity [27] of these tests is poor. Venous Po_2 measurement during handgrip testing has high specificity, and is therefore a reasonable screening test where available [28,29], but it usually complements the investigations described in this section.

Other non-invasive tests have limited ability to identify mitochondrial disorders in most situations, but they may rule out alternative diagnoses. Serum lactate and pyruvate measurement, either at rest or post-exercise, is usually within normal ranges in adult-onset mitochondrial disorders. Serum and urine amino acid, organic acid, and carnitine profiles occasionally have non-specific abnormalities in patients with mitochondrial disorders (respectively, elevated alanine, elevated Krebs cycle intermediates, and abnormal fatty acid oxidation). The results of these investigations will vary depending on sample handling as well as the laboratory measurement method. Elevated lactate in the central nervous system may be demonstrated by direct measurement with lumbar puncture, although cerebrospinal fluid (CSF) lactate is also affected by the presence of blood in the CSF and time from collection, and is elevated in other conditions causing altered mental status (bacterial and fungal meningitis). Indirectly, lactate may be measured using magnetic resonance (MR) spectroscopy, although again there is variability in measurement methods, and findings are usually within the normal range for adult-onset disorders. However, extremely high lactate (more than ten times the upper limit of normal) in CSF or blood from a child is highly suggestive of a mitochondrial disorder.

The field of genetic diagnosis in mitochondrial disorders has advanced rapidly with the development of high-throughput sequencing technologies. This can be applied to the sequencing of mtDNA by customized capture of mtDNA sequences, but has been most beneficial for nuclear gene defects using exome sequencing.

This has identified new nuclear genes for mitochondrial syndromes [30,31], and expanded the phenotypic spectrum of particular nuclear gene defects [32]. At present next-generation sequencing is used for research purposes only, although it is only natural that this technology will eventually be applied for diagnostic purposes, given the broad variety of genetic aetiologies for many of the genetic syndromes.

Clinical management

Diagnostic testing which addresses the dysfunction of multiple organ systems in patients with a mitochondrial myopathy must be tailored depending on each patient's symptoms and signs (see Table 30.1). However, certain organ systems should be discussed in more detail because they influence patient management. It is important to identify cardiac complications with electrocardiogram and echocardiogram, and depending on the patient's syndrome screening tests may be needed at regular intervals. Patients with Kearns–Sayre syndrome (KSS), MERRF, and MELAS syndromes appear to be most likely to develop progressive cardiac disease [33], although optimal screening recommendations do not exist for these syndromes, or others. Cardiac conduction defects can be fatal if untreated, and are addressed with cardiac pacemakers and/or antiarrhythmics [34]. Cardiomyopathy may be treated with angiotensin-converting enzyme (ACE) inhibitors and beta blockers and cardiac transplantation in specially selected cases [35]. Ptosis in PEO can become disabling if the eyelids obstruct vision, and surgical treatment with levator palpebrae superioris resection or frontalis slings is possible. Endocrine investigations may identify diabetes mellitus, hypothyroidism, or growth hormone deficiency, all of which are treatable. Patients with hearing or visual symptoms should be investigated in order to prescribe appropriate aids if required. There is growing international experience using cochlear implants, which appear to be highly effective for the post-lingual deafness that develops as part of mitochondrial disease [36].

Dysphagia is common in several mitochondrial syndromes [37] and improvement is possible with dietary modification.

Treatment of mitochondrial disorders overwhelmingly concentrates on supportive therapy and symptomatic management of disease complications. However, there was recently a double-blind, randomized, placebo-controlled trial of idebenone in LHON, in which visual function stabilized in patients who had discordant visual acuity at entry to the study [38]. These patients may have been earlier in the course of their disease, and this suggests that treatment with idebenone may be useful early in the condition. These findings are supported by extensive retrospective case series analysis; however, further evidence is required to establish the efficacy of this agent.

All patients with a predominantly myopathic presentation should have muscle CoQ_{10} measurements performed, because patients with biosynthetic defects of CoQ_{10} are reported to respond to CoQ_{10} supplementation [39].

For patients with myopathy, there is accumulating evidence that various forms of exercise therapy are beneficial for numerous end points, including strength, fatigue, and quality of life. Aerobic [40,41], endurance [42,43], and resistance [44] training programmes have been studied. Exercise therapy may simply reverse the deconditioning, which is a common feature of many muscle diseases, or it is possible the exercise affects the underlying pathology (or a combination of these effects).

Data from a single group of investigators suggest L-arginine as therapy for MELAS—for both the acute stroke-like episodes and for chronic therapy to prevent further events [45]. The data should be interpreted with caution because they are not blinded and all originate from the same investigators. A separate study suggested L-arginine may be useful in mitochondrial cardiomyopathy [46]. This agent could be beneficial and should be studied in a prospective, randomized, blinded, controlled trial.

Otherwise, there has been no demonstration of any clinically beneficial disease-modifying therapy in mitochondrial diseases, which was the conclusion reached in a recent Cochrane review of the topic [47]. Therapeutic agents to date have focused on various nutritional supplements, including carnitine [48], creatine [49–51], CoQ_{10} [52,53], cysteine [54], dichloroacetate [52,55–58], dimethylglycine [59], and a combination of creatine, CoQ_{10}, and lipoic acid [60], which have been evaluated in controlled trials. Various other agents including ascorbate and menadione, a high-fat diet, magnesium, nicotinamide, and succinate have appeared in case reports but further study would be required to indicate whether they are beneficial. The most commonly used of these supplements is CoQ_{10}, which is prescribed by some specialist physicians in the UK National Health Service and can be bought from health food suppliers. We reiterate that all randomized controlled trials of CoQ_{10} in mitochondrial disease have failed to demonstrate any benefit of this agent, even at an elevated dosage of 1200 mg day^{-1} [61]. However, CoQ_{10} is commonly prescribed because its effects may be difficult to measure in clinical trials, it generally has no adverse reactions, and it may also have a placebo effect. The situation in which CoQ_{10} should always be prescribed is for patients with defects of CoQ_{10} biosynthesis: there is a very strong biological rationale for treatment benefit (although due to the rarity of these conditions it is unlikely a high-quality clinical trial will address this question formally).

Other important management issues involve the avoidance of precipitating factors in mitochondrial diseases. Valproic acid interferes with mitochondrial function and can aggravate mitochondrial myopathy symptoms [62]. Valproate-induced hepatotoxicity may be more common in patients with mitochondrial myopathy [63,64], which in some cases is modulated by genetic variation in POLG [65]. However, it has been our clinical experience that patients with mitochondrial syndromes may use valproate safely if they are adequately monitored, and this is appropriate if valproate provides better seizure control. Antiretroviral agents, particularly nucleotide reverse transcriptase inhibitors, cause reversible and dose-dependent mitochondrial toxicity [66]. Certain agents have lower mitochondrial toxicity [67], and should be used preferentially. Small series have documented the development of PEO-like syndromes in patients on antiretrovirals [68–70], although whether this is due to an unmasking effect or whether the disease is caused by cumulative mitochondrial toxicity requires further study (although a recent study hypothesized that HIV and antiretrovirals induced clonal expansion of deleted mtDNA molecules). Statin medications are thought to interfere with mitochondrial function [71], although the mechanisms remain unclear. Ten per cent of patients who receive statins develop muscle symptoms [72], and statins have been reported to unmask symptoms in asymptomatic mitochondrial myopathy patients [73]. These agents have also been reported in association with syndromes resembling PEO [74,75]. In theory they should be used cautiously in mitochondrial myopathy, but again our clinical experience suggests these agents are safe when used with proper clinical monitoring and regular creatine kinase (CK) measurements. The use of anaesthetic agents is an unresolved issue in mitochondrial disorders, with several case reports documenting individual adverse reactions. Decisions regarding these agents should probably be made on a case-by-case basis in consultation with an anaesthetist, with special consideration for the patient's general condition, respiratory muscle, and cardiac function.

Finally, it is important for all patients with mitochondrial syndromes to receive genetic counselling, and in this respect it is especially important to establish a genetic diagnosis. When the genetic aetiology is known, patients and their family members can make informed decisions about whether to have biological children of their own and, if so, whether reproductive technologies will be employed. Available methods include preimplantation genetic diagnosis; pronuclear transfer has been achieved on an experimental basis and this reduces or may eliminate the risk of transmission of mtDNA defects.

The clinical outcome of mitochondrial disorders is dependent on the individual syndrome, and because of the rarity of some of these conditions the natural history is not fully known. This chapter continues with summary descriptions of the major clinical syndromes.

Leber hereditary optic neuropathy (LHON)

LHON is caused by mtDNA mutations and is a disease with variable penetrance [76]. Male carriers of the mutation have a fivefold increased risk of developing the disease compared with female carriers. Acquired mitochondrial toxicity from cigarettes and alcohol may also affect disease expression [77]. Patients typically present in early adulthood with unilateral visual loss, consisting of an enlarging central scotoma; within months the second eye becomes involved. The visual loss is typically subacutely progressive until the disease stabilizes with severe bilateral visual loss; patients may then have some marginal improvement in visual acuity and this is more common in patients with mutations m.14484T>C and m.11778G>A. Ultimately, most patients remain legally blind [76].

Other neurological features may coexist with LHON, but these are rare and include peripheral neuropathy or movement disorder. Typically these additional features do not contribute significantly to patient disability. The coexistence of a multiple sclerosis-like illness with LHON has been reported, and it remains undetermined whether there may be a relationship between these conditions or whether the co-occurrence is coincidental [78].

Three genetic mutations of mtDNA cause 90% of cases of LHON in patients of European extraction (m.11778G>A is most common, followed by m.3460G>A and m.14484T>C). These can be detected in DNA from blood leucocytes, making a simple genetic test the best means to confirm the diagnosis [79]. Clinically relevant LHON mtDNA mutations are always detectable in blood. The genetic mutations causing LHON are in mtDNA genes coding for components of complex I, and in most cases a complex I defect can be detected with respiratory chain enzyme analysis from muscle biopsy (although a muscle biopsy is rarely performed for diagnostic purposes). Abnormalities may also be demonstrated with MR spectroscopy [80]. When a high suspicion for LHON exists in the context of negative genetic testing, other mutations have been reported and may be detectable with complete mtDNA sequencing.

Management of LHON should include consideration of treatment with idebenone, which has been demonstrated to stabilize the visual deficit in patients with discordant visual acuity (Class II evidence from a single trial) [38]. Patients should be appropriately referred according to local regulations for assessment of driving capability and benefits relating to legal blindness. Referrals to genetic counselling should be made given the potential implications for other family members who may carry the mutation, or for prenatal diagnosis.

Progressive external ophthalmoplegia (PEO)

PEO is an ocular myopathy characterized by a gradual onset of ophthalmoparesis and ptosis. This condition should probably be considered a syndrome rather than a disease unto itself on account of its extensive phenotypic variability (may be pure PEO or present with dysfunction in multiple organ systems), variability in age of onset (early childhood to late adulthood), and massive heterogeneity of genetic causes (mtDNA point mutations, single large-scale mtDNA deletions, or nuclear gene defects causing secondary mtDNA defects). To complicate matters further, ocular myopathy is a component of the clinical presentation of various other mitochondrial syndromes (MELAS, MERRF, KSS, MNGIE, and ANS discussed in this chapter and other diseases which are not primary respiratory chain disorders, such as dominant optic atrophy due to OPA1 mutation).

Certain general principles apply in PEO. Onset of PEO in childhood tends to have a more severe phenotype with regard to the ocular myopathy, and is more likely to be complicated by dysfunction in other organ systems, particularly the cardiac system. Many of these cases are caused by single large-scale mtDNA deletions and exist on a phenotypic spectrum with patients having KSS. PEO in adulthood generally has a more slowly progressive ocular myopathy

and more benign course, with a milder severity and different pattern of multisystem dysfunction [17].

On clinical examination patients with PEO have bilateral ptosis, multidirectional ophthalmoparesis, and slow saccades. Other ocular findings depend on aetiology, such as pigmentary retinopathy in PEO due to single large-scale deletions, or optic atrophy in PEO due to OPA1 mutation.

Diagnostic tests include the finding of RRFs and/or COX-negative fibres in most cases on muscle biopsy. Genetic testing for mtDNA defects must be performed on muscle DNA since the abnormalities are usually absent in leucocyte DNA. Testing of mtDNA should include long PCR and/or Southern blot for mtDNA deletions, mtDNA sequencing for point mutations, and sequencing of nuclear genes including POLG1, POLG2, SLC25A4 (ANT1), C10orf2 (PEO1), RRM2B, TK2, and OPA1. Neuroimaging can incidentally demonstrate volume loss of the extraocular muscles [81], or non-specific white matter signal abnormalities [82]. Elevated lactate is occasionally demonstrated on testing of serum at rest and/or post-exercise, or with MR spectroscopy.

Treatment of PEO includes management of secondary complications of the disease. The most disabling component of the ocular myopathy is ptosis, which can be treated with oculoplastic procedures such as levator palpebrae muscle resection or the insertion of slings connected to the frontalis muscle.

Mitochondrial DNA deletion syndromes

These disorders exist on a disease spectrum and include (in order of decreasing clinical severity) Pearson syndrome, KSS, and some cases of PEO (those caused by single mtDNA deletions) [83]. Isolated mitochondrial myopathy can also be caused by single large-scale mtDNA deletions, but like PEO it is genetically heterogeneous.

KSS is the syndrome of PEO and pigmentary retinopathy prior to the age of 20, accompanied by cardiac conduction defects, cerebellar ataxia, and/or elevated CSF protein. Various other combinations of organ dysfunction frequently coexist, particularly sensorineural hearing loss and diabetes mellitus. Most cases are caused by single large-scale mtDNA deletions (most frequently, the 'common deletion' m.8470-13446del4977).

Genetic testing on mtDNA, as in PEO, should be performed on DNA extracted from muscle. Other diagnostic testing is as for PEO, except that when KSS is suspected it should always include further testing to confirm the diagnosis and identify the common treatable complications, specifically electrocardiogram and echocardiogram, fasting glucose, hearing tests, and CSF analysis.

There is no disease-modifying therapy for KSS, and again treatment focuses on the management of secondary complications. Particularly pertinent are the cardiac manifestations, which may require management with cardiac pacemakers, antiarrhythmics, ACE inhibitors, or in severe and specially selected cases, cardiac transplantation.

Pearson syndrome is an infantile onset disorder including sideroblastic anaemia and pancreatic exocrine failure [84]. The condition is usually fatal in infancy, although patients who survive develop a syndrome resembling a severe form of KSS. Bone marrow biopsy is diagnostic and demonstrates ringed sideroblasts and normoblasts with iron deposition within mitochondria. The pancreatic failure causes steatorrhoea. Leucocyte DNA is suitable for the purposes of genetic testing for Pearson syndrome because the mtDNA deletion is present at high levels in this tissue.

Mitochondrial encephalomyopathy with lactic acidosis and stroke-like episodes (MELAS)

MELAS syndrome has a heterogeneous clinical presentation. The onset of symptoms is typically in childhood or early adulthood. Clinical features may include episodes of encephalopathy, proximal myopathy, cardiomyopathy, lactic acidosis, stroke-like episodes (preferentially affecting the occipital lobes and not respecting typical vascular distributions; Fig. 30.2), migraine headaches, epilepsy, hearing loss, and endocrinopathy [85]. These comorbidities may cause significant disability and a shortened lifespan, usually due to cardiac dysfunction or seizures/encephalopathy [86]. The syndrome is caused by mutations of mtDNA-encoded tRNAs, specifically by the m.3243A>G mutation in 80% of cases.

Diagnosis of MELAS is confirmed by genetic testing, and the mutation can be detected from blood, urine sediment, or muscle. The heteroplasmy level of the 3243A>G mutation from urine samples may have prognostic significance and be correlated with phenotypic severity [8]. Other tests providing evidence for MELAS include muscle biopsy, which characteristically demonstrates RRFs and strongly SDH-reactive blood vessels. Respiratory chain enzyme analysis performed using muscle tissue can be normal or demonstrate non-specific abnormalities. Magnetic resonance imaging (MRI) of the brain is useful during stroke-like events to reveal regions of T_2 signal abnormality, usually predominantly

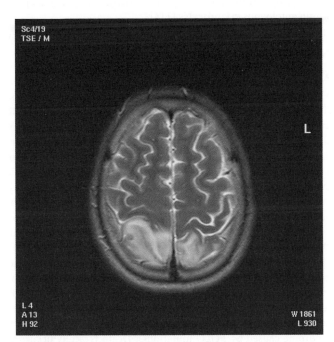

Fig. 30.2 This transverse axial image from a T_2-weighted magnetic resonance imaging (MRI) scan demonstrates high signal abnormality posteriorly, involving portions of both the posterior and middle cerebral artery vascular territories. This type of lesion, which is posterior-predominant and does not respect vascular boundaries, is a typical MRI finding in the stroke-like episodes of MELAS (mitochondrial encephalomyopathy with lactic acidosis and stroke-like episodes) syndrome.

in the occipital lobes and not respecting typical vascular boundaries [87].

Management of MELAS pertains mainly to the identification and treatment of disease complications [88]. There is no proven disease-modifying therapy available, although two non-blinded studies from the same investigators demonstrated a benefit of L-arginine for the prevention and acute treatment of stroke-like episodes [45]. Genetic counselling is recommended for women with the mutation, who are at risk of transmitting the disease to their offspring.

Myoclonic epilepsy with ragged-red fibres (MERRF)

This syndrome classically presents as one of the progressive myoclonic epilepsy (PME) syndromes. As in the other PMEs, patients have normal early development until the onset of generalized myoclonic jerks, generalized seizures, and other neurological dysfunction. In the case of MERRF, the syndrome includes myoclonus, generalized epilepsy, ataxia, and RRFs on muscle biopsy [89]. Patients usually also develop other multisystem complications of mitochondrial disease, although cardiac dysfunction deserves a special mention because it is common in this syndrome, treatable, and a cause of early morbidity and mortality [90].

The genetic aetiology of about 90% of MERRF cases is mutations of the mitochondrially encoded *TRNK* gene (most often m.8344A>G) [91], and the remaining cases are caused by other mutations of mtDNA. The mutation is best detected from muscle DNA but is also detectable from skin biopsy, urine sediment, and leucocyte DNA. Serum lactate is often elevated. Analysis of the CSF can show elevated lactate and/or mildly elevated protein. Muscle biopsy demonstrates RRFs and COX-negative fibres. An electroencephalogram (EEG) reveals slow background activity, generalized epileptiform abnormalities, and occasionally a photoparoxysmal response [92]. MRI is similarly non-specific and may show generalized loss of cerebral and cerebellar volume.

Treatment includes lifelong anticonvulsant therapy with agents that can control both the myoclonic and generalized seizures. There are no trials demonstrating preferred treatment, although there are theoretical contraindications to the use of valproic acid (due to the development of carnitine deficiency) [93]. However, in our experience valproic acid may be the only agent providing adequate seizure control, and it has been used without aggravating the syndrome in several reported cases. Supplementation with L-carnitine while on therapy with valproic acid has been advocated. In our experience levetiracetam provides good control of myoclonic seizures and is an alternative to valproic acid.

Leigh syndrome

Leigh syndrome has its onset in infancy and is sometimes precipitated by a viral illness. Diagnostic criteria have been suggested for this condition [94], including the presence of progressive disease with brainstem and cerebellar signs (movement disorder, hypotonia, ataxia), elevated lactate in blood or CSF, and characteristic MRI [95] or neuropathological abnormalities of the basal ganglia and brainstem. Commonly associated features include central respiratory failure, developmental delay, seizures, and pigmentary retinopathy [96].

Muscle histopathology is of limited value in this condition, although muscle tissue is essential for the analysis of RCEs. The identification of individual RCE complex defects can guide the direction of genetic investigation, which includes a lengthy and expanding list of nDNA defects and mtDNA point mutations [96]. MRI abnormalities are present in most patients and may be visible preclinically with diffusion-weighted imaging [97]. About one-third of cases of Leigh syndrome are caused by mtDNA mutations, and of these, mutations in *MTATP6* are most common. Prognosis is not predictable based upon the genetic aetiology. In most cases the condition is fatal within a year of onset although massive variation in clinical phenotype exists [98], and presentation can rarely occur even in advanced age [99].

Neurogenic muscle weakness, ataxia, and retinitis pigmentosa (NARP) syndrome

NARP is on a disease spectrum with Leigh syndrome, and these conditions share a common genetic aetiology in the form of mutations in the mitochondrially encoded *MTATP6* gene (although note that the genetic aetiology for Leigh syndrome is usually due to one of a myriad of nDNA defects) [100]. NARP is defined by childhood onset of sensorimotor neuropathy, ataxia, and pigmentary retinopathy [101], accompanied by learning disability, and other milder features of Leigh syndrome such as movement disorder or cardiac dysfunction. Most cases are caused by mutations at position m.8993. Mutations in the *MTATP6* gene are part of an even broader disease spectrum that also includes adult-onset spasticity [102] and ataxia [103,104].

Ataxia–neuropathy syndromes (ANS)

The ANS comprise disorders that are typically caused by nuclear gene defects and have been previously designated as: spinocerebellar ataxia with epilepsy; myoclonic epilepsy, myopathy, sensory ataxia (MEMSA) [105]; sensory ataxia, neuropathy, dysarthria, ophthalmoplegia (SANDO) [106]; and mitochondrial recessive ataxia syndrome (MIRAS) [105]. The various syndromes have in common the presence of sensory or sensorimotor neuropathy, cerebellar ataxia, and variable degrees of other central nervous dysfunction, PEO, and involvement of other organ systems. The age of onset, severity, and prognosis can be quite variable, although in general patients with earlier onset, and seizure disorders, tend to have worse outcomes.

Mitochondrial neurogastrointestinal encephalopathy (MNGIE) disease

MNGIE is characterized by diffuse gastrointestinal neuropathy and myopathy and demyelinating peripheral neuropathy. The age of onset is typically in childhood or early adulthood. The dominant clinical feature of this disease is the presence of severe gastrointestinal dysmotility throughout the gastrointestinal tract, due to atrophy of smooth muscle and autonomic nervous system dysfunction. Patients develop symptoms due to oesophageal dysmotility (dysphagia), gastroparesis (nausea, vomiting, early satiety), and intestinal hypomotility (malabsorption, diarrhoea, constipation).

Symptoms may also be episodic in the form of abdominal pain or pseudo-obstruction [107]. Ultimately, cachexia develops as a consequence of the combined gastrointestinal dysfunction, and patients have a shortened lifespan of only two to four decades after the onset of disease.

The demyelinating sensorimotor peripheral neuropathy affects the distal lower extremities first and most commonly manifests as foot drop, sensory ataxia, and/or neuropathic pain. Myopathy is also a common associated feature, in the form of external ophthalmoplegia and ptosis.

The disease is caused by homozygous or compound heterozygous mutations in thymidine phosphorylase (*TYMP*), although MNGIE-like syndromes have been described in patients with mtDNA (108) and other nDNA mutations (*POLG* [109] and *RRM2B* [110]). Diagnostic testing includes elevations in serum thymidine and deoxyuridine concentrations, a secondary effect of markedly reduced thymidine phosphorylase activity. Muscle biopsy demonstrates RRFs and COX-negative fibres. Leucoencephalopathy is present on MRI.

Treatment includes the management of secondary complications of the disease, and genetic counselling. There is no disease-modifying therapy at present, although experimental interventions to replace thymidine phosphorylase activity are under investigation. Allogeneic bone marrow transplantation corrects the biochemical defects [111] and appears to produce improvement in gastrointestinal symptoms [112], but would appear to carry a high mortality risk [112]. Other possible treatment options that have been trialled in other enzyme deficiency diseases and could be attempted for MNGIE include gene therapy and various delivery options for enzyme replacement therapy [113]. One avenue for the latter option includes encapsulated thymidine phosphorylase within autologous erythrocytes [114].

Mitochondrial DNA depletion syndromes

Mitochondrial DNA depletion syndromes are caused by recessive nuclear gene mutations, and are fatal disorders with onset in infancy and severely decreased mtDNA content in cells. The major clinical presentations include two major phenotypes, either severe diffuse myopathy or a hepatocerebral syndrome (which consists of a disease continuum ranging from more marked cerebral or hepatic involvement, or both; other features such as diffuse myopathy, metabolic derangements, and seizures are often present). The myopathic form is caused by mutations in *TK2* and *RRM2B* [115,116], whereas hepatocerebral syndromes are caused by mutations in *DGUOK*, *MPV17*, *POLG*, *PEO1*, *SUCLA2*, or *SUCLG1* [117–120]. The common mechanism for all the genetic lesions would appear to be dysfunction in mtDNA replication and/or maintenance of the mtDNA nucleotide supply. The use of valproic acid is particularly contraindicated in these disorders as it exacerbates hepatic failure (as is also the case for Alpers syndrome, another hepatocerebral syndrome caused by *POLG* mutations). Death typically occurs in infancy or early childhood due to liver or respiratory failure.

References

1. Martin LJ. Biology of mitochondria in neurodegenerative diseases. *Prog Mol Biol Transl Sci* 2012; **107**: 355–415.

2. Witte ME, Geurts JJ, de Vries HE, van der Valk P, van Horssen J. Mitochondrial dysfunction: a potential link between neuroinflammation and neurodegeneration? *Mitochondrion* 2010; **10**: 411–18.

3. Westermann B. Mitochondrial fusion and fission in cell life and death. *Nat Rev Mol Cell Biol* 2010; **11**: 872–84.

4. Chinnery PF, Johnson MA, Wardell TM, et al. The epidemiology of pathogenic mitochondrial DNA mutations. *Ann Neurol* 2000; **48**: 188–93.

5. Elliott HR, Samuels DC, Eden JA, Relton CL, Chinnery PF. Pathogenic mitochondrial DNA mutations are common in the general population. *Am J Hum Genet* 2008; **83**: 254–60.

6. Chinnery PF, DiMauro S, Shanske S, et al. Risk of developing a mitochondrial DNA deletion disorder. *Lancet* 2004; **364**: 592–6.

7. DiMauro S, Schon EA. Mitochondrial DNA mutations in human disease. *Am J Med Genet* 2001; **106**: 18–26.

8. Whittaker RG, Blackwood JK, Alston CL, et al. Urine heteroplasmy is the best predictor of clinical outcome in the m.3243A>G mtDNA mutation. *Neurology* 2009; **72**: 568–9.

9. Greaves LC, Yu-Wai-Man P, Blakely EL, et al. Mitochondrial DNA defects and selective extraocular muscle involvement in CPEO. *Invest Ophthalmol Vis Sci* 2010; **51**: 3340–6.

10. Pfeffer G, Waters PJ, Maguire J, Vallance HD, Wong VA, Mezei MM. Levator palpebrae biopsy and diagnosis of progressive external ophthalmoplegia. *Can J Neurol Sci* 2012; **39**: 520–4.

11. Eshaghian J, Anderson RL, Weingeist TA, Hart MN, Cancilla PA. Orbicularis oculi muscle in chronic progressive external ophthalmoplegia. *Arch Ophthalmol* 1980; **98**: 1070–3.

12. Almousa R, Charlton A, Rajesh ST, Sundar G, Amrith S. Optimizing muscle biopsy for the diagnosis of mitochondrial myopathy. *Ophthal Plast Reconstr Surg* 2009; **25**: 366–70.

13. Bernier FP, Boneh A, Dennett X, Chow CW, Cleary MA, Thorburn DR. Diagnostic criteria for respiratory chain disorders in adults and children. *Neurology* 2002; **59**: 1406–11.

14. Taylor RW, Schaefer AM, Barron MJ, McFarland R, Turnbull DM. The diagnosis of mitochondrial muscle disease. *Neuromuscul Disord* 2004; **14**: 237–45.

15. Hasegawa H, Matsuoka T, Goto Y, Nonaka I. Strongly succinate dehydrogenase-reactive blood vessels in muscles from patients with mitochondrial myopathy, encephalopathy, lactic acidosis, and stroke-like episodes. *Ann Neurol* 1991; **29**: 601–5.

16. Bernier FP, Boneh A, Dennett X, Chow CW, Cleary MA, Thorburn DR. Diagnostic criteria for respiratory chain disorders in adults and children. *Neurology* 2002; **59**: 1406–11.

17. Pfeffer G, Sirrs S, Wade NK, Mezei MM. Multisystem disorder in late-onset chronic progressive external ophthalmoplegia. *Can J Neurol Sci* 2011; **38**: 119–23.

18. Schaefer AM, Blakely EL, Griffiths PG, Turnbull DM, Taylor RW. Ophthalmoplegia due to mitochondrial DNA disease: the need for genetic diagnosis. *Muscle Nerve* 2005; **32**: 104–7.

19. Wibrand F, Jeppesen TD, Frederiksen AL, et al. Limited diagnostic value of enzyme analysis in patients with mitochondrial tRNA mutations. *Muscle Nerve* 2010; **41**: 607–13.

20. Medja F, Allouche S, Frachon P, et al. Development and implementation of standardized respiratory chain spectrophotometric assays for clinical diagnosis. *Mitochondrion* 2009; **9**: 331–9.

21. van den Heuvel LP, Smeitink JA, Rodenburg RJ. Biochemical examination of fibroblasts in the diagnosis and research of oxidative phosphorylation (OXPHOS) defects. *Mitochondrion* 2004; **4**: 395–401.

22. Rotig A, Appelkvist EL, Geromel V, et al. Quinone-responsive multiple respiratory-chain dysfunction due to widespread coenzyme Q10 deficiency. *Lancet* 2000; **356**: 391–5.

23. Ogasahara S, Engel AG, Frens D, Mack D. Muscle coenzyme Q deficiency in familial mitochondrial encephalomyopathy. *Proc Natl Acad Sci USA* 1989; **86**: 2379–82.

24. Tarnopolsky M. Exercise testing as a diagnostic entity in mitochondrial myopathies. *Mitochondrion* 2004; **4**: 529–542.

25. Dandurand RJ, Matthews PM, Arnold DL, Eidelman DH. Mitochondrial disease. Pulmonary function, exercise performance, and blood lactate levels. *Chest* 1995; **108**: 182–9.

26. Hammaren E, Rafsten L, Kreuter M, Lindberg C. Modified exercise test in screening for mitochondrial myopathies—adjustment of workload in relation to muscle strength. *Eur Neurol* 2004; **51**: 38–41.

27. Jeppesen TD, Olsen D, Vissing J. Cycle ergometry is not a sensitive diagnostic test for mitochondrial myopathy. *J Neurol* 2003; **250**: 293–9.

28. Jensen TD, Kazemi-Esfarjani P, Skomorowska E, Vissing J. A forearm exercise screening test for mitochondrial myopathy. *Neurology* 2002; **58**: 1533–8.

29. Taivassalo T, Abbott A, Wyrick P, Haller RG. Venous oxygen levels during aerobic forearm exercise: An index of impaired oxidative metabolism in mitochondrial myopathy. *Ann Neurol* 2002; **51**: 38–44.

30. Wortmann SB, Vaz FM, Gardeitchik T, et al. Mutations in the phospholipid remodeling gene SERAC1 impair mitochondrial function and intracellular cholesterol trafficking and cause dystonia and deafness. *Nat Genet* 2012; **44**: 797–802.

31. Galmiche L, Serre V, Beinat M, et al. Exome sequencing identifies MRPL3 mutation in mitochondrial cardiomyopathy. *Hum Mutat* 2011; **32**: 1225–31.

32. Tyynismaa H, Sun R, Ahola-Erkkila S, et al. Thymidine kinase 2 mutations in autosomal recessive progressive external ophthalmoplegia with multiple mitochondrial DNA deletions. *Hum Mol Genet* 2012; **21**: 66–75.

33. Wahbi K, Larue S, Jardel C, et al. Cardiac involvement is frequent in patients with the m.8344A>G mutation of mitochondrial DNA. *Neurology* 2010; **74**: 674–7.

34. Polak PE, Zijlstra F, Roelandt JR. Indications for pacemaker implantation in the Kearns–Sayre syndrome. *Eur Heart J* 1989; **10**: 281–2.

35. Bhati RS, Sheridan BC, Mill MR, Selzman CH. Heart transplantation for progressive cardiomyopathy as a manifestation of MELAS syndrome. *J Heart Lung Transplant* 2005; **24**: 2286–9.

36. Sinnathuray AR, Raut V, Awa A, Magee A, Toner JG. A review of cochlear implantation in mitochondrial sensorineural hearing loss. *Otol Neurotol* 2003; **24**: 418–26.

37. Read JL, Whittaker RG, Miller N, et al. Prevalence and severity of voice and swallowing difficulties in mitochondrial disease. *Int J Lang Commun Disord* 2012; **47**: 106–11.

38. Klopstock T, Yu-Wai-Man P, Dimitriadis K, et al. A randomized placebo-controlled trial of idebenone in Leber's hereditary optic neuropathy. *Brain* 2011; **134**: 2677–86.

39. Gempel K, Topaloglu H, Talim B, et al. The myopathic form of coenzyme Q10 deficiency is caused by mutations in the electron-transferring-flavoprotein dehydrogenase (ETFDH) gene. *Brain* 2007; **130**: 2037–44.

40. Jeppesen TD, Schwartz M, Olsen DB, et al. Aerobic training is safe and improves exercise capacity in patients with mitochondrial myopathy. *Brain* 2006; **129**: 3402–12.

41. Taivassalo T, De Stefano N, Argov Z, et al. Effects of aerobic training in patients with mitochondrial myopathies. *Neurology* 1998; **50**: 1055–60.

42. Taivassalo T, Gardner JL, Taylor RW, et al. Endurance training and detraining in mitochondrial myopathies due to single large-scale mtDNA deletions. *Brain* 2006; **129**: 3391–401.

43. Cejudo P, Bautista J, Montemayor T, et al. Exercise training in mitochondrial myopathy: a randomized controlled trial. *Muscle Nerve* 2005; **32**: 342–50.

44. Murphy JL, Blakely EL, Schaefer AM, et al. Resistance training in patients with single, large-scale deletions of mitochondrial DNA. *Brain* 2008; **131**: 2832–40.

45. Koga Y, Akita Y, Nishioka J, et al. L-arginine improves the symptoms of strokelike episodes in MELAS. *Neurology* 2005; **64**: 710–12.

46. Arakawa K, Kudo T, Ikawa M, et al. Abnormal myocardial energy-production state in mitochondrial cardiomyopathy and acute response to L-arginine infusion. C-11 acetate kinetics revealed by positron emission tomography. *Circ J* 2010; **74**: 2702–11.

47. Pfeffer G, Majamaa K, Turnbull DM, Thorburn D, Chinnery PF. Treatment for mitochondrial disorders. *Cochrane Database Syst Rev* 2012; **4**: CD004426.

48. Gimenes AC, Napolis LM, Silva NL, et al. The effect of L-carnitine supplementation on respiratory muscle strength and exercise tolerance in patients with mitochondrial myopathies [abstract]. *Eur Respir J* 2007; **51** (Suppl): 21S [E297].

49. Kornblum C, Schroder R, Muller K, et al. Creatine has no beneficial effect on skeletal muscle energy metabolism in patients with single mitochondrial DNA deletions: a placebo-controlled, double-blind 31P-MRS crossover study. *Eur J Neurol* 2005; **12**: 300–9.

50. Klopstock T, Querner V, Schmidt F, et al. A placebo-controlled crossover trial of creatine in mitochondrial diseases. *Neurology* 2000; **55**: 1748–51.

51. Tarnopolsky MA, Roy BD, MacDonald JR. A randomized, controlled trial of creatine monohydrate in patients with mitochondrial cytopathies. *Muscle Nerve* 1997; **20**: 1502–9.

52. Stacpoole PW, Kerr DS, Barnes C, et al. Controlled clinical trial of dichloroacetate for treatment of congenital lactic acidosis in children. *Pediatrics* 2006; **117**: 1519–31.

53. Bresolin N, Doriguzzi C, Ponzetto C, et al. Ubidecarenone in the treatment of mitochondrial myopathies: a multi-center double-blind trial. *J Neurol Sci* 1990; **100**: 70–8.

54. Mancuso M, Orsucci D, Logerfo A, et al. Oxidative stress biomarkers in mitochondrial myopathies, basally and after cysteine donor supplementation. *J Neurol* 2010; **257**: 774–81.

55. Kaufmann P, Engelstad K, Wei Y, et al. Dichloroacetate causes toxic neuropathy in MELAS: a randomized, controlled clinical trial. *Neurology* 2006; **66**: 324–30.

56. De Stefano N, Matthews PM, Ford B, Genge A, Karpati G, Arnold DL. Short-term dichloroacetate treatment improves indices of cerebral metabolism in patients with mitochondrial disorders. *Neurology* 1995; **45**: 1193–8.

57. Vissing J, Gansted U, Quistorff B. Exercise intolerance in mitochondrial myopathy is not related to lactic acidosis. *Ann Neurol* 2001; **49**: 672–6.

58. Duncan GE, Perkins LA, Theriaque DW, Neiberger RE, Stacpoole PW. Dichloroacetate therapy attenuates the blood lactate response to submaximal exercise in patients with defects in mitochondrial energy metabolism. *J Clin Endocrinol Metab* 2004; **89**: 1733–8.

59. Liet JM, Pelletier V, Robinson BH, et al. The effect of short-term dimethylglycine treatment on oxygen consumption in cytochrome oxidase deficiency: a double-blind randomized crossover clinical trial. *J Pediatr* 2003; **142**: 62–6.

60. Rodriguez MC, MacDonald JR, Mahoney DJ, Parise G, Beal MF, Tarnopolsky MA. Beneficial effects of creatine, CoQ10, and lipoic acid in mitochondrial disorders. *Muscle Nerve* 2007; **35**: 235–42.

61. Glover EI, Martin J, Maher A, Thornhill RE, Moran GR, Tarnopolsky MA. A randomized trial of coenzyme Q10 in mitochondrial disorders. *Muscle Nerve* 2010; **42**: 739–48.

62. Lin CM, Thajeb P. Valproic acid aggravates epilepsy due to MELAS in a patient with an A3243G mutation of mitochondrial DNA. *Metab Brain Dis* 2007; **22**: 105–9.

63. Krahenbuhl S, Brandner S, Kleinle S, Liechti S, Straumann D. Mitochondrial diseases represent a risk factor for valproate-induced fulminant liver failure. *Liver* 2000; **20**: 346–8.

64. McFarland R, Hudson G, Taylor RW, et al. Reversible valproate hepatotoxicity due to mutations in mitochondrial DNA polymerase gamma (POLG1). *Arch Dis Child* 2008; **93**: 151–3.

65. Stewart JD, Horvath R, Baruffini E, et al. Polymerase gamma gene POLG determines the risk of sodium valproate-induced liver toxicity. *Hepatology* 2010; **52**: 1791–6.

66. Venhoff N, Setzer B, Melkaoui K, Walker UA. Mitochondrial toxicity of tenofovir, emtricitabine and abacavir alone and in combination with additional nucleoside reverse transcriptase inhibitors. *Antivir Ther* 2007; **12**: 1075–85.

67. Ananworanich J, Nuesch R, Cote HC, et al. Changes in metabolic toxicity after switching from stavudine/didanosine to tenofovir/lamivudine—a Staccato trial substudy. *J Antimicrob Chemother* 2008; **61**: 1340–3.

68. Dinges WL, Witherspoon SR, Itani KM, Garg A, Peterson DM. Blepharoptosis and external ophthalmoplegia associated with long-term antiretroviral therapy. *Clin Infect Dis* 2008; **47**: 845–52.

69. Zannou DM, Azon-Kouanou A, Bashi BJ, et al. Mitochondrial toxicity: a case of palpebral ptosis in a woman infected by HIV and treated with HAART including zidovudine [in French]. *Bull Soc Pathol Exot* 2009; **102**: 97–8.

70. Pfeffer G, Cote HC, Montaner JS, Li CC, Jitratkosol M, Mezei MM. Ophthalmoplegia and ptosis: mitochondrial toxicity in patients receiving HIV therapy. *Neurology* 2009; **73**: 71–2.

71. Sirvent P, Bordenave S, Vermaelen M, et al. Simvastatin induces impairment in skeletal muscle while heart is protected. *Biochem Biophys Res Commun* 2005; **338**: 1426–34.

72. Bruckert E, Hayem G, Dejager S, Yau C, Begaud B. Mild to moderate muscular symptoms with high-dosage statin therapy in hyperlipidemic patients—the PRIMO study. *Cardiovasc Drugs Ther* 2005; **19**: 403–14.

73. Baker SK, Vladutiu GD, Peltier WL, Isackson PJ, Tarnopolsky MA. Metabolic myopathies discovered during investigations of statin myopathy. *Can J Neurol Sci* 2008; **35**: 94–7.

74. Elsais A, Lund C, Kerty E. Ptosis, diplopia and statins: an association? *Eur J Neurol* 2008; **15**: e90–e91.

75. Fraunfelder FW, Richards AB. Diplopia, blepharoptosis, and ophthalmoplegia and 3-hydroxy-3-methyl-glutaryl-CoA reductase inhibitor use. *Ophthalmology* 2008; **115**: 2282–5.

76. Yu-Wai-Man P, Griffiths PG, Hudson G, Chinnery PF. Inherited mitochondrial optic neuropathies. *J Med Genet* 2009; **46**: 145–58.

77. Kirkman MA, Yu-Wai-Man P, Korsten A, et al. Gene-environment interactions in Leber hereditary optic neuropathy. *Brain* 2009; **132**: 2317–26.

78. Palace J. Multiple sclerosis associated with Leber's hereditary optic neuropathy. *J Neurol Sci* 2009; **286**: 24–7.

79. Man PY, Griffiths PG, Brown DT, Howell N, Turnbull DM, Chinnery PF. The epidemiology of Leber hereditary optic neuropathy in the north east of England. *Am J Hum Genet* 2003; **72**: 333–9.

80. Lodi R, Carelli V, Cortelli P, et al. Phosphorus MR spectroscopy shows a tissue specific in vivo distribution of biochemical expression of the G3460A mutation in Leber's hereditary optic neuropathy. *J Neurol Neurosurg Psychiatry* 2002; **72**: 805–7.

81. Ortube MC, Bhola R, Demer JL. Orbital magnetic resonance imaging of extraocular muscles in chronic progressive external ophthalmoplegia: specific diagnostic findings. *J AAPOS* 2006; **10**: 414–18.

82. Saneto RP, Friedman SD, Shaw DW. Neuroimaging of mitochondrial disease. *Mitochondrion* 2008; **8**: 396–413.

83. DiMauro S, Hirano M. Mitochondrial DNA deletion syndromes. In: Pagon RA, Bird TD, Dolan CR, Stephens K, Adam MP (ed) *GeneReviews*™ [Internet] Seattle, WA: University of Washington, Seattle, **17** December 2003, updated 3 May 2011. Available at: <http://www.ncbi.nlm.nih.gov/books/NBK1203/>.

84. Rotig A, Cormier V, Blanche S, et al. Pearson's marrow-pancreas syndrome. A multisystem mitochondrial disorder in infancy. *J Clin Invest* 1990; **86**: 1601–8.

85. Kaufmann P, Engelstad K, Wei Y, et al. Protean phenotypic features of the A3243G mitochondrial DNA mutation. *Arch Neurol* 2009; **66**: 85–91.

86. Majamaa-Voltti K, Turkka J, Kortelainen ML, Huikuri H, Majamaa K. Causes of death in pedigrees with the 3243A>G mutation in mitochondrial DNA. *J Neurol Neurosurg Psychiatry* 2008; **79**: 209–11.

87. Ito H, Mori K, Kagami S. Neuroimaging of stroke-like episodes in MELAS. *Brain Dev* 2011; **33**: 283–8.

88. Sproule DM, Kaufmann P. Mitochondrial encephalopathy, lactic acidosis, and strokelike episodes: basic concepts, clinical phenotype, and therapeutic management of MELAS syndrome. *Ann NY Acad Sci* 2008; 1142: 133–58.

89. Silvestri G, Ciafaloni E, Santorelli FM, et al. Clinical features associated with the A→G transition at nucleotide 8344 of mtDNA ('MERRF mutation'). *Neurology* 1993; **43**: 1200–6.

90. Wahbi K, Larue S, Jardel C, et al. Cardiac involvement is frequent in patients with the m.8344A>G mutation of mitochondrial DNA. *Neurology* 2010; **74**: 674–7.

91. Shoffner JM, Lott MT, Lezza AM, Seibel P, Ballinger SW, Wallace DC. Myoclonic epilepsy and ragged-red fiber disease (MERRF) is associated with a mitochondrial DNA tRNA(Lys) mutation. *Cell* 1990; **61**: 931–7.

92. Thompson PD, Hammans SR, Harding AE. Cortical reflex myoclonus in patients with the mitochondrial DNA transfer RNA(Lys)(8344) (MERRF) mutation. *J Neurol* 1994; **241**: 335–40.

93. Finsterer J, Segall L. Drugs interfering with mitochondrial disorders. *Drug Chem Toxicol* 2010; **33**: 138–51.

94. Rahman S, Blok RB, Dahl HH, et al. Leigh syndrome: clinical features and biochemical and DNA abnormalities. *Ann Neurol* 1996; **39**: 343–51.

95. Arii J, Tanabe Y. Leigh syndrome: serial MR imaging and clinical follow-up. *Am J Neuroradiol* 2000; **21**: 1502–9.

96. Finsterer J. Leigh and Leigh-like syndrome in children and adults. *Pediatr Neurol* 2008; **39**: 223–35.

97. Kumakura A, Asada J, Okumura R, Fujisawa I, Hata D. Diffusion-weighted imaging in preclinical Leigh syndrome. *Pediatr Neurol* 2009; **41**: 309–11.

98. Debray FG, Lambert M, Lortie A, Vanasse M, Mitchell GA. Long-term outcome of Leigh syndrome caused by the NARP-T8993C mtDNA mutation. *Am J Med Genet A* 2007; **143A**: 2046–51.

99. McKelvie P, Infeld B, Marotta R, Chin J, Thorburn D, Collins S. Late-adult onset Leigh syndrome. *J Clin Neurosci* 2012; **19**: 195–202.

100. Holt IJ, Harding AE, Petty RK, Morgan-Hughes JA. A new mitochondrial disease associated with mitochondrial DNA heteroplasmy. *Am J Hum Genet* 1990; **46**: 428–33.

101. Ortiz RG, Newman NJ, Shoffner JM, Kaufman AE, Koontz DA, Wallace DC. Variable retinal and neurologic manifestations in patients harboring the mitochondrial DNA 8993 mutation. *Arch Ophthalmol* 1993; **111**: 1525–30.

102. Verny C, Guegen N, Desquiret V, et al. Hereditary spastic paraplegia-like disorder due to a mitochondrial ATP6 gene point mutation. *Mitochondrion* 2011; **11**: 70–5.

103. Craig K, Elliott HR, Keers SM, et al. Episodic ataxia and hemiplegia caused by the 8993T→C mitochondrial DNA mutation. *J Med Genet* 2007; **44**: 797–9.

104. Pfeffer G, Blakely EL, Alston CL, et al. Adult-onset spinocerebellar ataxia syndromes due to MTATP6 mutations. *J Neurol Neurosurg Psychiatry* 2012; **83**: 883–6.

105. Rahman S. Mitochondrial disease and epilepsy. *Dev Med Child Neurol* 2012; **54**: 397–406.

106. Van Goethem G, Martin JJ, Dermaut B, et al. Recessive POLG mutations presenting with sensory and ataxic neuropathy in compound heterozygote patients with progressive external ophthalmoplegia. *Neuromuscul Disord* 2003; **13**: 133–42.

107. Hirano M, Silvestri G, Blake DM, et al. Mitochondrial neurogastrointestinal encephalomyopathy (MNGIE): clinical, biochemical, and genetic features of an autosomal recessive mitochondrial disorder. *Neurology* 1994; **44**: 721–7.

108. Horvath R, Bender A, Abicht A, et al. Heteroplasmic mutation in the anticodon-stem of mitochondrial tRNA(Val) causing MNGIE-like gastrointestinal dysmotility and cachexia. *J Neurol* 2009; **256**: 810–15.

109. Tang S, Dimberg EL, Milone M, Wong LJ. Mitochondrial neurogastrointestinal encephalomyopathy (MNGIE)-like phenotype: an expanded clinical spectrum of POLG1 mutations. *J Neurol* 2012; **259**: 862–8.

110. Shaibani A, Shchelochkov OA, Zhang S, et al. Mitochondrial neurogastrointestinal encephalopathy due to mutations in RRM2B. *Arch Neurol* 2009; **66**: 1028–32.

111. Hirano M, Marti R, Casali C, et al. Allogeneic stem cell transplantation corrects biochemical derangements in MNGIE. *Neurology* 2006; **67**: 1458–60.

112. Filosto M, Scarpelli M, Tonin P, et al. Course and management of allogeneic stem cell transplantation in patients with mitochondrial neurogastrointestinal encephalomyopathy. *J Neurol* 2012; **259**: 2699–706.

113. Lara MC, Valentino ML, Torres-Torronteras J, Hirano M, Marti R. Mitochondrial neurogastrointestinal encephalomyopathy (MNGIE): biochemical features and therapeutic approaches. *Biosci Rep* 2007; **27**: 151–63.

114. Moran N, Bax BE, Bain MD. Erythrocyte entrapped thymidine phosphorylase (EE-TP) therapy for mitochondrial neurogastrointestinal encephalomyopathy (MNGIE). *J Neurol Neurosurg Psychiatry* 2012; **83**(e1): doi: 10.1136/jnnp-2011-301993.141.

115. Bourdon A, Minai L, Serre V, et al. Mutation of RRM2B, encoding p53-controlled ribonucleotide reductase (p53R2), causes severe mitochondrial DNA depletion. *Nat Genet* 2007; **39**: 776–80.

116. Saada A, Shaag A, Mandel H, Nevo Y, Eriksson S, Elpeleg O. Mutant mitochondrial thymidine kinase in mitochondrial DNA depletion myopathy. *Nat Genet* 2001; **29**: 342–4.

117. Sarzi E, Bourdon A, Chretien D, et al. Mitochondrial DNA depletion is a prevalent cause of multiple respiratory chain deficiency in childhood. *J Pediatr* 2007; **150**: 531–4, 534.e1–6.

118. Spinazzola A, Viscomi C, Fernandez-Vizarra E, et al. MPV17 encodes an inner mitochondrial membrane protein and is mutated in infantile hepatic mitochondrial DNA depletion. *Nat Genet* 2006; **38**: 570–5.

119. Ostergaard E, Christensen E, Kristensen E, et al. Deficiency of the alpha subunit of succinate-coenzyme A ligase causes fatal infantile lactic acidosis with mitochondrial DNA depletion. *Am J Hum Genet* 2007; **81**: 383–7.

120. Mandel H, Szargel R, Labay V, et al. The deoxyguanosine kinase gene is mutated in individuals with depleted hepatocerebral mitochondrial DNA. *Nat Genet* 2001; **29**: 337–41.

CHAPTER 31

Skeletal muscle channelopathies

Emma Matthews and Michael G. Hanna

The skeletal muscle channelopathies comprise a group of rare inherited neuromuscular disorders. They derive their name from the fact that each is due to dysfunction of an ion channel present in the sarcolemma of skeletal muscle. These ion channels regulate the electrical excitability of the muscle membrane such that in health muscle contraction and relaxation occur in a controlled and timely manner in response to appropriate stimulation.

The skeletal muscle channelopathies can be divided into two broad groups. In the first the predominant problem is an inexcitable muscle membrane that manifests clinically as episodes of severe muscle weakness or paralysis. This group is known as the periodic paralyses. In the second, the muscle membrane is hyperexcitable, observed clinically as myotonia (delayed muscle relaxation after contraction). This group is known as the non-dystrophic myotonias.

The periodic paralyses

The inherited periodic paralyses consist of three disorders: hypokalaemic periodic paralysis, hyperkalaemic periodic paralysis, and Andersen–Tawil syndrome. The exact incidence of the periodic paralyses is unknown but hypokalaemic periodic paralysis is thought to be the most common with an estimated incidence of 1 in 100 000 [1] and Andersen–Tawil syndrome the rarest of the three [2].

A fourth entity, normokalaemic periodic paralysis, has previously been described in the literature. Fluctuations in serum potassium levels during paralytic attacks are what originally gave rise to the distinction of hypokalaemic periodic paralysis and hyperkalaemic periodic paralysis. Although rising or decreasing serum potassium levels do occur these can be mild and the absolute value does not always fall outwith the normal range. As a result, taken in isolation, a serum potassium level is not always helpful diagnostically. With the availability of genetic testing many cases of reported normokalaemic periodic paralysis have subsequently been shown to be sodium channel disorders, and thus a form of hyperkalaemic periodic paralysis [3].

Hypokalaemic periodic paralysis

Hypokalaemic periodic paralysis is characterized by episodes of flaccid skeletal muscle paralysis associated with low serum potassium levels during the attack. As a result precipitators to attacks include factors that will lower serum potassium, e.g. eating a large carbohydrate meal or rest after exertion. It can present at any age

from the first to the third decade [4] but typically will present in the teenage years. The paralysis affects skeletal muscle, predominantly the limb muscles, although occasionally respiratory muscles may be involved [5,6]. Attacks usually take place during the night or early morning and last for several hours or even days (see Table 31.1). In severe cases attacks may last weeks and in some it is several months before full muscle strength is completely restored. Hypokalaemic periodic paralysis does not affect cardiac muscle directly but low serum potassium levels in the ictal phase may cause secondary cardiac dysfunction [5,7,8].

Thyrotoxic periodic paralysis

This is a rare but important differential for hypokalaemic periodic paralysis. It is a condition in which attacks of muscle paralysis that are clinically indistinguishable from hypokalaemic periodic paralysis occur in the presence of thyrotoxicosis. The elevation of thyroid hormones may be relatively mild without any obvious symptoms or signs of thyrotoxicosis, so it is important to have a high index of suspicion for this condition [9]. It is most common amongst Asian males, usually between the ages of 20 and 40 years. Treatment of the thyroid dysfunction will prevent any further attacks of paralysis. This was considered to be a sporadic condition, but recent evidence has indicated a genetic component in a significant number of cases [10].

Hyperkalaemic periodic paralysis

Hyperkalaemic periodic paralysis is characterized by episodes of skeletal muscle weakness in association with high serum potassium levels. Precipitating factors include ingestion of potassium-rich foods, particularly fruits, e.g. tomatoes and bananas. As with hypokalaemic periodic paralysis onset can be at any age from the first to the third decade but is typically younger than in hypokalaemic periodic paralysis, most frequently presenting in the first decade [4]. Attacks of skeletal muscle weakness are also shorter, commonly lasting minutes to hours, and occurring at any time of the day [2].

In addition to muscle weakness or paralysis, myotonia can occur in hyperkalaemic periodic paralysis. Myotonia is delayed muscle relaxation after contraction, and this will often be described as a feeling of stiffness in the muscles with or without myalgia. Hyperkalaemic periodic paralysis is primarily a paralytic disorder, however, and while myotonia may occur it is not the predominant feature. As such, patients may not spontaneously complain of symptoms suggestive of myotonia or will mention them as minimal, and

Table 31.1 Clinical features of the periodic paralyses

	Hyperkalaemic periodic paralysis	Hypokalaemic periodic paralysis	Andersen–Tawil syndrome
Causative gene	SCN4A	CACNA1S, SCN4A	KCNJ2
Inheritance	Autosomal dominant	Autosomal dominant	Autosomal dominant
Episodic skeletal muscle paralysis	Yes	Yes	Yes
Duration of paralysis	Commonly minutes to hours	Commonly hours to days	Variable, minutes to days
Ictal potassium levels	High	Low	Low, high, or normal
Precipitators of paralysis	Potassium-rich foods, rest after exercise	Large carbohydrate load, rest after exercise	Dependent on ictal potassium
Typical time of attacks	Any time of day	During night or early morning	Any—dependant on ictal potassium
Cardiac conduction defects	Only those attributable to severe hyperkalaemia; resolve with restoration of normal potassium values	Only those attributable to severe hypokalaemia; resolve with restoration of normal potassium values	Common, especially abnormal u waves, prolonged QUc interval, and ventricular arrhythmias, irrespective of potassium levels
Dysmorphic features	No	No	Common, especially short stature, mandibular hypoplasia, clinodactyly, and low-set ears

if hyperkalaemic periodic paralysis is suspected it is important to enquire about these.

As with hypokalaemic periodic paralysis, hyperkalaemic periodic paralysis does not inherently affect cardiac muscle but arrhythmia may be precipitated by the ictal phase of raised serum potassium.

Andersen–Tawil syndrome

Andersen–Tawil syndrome comprises a triad of episodic skeletal muscle paralysis, dysmorphic features, and cardiac conduction defects [11,12]. Two out of three features are considered adequate for clinical diagnosis. It is the only skeletal muscle channelopathy to directly affect organs other than skeletal muscle. The paralysis is most commonly of a hypokalaemic periodic paralysis phenotype but normal or high potassium levels have been reported during attacks [13]. The dysmorphic features can include mandibular micrognathia, short stature, clinodactyly, syndactyly, hypertelorism or hypotelorism, low-set ears, a broad forehead, and a high arched palate [11–14] but can be very subtle and easily missed, e.g. the patient may not strike you as of particularly short stature when they attend clinic by themselves but it is important to ask how they compare in height to other members of their family.

Likewise there are often no cardiac symptoms, and unless an ECG is performed for unrelated circumstances or a diagnosis of Andersen–Tawil syndrome is considered the cardiac conduction defects are often undetected. For these reasons hypokalaemic periodic paralysis may be the only obvious presentation and some individuals may be clinically misdiagnosed. This can have significant consequences because, although rare, sudden death may occur [12–15]. Conduction defects described include abnormal u waves, a prolonged QUc interval, a prolonged QTc interval, bigeminy, and bidirectional VT.

Clinical examination in the periodic paralyses

The periodic paralyses are episodic disorders. Commonly the clinical examination of a patient with periodic paralysis is performed on a day when no symptoms and consequently no signs are present. However, it is useful to specifically consider some pertinent features:

♦ In between attacks the examination is typically normal.

♦ Are there any dysmorphic features? Is this a case of Andersen–Tawil syndrome?

♦ Is there any evidence of myotonia, e.g. lid lag, delayed eye opening after forceful closure, or delayed hand opening after forceful grip?

♦ If presenting some years after the first onset of symptoms, a proximal myopathy may be present.

♦ Are there any features of thyrotoxicosis?

If a patient is examined during an attack, it is a flaccid paralysis or weakness that occurs, with loss of deep tendon reflexes. Vague sensory symptoms are occasionally reported but sensory loss on examination is not in keeping with a diagnosis of periodic paralysis and if present reflects an alternative or additional pathology.

Investigations

Blood tests

Routine haematological and biochemical tests are generally unremarkable with the exception of deranged intra-ictal potassium levels and occasionally raised serum creatine kinase.

Serum potassium levels are characteristically low during an attack of muscle weakness in hypokalaemic periodic paralysis and elevated in hyperkalaemic periodic paralysis. The potassium value can increase or decrease with respect to the baseline, but may remain ultimately within the normal range. For this reason it is ideal to record a potassium level before, during, and after an attack but this is seldom feasible in clinical practice.

Creatine kinase may be chronically elevated in the periodic paralyses [16] but the increase is generally modest (<1000 IU L^{-1}) and values above this raise suspicion of other aetiologies.

Periodic paralysis associated with thyrotoxicosis is most common in Asian populations [9] but thyroid function tests should always be undertaken as it is important not to miss this treatable disease.

Electrophysiological testing

Basic electrophysiological testing can provide additional clues to a diagnosis of periodic paralysis, including the presence of myotonia in hyperkalaemic periodic paralysis and non-specific myopathic features. The ability to diagnose periodic paralysis is significantly improved by the use of more advanced neurophysiological techniques including short and long (McManis) exercise tests [17,18]. The exercise tests in essence are designed to 'exercise' or 'work' the muscles to establish if an episode of abnormal muscle weakness can be produced. This is usually done by asking the patient to abduct their little finger against resistance, and is reflected electrophysiologically by recording a decline in the compound muscle action potential (CMAP) amplitude of abductor digit minimi.

As a general guide, in the periodic paralyses there is no significant reduction in CMAP during the short exercise test. The long exercise or McManis test is usually positive in the periodic paralyses (Fig. 31.1), although a minority of patients with a genetically confirmed diagnosis can have a normal test [19]. A positive McManis test is defined as a 40% or greater reduction in CMAP. Although useful in diagnosing periodic paralysis per se a positive McManis test generally does not differentiate between hypokalaemic periodic paralysis, hyperkalaemic periodic paralysis, or Andersen–Tawil syndrome. There are minor differences between the groups electrophysiologically, particularly in the short exercise test, but this is often only performed in specialist centres [19].

Detailed electrophysiological testing undoubtedly enhances the ability to diagnose periodic paralysis and in specialist centres may point towards the specific subgroup, but these are ultimately not diagnostic tests. It must also be considered that a McManis test can take up to 50 min to perform which can limit its usefulness due to lack of resources or patient inability to tolerate the test.

Genetic testing

Hypokalaemic periodic paralysis can be caused by dysfunction of one of two voltage-gated ion channels that reside in the skeletal muscle membrane. The majority of cases are due to abnormal functioning of the dihydropyridine receptor (voltage-gated calcium channel, $Ca_V1.1$) which is coded for by the *CACNA1S* gene [20,21]. A minority of cases are caused by dysfunction of the voltage-gated sodium channel, $Na_V1.4$, coded for by the *SCN4A* gene [22]. Up to 90% of cases of hypokalaemic periodic paralysis occur due to mutations in specific portions of either $Ca_V1.1$ or $Na_V1.4$ known as the 'voltage sensors' [23]. As a result routine diagnostic genetic analysis may only include these portions.

Hyperkalaemic periodic paralysis is a sodium channel disorder due to mutations in the *SCN4A* gene. Certain mutations are common, e.g. T704M, but mutations can be found throughout the length of the gene and diagnostic testing should analyse all coding regions if common mutations are not initially identified.

Andersen–Tawil syndrome occurs due to mutations of the *KCNJ2* gene which codes for the voltage-gated inward rectifying potassium channel, $K_{ir}2.1$ [24]. Genetic testing is the diagnostic test for these disorders but a minority of patients do not have a mutation in any of these genes, suggesting that undiscovered disease-causing genes may exist.

All of the primary periodic paralyses are autosomal dominant disorders, i.e. only one abnormal gene copy is required for clinical manifestation of the disease. The children of affected patients will each have a 50% chance of inheriting the mutant gene. A lack of positive family history may occur in sporadic cases where neither parent may be affected or with the phenomenon of reduced penetrance [4,25,26]. In these cases a patient or one of their parents will appear to be clinically unaffected but genetic testing will confirm they have a mutation. They may not complain of any symptoms of periodic paralysis but sometimes they will have dismissed vague symptoms such as occasional myalgia or minimal temporary weakness, and it is important to consider their history carefully. Even if clinically asymptomatic a McManis test can be positive. Ultimately, a lack of positive family history should not deter one from a diagnosis of periodic paralysis.

Other investigations

Prior to widely available electrophysiological and genetic testing, provocative tests were used in the diagnosis of the periodic paralyses. These aimed to induce either a hypokalaemic or hyperkalaemic state with observable paralysis by infusing either intravenous

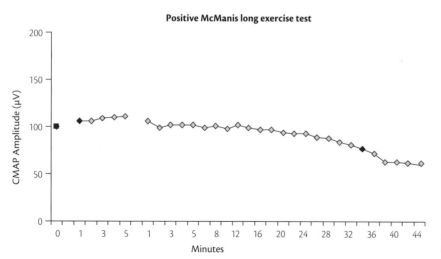

Positive McManis long exercise test

Fig. 31.1 Example of a positive McManis test in a patient with hypokalaemic periodic paralysis.

insulin/glucose or potassium. These tests were performed in hospital under close monitoring but the risks of inducing an aberrant potassium level are not insignificant.

Muscle biopsies were also frequently performed in the past. Non-specific changes including vacuolar formation and tubular aggregates lend support to a diagnosis [4] but are not specific to these disorders and do not differentiate between the subgroups of periodic paralysis.

Neither provocative testing nor muscle biopsy is currently necessary or recommended in the investigation of a patient with possible periodic paralysis.

Treatment

Symptom severity is very variable in the periodic paralyses. If mild, patients may opt to manage their symptoms by lifestyle modification and the avoidance of precipitating factors alone. None of the treatments used in the periodic paralyses have been subjected to large-scale randomized controlled trials [27]. However, if treatment is considered necessary, available therapies for hypokalaemic periodic paralysis include potassium supplements or potassium-sparing diuretics such as spironolactone. Thiazide diuretics may be beneficial in hyperkalaemic periodic paralysis. Inhaled salbutamol if taken at the onset of a hyperkalaemic attack may help to abort it or limit its duration [28].

Carbonic anhydrase inhibitors including acetazolamide or dichlorphenamide are the mainstay of treatment for all the periodic paralyses, although the mechanism of therapeutic benefit is unknown. Acetazolamide use can be limited by paraesthesia. There is some evidence in hypokalaemic periodic paralysis that the specific genotype may influence treatment response and that a small subgroup of patients may not respond to acetazolamide or even find it detrimental [29]. This emphasizes the importance of obtaining a genetic diagnosis where possible. Carbonic anhydrase inhibitors are reported to reduce the severity, duration, or frequency of paralytic attacks [30]. The natural history of these disorders, however, is that the frequency of attacks does tend to diminish with increasing age which allows scope for considering an attempt to withdraw therapy if desired. There are some case reports of carbonic anhydrase inhibitors inhibiting the development of proximal myopathy, but this is not substantiated [31]. Carbonic anhydrase inhibitors can be associated with the development of renal calculi, and renal ultrasound screening is recommended on an annual basis.

The periodic paralysis of Andersen–Tawil syndrome can be treated using the same therapies. Any cardiological treatment is determined by electrocardiogram (ECG) changes or the presence of arrhythmia on ambulatory testing and cardiac symptoms. Specialist cardiology advice is essential. Pharamacological control of ventricular arrhythmias can be difficult, although flecainide is commonly used [32]. Whilst drug treatment may reduce the frequency of arrhythmia, however, there is no evidence it prevents sudden death [33]. Implantable devices may be needed.

The mainstay of treatment of thyrotoxic periodic paralysis is to induce a euthyroid state as this will abolish the associated paralytic attacks [9].

Treatment of acute attacks of paralysis

Total body potassium during an attack of muscle weakness is normal but the distribution is displaced, e.g. in hypokalaemic periodic paralysis the serum potassium is low because the majority of potassium ions are being held intracellularly. This is an important consideration as equilibrium will be restored by the body as the attack diminishes. Thus if potassium supplementation is given in an attack of hypokalaemic periodic paralysis a subsequent high serum potassium level may be induced and could have adverse cardiac consequences [34].

Replacing or attempting to reduce serum potassium levels should only be considered if there are detrimental ECG changes during an attack of muscle weakness, or there is weakness of respiratory muscles leading to respiratory failure (a rare event). ECG and serum potassium monitoring are mandatory.

Development of future therapies

Recent anecdotal evidence suggests that despite being regarded as the mainstay of treatment for hypokalaemic periodic paralysis acetazolamide is only effective in 50–60% of patients [29]. The efficacy in hyperkalaemic periodic paralysis is not known. A trial is currently open comparing dichlorphenamide with placebo in both hypo- and hyperkalaemic periodic paralysis. Recent studies into the pathomechanism of hypokalaemic periodic paralysis took note of the specificity of mutations to the voltage sensors of the dysfunctional ion channel, and an aberrant ion current has been shown to be produced by these mutations [35–37]. Future therapies may target and block this current, but at present none with this action exist. A secondary consequence of the dysfunctional calcium or sodium channels in hypokalaemic periodic paralysis is to reduce the inward rectifying potassium channel current; early preliminary studies did suggest that potassium channel activators may be beneficial but development of these as a therapy has never really advanced [38].

The non-dystrophic myotonias

The non-dystrophic myotonias comprise three disorders: paramyotonia congenita, sodium channel myotonia (including potassium- and cold-aggravated myotonias), and myotonia congenita. The predominant symptom in each is myotonia, although variable muscle weakness or paralysis can additionally occur (see Table 31.2). Unlike myotonic dystrophy none of these disorders have systemic features. The exact incidence is unknown but estimates range from 1 in 100 000 to 7 in 100 000 [39].

Paramyotonia congenita

Eulenberg first described paramyotonia congenita in 1886. It is a sodium channel disorder due to mutations in the *SCN4A* gene but is considered separately from the sodium channel myotonias due to the presence of episodic muscle weakness, which differentiates it from this group. Symptoms can be present from birth and parents may note facial myotonia, especially if the infant is washed with cool water [40]. Symptoms are generally noted by the patient themselves within their first decade [41,42], often when they attend primary school. Characteristic symptoms are myotonia, especially of the hand and facial muscles, that is exacerbated by a cold environment or by repetitive muscle action. Conversely a warm environment often alleviates the myotonia and there is frequently a seasonal variation to the severity of the disease. Cold is the most significant exacerbator of the myotonia, and most patients will volunteer this when asked what makes their symptoms worse. A common story is struggling to change clothes in a cold changing room

Table 31.2 Common clinical features and electrophysiological patterns of the subgroups of non-dystrophic myotonia

	Recessive myotonia congenita	Dominant myotonia congenita	Paramyotonia congenita	Sodium channel myotonia
Inheritance	Recessive	Dominant	Dominant	Dominant
Causative gene	CLCN1	CLCN1	SCN4A	SCN4A
Myotonia distribution	Lower limbs more than upper limbs	Upper limbs more than lower limbs. Facial muscles may be involved	Upper limbs and face more than lower limbs	Upper limbs, face, extraocular, more than lower limbs
Myotonia cold sensitivity	None or minimal	None or minimal	Yes—often dramatic	Variable—ranging from none to severe
Warm-up phenomenon	Present	Present	Absent	May be present
Paradoxical myotonia	Absent	Absent	Present	May be present
Delayed onset myotonia after exercise*	Absent	Absent	Absent	May be present. Characteristic of myotonia fluctuans
Episodic muscle weakness	Common, develops on initiation of movement but transient and improves rapidly	Uncommon	Common, often exacerbated by cold and/or exercise and frequently prolonged for several hours	Not reported
Eyelid myotonia	Infrequent	Infrequent	Common	Common
SET without cooling	Early decrement in CMAP with rapid recovery. Decrement reduces with repetition	Little or no decrement in CMAP	Gradual and persistent reduction in CMAP enhanced by repetition	No significant change of the CMAP from baseline†
SET with cooling	Cooling has little further effect	Early decrement with rapid recovery and reduction with repetition may be seen	Gradual and persistent reduction in CMAP enhanced further by cooling	No significant change of the CMAP from baseline†
Fournier pattern	II	II/III	I	III

*Myotonia typically develops after a short period of exercise, e.g. 10 min, or on resting after a period of exercise.
†Note: this same pattern may be observed in dominant MC.
SET, short exercise test; CMAP, compound muscle action potential. This is re-used with permission from: The non-dystrophic myotonias: molecular pathogenesis, diagnosis and treatment. Matthews E, Fialho D, Tan SV, Venance SL, Cannon SC, Sternberg D, Fontaine B, Amato AA, Barohn RJ, Griggs RC, Hanna MG; CINCH Investigators. Brain. 2010 Jan;133(Pt 1):9–22

after swimming in a cool pool because their hands were stiff (due to myotonia).

The myotonia itself generally resolves within 1–2 min (although it may take longer on a cold day) but a muscle that has been afflicted can subsequently become weak or even paralysed for several hours. Terms commonly used to describe the myotonic symptoms include the muscle feeling 'stiff' or 'stuck'. Sometimes it is hard for the patient to accurately define the symptom, and descriptors may be vaguer including 'a feeling that the muscles don't work properly'. Myalgia is relatively common and can occur exclusively with the myotonia or in isolation.

The sodium channel myotonias

This can be the hardest group of the non-dystrophic myotonias to characterize. The key feature is that they are purely myotonic disorders and muscle weakness or paralysis does not occur. They are due to mutations of the same gene as paramyotonia congenita (the SCN4A gene). Symptoms also can be present from birth and usually within the first decade. The myotonia predominantly affects the face and hand muscles as with paramyotonia congenita, but the legs are more frequently affected than in paramyotonia congenita [39]. In contrast, while the myotonia may be exacerbated by repetition it may also *improve* with repetition, displaying the 'warm up'

phenomenon [42] that at one time was thought to exclusively characterize myotonia congenita. Many individual phenotypes have been described that now collectively come under the umbrella term 'sodium channel myotonia'. These include the potassium-aggravated myotonias (acetazolamide-responsive myotonia congenita [43,44], myotonia fluctuans [45,46], and myotonia permanens [47,48]). The myotonia of the potassium-aggravated myotonias is significantly exacerbated by potassium ingestion but not by a cold environment. Other phenotypes are cold sensitive [49,50].

Overall the age of onset and distribution of myotonia is generally similar to that in paramyotonia congenita although the lower limbs can be more significantly affected. The myotonia itself displays overlapping features of paramyotonia congenita and myotonia congenita in that it can be paradoxical or display warm up. Exacerbating factors can include potassium and/or cold but may vary.

Myotonia congenita

The age of onset of myotonia congenita is commonly also in the first decade, although it can be a few years later than paramyotonia congenita [42]. Overall there is a relatively wide spectrum from the first to the fourth decade. The distribution of myotonia also varies, and lower limbs tend to be most severely affected. Affected patients may also have a 'Herculean' appearance due to muscle hypertrophy, and this is often best seen in the calves [51]. It is important to enquire about physical activity because the significance of a muscular physique may be overlooked in young patients if it is assumed that it reflects an active lifestyle. The typical feature of the myotonia is the warm up phenomenon where it can be seen to improve with repetitive muscle action. The myotonia is often worst when attempting to move after a period of rest, and a typical description includes rising from a seat on public transport but missing the stop due to being unable to 'move fast enough' to get off before the doors close. A transient muscle weakness can also occur after a period of rest and for unknown reasons this also improves with activity. A cold environment may exacerbate the myotonia of myotonia congenita but this is variable and it is not as prominent as in paramyotonia congenita.

Myotonia congenita is the only skeletal muscle channelopathy that can be inherited in either a dominant (Thomson disease [52]) or recessive manner (Becker disease [53]), both involving the voltage-gated chloride channel ClC-1. Symptoms of the recessive form tend to be more severe, and of earlier onset, than the dominant form [51]. Transient weakness is often absent in dominant cases and it can be very difficult to differentiate this clinically from sodium channel myotonia.

In all of the non-dystrophic myotonia subgroups, as with the periodic paralyses, a proximal myopathy can develop [53–55].

Clinical examination of the non-dystrophic myotonias

On general inspection a muscular physique may be evident, commonly in the calves and beyond what would be expected for the patient's level of physical activity. The myotonia that occurs in the non-dystrophic myotonias is sensitive to changes in temperature. This is most obvious and pronounced in paramyotonia congenita but can apply to any of the subgroups. Nearly always there is some evidence of myotonia when the patient is examined but if examined in the summer in a hot clinic room it can rarely be absent or, more likely, minimal and missed by an inexperienced physician [41]. A proximal myopathy may be present.

The myotonia is best seen by examining for lid lag, myotonia of orbicularis oculi, hand grip myotonia, and percussion myotonia of the thenar eminence. If present each muscle action should be repeated two or three times at least to establish if the myotonia is improving (warm up) with repetition or worsening. Another useful way of assessing this is to ask the patient to rise from a chair, walk across the clinic room, sit down, and then repeat the exercise. In myotonia congenita they can be particularly stiff and slow when first attempting to rise from the chair and walk but this can be seen to become easier and they walk more quickly with each attempt.

A more formal timed 10-m walk can be performed, but in practice this is usually reserved for clinical trials.

There are a number of general points to consider when examining a patient displaying myotonia:

- In paramyotonia congenita the myotonia is paradoxical and will worsen with repetitive muscle action.

- In myotonia congenita the myotonia will display a warm-up phenomenon and improve with repetitive muscle action.

- In sodium channel myotonia the myotonia may be paradoxical or show warm up or display both features.

- If a cold environment is volunteered as a severe precipitating factor for the myotonia this suggests paramyotonia congenita.

- If the patient has a muscular physique, consider myotonia congenita.

- By far and away the commonest cause of myotonia is myotonic dystrophy. In mild cases the myotonia may be pronounced but dystrophic features (i.e. weakness) are absent.

Investigations

Blood tests

In general blood tests have no specific role in the investigation of non-dystrophic myotonia. The serum creatine kinase, as in the periodic paralyses, may be minimally raised, but is generally less than 1000 IU L^{-1} [51,54,56]. Very high levels suggest an alternative or additional pathology.

Electrophysiological tests

Basic testing is useful to confirm the presence of myotonia. More advanced neurophysiological techniques include the short and long exercise tests. In the periodic paralyses, the long exercise test is the most helpful. In the non-dystrophic myotonias it is the short exercise test that provides the most information. To be fully informative this test must be performed three times (repeat short exercise test) at room temperature and then repeated with the hand cooled to 20ºC by being placed in iced water.

If performed in this way, specific patterns emerge, termed Fournier patterns I, II, and III [57,58] (see Fig. 31.2). The repeat short exercise test is a test of muscle strength (not myotonia) and reflects electrophysiologically what the patient describes and what can often be demonstrated clinically.

- Pattern I: a fall in CMAP (reflecting muscle weakness) that is progressively worse with each repetition and enhanced further if the muscle is cooled. This pattern is seen in paramyotonia congenita.

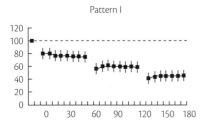
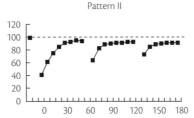
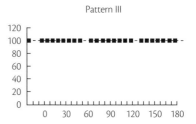

Fig. 31.2 Illustrations of the electromyograph patterns described in typical examples of each of the non-dystrophic myotonia subgroups. (Modified with permission from *Annals of Neurology* 2006.)

♦ Pattern II: a fall in CMAP (reflecting an initial muscle weakness) that rapidly recovers—the change becomes less evident with each repetition (reflecting an improvement in muscle strength each time). This is indicative of myotonia congenita, particularly the recessive form.

♦ Pattern III: no change in CMAP from the baseline during any of the repetitions or when the muscle is cooled (reflecting an absence of muscle weakness). This pattern is seen in sodium channel myotonia and sometimes in dominant myotonia congenita.

These are useful techniques but are not always readily available outside of specialist centres. Also these are the patterns seen in typical examples of each subgroup but there can be significant overlap and variability so they are not diagnostic in isolation.

Genetic testing

Two genes are routinely tested in the non-dystrophic myotonias. The *CLCN1* gene codes for the voltage-gated chloride channel ClC-1. This is dysfunctional in myotonia congenita [59,60]. Myotonia congenita is the only skeletal muscle channelopathy to be inherited in either an autosomal dominant or autosomal recessive fashion. Mutations of the *SCN4A* gene are responsible for paramyotonia congenita and sodium channel myotonia [47,48]. These are both autosomal dominant disorders. Mutations occur throughout the length of both genes and ideally the entire gene requires sequencing if a diagnosis of non-dystrophic myotonia is suspected. Gene 'hotspots' do exist, however, for *SCN4A* (exons 22 and 24) and initial sequencing of just these two exons will capture the majority of cases of paramyotonia congenita and sodium channel myotonia.

There is significant overlap of both the clinical and EMG features of sodium channel myotonia and dominant myotonia congenita. A useful clue to help in differentiation can be eyelid myotonia.

It can occur in either condition but is more indicative of sodium channel myotonia and would direct sequencing to *SCN4A* first [19,42]. However, if either of these conditions is suspected and gene sequencing of one gene is negative the other gene should be screened. When present, the systemic features and distal weakness of myotonic dystrophy Type 1 (DM1) allow for easy distinction from the non-dystrophic myotonias. Early presentations of DM1, however, in the teenager or young adult (i.e. at a similar age to when patients with non-dystrophic myotonia may first come to medical attention), may only demonstrate myotonia without weakness or systemic features. Myotonic dystrophy is covered elsewhere but a diagnosis of DM1 or DM2 should always be considered if myotonia congenita is suspected and genetic analysis is negative (see Fig. 31.3).

Treatment

As with the periodic paralyses, some patients will opt for lifestyle modification and the avoidance of factors that provoke myotonia as much as possible rather than consider pharmacological therapies. There are no currently available drugs that directly target the dysfunctional ClC-1 channel in myotonia congenita. There is a lack of evidence form randomized controlled trials for any of the available therapies and recommendations are based upon case reports and clinical experience [61].

Currently the first line drugs are the Class I antiarrhythmics. Although there is a lack of trial evidence, benefit from both flecainide and propafenone has been described in case studies [62,63]. However, the most effective and tolerated drug seems to be mexiletine. Although it is a sodium channel blocker it is also reported to have benefit in myotonia congenita [64]. There is further evidence of its effectiveness as an antimyotonic agent in DM1 patients [65].

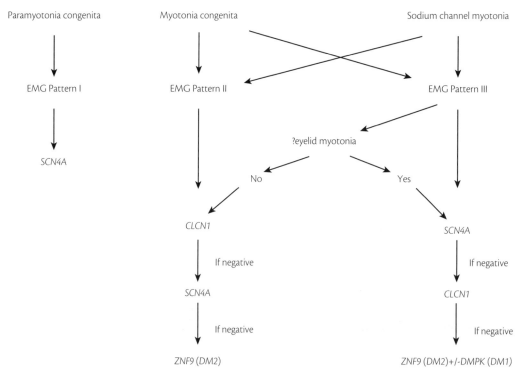

Fig. 31.3 Diagnostic algorithm for combining clinical diagnosis with electrophysiological results to assist genetic analysis. Disease-causing genes are *SCN4A*, *CLCN1*, *ZNF9*, and *DMPK*; EMG, electromyograph; DM1/2, myotonic dystrophy Type 1/2. (Modified with permission from *Annals of Neurology* 2011.)

A randomized double-blind placebo-controlled clinical trial of mexiletine in non-dystrophic myotonia is currently under way. As with all antiarrhymics, mexiletine can also be pro-arrhythmic and an ECG and cardiac history should be taken prior to commencing treatment. If there is any uncertainty over its safe use in an individual, cardiological review should be sought.

Despite being a favoured treatment for non-dystophic myotonia, mexiletine is not a first-line antiarrhythmic agent. In 2009, the only manufacturer with a licence to supply mexiletine in the UK ceased production as overall demand for the drug was low. It is still manufactured in Canada, and special arrangements can be made via UK hospital pharmacies for mexiletine to be imported for supply to patients with non-dystrophic myotonia. Even in Canada, however, there is a risk that manufacture may cease in the future. As a result, some of the other Class I antiarrhythmics, e.g. flecainide, may become increasingly used instead, although cardiotoxicity may limit their use in certain patients.

There are small series and case reports describing benefit from the carbonic anhydrase inhibitor acetazolamide [43,66] which is widely used as a treatment for periodic paralysis. This is not generally the first choice for the non-dystrophic myotonias but may be tried if other therapies are ineffective or if antiarrhythmics are contraindicated.

Historical treatments have included quinine, procainamide, prednisolone, phenytoin, and lignocaine but none of these are currently recommended. Tocainide, a lignocaine derivative, seemed a promising therapy but was withdrawn from the market following reports of potentially fatal agranulocytosis [39].

Development of future therapies

Several possibilities for newer therapies are on the horizon. Analogues of tocainide have shown promising results *in vitro* and remain an area for potential development if the side effect profile is acceptable. Techniques targeting dysfunctional ClC-1 channels are also being explored, including exon skipping, *trans*-splicing, and protein trafficking [39].

Preganancy and labour in the skeletal muscle channelopathies

There is some evidence that hormones may detrimentally influence the severity of symptoms in the skeletal muscle channelopathies [67]. Symptoms are often reported as being more severe during pregnancy. The skeletal muscle channelopathies themselves have no adverse effect on fetal development, although some consideration may be given to the risk of injury should an attack of muscle paralysis or myotonia provoke a fall.

There is no absolute contraindication to a spontaneous vaginal delivery and many women with skeletal muscle channelopathies do give birth this way successfully. There is a small risk that the stress of labour, particularly if it is prolonged, may provoke an attack of muscle weakness or paralysis, so overall while a trial of labour may be attempted, prolonged labour should be avoided.

Neonatal complications of paramyotonia congenita and sodium channel myotonia

Since Eulenberg's first description of paramyotonia congenita it has been recognized that infants can display myotonia. In recent years more significant neonatal presentations have been reported. The most significant includes a fatal case that involved myotonia of the respiratory muscles with the infant ultimately dying from respiratory failure [68]. Other cases of severe laryngospasm and stridor have subsequently emerged [69,70]. All these cases had different *SCN4A* mutations and no specific phenotype–genotype link was evident. Importantly there was generally a positive response to treatment with mexiletine.

A less severe phenotype of neonatal hypotonia with variable feeding and respiratory difficulties has been described in a number of families all carrying the same *SCN4A* mutation, I693T [71]. These infants were floppy at birth or within 24 h of delivery. Some required nasogastric tube feeding as they were unable to adequately suckle. Respiratory compromise was generally mild and supplemental oxygen only was given. With this supportive care, all cases spontaneously improved.

It is important to be aware of neonatal or infantile presentations of non-dystrophic myotonia in order to counsel expectant mothers (including unaffected partners of affected males) appropriately and to provide essential information to the relevant paediatric and obstetric teams who may be involved.

Overall, labour in skeletal muscle channelopathy should be considered of relatively high risk and managed in a centre that has appropriate senior obstetric, paediatric, and anaesthetic services available.

Natural history and morbidity

In all the skeletal muscle channelopathies there is a decline in the frequency of paralytic or myotonic attacks with increasing age. Patients often find it harder to define discrete episodes of muscle weakness but may still report fluctuations in muscle strength. A fixed proximal myopathy of varying severity commonly develops. This may be sufficiently mild that the patient is not functionally limited and it is only evident on clinical examination, or severe enough for a wheelchair and home modification to be required. Whether the myopathy that develops is directly related to the number or severity of attacks of muscle paralysis or myotonia is not clear, although evidence suggests it may not be [16,72]. Consequently it is unclear if treatment aimed at reducing these attacks would have any effect on minimizing the development of myopathy. There is some anecdotal evidence that carbonic anhydrase inhibitors may prevent myopathy, but the mechanism by which they may do this is unclear and this benefit is unsubstantiated. It will be important to clarify this issue as many patients opt for non-pharmacological management of their symptoms. However, if current (or future) therapies can minimize myopathy, regardless of their effect on episodic symptoms, this would direct advice regarding the initiation of therapy.

There are virtually no data available on the morbidity or effect on quality of life of the skeletal muscle channelopathies. It is not infrequent that it takes years for a diagnosis to be made and many patients will have been to multiple clinics, often being mislabelled with fibromyalgia or non-organic illness. Emerging evidence suggests that pain is an under-recognized feature in the non-dystrophic myotonias that requires more consideration [73]. Pain may occur with myotonia or in isolation, but as at least some of the pain is usually linked to myotonia it is likely that this aspect will respond to mexiletine therapy although there is no trial evidence currently available to support this.

Practical issues are often also overlooked. Cold is such a severe exacerbator of symptoms in paramyotonia congenita that some patients dread the winter months and have their central heating on for the majority of the time. This can cause significant expense for which they may be able to receive financial aid.

References

1. Fontaine B. Primary periodic paralysis and muscle sodium channel. *Adv Nephrol Necker Hosp* 1994; **23**: 191–7.

2. Venance SL, Cannon SC, Fialho D, et al. The primary periodic paralyses: diagnosis, pathogenesis and treatment. *Brain* 2006; **129**: 8–17.

3. Chinnery PF, Walls TJ, Hanna MG, Bates D, Fawcett PR. Normokalemic periodic paralysis revisited: does it exist? *Ann Neurol* 2002; **52**: 251–2.

4. Miller TM, as da Silva MR, Miller HA, et al. Correlating phenotype and genotype in the periodic paralyses. *Neurology* 2004; **63**: 1647–55.

5. Kil TH, Kim JB. Severe respiratory phenotype caused by a de novo Arg528Gly mutation in the CACNA1S gene in a patient with hypokalemic periodic paralysis. *Eur J Paediatr Neurol* 2010; **14**: 278–81.

6. Arzel-Hezode M, Sternberg D, Tabti N, et al. Homozygosity for dominant mutations increases severity of muscle channelopathies. *Muscle Nerve* 2010; **41**: 470–7.

7. Kim JB, Lee KY, Hur JK. A Korean family of hypokalemic periodic paralysis with mutation in a voltage-gated calcium channel (R1239G). *J Korean Med Sci* 2005; **20**: 162–5.

8. Hecht ML, Valtysson B, Hogan K. Spinal anesthesia for a patient with a calcium channel mutation causing hypokalemic periodic paralysis. *Anesth Analg* 1997; **84**: 461–4.

9. Kung AW. Clinical review: thyrotoxic periodic paralysis: a diagnostic challenge. *J Clin Endocrinol Metab* 2006; **91**: 2490–5.

10. Ryan DP, da Silva MR, Soong TW, et al. Mutations in potassium channel Kir2.6 cause susceptibility to thyrotoxic hypokalemic periodic paralysis. *Cell* 2010; **140**: 88–98.

11. Andersen ED, Krasilnikoff PA, Overvad H. Intermittent muscular weakness, extrasystoles, and multiple developmental anomalies. A new syndrome? *Acta Paediatr Scand* 1971; **60**: 559–64.

12. Tawil R, Ptacek LJ, Pavlakis SG, et al. Andersen's syndrome: potassium-sensitive periodic paralysis, ventricular ectopy, and dysmorphic features. *Ann Neurol* 1994; **35**: 326–30.

13. Davies NP, Imbrici P, Fialho D, et al. Andersen–Tawil syndrome: new potassium channel mutations and possible phenotypic variation. *Neurology* 2005; **65**: 1083–9.

14. Haruna Y, Kobori A, Makiyama T, et al. Genotype-phenotype correlations of KCNJ2 mutations in Japanese patients with Andersen–Tawil syndrome. *Hum Mutat* 2007; **28**: 208.

15. Zhang L, Benson DW, Tristani-Firouzi M, et al. Electrocardiographic features in Andersen–Tawil syndrome patients with KCNJ2 mutations: characteristic T-U-wave patterns predict the KCNJ2 genotype. *Circulation* 2005; **111**: 2720–6.

16. Links TP, Zwarts MJ, Wilmink JT, Molenaar WM, Oosterhuis HJ. Permanent muscle weakness in familial hypokalaemic periodic paralysis. Clinical, radiological and pathological aspects. *Brain* 1990; **113**: 1873–89.

17. Streib EW SSYT. Transient paresis in myotonic syndromes: a simplified electrophysiologic approach. *Muscle Nerve* 1982; **5**: 719–23.

18. McManis PG, Lambert EH, Daube JR. The exercise test in periodic paralysis. *Muscle Nerve* 1986; **9**: 704–10.

19. Tan SV, Matthews E, Barber M, et al. Refined exercise testing can aid DNA-based diagnosis in muscle channelopathies. *Ann Neurol* 2011; **69**: 328–40.

20. Ptacek LJ, Tawil R, Griggs RC, et al. Dihydropyridine receptor mutations cause hypokalemic periodic paralysis. *Cell* 1994; **77**: 863–8.

21. Jurkat-Rott K, Lehmann-Horn F, Elbaz A, et al. A calcium channel mutation causing hypokalemic periodic paralysis. *Hum Mol Genet* 1994; **3**: 1415–19.

22. Bulman DE, Scoggan KA, van Oene MD, et al. A novel sodium channel mutation in a family with hypokalemic periodic paralysis. *Neurology* 1999; **53**: 1932–6.

23. Matthews E, Labrum R, Sweeney MG, et al. Voltage sensor charge loss accounts for most cases of hypokalemic periodic paralysis. *Neurology* 2009; **72**: 1544–7.

24. Plaster NM, Tawil R, Tristani-Firouzi M, et al. Mutations in Kir2.1 cause the developmental and episodic electrical phenotypes of Andersen's syndrome. *Cell* 2001; **105**: 511–19.

25. Elbaz A, Vale-Santos J, Jurkat-Rott K, et al. Hypokalemic periodic paralysis and the dihydropyridine receptor (CACNL1A3): genotype/phenotype correlations for two predominant mutations and evidence for the absence of a founder effect in 16 caucasian families. *Am J Hum Genet* 1995; **56**: 374–80.

26. Fouad G, Dalakas M, Servidei S, et al. Genotype–phenotype correlations of DHP receptor alpha 1-subunit gene mutations causing hypokalemic periodic paralysis. *Neuromuscul Disord* 1997; **7**: 33–8.

27. Sansone V, Meola G, Links TP, Panzeri M, Rose MR. Treatment for periodic paralysis. *Cochrane Database Syst Rev* 2008; **1**: CD005045.

28. Hanna MG, Stewart J, Schapira AH, Wood NW, Morgan-Hughes JA, Murray NM. Salbutamol treatment in a patient with hyperkalaemic periodic paralysis due to a mutation in the skeletal muscle sodium channel gene (SCN4A). *J Neurol Neurosurg Psychiatry* 1998; **65**: 248–50.

29. Matthews E, Portaro S, Ke Q, et al. Acetazolamide efficacy in hypokalemic periodic paralysis and the predictive role of genotype. *Neurology* 2011; **77**: 1960–4.

30. Tawil R, McDermott MP, Brown R, Jr, et al. Randomized trials of dichlorphenamide in the periodic paralyses. Working Group on Periodic Paralysis. *Ann Neurol* 2000; **47**: 46–53.

31. Griggs RC, Engel WK, Resnick JS. Acetazolamide treatment of hypokalemic periodic paralysis. Prevention of attacks and improvement of persistent weakness. *Ann Intern Med* 1970; **73**: 39–48.

32. Sansone V, Tawil R. Management and treatment of Andersen–Tawil syndrome (ATS). *Neurotherapeutics* 2007; **4**: 233–7.

33. Tristani-Firouzi M, Etheridge SP. Kir 2.1 channelopathies: the Andersen–Tawil syndrome. *Pflugers Arch* 2010; **460**: 289–94.

34. Ahmed I, Chilimuri SS. Fatal dysrhythmia following potassium replacement for hypokalemic periodic paralysis. *West J Emerg Med* 2010; **11**: 57–9.

35. Sokolov S, Scheuer T, Catterall WA. Gating pore current in an inherited ion channelopathy. *Nature* 2007; **446**: 76–8.

36. Struyk AF, Cannon SC. A Na+ channel mutation linked to hypokalemic periodic paralysis exposes a proton-selective gating pore. *J Gen Physiol* 2007; **130**: 11–20.

37. Cannon SC. Voltage-sensor mutations in channelopathies of skeletal muscle. *J Physiol* 2010; **588**: 1887–95.

38. Matthews E, Hanna MG. Muscle channelopathies: does the predicted channel gating pore offer new treatment insights for hypokalaemic periodic paralysis? *J Physiol* 2010; **588**: 1879–86.

39. Matthews E, Fialho D, Tan SV, et al. The non-dystrophic myotonias: molecular pathogenesis, diagnosis and treatment. *Brain* 2010; **133**: 9–22.

40. Eulenberg A. Ueber eine Familiäre, durch 6 Generationen verfolbare form Congenitaler Paramyotonie. *Neurol Centralblatt* 1886; **12**: 265–72.

41. Matthews E, Tan SV, Fialho D, et al. What causes paramyotonia in the United Kingdom? Common and new SCN4A mutations revealed. *Neurology* 2008; **70**: 50–3.

42. Trip J, Drost G, Ginjaar HB, et al. Redefining the clinical phenotypes of non-dystrophic myotonic syndromes. *J Neurol Neurosurg Psychiatry* 2009; **80**: 647–52.

43. Trudell RG, Kaiser KK, Griggs RC. Acetazolamide-responsive myotonia congenita. *Neurology* 1987; **37**: 488–91.

44. Ptacek LJ, Tawil R, Griggs RC, et al. Sodium channel mutations in acetazolamide-responsive myotonia congenita, paramyotonia

congenita, and hyperkalemic periodic paralysis. *Neurology* 1994; **44**: 1500–3.

45. Ricker K, Lehmann-Horn F, Moxley RT, III. Myotonia fluctuans. *Arch Neurol* 1990; **47**: 268–72.

46. Ricker K, Moxley RT, III, Heine R, Lehmann-Horn F. Myotonia fluctuans. A third type of muscle sodium channel disease. *Arch Neurol* 1994; **51**: 1095–102.

47. McClatchey AI, Van den Burgh P, Pericak-Vance MA, et al. Temperature-sensitive mutations in the III–IV cytoplasmic loop region of the skeletal muscle sodium channel gene in paramyotonia congenita. *Cell* 1992; **68**: 769–74.

48. Lerche H, Heine R, Pika U, et al. Human sodium channel myotonia: slowed channel inactivation due to substitutions for a glycine within the III–IV linker. *J Physiol* 1993; **470**: 13–22.

49. Heine R, Pika U, Lehmann-Horn F. A novel SCN4A mutation causing myotonia aggravated by cold and potassium. *Hum Mol Genet* 1993; **2**: 1349–53.

50. Koch MC, Baumbach K, George AL, Ricker K. Paramyotonia congenita without paralysis on exposure to cold: a novel mutation in the SCN4A gene (Val1293Ile). *Neuroreport* 1995; **6**: 2001–4.

51. Fialho D, Schorge S, Pucovska U, et al. Chloride channel myotonia: exon 8 hot-spot for dominant-negative interactions. *Brain* 2007; **130**: 3265–74.

52. Thomsen J. Tonische Krampfe in willkurlich beweglichen Muskeln in Folge von ererbter psychischer Disposition. *Arch Psychiatr Nervenkrankheit* 1876; **6**: 702–18.

53. Becker PE. *Myotonia Congenita and Syndromes Associated with Myotonia*. Stuttgart: Georg Thieme Verlag, 1977.

54. Plassart E, Eymard B, Maurs L, et al. Paramyotonia congenita: genotype to phenotype correlations in two families and report of a new mutation in the sodium channel gene. *J Neurol Sci* 1996; **142**: 126–33.

55. Nagamitsu S, Matsuura T, Khajavi M, et al. A 'dystrophic' variant of autosomal recessive myotonia congenita caused by novel mutations in the CLCN1 gene. *Neurology* 2000; **55**: 1697–703.

56. Colding-Jorgensen E, Duno M, Vissing J. Autosomal dominant monosymptomatic myotonia permanens. *Neurology* 2006; **67**: 153–5.

57. Fournier E, Arzel M, Sternberg D, et al. Electromyography guides toward subgroups of mutations in muscle channelopathies. *Ann Neurol* 2004; **56**: 650–61.

58. Fournier E, Viala K, Gervais H, et al. Cold extends electromyography distinction between ion channel mutations causing myotonia. *Ann Neurol* 2006; **60**: 356–65.

59. George AL, Jr, Crackower MA, Abdalla JA, Hudson AJ, Ebers GC. Molecular basis of Thomsen's disease (autosomal dominant myotonia congenita). *Nat Genet* 1993; **3**: 305–10.

60. Koch MC, Steinmeyer K, Lorenz C, et al. The skeletal muscle chloride channel in dominant and recessive human myotonia. *Science* 1992; **257**: 797–800.

61. Trip J, Drost G, van Engelen BG, Faber CG. Drug treatment for myotonia. *Cochrane Database Syst Rev* 2006; **1**: CD004762.

62. Rosenfeld J, Sloan-Brown K, George AL, Jr. A novel muscle sodium channel mutation causes painful congenital myotonia. *Ann Neurol* 1997; **42**: 811–14.

63. Alfonsi E, Merlo IM, Tonini M, et al. Efficacy of propafenone in paramyotonia congenita. *Neurology* 2007; **68**: 1080–1.

64. Leheup B, Himon F, Morali A, Brichet F, Vidailhet M. [Value of mexiletine in the treatment of Thomsen–Becker myotonia]. *Arch Fr Pediatr* 1986; **43**: 49–50.

65. Logigian EL, Martens WB, Moxley RT, et al. Mexiletine is an effective antimyotonia treatment in myotonic dystrophy type 1. *Neurology* 2010; **74**: 1441–8.

66. Ferriby D, Stojkovic T, Sternberg D, Hurtevent JF, Hurtevent JP, Vermersch P. A new case of autosomal dominant myotonia associated with the V1589M missense mutation in the muscle sodium channel gene and its phenotypic classification. *Neuromuscul Disord* 2006; **16**: 321–4.

67. Fialho D, Kullmann DM, Hanna MG, Schorge S. Non-genomic effects of sex hormones on CLC-1 may contribute to gender differences in myotonia congenita. *Neuromuscul Disord* 2008; **18**: 869–72.

68. Gay S, Dupuis D, Faivre L, et al. Severe neonatal non-dystrophic myotonia secondary to a novel mutation of the voltage-gated sodium channel (SCN4A) gene. *Am J Med Genet A* 2008; **146**: 380–3.

69. Lion-Francois L, Mignot C, Vicart S, et al. Severe neonatal episodic laryngospasm due to de novo SCN4A mutations: a new treatable disorder. *Neurology* 2010; **75**: 641–5.

70. Matthews E, Manzur AY, Sud R, Muntoni F, Hanna MG. Stridor as a neonatal presentation of skeletal muscle sodium channelopathy. *Arch Neurol* 2011; **68**: 127–9.

71. Matthews E, Guet A, Mayer M, et al. Neonatal hypotonia can be a sodium channelopathy: recognition of a new phenotype. *Neurology* 2008; **71**: 1740–2.

72. Buruma OJ, Bots GT. Myopathy in familial hypokalaemic periodic paralysis independent of paralytic attacks. *Acta Neurol Scand* 1978; **57**: 171–9.

73. Trip J, de Vries J, Drost G, Ginjaar HB, van Engelen BG, Faber CG. Health status in non-dystrophic myotonias: close relation with pain and fatigue. *J Neurol* 2009; **256**: 939–47.

CHAPTER 32

Idiopathic inflammatory myopathies

Marianne de Visser and Anneke J. van der Kooi

Introduction

Classification

There is ongoing controversy about the classification of idiopathic inflammatory myopathies (IIM). In 1975, Bohan and Peter were the first to establish diagnostic criteria for polymyositis (PM) and dermatomyositis (DM) [1]. Their criteria for polymyositis included the following:

1. symmetrical weakness of the limb-girdle muscles worsening across weeks and months;

2. elevated activity of serum creatine kinase;

3. the electromyographic triad of small-amplitude, short-duration polyphasic motor unit action potentials; fibrillations, positive sharp waves, and increased insertional irritability; and spontaneous, bizarre high-frequency discharges; and

4. muscle biopsy abnormalities (i.e. degeneration and regeneration of muscle fibres, necrosis, phagocytosis, perifascicular atrophy, and an interstitial infiltrate of mononuclear cells).

According to these criteria, skin features, i.e. lilac discoloration of the eyelids, a Gottron sign, and erythematous dermatitis of the knees, elbows, upper part of the torso, face, and neck, were the only distinction between DM and PM. Sporadic inclusion body myositis (sIBM) was first reported in 1971 [2].

In the 1980s Engel and Arahata observed that in both PM and sIBM non-necrotic muscle fibres are injured by autoinvasive T8+ cells that act in concert with macrophages [3]. In 1995 diagnostic criteria mainly relying on histopathological features were proposed for sIBM [4]. For a diagnosis of definite sIBM the patient should exhibit the following features: inflammatory myopathy characterized by mononuclear cell invasion of non-necrotic muscle fibres, vacuolated muscle fibres, and amyloid deposits within muscle fibres.

The Bohan and Peter criteria were found to have a low specificity and therefore fail to distinguish IIM from sIBM and non-inflammatory myopathies, including limb muscular dystrophies with a similar distribution of weakness, e.g. dysferlinopathies which may be associated with cellular infiltrates [5,6]. In addition, the concept of PM as such was challenged, since the histopathological picture was considered to be very rare [7,8].

Over the years, IIM had been classified by rheumatologists according to the Bohan and Peter criteria and by neurologists on the basis of histopathological and immunohistochemical findings [3]. A recent attempt to reconcile these two classifications was made during a workshop under the auspices of the European Neuromuscular Centre (ENMC) [9] in which two immune-mediated disease entities were also added to PM, DM, and sIBM, namely necrotizing autoimmune myopathy (NAM) and non-specific or overlap myositis. Both are only present in adults and have subacute or insidious onset, progressive symmetrical proximal weakness, no skin abnormalities, and elevated serum creatine kinase (CK) activity. In NAM serum CK is usually grossly increased. NAM is distinguished from the other IIMs by the absence of prominent inflammatory infiltrates and with macrophages rather than T-cells being the effector cells [10]. Because NAM is potentially amenable to treatment, it is important to distinguish NAM from other causes of muscle necrosis, such as rhabdomyolysis, muscular dystrophies, endocrinopathies, medications, and toxins. Non-specific or overlap myositis shows perivascular, perimysial inflammatory cell infiltrates or scattered CD8+ T-cells that do not clearly surround or invade muscle fibres [7,8]. The ENMC classification also includes the entity of amyopathic dermatomyositis, in the past also termed 'dermatomyositis sine myositis' and now recognized as 'clinically amyopathic dermatomyositis' (CADM) (11).

In a study aimed at assessing the performance of the ENMC criteria against the main previously published criteria [1,12–14] using the specialist consultant diagnosis as the gold standard, the ENMC criteria were found to be more specific for IIM than the older classification criteria but had the lowest sensitivity due to stringent exclusion criteria [6]. Figure 32.1 depicts the current classification taking all these considerations into account.

In 2011 Pestronk took another view on the classification of IIM by describing the light microscopic findings and correlating these with the clinical picture [15].

Pathogenesis

By definition, the causes of the IIMs remain unknown. Evidence supporting a role for the immune system in the pathogenesis of IIMs includes the findings that some patients have multiple autoimmune disorders [16], autoantibodies are characteristic of certain phenotypes [17], T-cell-mediated myocytotoxicity or complement-mediated microangiopathy is seen in particular clinical phenotypes [18], polymorphic immune response genes are primary genetic risk factors [19], and immunotherapies often result in a clinical response. Data from similar autoimmune diseases support the hypothesis that these conditions result from chronic immune activation after exposure to environmental risk factors in individuals with a predisposing genetic background [20,21].

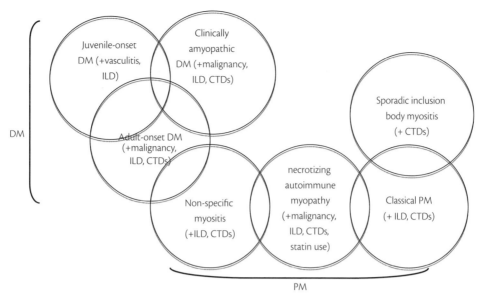

Fig. 32.1 Classification of the idiopathic inflammatory myopathies based on clinical and histopathological features, and associated disorders: DM, dermatomyositis; PM, polymyositis; CTD, connective tissue disorder; ILD, interstitial lung disease.

Different IIM phenotypes

Dermatomyositis (Box 32.1)

Clinical features

DM is characterized by a rash which occurs (months) prior to or together with muscle weakness. The onset of weakness is typically

---

Box 32.1 A case of dermatomyositis

A 48-year-old woman was referred because of progressive muscle weakness over 8 months. Subsequently she developed a skin rash and dysphagia and she complained of myalgia and arthralgia. At the time of referral she was barely able to climb stairs and she fell frequently.

Three months prior to referral she was diagnosed with breast cancer, for which she underwent surgery followed by radiotherapy and chemotherapy.

On examination she was found to have characteristic skin changes, including heliotrope erythema in the face, Gottron papules (Fig. 32.2a) and V-sign (Fig. 32.2b).

She had a dropped head due to weakness of the neck extensor muscle, and in addition the neck flexors and proximal muscles of the arms and legs were affected (varying from Medical Research Council grade 2 to 4). She had a waddling gait and a positive Gowers sign. There was limited mobility in the shoulder joints.

Since the dermatological features were characteristic we refrained from ancillary investigations and a diagnosis of dermatomyositis was established.

Prednisone, 100 mg per day, was prescribed for 6 weeks and subsequently the medication was tapered. In addition she received osteoporosis prophylaxis.

She came quickly into remission and did not relapse when the prednisone was further tapered. However, she developed painful calcifications at various sites of the legs.

---

subacute (over several weeks), although it can develop abruptly (over days) or insidiously (over months) [22]. Children are more likely to present with an insidious onset of muscle weakness and myalgias, often preceded by fatigue and low-grade fever. The five weakest muscle groups for all three IIM clinical groups, including DM, juvenile (J) DM and PM, are the hip flexors, hip extensors, hip abductors, neck flexors, and shoulder abductors. Patients with JDM have the least overall weakness among the three clinical groups. Neck flexors are the weakest muscle group in JDM [23].

Characteristic skin manifestations include a heliotropic (purple) periorbital oedema, erythematous dermatitis over the dorsum of the hands (Gottron papules or macules; Fig. 32.2a) and below the knee (the Gottron sign), and an erythematous rash on the face, neck, and anterior chest (V sign) (Fig. 32.2b) or back and shoulders (shawl sign). Periungual telangiectasia may be evident.

Dysphagia is observed in about 30% of the cases. Involvement of the pharyngeal and tongue muscles may result in dysarthria or speech delay in children [22].

Childhood-onset DM can be associated with vasculopathy of the gut leading to gastrointestinal bleeding.

Interstitial lung disease (ILD) complicates at least 10% of adult DM and can also occur in childhood cases [22]. ILD may lead to life-threatening complications, i.e. ventilatory failure, secondary pulmonary arterial hypertension, or cor pulmonale. It has been shown that once pulmonary involvement is recognized in DM, the 5-year mortality rate ranges from 0 to 55% [24].

Nearly 60% of ILD patients have antisynthetase syndrome. Antisynthetase syndrome is a unique clinical syndrome which includes myositis, ILD, non-erosive arthritis, fever, and mechanic's hands (the skin on the hands and fingers is dry and cracked) [25].

Calcifications in the subcutaneous tissues occur in 25% of children but are uncommon in adults with DM [21]. Cutaneous calcinosis tends to develop over pressure points (buttocks, knees, elbows) and presents as painful, hard nodules [22]. Myalgia is a frequently occurring symptom in both JDM and PM. Rhabdomyolysis can rarely occur with dermatomyositis [26].

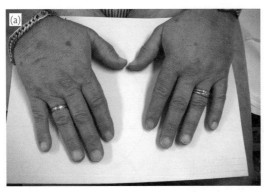 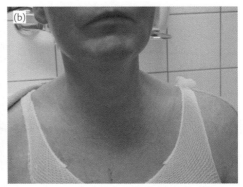

Fig. 32.2 (a) Characteristic skin feature in a patient with dermatomyositis: erythematous dermatitis over the dorsum of the hands (Gottron papules or macules). (b) Characteristic skin feature in a patient with dermatomyositis: erythematous rash on the face, neck, and anterior chest (V sign). (See also figure in colour plate section)

In CADM or dermatomyositis sine myositis [11] patients do not develop muscle weakness. A proportion of these patients develop classical DM in which the skin features concur with muscle weakness. As in classical DM, CADM may be associated with ILD. CADM can also occur in children. In general, juvenile-onset CADM seems to carry a low risk of developing systemic involvement and has a good prognosis.

There is an increased incidence for an underlying malignancy in adult DM (and also CADM) ranging from 6–45%, and thus DM can be considered as a paraneoplastic condition [7,27–30]. While detection of an underlying neoplasm can precede or follow the diagnosis of DM, most malignancies are identified within 3 years of the presentation of myositis. All types of malignancy, including lymphomas and solid tumours, can be found. Patients should be screened for the presence of ovarian, lung, breast, and gastrointestinal cancer by detailed history, physical examination, and imaging studies of chest, abdomen, and pelvis after the diagnosis has been established and annually for 3 years after diagnosis.

Diagnosis

In patients with characteristic skin features (Gottron papules/sign in combination with heliotrope erythema or Gottron papules/sign or heliotrope erythema in combination with erythema at specific sites of the body) the clinical picture suffices and no ancillary investigations have to be performed since specificity is 90.7–99.6% and sensitivity 62–74.2% [13].

Serum CK activity

Serum CK activity is elevated in 20–90% of DM patients, varying from two to more than ten times the normal value [12,30]. Patients with the classical form of DM more often have elevated serum CK than patients with amyopathic DM.

Myositis-specific autoantibodies (MSAs)

MSAs are directed to specific proteins found in both the nuclear and cytoplasmic regions of the cell. Anti-Mi-2 autoantibodies occur exclusively in patients with dermatomyositis (in 20–30% of adult patients) and are associated with mild muscle involvement, rashes in the V-region of the neck and over the shoulders in a shawl distribution, and cuticular overgrowth [31]. These antibodies are found in 6% of JDM patients [31a]. The anti-155/140 (transcriptional intermediary factor 1-gamma, TIF1-γ) autoantibody, though highly specific for DM, is found in approximately 15% of DM patients. Anti-155/140 (TIF1-γ) positive patients have a markedly higher rate of malignancy than DM patients who are negative for this antibody [32,33]. Interestingly, anti-155/140 (TIF1-γ) is also found in patients with JDM (23%), which is remarkable because the presence of other MSAs in JDM is rare and JDM is never associated with malignancy. Instead JDM patients with anti-155/140 (TIF1-γ) autoantibodies had significantly more cutaneous involvement (Gottron papules, ulceration and oedema) [34]. Anti-CADM-140 (melanoma differentiation-associated gene 5, MDA5) antibody is highly specific to CADM and is associated with rapidly progressive ILD in a Japanese population [35].

Electromyography

EMG is usually abnormal in active myositis but the findings are not specific. Short-duration, low-amplitude polyphasic action potentials can be found in almost 100% of patients with DM, PM, and sIBM, and 75% of patients have fibrillations and positive sharp waves. Long-duration motor unit potentials have been found in all three diagnostic groups and were not associated with disease duration [36]. These findings in conjunction with the frequent spontaneous activity may cause confusion and may be interpreted as consistent with a neurogenic disorder.

EMG can be helpful in distinguishing between a relapse of DM or PM and steroid myopathy, since spontaneous muscle fibre activity is not found in steroid myopathy [37].

Neuroimaging

MRI can demonstrate muscular oedema by showing areas of high signal intensity on short TI inversion recovery (STIR) (Fig. 32.3) and fat-suppressed T_2-weighted sequences, even in clinically asymptomatic muscles [38].

Skin biopsy

Skin biopsy is a relatively easy diagnostic procedure. Examination of a skin biopsy can support the diagnosis of dermatitis associated with dermatomyositis, and it can be helpful in the differential diagnosis with systemic lupus erythematosus (SLE) [39,40]. It should be taken from affected skin, and for comparison from normal skin as well. Small to moderate size mononuclear T-cell (CD4+) cellular infiltrates, vacuolization of basal keratocytes, upper dermal oedema, and epidermal atrophy are observed. All these changes and deposition of membrane attack complex (MAC) near the dermo-epidermal junction can also occur in SLE. The distinction between DM and SLE is the immunoglobulin deposit at the dermo-epidermal junction—the so-called lupus band test—in SLE, not DM, and the occlusion and reduction in the number of capillaries in DM, not SLE.

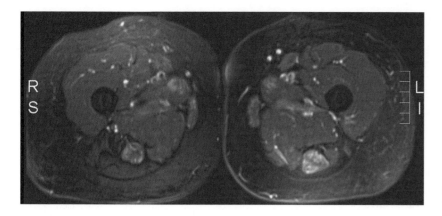

Fig. 32.3 Magnetic resonance image showing areas of high signal intensity on fat-suppressed T_2-weighted sequences in the thigh muscles of a patient with dermatomyositis.

Muscle biopsy

In patients with DM skin abnormalities, muscle biopsies demonstrate inflammatory infiltrates, mainly CD4+ T-cells, macrophages, plasmacytoid dendritic cells, and B-cells, which are confined to the perimysium (Fig. 32.4a), often around blood vessels, perifascicular muscle fibre atrophy (Fig. 32.4b), and scattered necrotic and regenerating muscle fibres [3,41–44]. Major histocompatibility complex type I (MHC I) is upregulated in perifascicular muscle fibres.

The earliest demonstrable histological abnormality in DM is deposition of the C5b-9 complement MAC on small blood vessels [42,43,45]. MAC precedes inflammation and other structural abnormalities in the muscle on light microscopy and is specific for DM. The subsequent necrosis of vessels results in a reduction in the capillary density (the number of capillaries per area of muscle) [43]. Microtubular inclusion in the endothelial cells, which can be observed at the ultrastructural level, is another early abnormality which may occur when the muscle tissue is relatively preserved

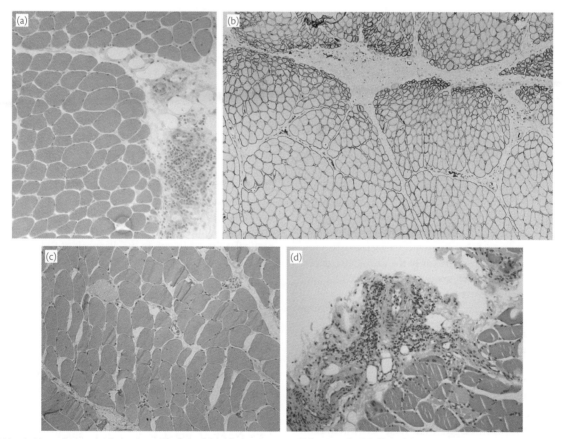

Fig. 32.4 (a) Muscle biopsy (haematoxylin–eosin stain) of an adult with dermatomyositis showing a large infiltrate of mononuclear cells in the perimysium and around the microvasculature. (b) Muscle biopsy (spectrin stain) from a child with dermatomyositis showing perifascicular muscle fibre atrophy. (c) Muscle biopsy (haematoxylin–eosin stain) of an adult with necrotizing autoimmune myopathy showing scattered necrotic muscle fibres sometimes undergoing phagocytosis. (d) Muscle biopsy of a patient with the antisynthetase syndrome showing a histological picture similar to that of dermatomyositis with mononuclear cell infiltrates at the perimysial site and surrounding blood vessels. In the perifascicular region necrotizing and regenerating muscle fibres are present. (See also figure in colour plate section)

[43]. Perifascicular atrophy is usually a late phenomenon and is more often seen in children than in adults.

Muscle biopsy is normal or shows non-specific changes in 10–20% of patients, even in those with clinically active disease. False negative findings may be due to sampling error caused by the scattered distribution of cell infiltrates, even if clinically affected muscles are chosen as biopsy sites [46–48].

Polymyositis (Boxes 32.2 and 32.3)

Clinical features

The term polymyositis is derived from the Greek word 'poly' which means 'many', thus 'inflammation of many muscles'. The clinical picture resembles that of DM except for the dermatological features which are absent in PM. There seem to be three subgroups of PM which all manifest with subacute onset of progressive proximal muscle weakness, and are determined by different histopathological pictures.

There is a rare form of classical PM, defined by endomysial inflammation with or without invasion of non-necrotic fibres by mononuclear cells and with or without perimysial or perivascular inflammation, and two subtypes which are much more frequent, i.e. non-specific or overlap myositis and NAM [9]. In classical PM, myalgia is found in half of the patients [49]. As in DM, ILD may occur and here too prognosis is unfavourable if there is pulmonary involvement.

Patients with non-specific or overlap myositis have a one in four chance of being diagnosed with an associated connective tissue disorder (CTD) [7], including scleroderma, Sjögren syndrome, SLE, rheumatoid arthritis (RA), the antisynthetase syndrome, and mixed connective tissue disorder (MCTD).

In NAM muscle weakness can be severe and associated with myalgia. In severe cases muscle weakness extends to the distal muscles and dysphagia is not uncommon [50,51]. Respiratory insufficiency

---

> **Box 32.2** A case of necrotizing autoimmune myopathy
>
> A 61-year-old Portuguese woman was referred because of progressive muscle weakness in her arms and legs over approximately 4 months and she had difficulty with swallowing solid food. Previous history revealed that she has been taking atorvastatin for 3 years prior to referral.
>
> On examination there was weakness of the deltoideus, triceps brachii, iliopsoas, and neck flexors (Medical Research Council grade 4). Otherwise there were no abnormalities.
>
> Ancillary investigations included an elevated serum creatine kinase activity (9982 IU L^{-1}) and magnetic resonance imaging showed hyperintensity in various thigh muscles (Fig. 32.5a). A myositis lineblot disclosed no myositis-specific antibodies. A muscle biopsy showed the picture of a necrotizing myopathy with scattered necrotizing muscle fibres (Fig. 32.4c), occasional regenerating fibres, and expression of major histocompatibility complex I in non-necrotic muscle fibres.
>
> She was treated with pulsed high-dose dexamethasone (6 months, one cycle per month) and muscle weakness resolved. However, she relapsed 7 months after the last cycle (mild muscle weakness and serum creatine kinase activity of 12 000 IU L^{-1}). Again she was started on dexamethasone and responded well.

> **Box 32.3** A patient with antisynthetase syndrome
>
> A 37-year-old man was referred because of decreased stamina, myalgia, and shortness of breath developing over a few weeks. On examination muscle weakness, proximal more than distal, and arms (Medical Research Council grade 2) more than legs (grade 4+), was found. Ancillary investigations included a markedly elevated serum creatine kinase activity of 16 864 IU L^{-1} (normal < 145), positive anti-ENA, anti-Jo, and anti-SSA. Computed tomography of the lungs showed abnormalities consistent with interstitial lung fibrosis.
>
> A muscle biopsy revealed perivascular mononuclear cells at perimysial sites predominantly composed of CD4-positive lymphocytes, and numerous necrotic and regenerating muscle fibres (Fig. 32.4d).
>
> He was diagnosed with an antisynthetase syndrome including a non-specific myositis.
>
> He was treated with daily high-dose prednisone (90 mg) and muscle weakness resolved. However, in June 2005 he relapsed so the prednisone dosage which had been tapered was increased and again he came into remission. Since then he had several relapses for which he was treated with pulsed methylprednisolone (intravenous), rituximab, and most recently methotrexate added to the prednisone dosage of 20 mg per day. During one of his relapses MRI was performed showing hyperintensity of the anterior thigh muscles and fascial hyperintensity of the posterior thigh muscles (Fig. 32.5b).

in the wake of NAM is extremely rare (personal communication). There is an association between cancer and NAM [27–29] and also with CTDs [7]. Recently, statin-induced NAM was reported [51].

Diagnosis

PM is characterized by a limb-girdle pattern of muscle weakness which necessitates distinction from other causes of a limb-girdle syndrome. In cases of a hereditary nature (e.g. dystrophies, acid maltase deficiency) there is usually very slowly progressive muscle weakness, in contrast to PM where there is subacute onset (i.e. less than a year). However, there are other myopathies with subacute onset and a limb-girdle pattern, e.g. toxic myopathies caused by particular drugs. Therefore the diagnosis of PM must rest on combined clinical and pathological criteria.

Serum CK activity

There is one paper showing robust data on serum CK in classical PM, since other previously described cohorts most likely have included sIBM patients and perhaps also patients with muscular dystrophies [49]. By far the majority of the PM patients had an elevated CK (range 50–13 254 IU L^{-1}, median 1015), which was markedly higher than in patients with sIBM or patients with the clinical picture of sIBM but without the canonical muscle biopsy findings.

In non-specific or overlap myositis serum CK is usually elevated (more than ten times the upper limit of normal) [7].

In NAM serum CK is usually markedly elevated, from 3000–25 000 IU L^{-1}, with a mean of 12 900 IU L^{-1} [51,52]. In statin-related NAM, serum CK has also been found in the high range of 958–45 000 IU L^{-1} (51), with the majority between 3000 and 8000 IU L^{-1}.

Myositis-specific autoantibodies

Autoantibodies against histidyl-tRNA synthetase (anti-Jo-1) are the most common myositis-specific autoantibodies and were recognized to identify a group of patients with the antisynthetase syndrome.

Other antibodies targeting a number of additional aminoacyl-tRNA synthetases (ARSs) have been identified, including those recognizing threonyl-tRNA synthetase (anti-PL-7), alanyl-tRNA synthetase (anti-PL-12), glycyl-tRNA synthetase (anti-EJ), isoleucyl-tRNA synthetase (anti-OJ), asparaginyl-tRNA synthetase (anti-KS), tyrosyl-tRNA synthetase, and phenylalanyl-tRNA synthetase (anti-Zo).

Anti-Jo-1 is found in 12.6–30% of myositis patients, and the other anti-ARS autoantibodies occur in about 1–5% of myositis patients [31,54]. Interestingly, the various antisynthetase antibodies seem to be mutually exclusive in that individual patients do not produce more than one [55]. MSAs, mostly anti-Jo-1,were found in 37% and 41%, of non-specific myositis and overlap myositis cases, respectively [7,8].

Patients with NAM may have anti-signal recognition particle (SRP) antibodies which are generally associated with severe clinical forms of the disease, particularly those with heart and lung involvement and resistance to steroid therapy [56–60].

An autoantibody recognizing 200- and 100-kDa proteins was recently found in subjects with NAM in whom prior use of statins [which lower cholesterol levels by specifically inhibiting 3-hydroxy-3-methylglutary coenzyme A reductase (HMGCR), a key enzyme in the cholesterol biosynthetic pathway] was a frequent observation [61]. Subsequently these antibodies were found to represent antibodies against the HMGCR protein [62]. In a quarter of the patients these antibodies were found in the absence of statin use.

Neuroimaging

MRI can demonstrate muscular oedema by showing areas of high signal intensity on STIR imaging (Fig. 32.5a,b) and fat-suppressed T_2-weighted sequences.

Muscle biopsy

In classical polymyositis, mononuclear cells are predominantly located in the endomysium and consist of predominantly CD8+ T-lymphocytes, plasma cells, myeloid dendritic cells, and macrophages. The lymphocytes surround and may also invade non-necrotic muscle fibres that express MHC I on the sarcolemma [49]. Thus, PM appears to be the result of a MHC I-restricted cytotoxic T-cell response against an (auto)antigen expressed by muscle fibres [41].

NAM is histologically characterized by necrotic muscle fibres as the predominant abnormal histological feature (Fig. 32.4c). Inflammatory cells are sparse or only slight at perivascular sites and perimysial infiltrate is not evident. Deposition of MAC on small blood vessels or thickened basement membrane (pipestem capillaries) may be seen at the ultrastructural level [27], but tubuloreticular inclusions in endothelial cells are uncommon or not evident. MHC I expression is variable [55].

In non-specific myositis the histopathological picture resembles that of DM showing perivascular cell infiltrates at perimysial sites predominantly composed of macrophages and plasmacytoid dendritic cells (Fig. 32.4d), and muscle fibre pathology may occur in perifascicular regions. Microtubular inclusions in endothelial cells can be found in a proportion of cases of non-specific myositis associated with a connective tissue disorder [64]. The histopathological picture has also been classified as immune myopathy with perimysial pathology [15].

Sporadic inclusion body myositis (Box 32.4)

The clinical picture differs from PM, with early weakness of distal muscles (especially the deep finger flexors), and greater weakness of quadriceps than iliopsoas muscles [65]. This is designated 'clinically defined sIBM', determined by characteristic clinical features only (with pathological features that are supportive of and not inconsistent with the diagnosis), whereas those patients with the canonical biopsy features (rimmed vacuoles, amyloid, filaments), with appropriate clinical features, represent 'pathologically defined sIBM' [65].

Clinical features

In sIBM weakness is often asymmetric, and predominantly presents in the quadriceps muscle (Fig. 32.6a), but also in distal muscles such as the deep finger flexor muscles (Fig. 32.6b), tibialis anterior, or calf muscles [66–68]. Swallowing difficulties may also be a presenting symptom in fewer than 10% of cases [69].

Facial weakness is observed in 40% of cases and is sometimes severe, with an inability to close the eyes (usually in females) [66,69–71]. Myalgia is not a feature of sIBM.

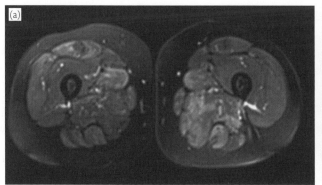
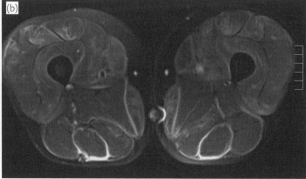

Fig. 32.5 (a) A magnetic resonance image (MRI) from a patient with necrotizing autoimmune myopathy, revealing hyperintensity in various muscles of the thigh. (b) MRI of a patient with antisynthetase syndrome revealing hyperintensity in various muscles of the thigh and also of the fascia, in particular of the hamstrings and the adductor magnus muscles.

In at least 20–30% of the patients sIBM is associated with systemic autoimmune or connective tissue disorders, including Sjögren syndrome and RA [49,72].

Serum CK activity

In sIBM serum CK is less than five times the normal value in 80% of patients, and it is only rarely up to more than 10 times the normal value [66].

Autoantibodies

An autoantibody against a 43-kDa muscle protein (anti-IBM-43) was recently identified for sIBM with a 52% sensitivity and 100% specificity [73].

Muscle imaging

T_1 abnormalities on MRI, indicating fatty replacement of muscle tissue in the flexor digitorum profundus, can help to distinguish between sIBM and PM/DM [68]. MRI may be helpful in selecting a suitable site for muscle biopsy and shows the selective involvement of the quadriceps muscles (Fig. 32.6a).

Muscle biopsy

The muscle pathology of sIBM typically demonstrates extensive endomysial inflammation, with inflammatory cells composed of macrophages and CD8+ cytotoxic/suppressor lymphocytes surrounding non-necrotizing myofibres (Fig. 32.7a) as in classical PM. There are small groups of atrophic fibres, eosinophilic cytoplasmic inclusions, and muscle fibres with one or more rimmed vacuoles (Fig. 32.7b) lined with granular material and immunostaining with antibodies directed against the nuclear proteins such as emerin, lamin A/C, valosin-containing protein (VCP), histone, and 43-kDa TAR DNA-binding protein, suggesting that a component of the rimmed vacuoles may be secondary to remnants of destroyed myonuclei [74]. On electron microscopy, 15–21 nm cytoplasmic and intranuclear tubulofilaments may be appreciated, although they can be difficult to find. Vacuolated fibres also contain cytoplasmic clusters of 6–10 nm amyloid-like fibrils [4]. Various 'Alzheimer characteristic proteins', e.g. β-amyloid, C- and N-terminal epitopes of β-amyloid precursor protein, hyperphosphorylated tau, prion protein (PrPc), apolipoprotein E, 1-antichymotrypsin, ubiquitin, and neurofilament heavy chain, have been reported in vacuolated muscle fibres using immunohistochemistry [75]. Although the invasion of non-necrotic myofibres by inflammatory cells has been frequently emphasized, the surrounding of myofibres by these cells without invasion is far more common [63]. In addition, there are many myeloid dendritic cells in the endomysium that appear to surround non-necrotic muscle fibres [76]. MHC I antigens are expressed on necrotic and non-necrotic muscle fibres.

There are also an increased number of ragged red fibres and cytochrome *c* oxidase (COX)-negative muscle fibres in sIBM (Fig. 32.7c) and large-scale mitochondrial DNA (mtDNA) deletions are more frequent in sIBM than in age-matched controls. COX-deficient muscle fibres are due to clonal expansion of mtDNA deletions and point mutations in segments of muscle fibres [77].

As has been mentioned before, there is an ongoing discussion about whether the presence of rimmed vacuoles is required for the diagnosis of sIBM. There are patients with a characteristic clinical picture of sIBM in whom the muscle biopsy shows the endomysial collections of CD8+ lymphocytes invading non-necrotic muscle fibres but where the rimmed vacuoles are lacking, even in repeat biopsies (see the case described in Box 32.4) [7,49]. Some consider these patients as a separate category called PM/sIBM [49].

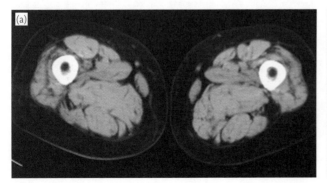
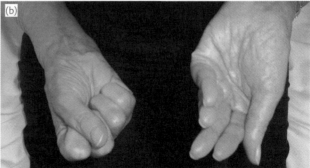

Fig. 32.6 (a) Computed tomography scan of a patient with inclusion body myositis (IBM) shows marked atrophy of the quadriceps femoris and in particular the vastus muscles. (b) Finger flexor weakness of the left hand in a patient with IBM.

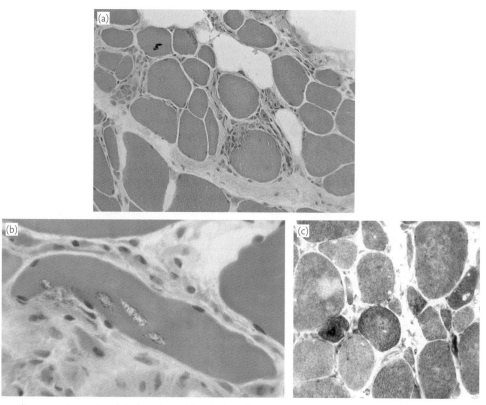

Fig. 32.7 (a) Muscle biopsy (haematoxylin–eosin stain) of a patient with sporadic inclusion body myositis (sIBM) showing endomysial collections of mononuclear cells surrounding and sometimes invading non-necrotic muscle fibres. (b) Muscle biopsy of a patient with IBM showing a muscle fibre with rimmed vacuoles. (c) Muscle bopsy (succinate dehydrogenase–cytochrome *c* oxidase stain) of a patient with sIBM showing an increased number of cytochrome *c* oxidase-negative muscle fibres which stain blue. (See also figure in colour plate section)

Prognosis for IIM

The prognosis for IIM is not well known since long-term outcome and prognostic factors vary widely.

Disease-related mortality rates in PM and DM are at least 10% [24,29,78]. Mortality is mostly related to cancer, especially during the first years after onset of treatment. Independent predictors for mortality are age at disease onset, the presence of cancer, and an elevated IgA level at diagnosis [78]. Other possible predictors of poor outcome are male sex, dysphagia, skin ulcers, long-standing symptoms prior to diagnosis or the start of therapy, subset of myositis, pulmonary (especially ILD) and cardiac involvement, including mainly left ventricular impairment, the presence of a low total protein and albumin level, and various myositis-specific antibodies. Coexistence of anti-Ro52 in anti-Jo1-positive patients is associated with a particular phenotype of PM/DM leading to more severe myositis/joint impairment, a symptomatic form of ILD, and an increased risk of cancer with a higher mortality rate. Moreover, anti-PL7/PL12 antibodies (antisynthetase antibodies) result in early and severe ILD and gastrointestinal complications; anti-SRP antibody is associated with an acute onset of refractory NAM. Finally, anti-155/140 (TIF1-γ) antibody is associated with malignancy in patients with adult DM, whereas the presence of anti-CADM-140 (MDA5) antibody is associated with amyopathic DM and rapidly progressive ILD [35].

There is no relation between the serum CK activity at disease onset and the outcome. However, in the individual patient who has been in remission a rise in serum CK activity may herald a relapse.

Favourable long-term outcome occurs in 18–90% of patients. A monocyclic disease course was seen in 15–48% of patients [78]. During the first 2–5 years 30–80% of patients with DM, PM, and PM in combination with a connective tissue disorder will show a relapse [78]. In the long term, 80% of patients with myositis have a chronic continuous or polycyclic disease course with major effects on perceived disability and quality of life, despite regained muscle strength [29], although others report that after a median of 7.5 years of follow-up most patients (86%) had no disease activity and 83% had no disability [78].

JDM has a low mortality rate. Functional outcome is greatly influenced by the presence of calcinosis and early diagnosis and treatment lead to a favourable outcome [79].

During pregnancy, spontaneous abortions, intrauterine fetal death, and early birth occur more frequently [80]. Relapses of myositis occur in some patients in the third trimester of the pregnancy or post-partum [81].

Sporadic IBM was believed to be a rather mild disorder; however, it was recently shown that sIBM is an extremely disabling disorder, albeit with normal life expectancy [82,83]. However, death is significantly more often caused by pneumonia, which may be contributed to aspiration from the associated dysphagia, and thus has an indirect relationship to the disease. Patients become wheelchair-dependent approximately 15 years after onset of the disease [82,83]. The decline in functional disability has profound impact on the quality of life [84].

Management of IIM

The inflammatory myopathies, sIBM excluded, are amenable to immunosuppressive and immunomodulation therapies. The general opinion is that patients with muscle weakness need treatment, albeit that the occasional patient with spontaneous recovery has been described [85]. The goals of therapy are to improve activities of daily living by increasing muscle strength, and to resolve other symptoms and signs such as dyspnoea, rash, and arthralgia.

Treatment remains difficult for sIBM because both T-cell mediated cytotoxicity and a degenerative process appear to coexist from the outset. Although early on some patients may have a partial response to steroids or intravenous immunoglobulin (IVIg), they soon become unresponsive and the disease progresses [86]. A recently published evidence-based guideline showed that there is insufficient evidence to support or refute the use of IVIg in treating sIBM [87].

Improvements in treatment for IIM are hampered by difficulty in the design of trials and the low incidence and prevalence of the disease. Outcome measures to be used in clinical trials in IIM include at present the core sets of outcome proposed by the International Myositis Assessment and Clinical Studies Group (IMACS) to assess three dimensions of myositis disease: disease activity (MYOACT), disease damage (MYODAM), and health related quality of life (SF-36) [88].

First-line treatment (corticosteroids)

High-dose prednisone (1–1.5 mg kg^{-1} prednisolone per day for at least 4 weeks) followed by slow tapering to prevent relapse is the treatment of first choice on an empirical basis for PM, non-specific or overlap myositis, (J)DM, and NAM; its effect has not been investigated in a randomized controlled trial (RCT) [41,89]. In NAM, sustained treatment with a combination of immunosuppressants is often required [7,10,50]. Comparison of oral dexamethasone pulse therapy versus daily prednisolone in adult patients with IIM (except sIBM) showed that although pulsed high-dose oral dexamethasone (40 mg daily on four consecutive days, six cycles of 28 days) is not superior to daily prednisolone as a first-line treatment, it is a good alternative as it has substantially fewer side effects [90]. In JDM intravenous methylprednisolone (once a day, 15–30 mg kg^{-1} on three consecutive days) can be considered as an alternative in the initial stage of treatment or in case of a relapse, albeit that concomitant treatment with oral steroids is nearly always needed [91].

During treatment with corticosteroids side effects such as weight gain, Cushingoid appearance, corticosteroid-induced myopathy, hypertension, glucose intolerance, cataracts, glaucoma, activation of peptic ulcers, increased susceptibility to infection, and, in children, growth arrest, should be monitored; osteoporosis prophylaxis, by dietary advice and the use of calcium, vitamin D supplements and biphosphonates, should be given. Dual-energy x ray absorptiometry (DEXA) is obtained at baseline and every 2 years while patients are receiving corticosteroids to assess bone loss. However, no solid evidence exists for this recommendation. In DM the affected skin needs protection against sunlight.

Second-line treatment

If corticosteroid treatment fails, or if the dose required to maintain remission is unacceptably high, various second-line treatments can be used, but most of these have not been appropriately investigated.

There is some evidence for azathioprine as an add-on therapy, with more improvement in functional disability and a requirement for less prednisone [92,93]. Methotrexate seems to have the same effect, with fewer side effects [94,95]. However, a Cochrane review concluded that the small number of randomized trials are inadequate to decide whether these agents are beneficial in dermatomyositis and polymyositis [89]. Based on one Class II study, IVIg is possibly effective for the treatment of non-responsive dermatomyositis in adults [87,96]. No benefit was shown for plasma exchange or leucapheresis [97].

Ciclosporin can also be of use in PM, DM, and JDM but the cost and potential side effects have limited its use in most myositis patients [98,99]. Mycophenelate mofetil might become a promising drug [100]. The evidence for intravenous cyclophosphamide is circumstantial [101].

Biological agents

Chronic immunosuppressive therapy is associated with significant side effects, and many patients remain (partially) refractory to treatment, thus novel therapeutic agents that are safe and effective would be highly desirable [102].

There are new biological agents in the form of monoclonal antibodies or fusion proteins targeting the following components and processes:

- B cells (rituximab), T cells (alemtuzumab, directed against the CD52 molecule), and T cell migration (fingolimod, an anti-T-cell-migration agent that traps lymphocytes in the lymphoid organs).
- Complement: eculizumab, a monoclonal antibody against C5, intercepts the formation of membranolytic attack complex and the subsequent generation of proinflammatory molecules.
- Tumour necrosis factor-α (TNF-α): available anti-TNF-α agents are those approved for rheumatoid arthritis and include etanercept, a TNF-α receptor fusion protein; infiximab, a chimeric anti-TNF-α monoclonal antibody; and adalimumab, a humanized anti-TNF-α agent.
- Interleukin 1 (IL1) receptor: an IL1 antagonist, anakinra, and disruptor of cellular adhesion, natalizumab, directed against the $\alpha4\beta1$ integrin on leucocytes, a fundamental molecule for adhesion and transmigration of T cells).

These drugs are potentially effective but have either been used in small uncontrolled series of refractory patients or are awaiting further investigation [102]. In a 52-week pilot study of etanercept compared with placebo in newly diagnosed and refractory DM patients, no statistically significant differences between treatment groups were found with regard to muscle strength and motor function but there was a possible steroid-sparing effect in the etanercept-treated patients [103]. Recently the efficacy and safety of rituximab have been assessed in 200 adult and paediatric patients with refractory PM or DM. More than 80% of the patients achieved the definition of improvement of the IMACS Group after 20 weeks irrespective of the timing (early or late, i.e. 8 weeks later) [104].

Non-pharmacological therapeutic interventions

Physical and occupation therapy along with aerobic exercise programmes help patients retain motor function, improve mobility, and prevent contractures. Patients with dysphagia may benefit from speech therapy. Dysphagia may be temporarily improved with oesophageal dilatation or cricopharyngeal myotomy. A very small number of patients may need a feeding tube, at least temporarily [105].

There is some evidence that in PM and DM creatine monohydrate combined with home exercise for 6 months improved muscle performance assessed both by functional tests reflecting the ability to undertake high-intensity muscular exercise and endurance work in comparison to exercise alone. This functional improvement was associated with increased muscle phosphocreatine levels measured by ^{31}P magnetic resonance spectroscopy. Creatine was well-tolerated [106,107].

A systematic review has been performed on the safety and efficacy of exercise training in adult patients with IIM [108]. Most of the included studies had a high selection and/or allocation bias. Despite the shortcomings, it was shown that exercise training in patients with IIM appears to be safe since disease activity and pain measures as used in the included studies did not worsen in any of the studies at a group level. Some studies even reported an improvement in disease activity measures [109–111]. Furthermore, the results of the included studies strongly indicate that exercise training provides benefits for muscle strength in sIBM [107] and DM/PM, but also benefits aerobic fitness [111–114]; activities of daily living improved significantly in patients with DM and PM [113,114].

References

1. Bohan A, Peter JB. Polymyositis and dermatomyositis (first of two parts). *N Engl J Med* 1975; **292**: 344–7.

2. Yunis EJ, Samaha FJ. Inclusion body myositis. *Lab Invest* 1971; **25**: 240–8.

3. Engel AG, Arahata K. Monoclonal antibody analysis of mononuclear cells in myopathies. II: Phenotypes of autoinvasive cells in polymyositis and inclusion body myositis. *Ann Neurol* 1984; **16**: 209–15.

4. Griggs RC, Askanas V, DiMauro S, et al. Inclusion body myositis and myopathies. *Ann Neurol* 1995; **38**: 705–13.

5. Nagaraju K, Rawat R, Veszelovszky E, et al. Dysferlin deficiency enhances monocyte phagocytosis: a model for the inflammatory onset of limb-girdle muscular dystrophy 2B. *Am J Pathol* 2008; **172**: 774–85.

6. Linklater H, Pipitone N, Rose MR, et al. Classification criteria for idiopathic inflammatory myositis: comparison of the performance of accepted criteria. *Rheumatology* 2009; **48** (Suppl 1): i74.

7. van der Meulen MF, Bronner IM, Hoogendijk JE, et al. Polymyositis: an overdiagnosed entity. *Neurology* 2003; **61**: 316–21.

8. Troyanov Y, Targoff IN, Tremblay JL, et al. Novel classification of idiopathic inflammatory myopathies based on overlap syndrome features and autoantibodies: analysis of 100 French Canadian patients. *Medicine (Baltimore)* 2005; **84**: 231–49.

9. Hoogendijk JE, Amato AA, Lecky BR, et al. 119th ENMC international workshop: trial design in adult idiopathic inflammatory myopathies, with the exception of inclusion body myositis, 10-12 October 2003, Naarden, The Netherlands. *Neuromuscul Disord* 2004; **14**: 337–45.

10. Liang C, Needham M. Necrotizing autoimmune myopathy. *Curr Opin Rheumatol* 2011; **23**: 612–19.

11. Sato S, Kuwana M. Clinically amyopathic dermatomyositis. *Curr Opin Rheumatol* 2010; **22**: 639–43.

12. Dalakas MC. Polymyositis, dermatomyositis and inclusion-body myositis. *N Engl J Med* 1991; **325**: 1487–98.

13. Tanimoto K, Nakano K, Kano S, et al. Classification criteria for polymyositis and dermatomyositis. *J Rheumatol* 1995; **22**: 668–74.

14. Targoff IN, Miller FW, Medsger TA, Jr, Oddis CV. Classification criteria for the idiopathic inflammatory myopathies. *Curr Opin Rheumatol* 1997; **9**: 527–35.

15. Pestronk A. Acquired immune and inflammatory myopathies: pathologic classification. *Curr Opin Rheumatol* 2011; **23**: 595–604.

16. Miller FW. Inflammatory myopathies: polymyositis, dermatomyositis, and related conditions. In: Koopman W, Moreland L (ed) *Arthritis and Allied Conditions: a Textbook of Rheumatology*, pp. 1593–620. Philadelphia, PA: Lippincott, Williams and Wilkins, 2005.

17. Betteridge ZE, Gunawardena H, McHugh NJ. Novel autoantibodies and clinical phenotypes in adult and juvenile myositis. *Arthritis Res Ther* 2011; **13**: 209–16.

18. Dalakas MC. Mechanisms of disease: signaling pathways and immunobiology of inflammatory myopathies. *Nat Clin Pract Rheumatol* 2006; **2**: 219–27.

19. O'Hanlon TP, Miller FW. Genetic risk and protective factors for the idiopathic inflammatory myopathies. *Curr Rheumatol Rep* 2009; **11**: 287–94.

20. Chinoy H, Lamb JA, Ollier WE, Cooper RG. Recent advances in the immunogenetics of idiopathic inflammatory myopathy. *Arthritis Res Ther* 2011; **13**: 216.

21. Rider LG, Miller FW. Deciphering the clinical presentations, pathogenesis, and treatment of the idiopathic inflammatory myopathies. *J Am Med Assoc* 2011; **305**: 183–90.

22. Amato AA, Greenberg SA. Inflammatory myopathies. *Continuum* 2006; **12**: 140–68.

23. Harris-Love MO, Shrader JA, Koziol D, et al. Distribution and severity of weakness among patients with polymyositis, dermatomyositis and juvenile dermatomyositis. *Rheumatology* 2009; **48**: 134–9.

24. Marie I, Hachulla E, Hatron PY, et al. Polymyositis and dermatomyositis: short term and longterm outcome, and predictive factors of prognosis. *J Rheumatol* 2001; **28**: 2230–7.

25. Marguerie C, Bunn CC, Beynon HL, et al. Polymyositis, pulmonary fibrosis and autoantibodies to aminoacyl-tRNA synthetase enzymes. *Q J Med* 1990; **77**: 1019–38.

26. Rose MR, Kissel JT, Bickley LS, Griggs RC. Sustained myoglobinuria: the presenting manifestation of dermatomyositis. *Neurology* 1996; **47**: 119–23.

27. Emslie-Smith AM, Engel AG. Necrotizing myopathy with pipestem capillaries, microvascular deposition of the complement membrane attack complex (MAC), and minimal cellular infiltration. *Neurology* 1991; **41**: 936–9.

28. Levin MI, Mozaffar T, Al-Lozi MT, Pestronk A. Paraneoplastic necrotizing myopathy: clinical and pathological features. *Neurology* 1998; **50**: 764–7.

29. Bronner IM, van der Meulen MF, de Visser M, et al. Long-term outcome in polymyositis and dermatomyositis. *Ann Rheum Dis* 2006; **65**: 1456–61.

30. Ang P, Sugeng MW, Chua SH. Classical and amyopathic dermatomyositis seen at the National Skin Centre of Singapore: a 3-year retrospective review of their clinical characteristics and association with malignancy. *Ann Acad Med Singapore* 2000; **29**: 219–23.

31. Mammen AL. Dermatomyositis and polymyositis: Clinical presentation, autoantibodies, and pathogenesis. *Ann NY Acad Sci* 2010; **1184**: 134–53.

31a. Wedderburn LR, McHugh NJ, Chinoy H, et al. Juvenile Dermatomyositis Research Group (JDRG). HLA class II haplotype and autoantibody associations in children with juvenile dermatomyositis and juvenile dermatomyositis-scleroderma overlap. *Rheumatology (Oxford)* 2007; **46**: 1786–91.

32. Kaji K, Fujimoto M, Hasegawa M, et al. Identification of a novel autoantibody reactive with 155 and 140 kDa nuclear proteins in patients with dermatomyositis: an association with malignancy. *Rheumatology* 2007; **46**: 25–8.

33. Targoff IN, Mamyrova G, Trieu EP, et al. A novel autoantibody to a 155-kd protein is associated with dermatomyositis. *Arthritis Rheum* 2006; **54**: 3682–9.

34. Gunawardena H, Wedderburn LR, North J, et al. Clinical associations of autoantibodies to a p155/140 kDa doublet protein in juvenile dermatomyositis. *Rheumatology* 2008; **47**: 324–8.

35. Sato S, Hirakata M, Kuwana M, et al. Autoantibodies to a 140-kd polypeptide, CADM-140, in Japanese patients with clinically amyopathic dermatomyositis. *Arthritis Rheum* 2005; **52**: 1571–6.

36. Blijham PJ, Hengstman GJD, Hama-Amin AD, Van Engelen BGM, Zwarts MJ. Needle electromyographic findings in 98 patients with myositis. *Eur Neurol* 2006; **55**: 183–8.

37. Sandstedt PE, Henriksson KG, Larrsson LE. Quantitative electromyography in polymyositis and dermatomyositis. *Acta Neurol Scand* 1982; **65**: 110–21.

38. Tomasová Studynková J, Charvát F, Jarosová K, Vencovsky J. The role of MRI in the assessment of polymyositis and dermatomyositis. *Rheumatology* 2007; **46**: 1174–9.

39. Crowson AN, Magro CM. The role of microvascular injury in the pathogenesis of cutaneous lesions of dermatomyositis. *Hum Pathol* 1996; **27**: 15–19.

40. Magro CM, Crowson AN. The immunofluorescent profile of dermatomyositis: a comparative study with lupus erythematosus. *J Cutan Pathol* 1997; **24**: 543–52.

41. Dalakas MC, Hohlfeld R. Polymyositis and dermatomyositis. *Lancet* 2003; **362**: 971–82.

42. Kissel JT, Halterman RK, Rammohan KW, Mendell JR. The relationship of complement-mediated microvasculopathy to the histologic features and clinical duration of disease in dermatomyositis. *Arch Neurol* 1991; **48**: 26–30.

43. Emslie-Smith AM, Engel AG. Microvascular changes in early and advanced dermatomyositis: a quantitative study. *Ann Neurol* 1990; **27**: 343–56.

44. Arahata K, Engel AG. Monoclonal antibody analysis of mononuclear cells in myopathies. I: Quantitation of subsets according to diagnosis and sites of accumulation and demonstration and counts of muscle fibers invaded by T cells. *Ann Neurol* 1984; **16**: 193–208.

45. Kissel JT, Mendell JR, Rammohan KW. Microvascular deposition of complement membrane attack complex in dermatomyositis. *N Engl J Med* 1986; **314**: 329–34.

46. Bohan A, Peter JB, Bowman RL, Pearson CM. Computer-assisted analysis of 153 patients with polymyositis and dermatomyositis. *Medicine (Baltimore)* 1977; **56**: 255–86.

47. Munsat T, Cancilla P. Polymyositis without inflammation. *Bull Los Angeles Neurol Soc* 1974; **39**: 113–20.

48. Bunch TW. Polymyositis: a case history approach to the differential diagnosis and treatment. *Mayo Clin Proc* 1990; **65**: 1480–97.

49. Chahin N, Engel AG. Correlation of muscle biopsy, clinical course, and outcome in PM and sporadic IBM. *Neurology* 2008; **70**: 418–24.

50. Bronner IM, Hoogendijk JE, Wintzen AR, et al. Necrotising myopathy, an unusual presentation of a steroid-responsive myopathy. *J Neurol* 2003; **250**: 480–5.

51. Grable-Esposito P, Katzberg HD, Greenberg SA, et al. Immune-mediated necrotizing myopathy associated with statins. *Muscle Nerve* 2010; **41**: 185–90.

52. Miller T, Al-Lozi MT, Lopate G, Pestronk A. Myopathy with antibodies to the signal recognition particle: clinical and pathological features. *J Neurol Neurosurg Psychiatry* 2002; **73**: 420–8.

53. Needham M, Mastaglia FL. Inclusion body myositis: current pathogenetic concepts and diagnostic and therapeutic approaches. *Lancet Neurol* 2007; **6**: 620–31.

54. Charles PJ, Lundberg IE, Paterson E, et al. Myositis associated autoantibodies detected using a novel recombinant protein blotting: clinical associations. *Ann Rheum Dis* 2010; **69** (Suppl 2): A9–A10.

55. Targoff IN. Laboratory testing in the diagnosis and management of idiopathic inflammatory myopathies. *Rheum Dis Clin North Am* 2002; **28**: 859–90, viii.

56. Targoff IN. Autoantibodies to aminoacyl-transfer RNA synthetases for isoleucine and glycine. Two additional synthetases are antigenic in myositis. *J Immunol* 1990; **144**: 1737–43.

57. Hengstman GJ, ter Laak HJ, Vree Egberts WT, et al. Anti-signal recognition particle autoantibodies: marker of a necrotising myopathy. *Ann Rheum Dis* 2006; **65**: 1635–8.

58. Reeves WH, Nigam SK, Blobel G. Human autoantibodies reactive with the signal-recognition particle. *Proc Natl Acad Sci USA* 1986; **83**: 9507–11.

59. Kao AH, Lacomis D, Lucas M, et al. Anti-signal recognition particle autoantibody in patients with and patients without idiopathic inflammatory myopathy. *Arthritis Rheum* 2004; **50**: 209–15.

60. Satoh T, Okano T, Matsui T, et al. Novel autoantibodies against 7SL RNA in patients with polymyositis/dermatomyositis. *J Rheumatol* 2005; **32**: 1727–33.

61. Christopher-Stine L, Casciola-Rosen LA, Hong G, et al. A novel autoantibody recognizing 200-kd and 100-kd proteins is associated with an immune-mediated necrotizing myopathy. *Arthritis Rheum* 2010; **62**: 2757–66.

62. Mammen AL, Chung T, Christopher-Stine L, et al. Autoantibodies against 3-hydroxy-3-methylglutaryl-coenzyme A reductase in patients with statin-associated autoimmune myopathy. *Arthritis Rheum* 2011; **63**: 713–21.

63. Greenberg SA. Inclusion body myositis. *Curr Opin Rheumatol* 2011; **23**: 574–8.

64. Bronner IM, Hoogendijk JE, Veldman H, et al. Tubuloreticular structures in different types of myositis: implications for pathogenesis. *Ultrastruct Pathol* 2008; **32**; 123–6.

65. Benveniste O, Hilton-Jones D. International Workshop on Inclusion Body Myositis held at the Institute of Myology, Paris, on 29 May 2009. *Neuromusc Disord* 2010; **20**: 414–21.

66. Felice KJ, North WA. Inclusion body myositis in Connecticut: observations in 35 patients during an 8-year period. *Medicine (Baltimore)* 2001; **80**: 320–7.

67. Peng A, Koffman BM, Malley JD, Dalakas MC. Disease progression in sporadic inclusion body myositis: observations in 78 patients. *Neurology* 2000; **55**: 296–8.

68. Sekul EA, Chow C, Dalakas MC. Magnetic resonance imaging of the forearm as a diagnostic aid in patients with sporadic inclusion body myositis. *Neurology* 1997; **48**: 863–6.

69. Badrising UA, Maat-Schieman MLC, van Houwelingen JC, et al. Inclusion body myositis. Clinical features and clinical course of the disease in 64 patients. *J Neurol* 2005; **252**: 1448–54.

70. Ringel SP, Kenny CE, Neville HE, Giorno R, Carry MR. Spectrum of inclusion body myositis. *Arch Neurol* 1987; **44**: 1154–7.

71. Amato AA, Gronseth GS, Jackson CE, et al. Inclusion body myositis: clinical and pathological boundaries. *Ann Neurol* 1996; **40**: 581–6.

72. Badrising UA, Schreuder GM, Giphart MJ, et al. Associations with autoimmune disorders and HLA class I and II antigens in inclusion body myositis. *Neurology* 2004; **63**: 2396–8.

73. Salajegheh M, Lam T, Greenberg SA. Autoantibodies against a 43 kDa muscle protein in inclusion body myositis. *PLoS One* 2011; **6**: e20266.

74. Amato AA, Barohn RJ. Inclusion body myositis: old and new concepts. *J Neurol Neurosurg Psychiatry* 2009; **80**: 1186–93.

75. Askanas V, Engel WK. Inclusion-body myositis, a multifactorial muscle disease associated with aging: current concepts of pathogenesis. *Curr Opin Rheumatol* 2007; **19**: 550–9.

76. Greenberg SA, Pinkus GS, Amato AA, Pinkus JL. Myeloid dendritic cells in inclusion-body myositis and polymyositis. *Muscle Nerve* 2007; **35**: 17–23.

77. Oldfors A, Moslemi AR, Jonasson L, et al. Mitochondrial abnormalities in inclusion-body myositis. *Neurology* 2006; **66** (Suppl 1): S49–S55.

78. Shu XM, Lu X, Xie Y, Wang GC. Clinical characteristics and favorable long-term outcomes for patients with idiopathic inflammatory myopathies: a retrospective single center study in China. *BMC Neurol* 2011; **11**: 143.

79. Huber AM, Lang B, LeBlanc CM, et al. Medium- and long-term functional outcomes in a multicenter cohort of children with juvenile dermatomyositis. *Arthritis Rheum* 2000; **43**: 541–9.

80. Vancsa A, Ponyi A, Constantin T, Zeher M, Danko K. Pregnancy outcome in idiopathic inflammatory myopathy. *Rheumatol Int* 2007; **27**: 435–9.

81. Gutierrez G, Dagnino R, Mintz G. Polymyositis/dermatomyositis and pregnancy. *Arthritis Rheum* 1984; **27**: 291–4.

82. Cox FM, Titulaer MJ, Sont JK, et al. A 12-year follow-up in sporadic inclusion body myositis: an end stage with major disabilities. *Brain* 2011; **134**: 3167–75.

83. Benveniste O, Leger JM. Inflammatory or necrotizing myopathies, myositides and other acquired myopathies, new insight in 2011. *Presse Med* 2011; **40**: e197–e198.

84. Sadjadi R, Rose MR. What determines quality of life in inclusion body myositis? *J Neurol Neurosurg Psychiatry* 2010; **81**: 1164–6.

85. van de Vlekkert J, Hoogendijk JE, Frijns CJ, de Visser M. Spontaneous recovery of dermatomyositis and unspecified myositis in three adult patients. *J Neurol Neurosurg Psychiatry* 2008; **79**: 729–30.

86. Dalakas MC. Immunotherapy of myositis: issues, concerns and future prospects. *Nat Rev Rheumatol* 2010; **6**: 129–37.

87. Patwa HS, Chaudhry V, Katzberg H, Rae-Grant AD, So YT. Evidence-based guideline: Intravenous immunoglobulin in the treatment of neuromuscular disorders: Report of the Therapeutics and Technology Assessment Subcommittee of the American Academy of Neurology. *Neurology* 2012; **78**: 1009–15.

88. Alexanderson H, Lundberg IE. Disease-specific quality indicators, outcome measures and guidelines in polymyositis and dermatomyositis. *Clin Exp Rheumatol* 2007; **25** (Suppl 47): 153–8.

89. Choy EH, Hoogendijk JE, Lecky B, Winer JB. Immunosuppressant and immunomodulatory treatment for dermatomyositis and polymyositis. *Cochrane Database Syst Rev* 2005; **3**: CD003643.

90. van de Vlekkert J, Hoogendijk JE, de Haan RJ, et al. Oral dexamethasone pulse therapy versus daily prednisolone in sub-acute onset myositis, a randomised clinical trial. *Neuromuscul Disord* 2010; **20**: 382–9.

91. Laxer RM, Stein LD, Petty RE. Intravenous pulse methylprednisolone treatment of juvenile dermatomyositis. *Arthritis Rheum* 1987; **30**: 328–34.

92. Bunch TW. Prednisone and azathioprine for polymyositis: long-term followup. *Arthritis Rheum* 1981; **24**: 45–8.

93. Bunch TW, Worthington JW, Combs JJ, Ilstrup DM, Engel AG. Azathioprine with prednisone for polymyositis. A controlled, clinical trial. *Ann Intern Med* 1980; **92**: 365–9.

94. Ramanan AV, Campbell-Webster N, Ota S, et al. The effectiveness of treating juvenile dermatomyositis with methotrexate and aggressively tapered corticosteroids. *Arthritis Rheum* 2005; **52**: 3570–8.

95. Villalba L, Hicks JE, Adams EM, et al. Treatment of refractory myositis: a randomized crossover study of two new cytotoxic regimens. *Arthritis Rheum* 1998; **41**: 392–9.

96. Dalakas MC, Illa I, Dambrosia JM, et al. A controlled trial of high-dose intravenous immune globulin infusions as treatment for dermatomyositis. *N Engl J Med* 1993; **329**: 1993–2000.

97. Miller FW, Leitman SF, Cronin ME, et al). Controlled trial of plasma exchange and leukapheresis in polymyositis and dermatomyositis. *N Engl J Med* 1992; **326**: 1380–4.

98. Grau JM, Herrero C, Casademont J, Fernandez-Sola J, Urbano-Marquez A. Cyclosporine A as first choice therapy for dermatomyositis. *J Rheumatol* 1994; **21**: 381–2.

99. Heckmatt J, Hasson N, Saunders C, et al. Cyclosporin in juvenile dermatomyositis. *Lancet* 1989; **1**(8646): 1063–6.

100. Chaudhry V, Cornblath DR, Griffin JW, O'Brien R, Drachman DB. Mycophenolate mofetil: a safe and promising immunosuppressant in neuromuscular diseases. *Neurology* 2001; **56**: 94–6.

101. Schnabel A, Reuter M, Gross WL. Intravenous pulse cyclophosphamide in the treatment of interstitial lung disease due to collagen vascular diseases. *Arthritis Rheum* 1998; **41**: 1215–20.

102. Dalakas MC. Inflammatory myopathies: management of steroid resistance. *Curr Opin Neurol* 2011; **24**: 457–62.

103. Muscle Study Group. A randomized, pilot trial of etanercept in dermatomyositis. *Ann Neurol* 2011; **70**: 427–36.

104. Oddis CV, Reed AM, Aggarwal R, et al. Rituximab in the treatment of refractory adult and juvenile dermatomyositis and adult polymyositis: a randomized, placebo-phase trial. *Arthritis Rheum* 2013; **65**: 314–24.

105. Amato AA, Barohn RJ. Evaluation and treatment of inflammatory myopathies. *J Neurol Neurosurg Psychiatry* 2009; **80**: 1060–8.

106. Chung YL, Alexanderson H, Pipitone N, et al. Creatine supplements in patients with idiopathic inflammatory myopathies who are clinically weak after conventional pharmacologic treatment: six-month, double-blind, randomized, placebo-controlled trial. *Arthritis Rheum* 2007; **57**: 694–702.

107. Kley RA, Tarnopolsky MA, Vorgerd M. Creatine for treating muscle disorders. *Cochrane Database Syst Rev* 2011; **2**: CD004760.

108. Habers GE, Takken T. Safety and efficacy of exercise training in patients with an idiopathic inflammatory myopathy—a systematic review. *Rheumatology* 2011; **50**: 2113–24.

109. Arnardottir S, Alexanderson H, Lundberg IE, Borg K. Sporadic inclusion body myositis: pilot study on the effects of a home exercise program on muscle function, histopathology and inflammatory reaction. *J Rehabil Med* 2003; **35**: 31–5.

110. Alexanderson H, Dastmalchi M, Esbjornsson-Liljedahl M, Opava CH, Lundberg IE. Benefits of intensive resistance training in patients with chronic polymyositis or dermatomyositis. *Arthritis Rheum* 2007; **57**: 768–77.

111. Nader GA, Dastmalchi M, Alexanderson H, et al. A longitudinal, integrated, clinical, histological and mRNA profiling study of resistance exercise in myositis. *Mol Med* 2010; **16**: 455–64.

112. Johnson LG, Collier KE, Edwards DJ, et al. Improvement in aerobic capacity after an exercise program in sporadic inclusion body myositis. *J Clin Neuromuscul Dis* 2009; **10**: 178–84.

113. Wiesinger GF, Quittan M, Aringer M, et al. Improvement of physical fitness and muscle strength in polymyositis/dermatomyositis patients by a training programme. *Br J Rheumatol* 1998; **37**: 196–200.

114. Wiesinger GF, Quittan M, Graninger M, et al. Benefit of 6 months long-term physical training in polymyositis/dermatomyositis patients. *Br J Rheumatol* 1998; **37**: 1338–42.

CHAPTER 33

Drug-induced neuromuscular disorders

Zohar Argov

Introduction

Drugs may produce adverse neuromuscular effects, either through direct myotoxicity or by interfering with the function of the neuromuscular synapse and the peripheral nerve (the latter will not be reviewed in this chapter). The possibility of a drug-induced neuromuscular disorder should be considered in the differential diagnosis for any patient with muscular symptoms while on drug therapy (including drug addicts). Since many such side effects are potentially reversible, early recognition is important in preventing residual damage. The clinical spectrum of drug-induced myopathies is very broad, thus a high degree of suspicion should be practised. In the case of many drugs the myopathic side effects are well documented; however, there are numerous medications for which a single case report is the only evidence for such a side effect and it should be regarded as a possibility only [1].

Drug-induced myopathies

The following clinical pathological syndromes have been observed.

Myalgia and increased serum creatine kinase

Myalgia and cramps, either at rest or aggravated by activity, may be induced by many medications. Transient increase of serum creatine kinase (CK) levels may accompany these symptoms, but asymptomatic elevation of CK (hyperCKaemia) may be the only sign of myotoxicity. It is not clear what level of drug-induced hyperCKaemia poses a risk to patients, but when pain accompanies a rise in CK the suspected medication should be stopped. Some medications may cause an increased CK level not through a myotoxic effect but by central nervous system effects leading to either increased muscle activity or muscle tone.

Myotonia

A small number of drugs may induce myotonia in humans [2], including colchicine, chloroquine, clofibric acid, and dichlorophenoxyacetate. A few drugs may exacerbate myotonia in an already diagnosed patient or rarely unmask previously undetected myotonia. Depolarizing muscle relaxants (e.g. suxamethonium), which can markedly exacerbate myotonia during general anaesthesia, should be avoided in patients with myotonia. The β2-adrenergic blockers (e.g. propranolol, pindolol) and the β2-adrenergic agonists (fenoterol and ritrodrine) can also aggravate myotonia.

Painful necrotizing myopathies

Several drugs can cause a necrotizing myopathy with symptoms evolving over a period of days to weeks. Myalgia and muscle tenderness can be prominent but weakness is usually the main complaint. The weakness may be limited to the proximal musculature, but can also be generalized. The serum CK level is elevated, sometimes markedly, and myoglobinuria may be detected. There is no clear dividing line between severe necrotizing myopathy and rhabdomyolysis and many medications can cause both. Since most of these cases are caused by the cholesterol-lowering agents this topic will be discussed separately.

Cholesterol-lowering agents
Statins
The drugs belonging to this group are currently the main lipid-lowering agents prescribed to more than 30 million people worldwide to reduce the risk of cardiovascular diseases [3,4]. Statins inhibit the function of 3-hydroxy-3-methylglutaryl coenzyme A reductase (HMGCR), the rate-limiting enzyme in cholesterol biosynthesis, causing a reduction in formation of mevalonate, which is an important intermediary metabolite in the synthesis of cholesterol. There are two general groups of statins—those metabolized through the cytochrome P450 system (via the CYP3A4 isoenzyme) and those that are not. These pharmacokinetic features affect the toxicity profile of statins, since other drugs metabolized through P450 will increase the risk for myotoxicity of the first group [4,5] (see Table 33.1).

It is estimated that 5–10% of patients discontinue statins because of muscle-related symptoms [4] but more formal evaluations of the prevalence differ widely in their results. Serious side effects defined as muscular symptoms with marked CK rise and hospitalization have been recorded in only four out of 127 000 patients on statins followed for more than 18 months [6]. However, if muscle symptoms of lesser severity are also calculated, then 8–9% of patients reported such side effects [7] and the risk rate for such symptoms tripled with time in the first year of use [8]. Also, differences between the various statin preparations in terms of risk of myopathy were found, with fluvastatin and pravastatin being of higher risk than rosuvastatin and atorvastatin [4]. In addition, some evidence suggests that a high statin dose, now recommended in some instances, carries a greater risk of myopathy [4].

An advisory committee report [9] defined four clinical presentations of statin myotoxicity: (1) statin myopathy (any muscle complaint); (2) myalgia (pain without hyperCKaemia); (3) myositis

Table 33.1 Drugs that potentially increase the risk for statin toxicity*

Azole antifungals
Cimetidine
Cyclosporine
Gemfibrozil and other fibrates
Macrolide antibiotics and erythromycin
Niacin
Nicotinic acid
Protease inhibitors (ritonavir)
Statins (combinations of two statins metabolized by CYP3A4 isoenzyme)
Tacrolimus
Verapamil

*Arranged alphabetically and not by frequency or severity.

(muscle symptoms with hyperCKaemia); (4) rhabdomyolysis (muscle symptoms with CK elevation above ten times the upper limit of normal). This subdivision is mainly used by non-neuromuscular specialists. It emphasizes non-specific complaints like muscle pain, yet ignores cases with asymptomatic hyperCKaemia [10]. The term myositis is also inaccurately defined since most patients with high CK do not have an inflammatory myopathy. In the neuromuscular clinic statin myotoxicity may have the following presentations:

1. Asymptomatic rise of serum CK which is usually mild (not more than five times the upper limit of normal or 1000 IU L^{-1}) and disappears after withdrawal of the statin. A subgroup in this category is exaggerated CK elevation after exercise in subjects on statins [11]. There is debate about when to stop statins in asymptomatic patients with a recorded CK elevation (whether it is determined to be a change from a pretreatment level or not).

2. Muscle pain (myalgia or cramps), usually but not always associated with hyperCKaemia. Some studies suggested that the rate of this complaint is similar in patients who are on a statin and those who are not [10,12] or is only modestly increased with statin usage [13]. Many large studies reported in the cardiological and lipid literature, together involving hundreds of thousands of patients, have relied on patient self-reporting without structured assessment of neuromuscular symptoms, without clinical examination to determine the presence or absence of weakness, and without a neuromuscular specialist being involved in the study.

3. Persistent muscle symptoms and high CK after withdrawal of the statin. This presentation seems less rare than was first thought and may represent a residual statin-induced myopathy or the presence of another neuromuscular condition unmasked by the statin [14]. In a subgroup of such patients evidence for a persistent or progressive myopathy was found. Up-regulation of major histocompatibility complex I (MHC I) expression was demonstrated in muscle biopsies, suggesting that the patients have a low-grade immune-mediated myopathy, probably induced by the statins [15].

4. Immune-mediated necrotizing myopathy. There seems to be an emerging recognition of a condition in which patients have a progressive myopathy with hyperCKaemia that responds only to aggressive immunotherapy [16]. In such patients signs appeared

with statin therapy which not only did not resolve upon withdrawal but continued to progress. The onset was subacute with myalgia, dysphagia, and arthralgia being the most frequent symptoms. Further support for the immune nature of this condition and its association with statins came with the identification of antibodies against a 100/200-kDa protein [17]. Ten of 16 patients had prolonged prior exposure to statins, a frequency much higher than in other inflammatory myopathies. MCH I up-regulation was demonstrated in only half of the biopsied patients, overlapping with a previously reported series [14]. The possibility that the 100-kDa autoantigen was HMGCR itself was studied in a cohort of 750 patients with apparent immune-mediated necrotizing myopathy and in 45 (6%) the presence of such antibody was demonstrated [18]. Of these 45 patients only 30 were exposed to statins (as expected most were over the age of 50 years). Thus, in a significant subgroup of adult patients with statin-associated myopathy, the statin-inhibited enzyme maybe the antigenic target of the autoimmune myopathy.

5. Rhabdomyolysis, which may be severe and even fatal. More than 3500 cases have been recorded in which rhabdomyolysis appeared in patients on statins [19] with an estimated mortality rate of 7.8% [10].

A higher susceptibility to the development of statin myopathy is associated with renal insufficiency, diabetes, and older age (>80 years) [20]. Also, it seems that professional athletes with a rigorous exercise programme are at risk for myotoxicity, as revealed by higher CK values in exercise-induced CK rise [20,21]. Much attention has been given recently to genetic factors which may increase the tendency toward statin-induced myopathy. Subjects with a single nucleotide polymorphism in the *SLCO1B1* gene were found to be more frequent among those with statin-induced myopathy [22,23]. This is not surprising because the gene encodes a hepatic statin transporter protein for almost all statins except fluvastatin [24]. Interestingly, however, there was no increase in this *SLCO1B1* polymorphism in the patients with possible HMGCR antibody-mediated myopathy [18].

A few metabolic myopathies were unmasked by statins, and these should be considered as possible contraindication for their use. The disorders reported to be revealed by statins are: myophosphorylase deficiency [25–27], carnitine palmitoyl transferase 2 deficiency (both homozygous and heterozygous individuals [25]), and mitochondrial encephalomyopathy with lactic acidosis and stroke [25,28,29]. Patients with known coenzyme Q10 deficiency are theoretically also at risk. Very rare conditions like acid maltase deficiency, rippling muscle disease, and susceptibility to malignant hyperthermia have also been suspected to be associated with statin myotoxicity [30]. However, caution should be used when considering these reports as proof of contraindication or increased risk. For almost 2 years the author has treated with a statin drug a young person with generalized mitochondrial myopathy (including progressive external ophthalmoplegia) and severe familial hyperlipidaemia associated with a high tendency to early atherosclerotic disease without there being a clinical change in the muscle disease. A view shared by several neuromuscular experts is that if a strong indication for statin use exists, patients with myopathies should not be denied this important treatment. Appropriate counselling of the patient and possibly stricter criteria for statin use are suggested, with an initial low dose and close monitoring during the early phases and during dose increases (by both clinical means and CK determination).

Importantly, a high baseline serum CK level without evidence for muscle disease on clinical examination has not been clearly shown to be a risk factor for statin myotoxicity [3,4,31]. The determination of CK levels before the onset of statin therapy is recommended by some experts but not others. However, such a determination can prevent a lot of confusion when the patient does report muscular symptoms and hyperCKaemia is first identified only after statins have been started. Currently statins have not been found to carry an extra risk in muscular dystrophies. It is not usually recommended to stop the statin if the rise in CK is less than three to five times the upper limit of normal (or of the pretreatment level) [9,31,32]. Another major decision is whether to reintroduce a statin after an episode of myotoxicity in patients with major cardiovascular risk. The preferred options in this situation are to commence another statin with a lower risk of myotoxicity (if indeed there is such an agent) or to reduce the dose of the statin to once every other day [33]. Switching therapy to another category of cholesterol-lowering agent such as ezetimibe, which inhibits the intestinal absorption of cholesterol, is recommended since the use of ezetimibe with a statin is probably not associated with a similar increased risk for myopathy [34], although is not fully safe either. One should be aware that this drug is currently more expensive than statins and arguably less effective (see Box 33.1)

The exact mechanism by which statins produce muscle damage is unknown but several hypotheses have been suggested (see [4,10,35] for review). The prevailing theory is that inhibition of protein prenylation and the induction of pro-apoptotic pathways are the main causes of statin myopathy but this remains controversial. As mentioned, a subgroup of statin-associated myopathy may be caused by triggering of an immune-mediated process against HMGCR [18]. This pathogenic mechanism remains to be proven as younger myositis patients who had not been exposed to statins also had such antibodies, suggesting that this might be an epiphenomenon in immune-mediated necrotizing myopathy.

Box 33.1 Typical scenarios and management advice to a patient on a statin who comes for consultation because of myalgia

1. Patient has normal creatine kinase (CK)
   Advice: discuss the severity of pain versus the need for a cholesterol-lowering agent. Examine for any weakness. If myalgia is tolerable continue and monitor CK every month. If not change to another statin or a different lipid-lowering drug.
2. Patient has either a very high CK (more than five time the normal value, tested after at least one day of relative rest) or weakness.
   Advice: stop statin immediately and follow. If the patient improves, continue to follow and refrain from statin usage. If not improved (or worse) perform biopsy. If rhabdomyolysis is found admit immediately and treat accordingly.
3. Patient deteriorates (increased weakness or CK levels) despite stopping statin.
   Advice: re-evaluate for other causes of muscle pain, weakness, and high CK. Perform biopsy if no immediate diagnosis emerges. Histological evaluation should include staining for markers for inflammation. Treat with high-dose steroids if immune-mediated myopathy is suspected.

Fibrates

Fibric acid derivatives are now widely used in treating hyperlipidaemia as a monotherapy or in combination with statins. This group of lipid-lowering agents has known myotoxic side effects and hyperCKaemia is common with their use [36]. A population-based cohort study concluded that the risk of developing a myopathy was six times greater in individuals taking a fibrate drug than in those taking a statin [37]. Necrotizing myopathy manifesting in myalgia and weakness with marked hyperCKaemia was reported with the use of the old and the new generation of fibrates [38,39]. Seventy-six patients who developed rhabdomyolysis (defined as CK levels more than ten times time the upper limit of normal) on fibrate therapy were reviewed [40]. Onset was usually a few weeks after introduction of fibrate. In most cases combination therapy with statins was prescribed but there were 23% on fibrate monotherapy. The two main drugs associated with rhabdomyolysis were gemfibrozil and bezafibrate. Withdrawal of the drug or dose reduction is usually followed by gradual recovery but readministration may lead to a recurrence of symptoms [39]. Death during rhabdomyolysis was recorded in 6% of the patients [40].

Nicotinic acid

A reversible myopathy characterized by severe muscle pain, cramping, and elevated CK can occur in patients taking nicotinic acid [41]. Rhabdomyolysis has been reported in patients taking nicotinic acid in combination with lovastatin [42], and the combination of nicotinic acid with a statin should therefore be avoided.

Ezetimibe

Myotoxic side effects have also been reported with this drug, although they are clearly milder and less frequent than with statins [43].

Other medications
Epsilon-aminocaproic acid

Myopathy is an uncommon complication of this antifibrinolytic agent given to patients with subarachnoid haemorrhage or hereditary angioneurotic oedema [44]. The myopathy usually develops after 4–6 weeks of treatment with daily doses over 18 g and may vary in severity from a mild self-limiting condition to severe rhabdomyolysis [45].

Emetine

A severe myopathy with weakness of the bulbar, neck, and proximal limb and trunk muscles may develop in individuals taking emetine for the treatment of amoebiasis or alcohol aversion therapy, or ipecac syrup as an emetic agent [46,47]. Serum CK activity is elevated up to 15-fold but may be normal. The drug also has cardiotoxic effects; it can cause left ventricular dysfunction and cardiac failure and may be fatal in some cases [47].

Cough suppressant

Reports of a proximal myopathy with muscle pain and hyperCKaemia in opiate addicts consuming large quantities of the cough suppressant Linctus Codeine appeared in Australia [49]. The myotoxicity was attributed to the cardiac glycosides scillarin A and B present in this medication [49].

Acute rhabdomyolysis

This is the most serious form of toxic myopathy encountered in clinical practice. It may occur following prolonged drug-induced coma (by self-intoxication or addiction), especially if associated with seizures or severe dyskinesia [50–53], after general anaesthesia if malignant hyperthermia occurs, in neuroleptic malignant syndrome, or as a severe side effect with one of a number of myotoxic drugs already discussed.

The condition is characterized by severe muscle pain and tenderness evolving over 24–48 h. Marked swelling of limb muscles may occur, leading at times to compartment syndromes. Serum CK values may be in the tens of thousands and myoglobinuria may lead to acute renal failure. Although the prognosis for recovery can be good, some patients die as a result of multiple organ failure and other complications.

Inflammatory myopathies

These are also painful myopathies associated with fibre necrosis but there is an additional element in this situation: the presence of inflammatory cell infiltration, considered to be a primary pathogenic event.

Polymyositis

A number of drugs have been associated with the development of polymyositis, dermatomyositis, or interstitial myositis (Table 33.2) (see [54]), but the causative role of the medication was not clear in all of them.

D-Penicillamine (DPA), used in the treatment of rheumatoid arthritis, progressive systemic sclerosis, or Wilson disease, has been known to induce an inflammatory myopathy indistinguishable from idiopathic polymyositis. The average dose of DPA used in reported cases was 600 mg day^{-1} and the average duration of treatment before development of the inflammatory myopathy was 12 months [55,56]. In most cases prompt improvement occurred after stopping DPA, but in some corticosteroids had to be administered. Myositis may reappear following a second course of DPA [55]. The development of myositis has been attributed to a disturbance of

Table 33.2 Drugs that can induce inflammatory myopathies*

Alfuzosin
Carbimazole
Cimetidine
D-penicillamine (DPA)
Hydralazine
Interferon-α
Leuprolide
Levodopa
L-tryptophan (contaminated)
Omeprazole
Penicillin
Phenytoin and mesantoin
Procainamide
Propylthiouracil
Terbinafine
Tumour necrosis factor alpha (TNFα) inhibitors
Statins
Vaccinations containing aluminium

*Arranged alphabetically and not by frequency or severity.

immunoregulation by the drug, which can also induce other autoimmune disorders. An association with HLA-B18, -B35, and -DR4 was reported in one series of cases, suggesting that there is a genetic predisposition [56].

More than two dozen patients with polymyositis that developed during interferon-α (INFα) treatment for chronic viral hepatitis or various malignancies were recently reviewed [57]. Most cases were of biopsy-proven inflammatory myopathy but in some only myopathy without inflammation was found. Improvement after withdrawal of INFα occurred in many but several patients needed immunomodulatory treatments. It is not clear if the known autoimmunity-inducing properties of INFα caused a disease de novo or unveiled a subclinical tendency for inflammatory myopathy in these patients.

An immune restoration inflammatory response (IRIS) is now more commonly seen, especially in early HIV treatment but also after stoppage of other immunomodulatory drugs. It should be borne in mind that there is one report of myositis as part of this syndrome [58].

Eosinophilia–myalgia syndrome

A syndrome of eosinophilia, myositis, and fasciitis was reported in the early 1990s in over 1500 patients in the United States taking certain preparations containing L-tryptophan [59]. It was characterized by severe myalgia, muscle tenderness, and hyperaesthesia with oedema and induration of the skin of the extremities resembling scleroderma and a marked peripheral blood eosinophilia [60]. The source of tryptophan preparation in the American cases was traced to a single manufacturer and the syndrome is now thought to have been due to a chemical contaminant [61].

Macrophagic myofasciitis

This syndrome was mainly recognized in France [62] manifesting with diffuse myalgia, arthralgia, and fatigue and responding to steroid therapy. It is now thought to have been caused by aluminium hydroxide which is a component of various intramuscularly injected vaccines [63]. Symptoms appeared immediately after the vaccination or were delayed by as much as a few months to a few years, The pathogenesis of this disorder is unclear.

Mitochondrial myopathy

A myopathy characterized by myalgia, fatigue, and proximal or generalized muscle weakness with hyperCKaemia has been described in patients treated with the nucleoside analogue zidovudine for acquired immunodeficiency syndrome (AIDS) but also with other agents belonging to this group [64,65]. The myopathy may improve when the drug is withdrawn. In some patients there is an associated AIDS-related inflammatory myopathy and it may be difficult to distinguish the two conditions. Muscle histology points to the mitochondrial basis of this condition with ragged-red fibres, cytochrome *c* oxidase-negative fibres, and abnormal mitochondria on electron microscopy. It was attributed to depletion of mitochondrial DNA but other mechanisms have also been suggested [66,67]. A case resembling chronic progressive ophthalmoplegia has also been reported with antiretroviral therapy [68].

Mitochondrial abnormalities and reduced cytochrome *c* oxidase activity have been observed in the myopathy induced by germanium, a constituent of a number of dietary supplements and elixirs [69]. A mitochondrial myopathy with ragged-red and cytochrome *c* oxidase-negative fibres and lipid accumulation has also been reported in patients taking statins [70,71]. These cases differ from the more common form of statin myopathy in having normal serum CK levels. These observations and the long list of drugs which can interfere with mitochondrial function [72] raise a difficult issue: should statins with their known mitochondrial inhibitory effects be avoided in patients with mitochondrial myopathies? There is no accepted policy and each patient should be evaluated separately, as discussed in the section on Statins.

Painless myopathies

Corticosteroid myopathy

Steroid myopathy is probably the most common drug-induced myopathy. It manifests with painless weakness and atrophy that develop insidiously (usually after weeks of continuous treatment), primarily in the hip and pelvic-girdle muscles. Fatigue is a frequent complaint. Moon face, hirsuitism, and weight gain frequently, but not always, accompany the muscle weakness. A condition called acute steroid myopathy developing especially in patients with status asthmaticus was described in the past, but currently it is believed to be part of the spectrum of critical illness myopathy (see section on Critical illness myopathy).

Symptomatic myopathy is more likely to develop in patients taking a higher steroid dose (daily doses of 40 mg of prednisone or the equivalent), but may occur at any dose after a prolonged period of treatment [73]. Electromyography shows a high incidence of subclinical myopathy [74]. Patients treated with fluorinated steroids (e.g. triamcinolone, dexamethasone) are more prone to develop myopathy [75]. An increased risk for the development of steroid myopathy is thought to occur in cancer patients, in people with asthma, and in older or inactive patients [76].

Serum CK levels are usually normal (or even lower than normal), and hyperCKaemia should alert the physician to the possibility of another diagnosis. Muscle biopsy shows selective Type 2 fibre atrophy, particularly of the Type 2B fibres.

The pathophysiology of steroid-induced muscle atrophy and weakness is not fully understood. The current prevailing hypothesis is that it results from a direct protein catabolic effect caused by decreasing protein synthesis and increasing proteolysis mediated via several signalling pathways (for review see [77]).

Corticosteroid myopathy is usually reversible if the drug is withdrawn shortly after the onset of symptoms or if the dose is quickly reduced. However, time to recovery even under such ideal circumstances maybe prolonged (weeks or more). Since steroid myopathy is a common problem and not all patients on steroids can be taken off them, various substances that could prevent or treat this complication have been investigated. Anabolic steroids, insulin growth factor and other growth hormones, branched chain amino acids, creatine, clenbuterol, and glutamine have all shown some promising results in animals but their effect in the human disease remains minimal or unproven [76,77]. Studies have shown that glucocorticoid-induced muscle atrophy and weakness can be partly prevented or reversed by a regular programme of physical training [78].

Hypokalaemic myopathy

Hypokalaemic myopathy may develop in patients with a severe drug-induced reduction in serum potassium. The weakness in such cases is usually generalized and may be associated with depressed tendon reflexes. The condition is usually painless, but myalgia may occur in the rapidly evolving cases. The main drugs with which this condition has been reported are diuretics, chlorthalidone, amphotericin B, carbenoxolone, lithium, and fluoroprednisolone containing nasal sprays, or with laxative abuse. Hypokalaemic myopathy may also develop in individuals who consume large quantities of liquorice or liquorice extracts, which are constituents of traditional Chinese medicines [79].

Autophagic myopathies

A large group of drugs with amphiphilic cationic properties have been shown to interfere with lysosomal digestion and to cause autophagic degeneration and accumulation of phospholipids in lysosomes [80]. With some of these medications (especially chloroquine and colchicine) myopathies are well documented but there are also rare reports with perhexiline [81], amiodarone [82], and vincristine [83].

Chloroquine and hydroxychloroquine

These antimalarial (and antirheumatic) drugs have been reported to cause a painless proximal myopathy, usually after prolonged administration (more than 6 months) [84,85]. Serum CK levels are normal or slightly elevated, and electromyography may show spontaneous activity with typical myopathic motor units [84]. Depression of tendon reflexes, mild sensory changes, and abnormal nerve conduction studies are often also found, pointing to an associated peripheral neuropathy. Histologically, the myopathy is characterized by autophagic vacuolar change in both major fibre types.

The prevalence of this myopathy (defined on the basis of histology and muscle enzyme disturbances) was prospectively evaluated. The accumulated prevalence was estimated to be around 12%, with about half of the patients showing some degree of weakness [85]. The myopathy is slowly reversible once the drug is withdrawn.

Colchicine

Marked, at times painful, neuromyopathy has been reported in more than 75 patients treated with colchicine over a prolonged period of administration or in the presence of renal insufficiency [86,88]. Serum CK levels are usually elevated 10- to 20-fold and electromyography reveals a mixed pattern of spontaneous activity with 'myopathic' units. Prompt recovery usually occurs on withdrawal of the drug.

Colchicine prevents the polymerization of tubulin into microtubules in a similar way to vincristine and may also cause an axonal neuropathy. Typical histological findings are those of small vacuoles ('autophagic' on electron microscopy) in muscle fibres, and central areas of altered staining in haematoxylin and eosin preparations with loss of enzyme activity resembling cores in histochemical preparations, but associated denervation changes may be found.

Alcoholic myopathy

Acute, subacute, and chronic forms of alcoholic myopathy are well documented [89] and although alcohol is not a medication its widespread usage merits a special description in this chapter devoted to toxic myopathies.

Alcohol is considered to be the most important cause of non-traumatic acute rhabdomyolysis in hospitalized patients [89]. Less severe cases with a predominantly proximal weakness may also be encountered. In some alcoholics, several attacks of acute myopathy may occur following alcohol binges. The prognosis for recovery after an attack is usually good. Transient asymptomatic hyperCKaemia can occur [90]. This is the most common form of myopathy in chronic alcoholics and is often subclinical [89]. Chronic progressive weakness and atrophy of the pelvic- and shoulder-girdle musculature is less common in alcoholics, and is usually associated with peripheral neuropathy. The serum CK level is normal. Electromyography shows myopathic potentials, or mixed myopathic and neuropathic changes in proximal limb muscles. The typical histological finding in biopsies from proximal limb muscles is Type 2 fibre atrophy [91]. This proximal myopathy may improve gradually with abstinence, and even the Type 2 fibre atrophy may be reversible [92].

Critical illness myopathy

Critical illness myopathy (CIM) is the term used for the syndrome of severe skeletal muscle weakness that develops in patients treated in intensive care units, usually with a combination of corticosteroids and non-depolarizing neuromuscular blocking agents. Numerous such cases have been reported and various other terms have been used for it, including acute quadriplegic myopathy and acute steroid myopathy. While most reported cases were treated with prolonged respiratory assistance, neuromuscular blockers, and steroids, many patients had only one of these agents and some others none [93]. Although the drugs may play some role in the development of CIM it is not now considered a pure drug-induced myopathy and will not be further dealt with in this chapter (see [94]).

Myasthenia aggravated by drugs

Several drugs can aggravate myasthenia gravis or other myasthenic syndromes (acquired and hereditary) through their blocking action at the neuromuscular synapse. This is the result of their basic pharmacology which induces a pre- or postsynaptic impairment of neuromuscular transmission. This side effect may manifest rapidly (hours to few days) or more slowly depending on the degree of blocking activity of the medication and the patient's condition. Rarely the same medications may unmask a previously undiagnosed myasthenia. A few medications may induce myasthenia via their immunomodulatory features. This *de novo* myasthenic syndrome takes usually a few months to develop. The list of drugs that may aggravate or unmask myasthenic conditions is increasing continuously (see Table 33.3, based on [95]). It is always important to monitor drug therapy in a patient with myasthenia who experiences deterioration and compare it with published reports on possible such side effects. However, the causative relationship between the drug and the deterioration is not always well established. This is especially true for the various antibiotics, since infection by itself can aggravate myasthenia. Not every listed drug is absolutely contraindicated in myasthenia (or other neuromuscular junction disorders) and the treating physician should exert common sense (associated with some extra caution) in the decision to start a listed medication.

An example of such a dilemma is the use of statins in myasthenic patients. There are a few reports about patients in whom statins have aggravated and even unmasked myasthenia [96–101]. The increased myasthenic symptoms appeared either early (1–2 weeks) after statin administration, suggesting a pharmacological blocking

Table 33.3 Drugs that may aggravate or induce myasthenia*

Antibiotics:
Ampicillin and imipenem
Aminoglycosides
Clarithromycin
Ciprofloxacin
Clindamycin
Colistin
Erythrpomycin
Lincomycin
Polymyxins
Tetracyclines

Antimicrobials:
Bretylium
Emetine
Imiquimod
Ritonavir

Cardiovascular:
Cibenzoline
Lidocaine (systemic)
Procainamide
Propranolol and other beta blockers
Quinidine
Verapamil

Psychoactive and neurological:
Chlorpromazine
Lithium
Phenytoin
Trihexyphenidyl
Trimethadione

Antirheumatic and immunomodulatory:
Chloroquine
Corticosteroids
Interferones
Penicillamine

Other medications:
Aprotinin
Contrast agents (iodinated)
Levonogestrel
Magnesium
Methoxyflurane
Pyrantal pamoate
Statins

*Arranged alphabetically in each group.

action, or were delayed by a few weeks to months. The increased myasthenic symptoms were severe enough to merit a change in the immune therapy and lasted for a few months in several of the reported patients. It should be noted that the myasthenic aggravation was not associated with symptoms of statin myopathy.

The mechanism of statin-aggravated myasthenia is unclear. Aggravation occurred in seropositive (antibodies to either acetylcholine receptor or to muscle-specific kinase) and seronegative myasthenia, suggesting a blockage of neuromuscular transmission. However, the length of the aggravation is not typical for a direct pharmacological action, which usually resolves few days after withdrawal of the offending medication. The most probable explanation for this side effect of statins is related to their immunomodulatory effects. The fact that in five patients a rechallenge with statins resulted in another aggravating episode strengthens the need for caution in the use of statins in myasthenic patients but currently this is not regarded as an absolute contraindication [95,102].

As in any drug-induced disorder, recognition and withdrawal of the suspected agent is the most important step in management. A few patients may develop a severe disease that will require increased immunosuppressive therapy. In acute severe drug-aggravated myasthenia, maintenance of respiratory function is essential and shortening the respirator time is a major goal. This can be achieved by agents that counteract the neuromuscular block induced by the offending drug. A positive response to edrophonium should be followed by neostigmine (1.0–2.5 mg intramuscularly). It should be repeated every 4 h if the edrophonium test remains positive. As combined pre- and postsynaptic block is common in drug-induced myasthenia, calcium infusions (one ampoule of calcium 10% given slowly) should be administered with the acetylcholinesterase inhibitors.

Avoidance of a possible drug complication in patients with myasthenia requires special consideration in two clinical situations: infection and elective operations. Myasthenic patients are prone to infection, mainly respiratory, and it is essential to achieve early control of the infection as it can aggravate the myasthenic condition. However, numerous antibiotics are known to impair neuromuscular transmission. If an ambulatory myasthenic patient needs antibiotics, it is mandatory to choose a 'safe' drug. Newer antibiotics that have not passed the time trial in myasthenia should not be regarded as safe even if there are no reports of drug-induced myasthenia concerning them. Myasthenic patients may require surgery, and a safe choice of anaesthetics is needed. Halothane may still be the best choice. Monitoring of the state of the neuromuscular junction by the 'train of four' method has long been practised by anaesthetists and is recommended for every patient with myasthenia during surgery and in the early postoperative period. Whenever possible, muscle relaxants should be avoided in myasthenia, especially the curariform agents.

Ten commandments in drug-induced myopathies

1. When in doubt stop the potential offending medication for at least 3 months.

2. Think of other potential emerging conditions (e.g. hypothyroid, low-grade myositis).

3. HyperCKaemia may be incidental—check several times after rest.

4. Identify patients 'at risk' for drug-induced disorders (e.g. liver or renal insufficiency).

5. Search the literature—many reports appear as Letters to the Editor only.

6. Electromyography is of little value in evaluating possible drug-induced myopathies.

7. Myalgia and fatigue are common in the general population.

8. A report to the drug company or regulatory bodies is not enough; alert the readership if strong new evidence exists even if not definite.

9. Rechallenge is sometimes the best way to prove a link, but is dangerous.

10. Treatment of severe drug-induced neuromuscular disorders may need more than simple drug withdrawal.

References

1. Kuncl RW. Agents and mechanisms of toxic myopathy. *Curr Opin Neurol* 2009; **22**: 506–15.

2. Kwiecinski H. Myotonia induced by chemical agents. *Crit Rev Toxicol* 1981; **8**: 279–310.

3. Baker SK, Samjoo IA. A neuromuscular approach to statin-related myotoxicity. *Can J Neurol Sci* 2008; **35**: 8–21.

4. Mamman AL, Amato A. Statin myopathy: a review of recent progress. *Curr Opin Rheumatol* 2010; **22**: 644–50.

5. Rowan C, Brinker AD, Nourjah P, et al. Rhabdomyolysis reports show interaction between simvastatin and CYP3AA inhibitors. *Pharmacoepidemiol Drug Saf* 2009; **18**: 301–9.

6. Garcia-Rodriguez LA, Massao-Gonzalez EL, Wallander MA, Johansson S. The safety of rosuvastatin in comparison with other statins in over 100,000 statin users in UK primary care. *Pharmacoepidemiol Drug Saf* 2008; **17**: 943–52.

7. Nichols GA, Koro CE. Does statin therapy initiation increase the risk for myopathy? An observational study of 32,225 diabetic and non diabetic patients. *Clin Ther* 2007; **29**: 1761–70.

8. Molokhia M, McKeigue P, Curcin V, Majeed A. Statin induced myopathy and myalgia: time trend analysis and comparison of risk associated with statin class from 1991–2006. *PLoS One* 2008; **3**: e2522.

9. Pasternak RC, Smith SC, Jr, Bairey-Merz CN, Grundy SM, Cleeman JI, Lenfant C. ACC/AHA/NHLBI clinical advisory on the use and safety of statins. *J Am Coll Cardiol* 2002; **40**: 567–72.

10. Thompson PD, Clarkson P, Karas RH. Statin-associated myopathy. *J Am Med Assoc* 2003; **289**: 1681–90.

11. Thompson PD, Nugent AM, Herbert PN. Increases in creatine kinase after exercise in patients treated with HMG Co-A reductase inhibitors. *J Am Med Assoc* 1990; **264**: 2992.

12. Armitage J, Bowan L, Collins R, Parish S, Torbert J and the MRC/BHF Heart Protection Study Collaborative Group. Effects of simvastatin 40 mg daily on muscle and liver adverse effects in a 5-year randomized placebo-controlled trial in 20,536 high-risk people. *BMC Clin Pharmacol* 2009; **9**: 6.

13. Buettner C, Davis RB, Leveille SG, et al. Prevalence of musculoskeletal pain and statin use. *J Gen Intern Med* 2008; **23**: 1182–6.

14. Echaniz-Laguna A, Mohr M, Tranchant C. Neuromuscular symptoms and elevated creatine kinase after statin withdrawal. *N Engl J Med* 2010; **362**: 564–5.

15. Needham M, Fabian V, Knezevic W, Panegryres P, Zilko P, Mastaglia FL. Progressive myopathy with up-regulationof MHC-I associated with statin therapy. *Neuromuscul Disord* 2007; **17**: 194–200.

16. Grable-Esposito P, Katzberg HD, Greenberg SA, et al. Immune-mediated necrotizing myopathy associated with statins. *Muscle Nerve* 2010; **41**: 185–90.

17. Christopher-Stine L, Casciola-Rosen L, Hong G, et al. A novel autoantibody recognizing 200 and 100 kDa proteins is associated with an immune-mediated necrotizing myopathy. *Arthritis Rheum* 2010; **62**: 2757–66.

18. Mammen AL, Chung T, Christopher-Stine L, et al. Autoantibodies against 3-hydroxy-3-methylglutaryl-coenzyme A reductase in patients with statin-associated autoimmune myopathy. *Arthritis Rheum* 2011; **63**: 713–21.

19. Omar MA, Wilson JP. FDA adverse event reports on statin-associated rhabdomyolysis. *Ann Pharmacother* 2002; **36**: 288–95.

20. Grundy SM. The issue of statin safety. Where do we stand? *Circulation* 2005; **111**: 3016–19.

21. Sinzinger H, O'Grady J. Professional athletes suffering from familial hypercholesterolaemia rarely tolerate statin treatment because of muscular problems. *Br J Clin Pharmacol* 2004; **57**: 525–8.

22. Armarenco P, Bogousslavsky J, Callahan A, et al. High dose atrovastatin after stroke or transient ischemic attack. *N Engl J Med* 2006; **355**: 789–99.

23. Voora D, Shah SH, Spasojevic I, et al. The SLCO1B1*5 genetic variant is associated with statin-induced side effects. *Am J Coll Cardiol* 2009; **54**: 1609–15.

24. Niemi M, Pasanen Mk, Neuvonen PJ. SLCO1B1 polymorphism and sex affect the pharmacokinetics of pravastatin but not fluvastation. *Clin Pharmacol Ther* 2006; **80**: 356–66.

25. Vladutiu GD, Simmons Z, Isackson PJ, et al. Genetic risk factors associated with lipid-lowering drug-induced myopathies. *Muscle Nerve* 2006; **34**: 153–62.

26. Lorenzoni PJ, Silvado CE, Scola RH, et al. McArdle disease with rhabdomyolysis induced by rosuvastatin: case report. *Arq Neuropsiquiatr* 2007; **65**: 834–7.

27. Livingstone C, Al Riyami S, Wilkins P, Ferns GA. McArdle's disease diagnosed following statin-induced myositis. *Ann Clin Biochem* 2004; **41**: 338–40.

28. Thomas JE, Lee N, Thompson PD. Statins provoking MELAS syndrome. A case report. *Euro Neurol* 2007; **57**: 232–5.

29. Tay SK, DiMauro S, Pang AY, et al. Myotoxicity of lipid-lowering agents in a teenager with MELAS mutation. *Pediatr Neurol* 2008; **39**: 426–8.

30. Ghatak A, Faheem O, Thompson PD. The genetics of statin-induced myopathy. *Atherosclerosis* 2010; **210**: 337–43.

31. Glueck CJ, Rawal B, Khan NA, et al. Should high creatine kinase discourage the initiation or continuance of statins for treatment of hypercholesterolemia? *Metabolism* 2009; **59**: 233–8.

32. Argov Z. Drug-induced myopathies. *Curr Opin Neurol* 2000; **13**: 541–5.

33. Backes JM, Venero CV, Gibson CA, et al. Effectiveness and tolerability of every-other-day rosuvastatin dosing in patients with prior statin intolerance. *Ann Pharmacotherap* 2008; **42**: 341–6.

34. Kashani A, Sallam T, Bheemreddy S, et al. Review of side-effect profile of combination ezetimibe and statin therapy in randomized clinical trials. *Am J Cardiol* 2008; **101**: 1606–13.

35. Ucar M, Mjorndal T, Dahlqvist R. HMG-CoA reductase inhibitors and myotoxicity. *Drug Saf* 2000; **22**: 441–57.

36. Baer AN, Wortmann RL. Myotoxicity associated with lipid-lowering drugs. *Curr Opin Rheumatol* 2007; **19**: 67–73.

37. Gaist D, Rodriguez LA, Huerta C, Hallas J, Sindrup SH. Lipid-lowering drugs and risk of myopathy: a population-based follow-up study. *Epidemiology* 2001; **12**: 565–9.

38. Langer T, Levy RI. Acute muscular syndrome associated with administration of clofibrate. *N Engl J Med* 1968; **279**: 856–8.

39. Magarian GJ, Lucas LM, Colley C. Gemfibrozil-induced myopathy. *Arch Intern Med* 1991; **151**: 1873–4.

40. Wu J, Song Y, Li H, Chen J. Rhabdomyolysis associated with fibrate therapy: review of 76 published cases and a new case report. *Eur J Pharmacol* 2009; **65**: 1169–74.

41. Litin SC, Anderson CF. Nicotinic acid-associated myopathy: a report of three cases. *Am J Med* 1989; **86**: 481–3.

42. Reaven P, Witztum JL. Lovastatin, nicotinic acid, and rhabdomyolysis. *Ann Intern Med* 1988; **109**: 597–8.

43. Florentin M, Liberopoulos EN, Elisaf MS. Ezetimibe-associated adverse effects: what the clinician needs to know. *Int J Clin Pract* 2008; **62**: 88–96.

44. Lane RJ, McLelland NJ, Martin AM, Mastaglia FL. Epsilon aminocaproic acid (EACA) myopathy. *Postgrad Med J* 1979; **55**: 282–5.

45. Mastaglia FL. Adverse effects of drugs on muscle. *Drugs* 1982; **24**: 304–21.

46. Bennett HS, Spiro AJ, Pollack MA, Zucker P. Ipecac-induced myopathy simulating dermatomyositis. *Neurology* 1982; **32**: 91–4.

47. Friedman EJ. Death from ipecac intoxication in a patient with anorexia nervosa. *Am J Psychiatry* 1984; **141**: 702–3.

48. Palmer EP, Guay AT. Reversible myopathy secondary to abuse of ipecac in patients with major eating disorders. *N Engl J Med* 1985; **313**: 1457–9.

49. Kennedy M. Cardiac glycoside toxicity. An unusual manifestation of drug addiction. *Med J Aust* 1981; **2**: 686, 688–9.

50. Gabow PA, Kaehny WD, Kelleher SP. The spectrum of rhabdomyolysis. *Medicine (Baltimore)* 1982; **61**: 141–52.

51. Grob D. Rhabdomyolysis and drug-related myopathies. *Curr Opin Rheumatol* 1990; **2**: 908–15.

52. Lazarus AL, Toglia JU. Fatal myoglobinuric renal failure in a patient with tardive dyskinesia. *Neurology* 1985; **35**: 1055–7.

53. Cogen FC, Rigg G, Simmons JL, Domino EF. Phencyclidine-associated acute rhabdomyolysis. *Ann Intern Med* 1978; **88**: 210–12.

54. Klopstock T. Drug-induced myopathies. *Curr Opin Neurol* 2008; **21**: 590–5.

55. Takahashi K, Ogita T, Okudaira H, Yoshinoya S, Yoshizawa H, Miyamoto T. D-penicillamine-induced polymyositis in patients with rheumatoid arthritis. *Arthritis Rheum* 1986; **29**: 560–4.

56. Carroll GJ, Will RK, Peter JB, Garlepp MJ, Dawkins RL. Penicillamine induced polymyositis and dermatomyositis. *J Rheumatol* 1987; **14**: 995–1001.

57. Stubgen JP. Interferon alpha and neuromuscular disorders. *J Neuroimmunol* 2006; **207**: 3–17.

58. Calza L Manfredi R Colangeli V, et al. Polymyositis associated with HIV infection during immune restoration induced by highly active antiretroviral therapy. *Clin Exp Rheumatol* 2004; **22**: 651–2.

59. Kaufman LD. Neuromuscular manifestations of the l-tryptophan-associated eosinophilia-myalgia syndrome. *Curr Opin Rheumatol* 1990; **2**: 896–900.

60. Varga J, Peltonen J, Uitto J, Jimenez S. Development of diffuse fasciitis with eosinophilia during L-tryptophan treatment: demonstration of elevated type I collagen gene expression in affected tissues. A clinicopathologic study of four patients. *Ann Intern Med* 1990; **112**: 344–51.

61. Belongia EA, Hedberg CW, Gleich GJ, et al. An investigation of the cause of the eosinophilia-myalgia syndrome associated with tryptophan use. *N Engl J Med* 1990; **323**: 357–65.

62. Gherardi RK, Coquet M, Cherin P, et al. Macrophagic myofasciitis lesions assess long-term persistence of vaccine-derived aluminium hydroxide in muscle. *Brain* 2001; **124**: 1821–31.

63. Gherardi RK, Authier FJ. Aluminum inclusion macrophagic myofasciitis: a recently identified condition. *Immunol Allergy Clin North Am* 2003; **23**: 699–712.

64. Dalakas MC, Illa I, Pezeshkpour GH, Laukaitis JP, Cohen B, Griffin JL. Mitochondrial myopathy caused by long-term zidovudine therapy. *N Engl J Med* 1990; **322**: 1098–105.

65. Dalaks MC. Toxic and drug-induced myopathies. *J Neurol Neurosurg Psychiatry* 2009; **80**: 832–8.

66. Arnaudo E, Dalakas M, Shanske S, Moraes CT, DiMauro S, Schon EA. Depletion of muscle mitochondrial DNA in AIDS patients with zidovudine-induced myopathy. *Lancet* 1991; **337**: 508–10.

67. Scruggs ER, Dirks Naylor AJ. Mechanisms of zidovudine-induced mitochondrial toxicity and myopathy. *Pharmacology* 2008; **82**: 83–8.

68. Pfeffer G, Cote HC Montaner JS, et al. Ophthalmoplegia and ptosis: mitochondrial toxicity in patients receiving HIV therapy. *Neurology* 2009; **73**: 71–2.

69. Tao SH, Bolger PM. Hazard assessment of germanium supplements. *Regul Toxicol Pharmacol* 1997; **25**: 211–19.

70. England JD, Walsh JC, Stewart P, Boyd I, Rohan A, Halmagyi GM. Mitochondrial myopathy developing on treatment with the HMG CoA reductase inhibitors—simvastatin and pravastatin. *Aust NZ J Med* 1995; **25**: 374–5.

71. Phillips PS, Haas RH, Bannykh S, et al. Statin-associated myopathy with normal creatine kinase levels. *Ann Intern Med* 2002; **137**: 581–5.

72. Finsterer J, Segall L. Drugs interfering with mitochondrial disorders. *Drugs Chemic Toxicol* 2010; **33**: 138–51.

73. Bowyer SL, LaMothe MP, Hollister JR. Steroid myopathy: incidence and detection in a population with asthma. *J Allergy Clin Immunol* 1985; **76**: 234–42.

74. Coomes EN. Corticosteroid myopathy. *Ann Rheum Dis* 1965; **24**: 465–72.

75. Dropcho EJ, Soong SJ. Steroid-induced weakness in patients with primary brain tumors. *Neurology* 1991; **41**: 1235–9.

76. Rodrigues Pereira RM, Freire de Carvalho J. glucocorticoid-induced myopathy. *Joint Bone Spine* 2011; **78**: 41–4.

77. Schakman O, Gilson H, Thissen JP. Mechanisms of glucocorticoid-induced myopathy. *J Endocrinol* 2008; **197**: 1–10.

78. Horber FF, Scheidegger JR, Grunig BE, Frey FJ. Thigh muscle mass and function in patients treated with glucocorticoids. *Eur J Clin Invest* 1985; **15**: 302–7.

79. Valeriano J, Tucker P, Kattah J. An unusual cause of hypokalemic muscle weakness. *Neurology* 1983; **33**: 1242–3.

80. Drenckhahn D, Lullmann-Rauch R. Experimental myopathy induced by amphiphilic cationic compounds including several psychotropic drugs. *Neuroscience* 1979; **4**: 549–62.

81. Tomlinson IW, Rosenthal FD. Proximal myopathy after perhexiline maleate treatment. *Br Med J* 1977; **1**(6072): 1319–20.

82. Fernando Roth R, Itabashi H, Louie J, Anderson T, Narahara KA. Amiodarone toxicity: myopathy and neuropathy. *Am Heart J* 1990; **119**: 1223–5.

83. Bradley WG, Lassman LP, Pearce GW, Walton JN. The neuromyopathy of vincristine in man. Clinical, electrophysiological and pathological studies. *J Neurol Sci* 1970; **10**: 107–31.

84. Mastaglia FL, Papadimitriou JM, Dawkins RL, Beveridge B. Vacuolar myopathy associated with chloroquine, lupus erythematosus and thymoma. Report of a case with unusual mitochondrial changes and lipid accumulation in muscle. *J Neurol Sci* 1977; **34**: 315–28.

85. Casado E, Gratacos J, Tolosa C, et al. Antimalarial myopathy: an underdiagnosed complication? Prospective longitudinal study of 119 patients. *Ann Rheum Dis* 2006; **65**; 385–90.

86. Riggs JE, Schochet SS, Jr, Gutmann L, Crosby TW, DiBartolomeo AG. Chronic human colchicine neuropathy and myopathy. *Arch Neurol* 1986; **43**: 521–3.

87. Kuncl RW, Duncan G, Watson D, Alderson K, Rogawski MA, Peper M. Colchicine myopathy and neuropathy. *N Engl J Med* 1987; **316**: 1562–8.

88. Wilbur K, Makowsky M. Colchicine myotoxicity: case report and literature review. *Pharmacotherapy* 2004; **24**: 1784–92.

89. Urbano-Marquez A, Fernandez-Sola J. Effects of alcohol on skeletal and cardiac muscle. *Muscle Nerve* 2004; **30**: 689–707.

90. Haller RG, Knochel JP. Skeletal muscle disease in alcoholism. *Med Clin North Am* 1984; **68**: 91–103.

91. Martin F, Ward K, Slavin G, Levi J, Peters TJ. Alcoholic skeletal myopathy, a clinical and pathological study. *Q J Med* 1985; **55**: 233–51.

92. Slavin G, Martin F, Ward P, Levi J, Peters T. Chronic alcohol excess is associated with selective but reversible injury to type 2B muscle fibres. *J Clin Pathol* 1983; **36**: 772–7.

93. Hoke A, Rewcastle NB, Zochodne DW. Acute quadriplegic myopathy unrelated to steroids or paralyzing agents: quantitative EMG studies. *Can J Neurol Sci* 1999 **26**: 325–9.

94. Latronico N, Bolton CF. Critical illness polyneuropathy and myopathy: a major cause of muscle weakness and paralysis. *Lancet Neurol* 2011; **10**: 931–41.

95. Argov Z. Treatment of myasthenia: nonimmune issues. *Curr Opin Neurol* 2009; **22**: 493–7.

96. Negvesky GJ, Kolsky MP, Laureno R, Yau TH. Reversible atrovastatin-associated external ophthalmoplegia, anti-acetylcholine receptor antibodies, and ataxia. *Arch Ophthalmol* 2000; **118**: 427–8.

97. Parmar B, Francis P, Ragge NK. Statins, fibrates and ocular myasthenia. *Lancet* 2002; **360**: 717.

98. Cartwright MS, Jeffery DR, Nuss GR, Donofrio P. Statin-associated exacerbation of myasthenia gravis. *Neurology* 2004; **63**: 2188.

99. Purvin V, Kawasaki A, Kyle H, et al. Statin-associated myasthenia gravis: report of 4 cases and review of the literature. *Medicine* 2006; **85**: 82–5.

100. De Sousa E, Howard J. More evidence for the association between statins and myasthenia gravis. *Muscle Nerve* 2008; **38**: 1085–6.

101. Oh SJ, Dhall R, Young A, et al. Statins may aggravate myasthenia gravis. *Muscle Nerve* 2008; **38**: 1101–7.

102. Gilhus NE. Is it safe to use statins in patients with myasthenia gravis? *Nat Neurol* 2009; **5**: 8–9.

CHAPTER 34

Endocrine myopathies

Merrilee Needham and Frank Mastaglia

Introduction

Neuromuscular problems can occur in a number of different endocrine disorders, and may occasionally be the presenting symptom or the clue that leads to a diagnosis. The possibility of an underlying endocrine disorder should be considered in patients presenting with myalgia, muscle cramps, weakness or fatigability, or with muscular atrophy or hypertrophy, and appropriate investigations should be carried out in the knowledge that the symptoms will usually be reversible once the endocrine disorder is corrected. An associated endocrinopathy should also be considered in individuals with other longer-standing neuromuscular disorders when there is an unexpected deterioration or acceleration of the condition. Muscle involvement occurs most frequently in patients with hyperthyroidism or hypothyroidism, but may also occur with parathyroid and adrenal cortical disorders, acromegaly, and diabetes mellitus [1].

Hypothyroid myopathy

Patients with hypothyroidism commonly complain of neuromuscular symptoms including myalgia, muscle stiffness, cramping, and weakness which usually resolve when thyroid replacement therapy is commenced [2]. However, some people with longer-standing untreated hypothyroidism develop a more severe proximal or more diffuse myopathy with markedly elevated serum creatine kinase (CK) levels, and myopathic electromyography (EMG) findings with prominent spontaneous potentials [3] resembling polymyositis [4]. Slowing in muscle contraction and relaxation ('pseudomyotonia') and delay in the relaxation phase of the tendon reflexes (the Woltman sign; 'hung-up reflexes'), classically the ankle jerk, is a useful confirmatory sign of hypothyroidism. Myoedema or the 'mounding' phenomenon may be demonstrable by direct percussion of the larger limb muscles in some patients and is electrically silent with EMG. Very rarely, adults with long-standing untreated hypothyroidism may develop a clinical picture characterized by painful muscle spasms on movement and diffuse muscular hypertrophy (Hoffman syndrome) (Fig. 34.1) [5]. A similar syndrome of diffuse muscular hypertrophy is documented in the older literature in children with untreated congenital hypothyroidism (Kocher–Debre–Semelaigne syndrome) but this no longer occurs with routine screening at birth. Hypothyroidism may also present with unexplained rhabdomyolysis [6] or with asymptomatic elevation of the serum CK level, and therefore needs to be considered in the differential diagnosis of unexplained hyperCKaemia. [7]. In addition, hypothyroidism may also predispose to the development of myopathy and rhabdomyolysis in patients taking cholesterol-lowering drugs, with both fibrates [8] and statins potentially unmasking a

previously undiagnosed hypothyroid myopathy [7]. Restoration of the euthyroid state is usually sufficient to result in the complete resolution of muscle symptoms in patients with hypothyroid myopathy, but the recovery period may be protracted in those with more severe long-standing myopathy.

The diagnosis of hypothyroid myopathy can usually be made on clinical grounds once the hypothyroidism has been confirmed biochemically (see Box 34.1). However, in patients who do not improve after treatment with thyroxine replacement or have atypical features, a muscle biopsy may be required to exclude other types of myopathy such as an immune-mediated myositis. The biopsy findings in hypothyroid myopathy are variable but are most commonly Type 1 hypertrophy and Type 2 fibre atrophy [4], reduced numbers of Type 2 fibres [9], and in some cases necrosis and regeneration of muscle fibres (Fig 34.2a) [3,10]. Other changes in long-standing cases include core-like areas which lack enzyme activity, stain with N-CAM antibodies [11], and contain

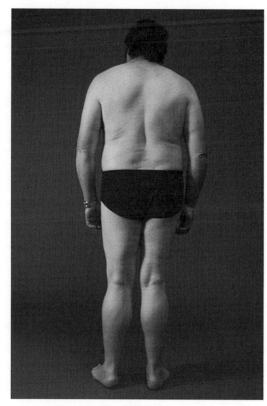

Fig. 34.1 Diffuse muscular hypertrophy in a 56-year-old man with severe hypothyroidism and Hoffman syndrome.

Box 34.1 Practice points: hypothyroid myopathy

♦ Clinically associated with myalgia, stiffness and cramping

♦ Occasionally associated with:
  • severe proximal myopathy
  • markedly elevated creatine kinase (CK)
  • 'myopathic' electromyogram with spontaneous activity
  • pseudomyotonia
  • 'hung-up' reflexes

♦ Consider hypothyroidism as a cause of:
  • asymptomatic hyperCKaemia
  • rhabdomyolysis
  • statin-induced myopathy

granulofilamentous material, and calcium deposits (Fig. 34.2b) [3]. Experimental animal studies have shown that the hypothyroid state causes a marked increase in the number of Type 1 (slow-twitch) fibres, with the conversion of fast to slow-twitch myosin isoforms [12].

Hyperthyroid myopathy

It is not uncommon to find subclinical weakness and atrophy in patients with long-standing untreated hyperthyroidism, and quantitative EMG studies have also shown a high incidence of subclinical myopathy [2]. However, only a small proportion of patients with hyperthyroidism develop a symptomatic myopathy, and this is rarely the presenting symptom [13]. The weakness is most prominent in proximal muscle groups, but in some cases it may be more diffuse; in severe cases the bulbar and respiratory muscles may also be affected [1]. Myalgia and muscle cramps are prominent in some cases and muscle fasciculations may also occur, but are uncommon. The association of fasciculations with bulbar symptoms and brisk tendon reflexes may lead to a mistaken diagnosis of motor neuron disease if hyperthyroidism is not considered [14]. The CK level is usually normal in patients with hyperthyroid myopathy and may even be below the normal range, but may be elevated in rare cases of thyroid storm. The muscle symptoms generally improve progressively after treatment of the hyperthyroid state; however, there have been reports of patients who developed a myopathy after a total thyroidectomy which was responsive to triiodothyronine (T3) [15], suggesting that a relative hypothyroid state may be sufficient to cause muscle symptoms.

The diagnosis is usually made clinically; recent advances in diagnostic imaging such as magnetic resonance elastography may be helpful but require further investigation [16]. Muscle biopsy is only required for the diagnosis of hyperthyroid myopathy in patients with atypical features, or if symptoms fail to improve after treatment of the hyperthyroidism. The biopsy findings in hyperthyroid myopathy are non-specific, including a variable degree of atrophy of Type 1 and Type 2 muscle fibres [9], increase in the size and number of mitochondria [17], and, in some cases, small interstitial

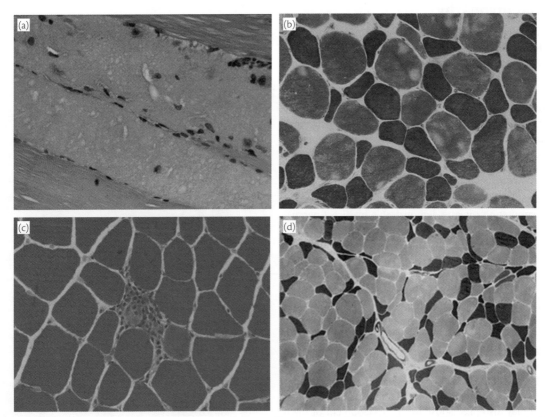

Fig. 34.2 (a) Myofibre necrosis in a case of hypothyroid myopathy. (b) Cores in myofibres and Type 2 fibre atrophy in a case of hypothyroid myopathy (ATPase, 9.4). (c) Single myofibre necrosis and inflammatory infiltrate in a case of hyperthyroid myopathy (haematoxylin and eosin). (d) Type 2 fibre atrophy in a case of corticosteroid myopathy (ATPase, 9.4). (See also figure in colour plate section)

lymphocytic infiltrates (Fig. 34.2c). Studies of experimental hyperthyroidism in rats have shown a reduction in number of Type 1 muscle fibres [12], which is associated with a switch in expression from slow to fast myosin isoforms [18].

Thyrotoxic periodic paralysis

A form of episodic paralysis with hypokalaemia, which closely resembles familial hypokalaemic periodic paralysis (HKPP), may occur in patients with hyperthyroidism, and can occasionally be the presenting symptom [19,20]. It most commonly occurs in association with Graves disease, but can also occur with thyroiditis, toxic multinodular goitre, and drug use (including thyroxine [21], amiodarone, and thyroxine-containing weight-loss supplements) [22]. Thyrotoxic periodic paralysis (TPP) is much more common in males, with a male:female ratio of approximately 20:1. The condition typically occurs in young Asian males and has been reported to occur in 5–13% of thyrotoxic Asian men [23,24]. Although TPP was considered to occur only in people of Asian origin, in recent years it has also been recognised increasingly in Western countries [21,23]. In contrast to familial HKPP, which is caused by mutations in the calcium channel (*CACN1AS*) or sodium channel (*SCN4A*) genes, no specific genetic basis has been identified for most cases of TPP [24]. However, an association with mutations in *KCNJ18*, which encodes a skeletal muscle-specific inwardly rectifying K(+) channel (Kir2.6), resulting in reduced activity of the channel has been reported in some patients [25,26]. This has been suggested to predispose to paradoxical depolarization of the sarcolemma when hypokalaemia occurs during attacks, leading to inactivation of the Na(+) channel and muscle inexcitability [25]. In addition, single nucleotide polymorphisms in the calcium channel alpha-1 subunit gene and certain human leucocyte antigen (HLA) haplotypes have been found in some Chinese and Japanese TPP patients [20,27], but not in the Na$^+$/K$^+$-ATPase genes [28]. The severity of the hyperthyroidism is variable, and in some cases of TPP the usual clinical signs of hyperthyroidism are absent, the diagnosis only being made when biochemical studies are performed. As in the primary form of HKPP, attacks of weakness are precipitated by meals with a high carbohydrate content or by alcohol, and may follow strenuous physical activity. They may also occur spontaneously, particularly on waking in the morning, and may last for several hours or, less often, for several days. The weakness initially affects the proximal limb and trunk muscles but in the more severe attacks it may progress to a profound flaccid quadriplegia. A feature that may lead to some diagnostic confusion is that in some cases of TPP the limb weakness is asymmetric, being more severe in muscles that were recently subjected to strenuous exercise. The severity of the weakness correlates with the degree of hypokalaemia [29], with K$^+$ levels of <3 mmol L^{-1} resulting from intracellular potassium shifts due to increased activity of the Na$^+$/K$^+$-ATPase pump [19]. The cause of this is uncertain, but a number of possible factors may contribute, including the direct effects of excessive thyroid hormone, an increased number and sensitivity of the β-adrenergic receptors, and an exaggerated insulin response to carbohydrate loading. In addition, androgens may increase the activity of this pump, which may help explain the male predominance [29,30]. A recent study comparing hyperthyroid Chinese men with and without TPP found significantly higher levels of testosterone and insulin (after a glucose load) despite lower levels of

thyroxine and free T3 in the cohort with TPP, providing further evidence for these theories [31].

Patients with TPP will often be admitted to hospital as a medical emergency during an acute attack. Treatment requires cautious intravenous or oral potassium replacement, with careful monitoring of the serum K$^+$ level to avoid rebound hyperkalaemia [23,32]. Phosphate infusions may also be necessary in patients with hypophosphataemia. Propranolol, a non-selective beta blocker, should also be commenced (3–4 mg kg^{-1} orally) to suppress the activity of the Na$^+$/K$^+$-ATPase pump; it is also effective in preventing further attacks of paralysis [23]. Control of the hyperthyroidisim by radioiodine, antithyroid drugs, or surgery will completely abolish further attacks [20,23]. However, patients should be advised to avoid known precipitating factors until the euthyroid state has been achieved, and any future thyroid hormone replacement should be monitored as attacks can recur with over-enthusiastic replacement (Box 34.2).

Thyroid ophthalmopathy

Thyroid ophthalmopathy is a serious condition caused by swelling of the contents of the orbit, leading to exophthalmos, hyperaemia and oedema of the eyelids and conjunctiva, diplopia, and, in severe cases, paresis of the extraocular muscles and compression of the optic nerve which can result in permanent visual loss if untreated. The condition is usually associated with Graves disease and less frequently with Hashimoto thyroiditis. Enlargement of the extraocular muscles, which is due to oedema, lymphocytic infiltration, and the proliferation of fibroblasts, can be demonstrated by computed tomography (CT) or magnetic resonance imaging (MRI) of the orbits in up to 70% of cases (Fig. 34.3), and tends to be symmetric [33]. However, oculomotor restriction due to infiltration only occurs in 10–15% of cases. The muscle most frequently affected is the inferior rectus [33].

Predisposing factors for Graves ophthalmopathy include smoking [34] and genetic factors such as specific polymorphisms in genes for interleukins 3, 4, 5, 10, and 12, transforming growth factor beta, interferon gamma, and tumour necrosis factor alpha [35–37]. In addition, thyroid-related eye disease has been reported to present shortly after cataract surgery, leading to serious sight-threatening complications [38], giving weight to the hypothesis that orbital trauma may also be a precipitant [33]. The pathogenesis is not known, but is thought to be due to a T-cell-mediated process against common antigen(s) shared by the orbital tissues and the thyroid

---

Box 34.2 Practice points: thyrotoxic periodic paralysis

- Clinically identical to familial hypokalaemic periodic paralysis
- Usually in association with Graves disease
- Males more often affected then females
- Attacks precipitated by high intake of carbohydrates, alcohol, or strenuous physical activity
- Judicious potassium replacement and beta blockers are effective therapy
- Control of hyperthyroidism effective in preventing future attacks.

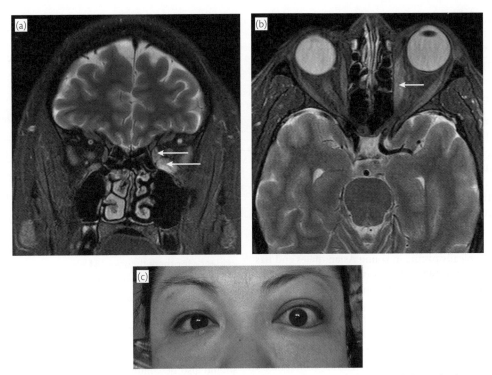

Fig. 34.3 (a) Coronal T_2 fat-suppressed magnetic resonance image (MRI) of the orbits of a young woman with Graves ophthalmopathy demonstrating swollen left inferior and medial rectus (arrows). (b) Axial T_2 MRI of the orbits of a young woman with Graves ophthalmopathy demonstrating swollen left medial rectus (arrow). (c) Photograph of the young woman with Graves ophthalmopathy affecting the left eye.

gland [39], with both the thyrotropin receptor on orbital fibroblasts and insulin-like growth factor receptor type 1 (IGF1R) being implicated as possible target antigens. The orbital fibroblasts are thought to be the primary target of the immune response because the fibrocytes express relevant autoantigens such as IGF1R and functional thyroid-stimulating hormone (TSH) receptors and differentially accumulate in the orbital tissue [40], but there is also some evidence for an antibody-dependent cell-mediated cytotoxic process involving extraocular muscle antigens [39]. In particular, there are serum autoantibodies associated with thyroid eye disease, including antibodies against the calcium-binding protein calsequestrin (CASQ) [41]. Moreover, persistently high levels of TSH receptor antibody are associated with a severe course of Graves orbitopathy [42], and the novel Mc4 thyroid-stimulating immunoglobulin is a functional indicator of activity and severity [43].

Treatment involves the administration of glucocorticoids systemically [44] or by intra-ocular injection [45] and correction of the associated thyroid abnormality. Other options in resistant cases include intravenous immunoglobulin, immunosuppressive agents (cyclosporine), somatostatin analogues (octreotide), and orbital radiotherapy [39,46]. Orbital decompression may be necessary in some cases and is useful in reducing proptosis, exposure keratopathy, congestive apex symptoms, and in improving cosmesis [47]. It can be combined with optic nerve decompression if vision is threatened. Total thyroid ablation combining surgery with radioiodine is increasingly being used for those with severe unresponsive ophthalmopathy in an effort to completely eliminate thyroid antigen, but studies supporting this approach are awaited [48]. Radioiodine has been reported to cause progression or *de novo* development of Graves ophthalmopathy, particularly in smokers, but this may be prevented with oral steroids [49]. Newer therapies which may be of interest, particularly rituximab that may counter pathogenic mechanisms of both hyperthyroidism and ophthalmopathy, need to be evaluated in randomized controlled trials [50–52].

Adrenal myopathies

Steroid myopathies occur in the presence of excess glucocorticoid, which is either endogenous [such as in Cushing syndrome or excess adrenocorticotropic hormone (ACTH)] or exogenous (such as oral or intravenous steroid therapy). In addition, it can also occur in patients with primary hyperaldosteronism (Conn syndrome) who can also develop HKPP [1,53]. Proximal myopathy is one of the most common symptoms in Cushing syndrome, being present in up to 80% of patients in some series [54]. Some patients can develop myopathy or worsen existing myopathy after adrenalectomy for treatment of Cushing syndrome due to excessive ACTH secretion (Nelson syndrome). The aetiopathogenesis is still not fully understood, but steroids are known to have complex effects, including impairment of protein synthesis as well as a catabolic effect on the muscle, possibly by stimulation of the ubiquitin–proteasome proteolytic pathway. Clinically it presents as a slowly progressive proximal myopathy affecting the lower limb muscles more than the upper limbs, particularly the quadriceps which are the most severely affected. The myopathy of Cushing syndrome can be associated with cardiac complications, including both hypertrophic and dilated cardiomyopathy [55]. The diagnosis is usually clinical, but is confirmed with the biopsy finding of Type 2 fibre atrophy (Fig. 34.2d). It has recently been suggested that low serum CK and myoglobin levels and reduced muscle fibre conduction velocity may be helpful in the diagnosis of steroid myopathy in Cushing syndrome [56] (Box 34.4).

Muscle symptoms can also occur in conditions of steroid depletion, with complaints of fatigue, muscle weakness, and cramping being common in patients with Addison disease. Occasionally patients may develop a more severe generalized myopathy which can involve the respiratory muscles, and which is reversible after cortisone replacement therapy [57]. The CK level is not usually elevated and the EMG and muscle biopsy findings are non-specific.

Hyperparathyroidism

Complaints of muscle weakness and fatigability may be the presenting symptoms in patients with primary hyperparathyroidism and some patients may develop a mild sensory peripheral neuropathy [58,59]. However, in modern clinical practice when the diagnosis of hyperparathyroidism is often made purely on biochemical grounds, many patients are asymptomatic. In two recent series myopathy was present in 47% of patients at presentation, but delayed diagnosis may have played a role in the number of symptomatic patients seen [60,61]. Reports in the older literature describe patients with a severe proximal myopathy and muscular atrophy, as well as other neurological abnormalities such as hyperreflexia, fasciculations of the tongue, and gait abnormalities [59,62] but such patients are now only rarely encountered in the West [1,63]. However, a recent series of cases from India suggested that the co-occurrence of primary hyperparathyroidism and vitamin D deficiency contributed to the high number of symptomatic cases seen, and described a case of such severe atrophy that the patient was misdiagnosed as suffering from spinal muscular atrophy, reinforcing the need to consider this diagnosis and to perform appropriate biochemical screening tests [61,64]. Patients with secondary hyperparathyroidism due to chronic renal failure may also develop a similar myopathy responsive to parathyroidectomy [65].

Studies of muscle function in patients with primary hyperparathyroidism have shown reduced muscle twitch and tetanic tension [63] and mildly impaired neuromuscular transmission in some cases [58]. Muscle biopsy findings reported in patients with a myopathy include non-selective fibre atrophy [62] and mild fibre-type grouping. However, in less severely affected cases the biopsy is usually normal [63].

Osteomalacia

Vitamin D deficiency is being increasingly recognized, and is present in between 40 and 100% of elderly Americans and Europeans [66,67]. It is associated with increasing age, skin pigmentation, obesity (due to sequestration in adipose tissue), distance from the equator, and insufficient exposure to sunlight, or can be due to an insufficient dietary intake or malabsorption of vitamin D. In addition it can also be due to abnormal vitamin D metabolism associated with renal tubular acidosis or anticonvulsant therapy [68,69] and high levels of fibroblast growth factor 23 (FGF23), which is a hormone secreted from osteocytes and acts on the kidney to reduce levels of serum phosphate and 1,25-dihydroxyvitamin D [70,71]. Osteomalacia in adults and in rickets in children can be associated with a painful proximal myopathy, often with disproportionate weakness of the gluteal muscles and a waddling gait, and with bone tenderness and pain on movement [1]. The frequency of myopathy in osteomalacia has varied from 73–97% in different series, and in

---

Box 34.3 Practice points: parathyroid and vitamin D-associated myopathies

- Hyperparathyroidism can be associated with proximal myopathy, muscle fatigability, and a sensory neuropathy
- Incidence of myopathy increased with combination of hyperparathyroidism and vitamin D deficiency.
- Osteomalacia (vitamin D deficiency) associated with a painful proximal myopathy often severely affecting the gluteal muscles
- Clues to vitamin D deficiency:
  - low serum phosphate
  - normal or raised serum calcium
  - raised alkaline phosphatase (ALP)
  - creatine kinase (CK) usually normal

---

one series the myopathy was the initial presenting problem in 30% of cases [69]. Secondary hyperparathyroidism is usually present and is an early sign of vitamin D deficiency (Box 34.3). It is usually also associated with low serum phosphate, normal or raised serum calcium, and a raised serum alkaline phosphatase level, which are useful screening tests. The serum CK level is usually normal. Muscle biopsy studies have shown atrophy of Type 2B fibres [72] and other minor non-specific changes [68,69]. Experimental vitamin D deficiency in rabbits was shown to be associated with reduced uptake of calcium by the sarcoplasmic reticulum and reduced troponin C levels [73].

The bone pain and weakness usually improve gradually after vitamin D supplements are commenced, and intakes of at least 1000 IU per day are required to maintain optimal vitamin D levels [74].

Hypoparathyroidism

Patients with hypocalcaemia due to hypoparathyroidism rarely develop a myopathy but commonly suffer from tetany, with associated muscle cramps and paraesthesiae. Reports in the older literature describe a myopathy with non-specific muscle biopsy changes and asymptomatic elevation of the serum CK and lactate dehydrogenase (LDH) activity, which recovered after administration of calcium and vitamin D supplements [75]. More recent cases reported a myopathy of variable severity in patients with idiopathic hypoparathyroidism resolving with calcium and vitamin D [76,77]. In experimental studies in rats prolonged hypocalcaemia has been shown to cause an elevated serum CK [78].

Box 34.4 Practice points: steroid myopathy

- Mild proximal myopathy, lower > upper limbs
- Quadriceps usually the most severely involved
- Creatine kinase (CK) level normal or low
- Low serum myoglobin levels
- Muscle biopsy shows Type 2 fibre atrophy

Pituitary disorders

Symptomatic complaints of weakness and fatigue are common in patients with acromegaly and some have mild proximal weakness even when the muscles are hypertrophied [79,80]. The CK level may be mildly elevated and EMG demonstrates a motor unit potential of reduced duration [80,81]. Muscle biopsy changes are non-specific, such as Type 1 and Type 2 fibre hypertrophy or atrophy, glycogen accumulation, muscle fibre necrosis, and in some cases tubular aggregates [82]. The mechanism of the myopathy has not been investigated but may be related to disturbed carbohydrate metabolism due to excess growth hormone and downstream effects mediated through insulin-like growth factor-1 (IGF-1), or to myocyte apoptosis as has been found in acromegalic cardiomyopathy [83].

The effects of growth hormone deficiency on skeletal muscle have not been investigated, but may contribute to the frequent complaints of muscular weakness and fatigue in patients with hypopituitarism and to the impaired muscle development in children. Growth hormone replacement in people with adult-onset deficiency results in a sustained increase in lean body mass and improvements in muscle strength [84].

Androgen deficiency

Androgens are known to be stimulators of muscle growth, and replacement of testosterone in men with hypogonadism restores muscle mass and power [85,86]. Men with either primary or secondary hypogonadism have reduced muscle strength and can show electromyographic evidence of myopathy [87,88]; in this group testosterone replacement results in increased muscle mass and strength, less body fat, and higher rates of protein synthesis [85,89].

Diabetes mellitus

People with poorly controlled diabetes may develop a focal ischaemic myopathy with infarction of the thigh muscles [90]. This presents with acute onset of muscle pain and swelling in the quadriceps or hamstring muscles, and the diagnosis can usually be confirmed with CT or muscle MRI without a muscle biopsy [91]. Ischaemic myopathy recovers spontaneously but may recur in the same leg or on the opposite side. This condition needs to be differentiated from diabetic amyotrophy which causes unilateral or bilateral painful proximal muscle weakness and atrophy in the lower limbs and is due to a proximal diabetic neuropathy or plexoradiculopathy, not a myopathy [92].

People with diabetes often take statins to reduce their risk of cardiovascular disease. However, an observational study found that myopathic symptoms occurred nearly twice as often in diabetic patients as in non-diabetics—although these myopathic symptoms were rarely severe or life-threatening and the risk of rhabdomyolysis was not significantly increased [93]. In addition, diabetes mellitus also occurs in association with mitochondrial myopathies [94], particularly in patients with the A3243G tRNA^{Leu} mutation [95,96]. It may also be associated with syndromes of partial or generalized lipodystrophy and myopathy [1].

References

1. Orrell RW. Endocrine myopathies. In: Mastaglia FL, Hilton-Jones D (ed) *Handbook of Clinical Neurology*, pp. 343–55. Oxford: Elsevier, 2007.

2. Duyff RF, Van den Bosch J, Laman DM, van Loon BJ, Linssen WH. Neuromuscular findings in thyroid dysfunction: a prospective clinical and electrodiagnostic study. *J Neurol Neurosurg Psychiatry* 2000; **68**: 750–5.

3. Mastaglia FL, Ojeda VJ, Sarnat HB, Kakulas BA. Myopathies associated with hypothyroidism: a review based upon 13 cases. *Aust NZ J Med* 1988; **18**: 799–806.

4. Madariaga MG. Polymyositis-like syndrome in hypothyroidism: review of cases reported over the past twenty-five years. *Thyroid* 2002; **12**: 331–6.

5. Turker H, Bayrak O, Gungor L, et al. Hypothyroid myopathy with manifestations of Hoffman's syndrome and myasthenia gravis. *Thyroid* 2008; **18**: 259–62.

6. Mouzouri H, El Omri N, Sekkach Y, et al. [Severe rhabdomyolysis revealing a myopathy linked to autoimmune hypothyroidism]. *Ann Endocrinol* 2009; **70**: 83–6.

7. Rush J, Danzi S, Klein I. Role of thyroid disease in the development of statin-induced myopathy. *The Endocrinologist* 2006; **16**: 279–85.

8. Lukjanowicz M, Trzcinska-Butkiewicz B, Brzosko M. [Fenofibrate—induced myopathy in a patient with undiagnosed hypothyroidism—case report and a review of the literature]. *Polsk Arch Med Wewn* 2006; **115**: 45–9.

9. Wiles CM, Young A, Jones DA, Edwards RH. Muscle relaxation rate, fibre-type composition and energy turnover in hyper- and hypo-thyroid patients. *Clin Sci (Lond)* 1979; **57**: 375–84.

10. Scott KR, Simmons Z, Boyer PJ. Hypothyroid myopathy with a strikingly elevated serum creatine kinase level. *Muscle Nerve* 2002; **26**: 141–4.

11. Modi G. Cores in hypothyroid myopathy: a clinical, histological and immunofluorescence study. *J Neurol Sci* 2000; **175**: 28–32.

12. Johnson MA, Olmo JL, Mastaglia FL. Changes in histochemical profile of rat respiratory muscles in hypo- and hyperthyroidism. *Q J Exp Physiol* 1983; **68**: 1–13.

13. Chen C-C, Chiu P-C, Shih C-H, Hsieh K-S. Proximal weakness of lower limbs as the sole presentation of hyperthyroidism: report of one case. *Acta Paediatr Taiwan* 2005; **46**: 91–3.

14. Shaw PJ, Bates D, Kendall-Taylor P. Hyperthyroidism presenting as pyramidal tract disease. *Br Med J* 1988; **297**: 1395–6.

15. Shaheen D, Kim CS. Myositis associated with the decline of thyroid hormone levels in thyrotoxicosis: a syndrome? *Thyroid* 2009; **19**: 1413–17.

16. Domire ZJ, McCullough MB, Chen Q, An K-N. Wave attenuation as a measure of muscle quality as measured by magnetic resonance elastography: initial results. *J Biomech* 2009; **42**: 537–40.

17. Lloreta J, Roquer J, Corominas JM, Serrano S. Hyperthyroid myopathy with mitochondrial paracrystalline rectangular inclusions. *Ultrastruct Pathol* 1996; **20**: 61–5.

18. Dulhunty AF. The rate of tetanic relaxation is correlated with the density of calcium ATPase in the terminal cisternae of thyrotoxic skeletal muscle. *Pflugers Arch* 1990; **415**: 433–9.

19. Kung AW, Lau KS, Cheung WM, Chan V. Thyrotoxic periodic paralysis and polymorphisms of sodium-potassium ATPase genes. *Clin Endocrinol* 2006; **64**: 158–61.

20. Lin SH. Thyrotoxic periodic paralysis. *Mayo Clin Proc* 2005; **80**: 99–105.

21. Hannon MJ, Behan LA, Agha A. Thyrotoxic periodic paralysis due to excessive L-thyroxine replacement in a Caucasian man. *Ann Clin Biochem* 2009; **46**: 423–5.

22. Akinyemi E, Bercovici S, Niranjan S, Paul N, Hemavathy B. Thyrotoxic hypokalemic periodic paralysis due to dietary weight-loss supplement. *Am J Ther* 2011; **18**: e81–3.

23. Kung AW. Clinical review: thyrotoxic periodic paralysis: a diagnostic challenge. *J Clin Endocrinol Metab* 2006; **91**: 2490–5.

24. Lien YH. A new diagnostic test for an old diagnostic challenge: thyrotoxic periodic paralysis. *Crit Care Med* 2006; **34**: 3053–4.

25. Cheng CJ, Lin SH, Lo YF, et al. Identification and functional characterization of Kir2.6 mutations associated with non-familial hypokalemic periodic paralysis. *J Biol Chem* 2011; **286**: 27425–35.

26. Puwanant A, Ruff RL, Puwanant A, Ruff RL. INa and IKir are reduced in Type 1 hypokalemic and thyrotoxic periodic paralysis. *Muscle Nerve* 2010; **42**: 315–27.

27. Kung AW, Lau KS, Fong GC, Chan V. Association of novel single nucleotide polymorphisms in the calcium channel alpha 1 subunit gene (Ca(v)1.1) and thyrotoxic periodic paralysis. *J Clin Endocrinol Metab* 2004; **89**: 1340–5.

28. Kung AW, Lau KS, Cheung WM, et al. Thyrotoxic periodic paralysis and polymorphisms of sodium-potassium ATPase genes. *Clin Endocrinol* 2006; **64**: 158–61.

29. Pothiwala P, Levine SN. Analytic review: thyrotoxic periodic paralysis: a review. *J Intensive Care Med* 2010; **25**: 71–7.

30. Guerra M, Rodriguez del Castillo A, Battaner E, Mas M. Androgens stimulate preoptic area Na+,K+-ATPase activity in male rats. *Neurosci Lett* 1987; **78**: 97–100.

31. Li W, Changsheng C, Jiangfang F, et al. Effects of sex steroid hormones, thyroid hormone levels, and insulin regulation on thyrotoxic periodic paralysis in Chinese men. *Endocrine* 2010; **38**: 386–90.

32. Shiang JC, Cheng CJ, Tsai MK, et al. Therapeutic analysis in Chinese patients with thyrotoxic periodic paralysis over 6 years. *Eur J Endocrinol* 2009; **161**: 911–16.

33. Bahn RS. Graves' ophthalmopathy. *N Engl J Med* 2010; **362**: 726–38.

34. Czarnywojtek A, Kurdybacha P, Florek E, et al. Smoking and thyroid diseases—what is new? *Przegl Lek* 2010; **67**: 1056–60.

35. Khalilzadeh O, Anvari M, Esteghamati A, et al. Genetic susceptibility to Graves' ophthalmopathy: the role of polymorphisms in anti-inflammatory cytokine genes. *Ophthalmic Genet* 2010; **31**: 215–20.

36. Anvari M, Khalilzadeh O, Esteghamati A, et al. Genetic susceptibility to Graves' ophthalmopathy: the role of polymorphisms in proinflammatory cytokine genes. *Eye (Lond)* 2010; **24**: 1058–63.

37. Zhu W, Liu N, Zhao Y, Jia H, Cui B, Ning G. Association analysis of polymorphisms in IL-3, IL-4, IL-5, IL-9, and IL-13 with Graves' disease. *J Endocrinol Invest* 2010; **33**: 751–5.

38. Yi BP, Leng SL, Kwang LB, Rootman J. Development of thyroid-related orbitopathy following cataract surgery. *Orbit* 2009; **28**: 383–7.

39. Bartalena L, Wiersinga WM, Pinchera A. Graves' ophthalmopathy: state of the art and perspectives. *J Endocrinol Invest* 2004; **27**: 295–301.

40. Douglas RS, Afifiyan NF, Hwang CJ, et al. Increased generation of fibrocytes in thyroid-associated ophthalmopathy. *J Clin Endocrinol Metab* 2010; **95**: 430–8.

41. de Haan S, Lahooti H, Morris O, Wall JR. Epitopes, immunoglobulin classes and immunoglobulin G subclasses of calsequestrin antibodies in patients with thyroid eye disease. *Autoimmunity* 2010; **43**: 698–703.

42. Eckstein A, Esser J, Mann K, Schott M. Clinical value of TSH receptor antibodies measurement in patients with Graves' orbitopathy. *Pediatr Endocrinol Rev* 2010; **7** (Suppl 2): 198–203.

43. Lytton SD, Ponto KA, Kanitz M, Matheis N, Kohn LD, Kahaly GJ. A novel thyroid stimulating immunoglobulin bioassay is a functional indicator of activity and severity of Graves' orbitopathy. *J Clin Endocrinol Metab* 2010; **95**: 2123–31.

44. Tambe K, Bhargava J, Tripathi A, Gregory M, Burns J, Sampath R. The role of intravenous methylprednisolone immunosuppression in the management of active thyroid eye disease. *Orbit* 2010; **29**: 227–31.

45. Alkawas AA, Hussein AM, Shahien EA. Orbital steroid injection versus oral steroid therapy in management of thyroid-related ophthalmopathy. *Clin Exp.Ophthalmol* 2010; **38**: 692–7.

46. Abboud M, Arabi A, Salti I, Geara F. Outcome of thyroid associated ophthalmopathy treated by radiation therapy. *Radiat Oncol* 2011; **6**: 46.

47. Chiarelli AG, De Min V, Saetti R, Fusetti S, Al Barbir H. Surgical management of thyroid orbitopathy. *J Plast Reconstr Aesthet Surg* 2010; **63**: 240–6.

48. Azzam I, Tordjman K. Clinical update: treatment of hyperthyroidism in Graves' ophthalmopathy. *Pediatr Endocrinol Rev* 2010; **7** (Suppl 2): 193–7.

49. Ponto KA, Zang S, Kahaly GJ. The tale of radioiodine and Graves' orbitopathy. *Thyroid* 2010; **20**: 785–93.

50. Hegedus L, Smith TJ, Douglas RS, Nielsen CH. Targeted biological therapies for Graves' disease and thyroid-associated ophthalmopathy. Focus on B-cell depletion with rituximab. *Clin Endocrinol* 2011; **74**: 1–8.

51. Bartalena L. The dilemma of how to manage Graves' hyperthyroidism in patients with associated orbitopathy. *J Clin Endocrinol Metab* 2011; **96**: 592–9.

52. Bartalena L, Lai A, Sassi L, et al. Novel treatment modalities for Graves' orbitopathy. *Pediatr Endocrinol Rev* 2010; **7** (Suppl 2): 210–16.

53. Atsumi T, Ishikawa S, Miyatake T, Yoshida M. Myopathy and primary aldosteronism: electron microscopic study. *Neurology* 1979; **29**: 1348–53.

54. Khaleeli AA, Edwards RH, Gohil K, et al. Corticosteroid myopathy: a clinical and pathological study. *Clin Endocrinol* 1983; **18**: 155–66.

55. Marazuela M, Aguilar-Torres R, Benedicto A, et al. Dilated cardiomyopathy as a presenting feature of Cushing's syndrome. *Int J Cardiol* 2003 **88**: 331–3.

56. Minetto MA, Lanfranco F, Botter A, et al. Do muscle fiber conduction slowing and decreased levels of circulating muscle proteins represent sensitive markers of steroid myopathy? A pilot study in Cushing's disease. *Eur J Endocrinol* 2011; **164**: 985–93.

57. Mier A, Laroche C, Wass J, Green M. Respiratory muscle weakness in Addison's disease. *Br Med J* 1988; **297**: 457–8.

58. Ljunghall S, Akerstrom G, Johansson G, Olsson Y, Stalberg E. Neuromuscular involvement in primary hyperparathyroidism. *J Neurol* 1984; **231**: 263–5.

59. Turken SA, Cafferty M, Silverberg SJ, et al. Neuromuscular involvement in mild, asymptomatic primary hyperparathyroidism. *Am J Med* 1989; **87**: 553–7.

60. George J, Acharya SV, Bandgar TR, et al. Primary hyperparathyroidism in children and adolescents. *Ind J Pediatr* 2010; **77**: 175–8.

61. Muthukrishnan J, Jha S, Modi KD, et al. Symptomatic primary hyperparathyroidism: a retrospective analysis of fifty one cases from a single centre. *J Assoc Physicians Ind* 2008; **56**; 503–7.

62. Patten BM, Bilezikian JP, Mallette LE, Prince A, Engel WK, Aurbach GD. Neuromuscular disease in primary hyperparathyroidism. *Ann Intern Med* 1974; **80**: 182–93.

63. Joborn C, Rastad J, Stalberg E, Akerstrom G, Ljunghall S. Muscle function in patients with primary hyperparathyroidism. *Muscle Nerve* 1989; **12**: 87–94.

64. Muthukrishnan J, Harikumar KV, Sangeeta J, Singh MK, Modi K, Harikumar KVS. Nerve, muscle or bone disease? Look before you leap. *Singapore Med J* 2009; **50**: e293–e294.

65. Adeniyi O, Agaba EI, King M, Servilla KS, Massie L, Tzamaloukas AH. Severe proximal myopathy in advanced renal failure. Diagnosis and management. *Afr J Med Med Sci* 2004; **33**: 385–8.

66. Bell DS, Bell DSH. Protean manifestations of vitamin D deficiency, part 1: the epidemic of deficiency. *South Med J* 2011; **104**: 331–4.

67. O'Malley G, Mulkerrin E. Vitamin D insufficiency: a common and treatable problem in the Irish population. *Ir J Med Sci* 2011; **180**: 7–13.

68. Mallette LE, Patten BM, Engel WK. Neuromuscular disease in secondary hyperparathyroidism. *Ann Intern Med* 1975; **82**: 474–83.

69. Russell JA. Osteomalacic myopathy. *Muscle Nerve* 1994; **17**: 578–80.

70. Razzaque MS, Razzaque MS (2011). Osteo-renal regulation of systemic phosphate metabolism. *IUBMB Life* **63**: 240–7.

71. Alon US. Clinical practice. Fibroblast growth factor (FGF)23: a new hormone. *Eur J Pediatr* 2011; **170**: 545–54.

72. Swash M, Schwartz MS, Sargeant MK. Osteomalacic myopathy: an experimental approach. *Neuropathol Appl Neurobiol* 1979; **5**: 295–302.

73. Pointon JJ, Francis MJ, Smith R. Effect of vitamin D deficiency on sarcoplasmic reticulum function and troponin C concentration of rabbit skeletal muscle. *Clin Sci (Lond)* 1979; **57**: 257–63.

74. Binkley N, Ramamurthy R, Krueger D. Low vitamin D status: definition, prevalence, consequences, and correction. *Endocrinol Metabol Clin North Am* 2010; **39**: 287–301.

75. Shane E, McClane KA, Olarte MR, Bilezikian JP. Hypoparathyroidism and elevated muscle enzymes. *Neurology* 1980; **30**: 192–5.

76. Syriou V, Kolitsa A, Pantazi L, et al. Hypoparathyroidism in a patient presenting with severe myopathy and skin rash. Case report and review of the literature. *Hormones* 2005; **4**: 161–4.

77. Nora DB, Fricke D, Becker J, et al. Hypocalcemic myopathy without tetany due to idiopathic hypoparathyroidism: case report. *Arq Neu Psiquiatr* 2004; **62**: 154–7.

78. Ishikawa T, Kanayama M, Oba T, Horie T. Hypocalcemic induced increase in creatine kinase in rats. *Pediatr Neurol* 1998; **18**: 326–30.

79. Khaleeli AA, Levy RD, Edwards RH, et al. The neuromuscular features of acromegaly: a clinical and pathological study. *J Neurol Neurosurg Psychiatry* 1984; **47**: 1009–15.

80. Mastaglia FL, Barwich DD, Hall R. Myopathy in acromegaly. *Lancet* 1970; **2**(7679): 907–9.

81. McNab TL, Khandwala HM, McNab TL, Khandwala HM. Acromegaly as an endocrine form of myopathy: case report and review of literature. *Endocrine Practice* 2005; **11**: 18–22.

82. Mastaglia FL. Pathological changes in skeletal muscle in acromegaly. *Acta Neuropathol (Berl)* 1973; **24**: 273–86.

83. Frustaci A, Chimenti C, Setoguchi M, et al. Cell death in acromegalic cardiomyopathy. *Circulation* 1999; **99**: 1426–34.

84. Svensson J, Sunnerhagen KS, Johannsson G. Five years of growth hormone replacement therapy in adults: age- and gender-related changes in isometric and isokinetic muscle strength. *J Clin Endocrinol Metabol* 2003; **88**: 2061–9.

85. Bhasin S, Storer TW, Berman N, et al. The effects of supraphysiologic doses of testosterone on muscle size and strength in normal men. *N Engl J Med* 1996; **335**: 1–7.

86. Bhasin S, Storer TW, Berman N, et al. Testosterone replacement increases fat-free mass and muscle size in hypogonadal men. *J Clin Endocrinol Metabol* 1997; **82**: 407–13.

87. Chauhan AK, Katiyar BC, Misra S, Thacker AK, Singh NK. Muscle dysfunction in male hypogonadism. *Acta Neurol Scand* 1986; **73**: 466–71.

88. Roy TA, Blackman MR, Harman SM, Tobin JD, Schrager M, Metter EJ. Interrelationships of serum testosterone and free testosterone index with FFM and strength in aging men. *Am J Physiol Endocrinol Metabol* 2002; **283**: E284–E294.

89. Brodsky IG, Balagopal P, Nair KS. Effects of testosterone replacement on muscle mass and muscle protein synthesis in hypogonadal men—a clinical research center study. *J Clin Endocrinol Metabol* 1996; **81**: 3469–75.

90. Kiers L. Diabetic muscle infarction: magnetic resonance imaging (MRI) avoids the need for biopsy. *Muscle Nerve* 1995; **18**: 129–30.

91. Huang BK, Monu JU, Doumanian J Diabetic myopathy: MRI patterns and current trends. *Am J Roentgenol* 2010; **195**; 198–204.

92. Said G, Elgrably F, Lacroix C, et al. Painful proximal diabetic neuropathy: inflammatory nerve lesions and spontaneous favorable outcome. *Ann Neurol* 1997; **41**: 762–70.

93. Nichols GA, Koro CE. Does statin therapy initiation increase the risk for myopathy? An observational study of 32,225 diabetic and nondiabetic patients. *Clin Ther* 2007; **29**; 1761–70.

94. Mechler F, Fawcett PR, Mastaglia FL, Hudgson P. Mitochondrial myopathy. *J Neurol Sci* 1981; **50**; 191–200.

95. Finsterer J. Genetic, pathogenetic, and phenotypic implications of the mitochondrial A3243G tRNALeu(UUR) mutation. *Acta Neurol Scand* 2007; **116**: 1–14.

96. Frederiksen AL, Jeppesen TD, Vissing J, et al. High prevalence of impaired glucose homeostasis and myopathy in asymptomatic and oligosymptomatic 3243A>G mitochondrial DNA mutation-positive subjects. *J Clin Endocrinol Metabol* 2009; **94**: 2872–9.

SECTION 7

Acute Neuromuscular Consults

CHAPTER 35

The neuromuscular emergency consult

Peter Connick and Maxwell S. Damian

Introduction: epidemiology of neuromuscular disease emergencies

Consults for neuromuscular emergencies are uncommon in hospital neurology practice, representing less than 2% of activity in a large Italian series [1] and less than 2% of referrals to a rapid-access neurology clinic in a UK hospital [2]. Neurologists are therefore required to be proficient and confident in the recognition and management of conditions that are encountered at low frequency in day-to-day practice.

Reflecting their relative infrequency in hospital neurology practice, neuromuscular emergencies are also an uncommon cause for admission to intensive care units (ICU), representing approximately 0.2–1.2% of all admissions [3,4]. Specialist neurological support is therefore required throughout the patient's admission in order to assist intensivists with monitoring and management, and to aid prognostication.

The range of diseases presenting as a neuromuscular emergency

Acute generalized weakness can occur due to disease affecting any part of the neuraxis. In the absence of features suggesting central nervous system disease, diagnostic consideration should include:

- lower motor neuronopathies
- motor polyradiculopathy and neuropathies
- neuromuscular junction disorders
- primary muscle disorders.

The general clinical approach and features of specific conditions are described in detail elsewhere in this volume; however, in the setting of the emergency neurology consult a prioritized approach is necessary to identify and urgently address life-threatening physiological compromise.

Prioritized approach to the patient with a neuromuscular emergency

A prioritized approach to the assessment of patients with a neuromuscular emergency requires the recognition and evaluation of life-threatening ventilatory failure and cardiac dysrhythmia in order to inform immediate decisions about the appropriate care environment, monitoring, and intervention. Comprehensive diagnostic evaluation forms a secondary objective, and targeted management may therefore need to be initiated based on the clinical working diagnosis pending the results of a further detailed diagnostic evaluation.

Pathophysiology of ventilatory failure in neuromuscular disease

Arterial hypoxaemia in patients with neuromuscular disease is the result of both hypoventilation and microatelectasis arising from the retention of secretions [5]; hypercapnia occurs only as a late feature and suggests impending respiratory arrest [3]. Hypoventilation in neuromuscular disease reflects both the severity and the distribution of weakness in respiratory muscles. In ascending neuromuscular diseases such as Guillain–Barré syndrome (GBS), diaphragmatic failure may be seen without significant compromise of intercostal and accessory respiratory muscles. In contrast, the reverse pattern may occur with a descending neuromuscular disease such as botulism. Patients with weak diaphragmatic function are particularly susceptible to decompensation in the supine position as gravitational assistance for caudal movement of the abdominal contents on inspiration is lost, and the efficiency of accessory muscle function is also reduced. Decompensation at night is therefore common in patients with diaphragmatic dysfunction, reflecting supine mechanical dysfunction compounded by the effect of the central respiratory drive during sleep being primarily directed through the phrenic nerves. In contrast, patients with preserved diaphragmatic function and impaired intercostal and accessory respiratory muscles may decompensate in the upright position as the abdominal contents are moved caudally by gravity, elongating and lowering the central diaphragm and rendering the peripheral fibres less efficient in elevation of the ribcage. Bulbar involvement may also be present as part of the primary disease process, contributing to respiratory impairment by limiting the clearance of secretions, in turn leading to an increased risk of upper airway obstruction or pulmonary aspiration.

Recognition of ventilatory failure in neuromuscular disease

Unlike ventilatory failure in primary cardiac or respiratory disease, patients with significant impairment of respiratory function due to neuromuscular disease can remain asymptomatic and appear well until rapid life-threatening decompensation occurs. Ventilatory failure must therefore be considered, and respiratory function specifically evaluated, in *all* patients in whom a neuromuscular disease is suspected. Detection can nevertheless be challenging, as the clinical findings in patients with respiratory compromise due to neuromuscular disease may be subtle.

Although breathlessness is a cardinal symptom of ventilatory failure in other settings, patients with neuromuscular disease may only exhibit breathlessness on talking or swallowing. Similarly, shallow breathing with increased heart and respiratory rate is characteristic but not universal; the absence of these features cannot therefore be used at the bedside to exclude significant ventilatory impairment. The pattern of respiratory muscle function, however, is helpful, and should be observed. In physiological conditions at rest, diaphragmatic movement performs the majority of the ventilatory function. This involves descent of the central fibres during inspiration—causing the abdomen to move anteriorly (outwards)—and elevation of the inferior ribcage by the peripheral fibres. Patients with diaphragmatic compromise but intact intercostal and accessory muscles therefore compensate during inspiration at rest by using accessory muscles of respiration (pectoral, scalene, sternocleidomastoid, levators of the nostrils). Diaphragmatic paralysis can also be observed by 'paradoxical abdominal movement'—indrawing of the abdominal wall on inspiration. In contrast, patients with impaired intercostal muscle function and preserved diaphragmatic function exhibit indrawing of the upper ribcage and intercostal spaces during inspiration due to loss of normal intercostal muscle tone. Auscultation of the chest is often unremarkable in patients with ventilatory impairment due to neuromuscular disease, although crepitations may be heard reflecting atelectasis, and transmitted upper airway noise may be present in patients with bulbar dysfunction.

The clinical evaluation of ventilatory function in patients with suspected neuromuscular disease is therefore highly dependent on bedside measurement of physiological parameters. Significant thresholds are readily remembered through the '20/30/40 rule' applicable to standard portable spirometry assessment [6]. Significant ventilatory dysfunction reflected by forced vital capacity (FVC) < 20 ml kg^{-1}, peak inspiratory pressure < 30 cmH$_2$O, or peak expiratory pressure < 40 cmH$_2$O should trigger critical care support. The objective of bedside assessment using spirometry is to detect significant hypoventilation *prior* to life-threatening decompensation that results in hypoxaemia detectable by pulse oximetry or arterial blood gas measurement.

Recognition of autonomic and cardiac dysfunction in patients with neuromuscular disease

Autonomic dysfunction is common in patients with acute neuromuscular disease, occurring in up to 60% of cases of GBS. Clinical manifestations include orthostatic hypotension, diabetes insipidus, ileus, and cardiac dysrhythmia that may require drug treatment and occasionally emergency pacing. Bedside assessment of postural blood pressures, together with heart rate and rhythm, is therefore essential in all patients with suspected neuromuscular disease. A standard 12-lead electrocardiogram (ECG) assessment should be reviewed as part of the initial neurological consult.

Choice of care environment for the acutely ill patient with neuromuscular disease

Given the potential for rapid decompensation of patients with neuromuscular disease, early discussion of all patients with critical care specialists is good practice. The involvement of intensivists during the dynamic phase of illness allows better management planning, and fosters a collaborative approach from the outset. Such an approach is particularly valuable given the relative infrequency with which neuromuscular disease reach critical care, and the relatively long periods of admission that are often required. Initial discussions should include immediate decisions about the most appropriate care environment and the thresholds for moving between intensive/high-dependency and ward-based care. We find that defining such thresholds based on objective measures of ventilatory and autonomic function is of particular utility for the care of ward-based patients during high-risk overnight periods when decompensation is common and staffing levels reduced. Where available, involvement of critical care outreach services can be invaluable to supporting the management of patients in this position on neurological units and elsewhere. Breach of either the '20/30/40 rule' or the presence of autonomic dysfunction can be used as a threshold to identify patients who should be managed in a critical care environment. The direction and rate of change in motor and ventilatory function should also be considered in the decision about an appropriate care environment.

Monitoring the acutely ill patient with neuromuscular disease

Regardless of the decision taken about the most appropriate care environment for the acutely ill patient with neuromuscular disease, advice from the neurological consult should include a specific plan for the type and frequency of ongoing monitoring required for motor, ventilatory, and cardiac function.

Regular neurological assessments need to be documented in a standardized manner that is comparable between different examiners, and uses gradings of power such as the Medical Research Council (MRC) score in a way that identifies meaningful changes—statements such as 'lower limb power 4/5 MRC' do not. The type of serial assessment needs to take into account whether weakness is fixed or fluctuating, i.e. documentation in myasthenic syndromes must include the number of repetitions or duration of testing until fatigue develops (i.e. testing according to standardized myasthenia scores).

Monitoring of respiratory function in acutely ill patients with neuromuscular disease is essential. Regular bedside assessment of vital capacity should ideally be supplemented with the more specific (although more dependent on cooperation and effort) measurement of mouth inspiratory and expiratory pressures. Nasal 'sniff' pressures can be used in patients with significant facial weakness who are unable to form a tight seal for conventional mouth spirometry.

ECG monitoring should be considered in bedbound patients with evidence of acute autonomic dysfunction as there are no reliable predictors for the risk of life-threatening autonomic complications.

Initiation of ventilatory support for acutely ill patients with neuromuscular disease

The decision to initiate ventilatory support in acutely ill patients with neuromuscular disease should be taken in the context of the underlying diagnosis and prognosis, together with knowledge of the patient's views. This can be particularly challenging in chronic neuromuscular disease where acute decompensation has occurred due to an intercurrent illness. Interdisciplinary communication between neurologists, intensivists, and relevant specialist physicians is essential in this setting to inform decisions that are necessarily based on the specific circumstances of individual cases. Similarly, decompensation of chronic neuromuscular disease due to progression of the primary disease process requires the neurologist to provide specialist input regarding the reversibility and prognosis of the underlying condition [7]. Although rare, this situation occasionally arises for patients in whom an underlying diagnosis has not previously been established. In such circumstances, the urgent need to reach an accurate diagnosis that will inform critical management decisions ranks amongst the most challenging scenarios encountered in neurological practice. Given the importance of diagnostic accuracy in this setting, definitive investigations must be expedited as they can be essential to inform immediate management decisions.

When a decision is taken that ventilatory support is required and appropriate, intubation should take place earlier rather than later [8]. Non-invasive bilevel positive airway pressure (BiPAP) ventilation, can be effective in patients with amyotrophic lateral sclerosis and myasthenia gravis, but may not be safe in progressing GBS [9]. Intubation is therefore preferable to BiPAP for patients with ventilatory failure due to GBS.

Tracheostomy for acutely ill patients with neuromuscular disease

The decision to perform tracheostomy should be based on the anticipated duration of requirement for ventilatory support, an understanding of the long-term prognosis, and the patient's views. A pulmonary function score (PFS) has been proposed to predict the requirement for prolonged ventilatory support and the need for tracheostomy in GBS. The PFS is calculated as the sum of the vital capacity and peak inspiratory and expiratory pressures. Lawn and Wijdicks report the use of this index in 37 ventilated GBS patients, where the day-12 PFS was higher than the day-1 PFS (ratio > 1) in all 10 patients ventilated for less than 3 weeks, whereas the pulmonary function ratio was < 1 in 19 of 27 patients ventilated for more than 3 weeks [10]. The sensitivity for requirement for tracheostomy using the PFS was therefore 70%, with a specificity of 100%. In contrast, myasthenic crisis often only requires a short period of ventilation, meaning that there is no requirement for early tracheostomy (i.e. before day 7). There is, however, a relatively high risk of reintubation, especially in patients with atelectasis, and the standard predictors of extubation success used in the ICU may not apply.

The decision to perform tracheostomy for the long-term ventilatory support of patients with chronic neuromuscular disease remains a significant practical and ethical clinical challenge, although improvement in the overall prognosis of chronic neuromuscular disease has resulted in practice moving towards a more aggressive approach for supportive care [11]. Prior discussion with patients who have chronic neuromuscular disease about the treatment options available for them in the event of possible future acute decompensation(s) is invaluable for informing difficult clinical decisions.

Detection and management of rhabdomyolysis in the acutely ill patient with neuromuscular disease

Muscle necrosis can complicate a variety of neuromuscular diseases in the setting of acute decompensation or intercurrent illness, resulting in the release of intracellular constituents into the blood and extracellular tissues [12]. The most commonly used serum markers are creatine kinase and lactate dehydrogenase, and plasma and urine myoglobin measurement are particularly useful in the early phase. Given the mortality rate of up to 8%, close monitoring is essential to prevent common complications of acute kidney injury (occurring in up to 33% of cases), compartment syndrome, cardiac dysrhythmias via electrolyte abnormalities, and disseminated intravascular coagulopathy [13]. Aggressive hydration and prompt correction of electrolyte abnormalities form the mainstay of treatment. In the pre-hospital setting, forced hydration with 1.5–2 L of sterile saline solution should be started immediately, followed by 1.5–2 L h^{-1}.

Summary

The neurological consult for an acutely ill patient with neuromuscular disease can occur in a variety of clinical settings, each with a differing emphasis. The priority is to identify and address potentially life-threatening physiological compromise, and indicate a pathway to more comprehensive diagnostic evaluation.

References

1. Falco FA, Sterzi R, Toso V, et al. The neurologist in the emergency department. An Italian nationwide epidemiological survey. *Neurol Sci* 2008; **29**: 67–75.
2. Chapman FA, Pope AE, Sorensen D, Knight RS, Al-Shahi Salman R. Acute neurological problems: frequency, consultation patterns and the uses of a rapid access neurology clinic. *J R Coll Physicians Edin* 2009; **39**: 296–300.
3. Hughes RA, Bihari D. Acute neuromuscular respiratory paralysis. *J Neurol Neurosurg Psychiatry* 1993; **56**: 334–43.
4. Simpson H, Clancy M, Goldfrad C, Rowan K. Admissions to intensive care units from emergency departments: a descriptive study. *Emerg Med J* 2005; **22**: 423–8.
5. Kelly BJ, Luce JM. The diagnosis and management of neuromuscular diseases causing respiratory failure. *Chest* 1991; **99**: 1485–94.
6. Rabinstein AA, Wijdicks EFM. Warning signs of imminent respiratory failure in neurological patients. *Semin Neurol* 2003; **23**: 97–104.
7. Shneerson JM. Is chronic respiratory failure in neuromuscular diseases worth treating? *J Neurol Neurosurg Psychiatry* 1996; **61**: 1–3.
8. Mehta S. Neuromuscular disease causing acute respiratory failure. *Respir Care* 2006; **51**: 1016–21, discussion 1021–3.
9. Wijdicks EFM, Roy TK. BiPAP in early Guillain–Barré syndrome may fail. *Can J Neurol Sci* 2006; **33**: 105–6.
10. Lawn ND, Wijdicks EF. Post-intubation pulmonary function test in Guillain-Barré syndrome. *Muscle Nerve* 2000; **23**: 613–16.
11. Ambrosino N, Carpenè N, Gherardi M. Chronic respiratory care for neuromuscular diseases in adults. *Eur Respir J* 2009; **34**: 444–51.
12. Cervellin G, Comelli I, Lippi G. Rhabdomyolysis: historical background, clinical, diagnostic and therapeutic features. *Clini Chem Lab Med* 2010; **48**: 749–56.
13. Bagley WH, Yang H, Shah KH. Rhabdomyolysis. *Intern Emerg Med* 2007; **2**: 210–18.

CHAPTER 36

Critical care of neuromuscular disorders

Maxwell S. Damian

Introduction—the intensive care unit in neuromuscular disease

Patients with neuromuscular disorders may require treatment on the intensive care unit (ICU) if they develop respiratory weakness, severe cardiomyopathy or arrhythmia, or, less frequently, acute rhabdomyolysis. Neuromuscular complications can also become a major aspect of multisystemic disease such as sepsis, vasculitis, or intoxication in the general ICU. Neuromuscular patients constitute only a small percentage of patients requiring critical care, but they often have a favourable prognosis for recovery, and problems may arise when ICU teams are unfamiliar with these disorders. Treatment in the ICU may be delayed when intensivists are reluctant to admit patients with degenerative muscle disease or muscular dystrophy because of perceived medical futility, or because there is inadequate understanding of how the need for ICU monitoring or treatment develops, e.g. in evolving myasthenic crisis. Patients with neuromuscular disorders may require long-term specialist care after weaning from the ventilator, and mortality after ICU treatment due to inadequate step-down care is surprisingly high [1].

Neuromuscular patients in the ICU fall into three broad groups:

1. patients undergoing treatment for specific acute neuromuscular diseases (e.g. Guillain–Barré syndrome, myasthenic crisis, inflammatory myopathy, rhabdomyolysis, or secondary toxic myopathies);

2. patients suffering from progression of chronic neuromuscular diseases (e.g. respiratory failure in muscular dystrophy or cardiac failure and dysrhythmia in cardiomyopathy); and

3. neuromuscular weakness developing during treatment in the ICU for another disease (e.g. 'ICU-acquired weakness').

The neurologist must understand practical aspects of management of the patient on the ICU, and be involved in treatment throughout the course, rather than just in weekly ward rounds, in order to contribute effectively to treatment.

ICU management of acute neuromuscular diseases

Guillain–Barré syndrome (GBS)

Some 30% of patients with GBS become bedbound, and about a third of these will need intubation. Patients with GBS are most often referred to the ICU for respiratory management. Autonomic dysregulation, which occurs in 60% of GBS patients, may cause life-threatening complications, and can be a reason for considering ICU admission even in the absence of respiratory failure.

Maximum weakness in GBS occurs after an average of 10 days, so most patients will have been hospitalized for some days before they require critical care, leaving enough time to plan for ICU admission. Relatively early admission is advisable, as patients left until frank respiratory decompensation occurs will have complications due to infection as a result of inadequate clearing of secretions or failure of airway protection owing to bulbar weakness. Bedbound patients are also most at risk of cardiac dysrhythmia or severe autonomic dysfunction, which may make emergency pacing necessary or cause extreme sensitivity to nursing manoeuvres or to commonplace ICU drugs. Death is mainly due to infection or cardiac arrhythmia and is therefore potentially avoidable.

On the ward patients who are at high risk can be identified by their initial rate of progression and through bedside monitoring protocols. Critical care outreach teams need neurological guidance on how to spot patients who are heading for intubation, even though their respiratory function might still be adequate, and ICU admission is best planned according to an agreed set of institutional criteria. Critical care transfers of a patient in extremis are always a sign of a lack of adequate forethought and planning. Monitoring on the ward with hand-held devices should include regular surveillance of vital capacity and inspiratory and expiratory mouth pressures, which are more specific for respiratory muscle weakness, although more dependent on cooperation. Patients with facial weakness can still provide nasal 'sniff' pressures. Critical values are a vital capacity below 20 ml kg^{-1}, peak inspiratory pressure below 30 cmH$_2$O, and peak expiratory pressure below 40 cmH$_2$O ('20/30/40'). Patients unable to walk 5 m (Hughes scale score ≥3) [2] require intensive monitoring; patients who do not pass the '20/30/40' test should be monitored in the ICU.

Non-invasive bilevel positive airway pressure (BiPAP) ventilation may not be a safe temporizing measure in evolving GBS [3], and early intubation and assist-control (AC) or synchronized intermittent mandatory ventilation (SIMV) with pressure support and positive end-expiratory pressure (PEEP) is advised. Fifty per cent of intubated patients require ventilation for over 3 weeks, but there is no clear benefit in early tracheotomy.

Orthostatic hypotension and symptomatic dysrhythmia indicate significant autonomic dysfunction in critical care. Such patients should have continuous electrocardiogram (ECG) monitoring, and should preferably be monitored on the ICU; emergency external pacing via chest pads must be readily available. Bedside autonomic tests, such as pulse frequency variation, Valsalva, or cold pressor responses, cannot accurately predict which patients are at particular risk; the eyeball pressure test [4] is now considered unsafe. Bradycardia/tachycardia syndrome may predict severe arrhythmia. Apart from dysrhythmia, autonomic dysfunction also causes labile blood pressure, adynamic ileus, or bladder dysfunction. The response to commonly used medications may be excessive in these patients; vasodilators and beta blockers in particular must be used with caution, likewise neostigmine or metoclopramide in bradycardic patients. The risk of autonomic complications remains even during the rehabilitation phase, and experience suggests that a significant number of deaths occur during the recovery phase after discharge from the ICU.

Younger survivors in particular have a chance of full recovery even after very prolonged ventilation, but up to 20% of all survivors retain a long-term disability. Mortality rates are commonly cited as 5–10%, but this applies to all cases of GBS and mortality Gravis Composite score [patients [5]. Mortality varies considerably between units, for reasons which are not yet clear, and bad outcomes may go unrecognized in units with a small volume of cases, which underlines the importance of systematic audit and of national registries.

Autoimmune myasthenia gravis and myasthenic crisis

The intensive care team is most often involved in the management of myasthenia gravis (MG) in myasthenic crisis, i.e. exacerbations in which airways or breathing are compromised. Myasthenic crisis most often occurs within 2 years of onset; later in the course crises may be precipitated by infection, thymoma recurrence, or inappropriate medication. In most patients with MG, even if the condition is ocular at onset, symptoms will become generalized and then may lead to severe weakness, including ventilatory failure. Patients with muscle-specific kinase (MuSK) antibody myasthenia often have bulbar and ventilatory rather than limb weakness and a more unpredictable course; they respond badly to pyridostimine. 'Cholinergic crisis' is a rare, second type of crisis which occurs due to excessive anticholinesterase medication (i.e. long-term treatment over 360 mg pyridostigmine daily), in which weakness is accompanied by cholinergic features such as miosis, bradycardia, increased bronchial secretions, cramps, fasciculations, abdominal pain, and diarrhoea. Treatment in some elderly patients may be complicated by features of both types of crisis (i.e. excessive bronchial secretions in a patient with weak cough and weak respiratory muscles).

The initial challenge is to recognize the impending myasthenic crisis early enough to put adequate protection in place if there is no longer the time for adjustment of immunosuppressive treatment to ward off deterioration. The team needs to monitor fatigability and not just initial strength, which means tests of sustained muscle contraction (e.g. using the Myasthenia Gravis Composite score [6]). The lack of fixed weakness initially seen in myasthenia can mislead the inexperienced examiner into underestimating disease severity. Other treatment principles include infection control, rehydration, and careful review of medication for drugs that may impair neuromuscular transmission (see Chapter 20)—the commonest errors are adding inappropriate antibiotics or sleeping tablets in elderly or borderline compensated patients.

On the ward, respiratory function, cough, swallowing, and oxygen saturation need to be checked frequently, and nursing and medical staff need to be trained to recognize deteriorating bulbar and respiratory capacity through increasingly nasal and staccato speech. Myasthenic crises have an erratic course, which needs to be taken into account when considering ICU admission. Intensive respiratory therapy and initial non-invasive BiPAP may help reduce the number of ventilator days or even avoid mechanical ventilation [7]. Once the patient is intubated, pyridostigmine is reintroduced gradually: 60 mg pyridostigmine orally is approximately equivalent to 2 mg of intravenous pyridostigmine, to 0.5 mg of intravenous neostigmine, and to 1–1.5 mg intramuscular or subcutaneous neostigmine, but requirements and toleration vary individually. High-dose steroids can be given in ventilated patients, as the potential transient exacerbation of weakness that may occur in response to initiation of steroids is not a concern. Often only a short period of ventilation is needed, meaning that there is no reason for early tracheostomy (i.e. before day 7). There is, however, a relatively high risk of reintubation, especially in patients with atelectasis or pre-existing additional lung disease, and the standard predictors of extubation success used on ICU are not reliable.

The choice of acute immunomodulatory treatment in myasthenic crisis is influenced by concomitant illness. Patients are often suffering from severe infections of the respiratory tract when admitted to the ICU. Treatment with intravenous immunoglobulin (IVIg) (0.4 g kg– for 5 days) is usually the first choice and has often been initiated before patients are admitted to the ICU. Plasma exchanges (PLEX) of four to six times 2–3 L each may have a more rapid beneficial effect, but cause some degree of acute immunosuppression and may be less well tolerated in patients with circulatory compromise. The principles of long-term immunotherapy are discussed in Chapter 20.

Other myasthenic syndromes

Congenital myasthenia (see Chapter 19) is due to an inherited defect affecting the neuromuscular junction. The defect can be pre- or postsynaptic, or can affect cholinesterase in the synaptic cleft. Most patients present in childhood with extraocular muscle involvement and proximal limb weakness. Some forms, e.g. choline acetyltransferase (ChAT) deficiency, are associated with episodic respiratory arrest which can be fatal and requires home monitoring for apnoea, but this tends to occur less frequently in adolescence and disappears before adulthood. Anticholinesterase drugs such as pyridostigmine help some forms, but exacerbate others. Other drugs that can be helpful in specific syndromes include 3,4-diaminopyridine (3,4-DAP), ephedrine, and selective serotonin reuptake inhibitors. It is extremely rare for such patients to require ICU admission in adult life.

Botulism is most often food borne and is an infrequent cause of a myasthenic syndrome, with some 930 cases per year worldwide, associated with a 5% mortality [8]. However, patients are disproportionately prone to require critical care due to frequent bulbar weakness, and less often respiratory failure. ICU monitoring is advised for all progressing cases, as respiratory weakness can develop rapidly [9]. Attempts may be made to remove unabsorbed botulinum toxin from the gut, although most of the toxin will have been absorbed in the upper intestine. Antitoxin may prevent progression and shorten ventilator dependency [10]. Further intensive care is supportive, and recovery may be very protracted. Although autonomic features such as blurred vision and altered heart rate variation are typical for botulism, life-threatening autonomic complications have not been reported.

The Lambert–Eaton myasthenic syndrome (LEMS) is disorder of the presynaptic neuromuscular junction in which antibodies against voltage-gated calcium channels (anti-VGCC) affect Ca^{2+} influx into the presynaptic terminals and thus reduce the Ca^{2+}-dependent release of acetylcholine quanta (see Chapter 21). Most patients suffer limb weakness affecting the legs more than the arms, up to half have some degree of bulbar dysfunction, and under 20% have respiratory weakness. ICU treatment is rarely needed, but if there is bulbar or respiratory compromise monitoring follows the same principles as in MG. Plasma exchanges should be instituted as soon as possible: 3,4-DAP may provide immediate benefit, and may head off the need for intubation. Excessive doses can cause seizures. Pyridostigmine can be helpful if 3,4-DAP is unavailable. A search for an underlying tumour, as well as antibody tests for associated autoimmune syndromes must go in parallel with treatment.

Acute muscle diseases causing severe weakness

Most muscle diseases cause chronic or subacute weakness, rather than acute or even fulminant paralysis. Therefore, ICU admission is more often necessary in advanced chronic disease than early in the course. However, there are a limited number of toxic–metabolic, inflammatory, and genetic muscle disorders, in which severe weakness leads to ICU treatment even before the diagnosis is made.

Acute rhabdomyolysis and toxic metabolic muscle disease

The most common causes of acute rhabdomyolysis are either toxic/drug-induced or physical (status epilepticus, trauma, or prolonged immobility). Table 36.1 lists the most common drugs and toxins recognized to cause rhabdomyolysis.

Physical or metabolic causes of rhabdomyolysis include ischaemia (including vasculitis), hypothermia, fever, immobility, and trauma. Acute rhabdomyolysis may be a presenting feature for undiagnosed underlying muscle disease, such as McArdle disease or other glycogen storage diseases, carnitine palmitoyltransferase deficiency, defects of oxidative phosphorylation and beta-oxidation, periodic paralyses, and disorders causing muscle hyperactivity such as malignant hyperthermia, heat stroke, and neuroleptic malignant syndrome. In such conditions, recurrent myoglobinuria can precede episodes of frank rhabdomyolysis. Inflammatory or paraneoplastic muscle conditions can occasionally cause rhabdomyolysis, in particular anti-MAS antibody or anti-signal recognition particle (SRP) antibody-associated myositis, fulminant paraneoplastic dermatomyositis, or acute necrotizing paraneoplastic myopathy.

Management of acute rhabdomyolysis centres on recognizing and removing the causative agent; avoiding acidosis, cardiovascular compromise and renal failure; and treatment of any underlying disease such as inflammatory muscle disease or vasculitis. The clinical examination may be limited by the patient's general condition, and electromyography (EMG) will often show unspecific myopathic changes; signs suggesting 'irritative myopathy' do not reliably mean the aetiology is inflammatory. Muscle magnetic resonance imaging (MRI) may help confirm a pattern of involvement, but often only shows unspecific diffuse oedema on fat-saturated sequences; however, as imaging is often more readily available than EMG it can help confirm the diagnosis early (Fig. 36.1). Muscle biopsy may

Table 36.1 Toxins and medications that can cause toxic myopathy and rhabdomyolysis

Toxins that can cause toxic myopathy and rhabdomyolysis:
- Amphetamines
- Chlorphenoxy insecticides
- Chromium picolinate
- Ciguatoxin
- Cocaine
- 20,25-diazacholesterol
- Ethanol
- Germanium
- Gossypol
- Haff disease (fish ingestion; buffalo fish in the United States, burbot in northern Europe)
- Hemlock; birds that eat water hemlock
- Heroin
- Insect bite (hornet, redback spider, wasp, African bee)
- Kidney beans
- Mushrooms (*Amanita phalloides, Tricholoma equestre/Tricholoma flavovirens*)
- Monensin
- Peanut oil
- Pentaborane
- Phencyclidine
- Snakebite (cobra, coral snake, taipan, viper, rattlesnake)
- Toluene
- Toxic oil (adulterated cheap olive oil)

Selected medications that cause myopathy and rhabdomyolysis:*
- **Amiodarone**
- Anti-tumour necrosis factor alpha agents
- Barium
- **Chloroquine**
- **Colchicine**
- **Corticosteroids**
- Ciclosporin
- **D-penicillamine**
- **Emetine**
- **Epsilon-aminocaproic acid**
- Gold
- **Interferon-α**
- Ipecacuanha
- Isotretinoin
- Lamotrigine
- **Lipid-lowering agents** (ezetimibe, fibrates, gemfibrocil, niacin/nicotinic acid)
- Lithium
- L-tryptophan
- **Perhexiline**
- Procainamide
- **Propofol**
- Proton pump inhibitors
- **Statins**
- Streptokinase
- Valproate (especially patients with carnitine palmitoyltransferase II deficiency)
- Vecuronium
- Vinca alkaloids
- **Zidovudine (AZT)**

*More commonly implicated substances are indicated in bold.

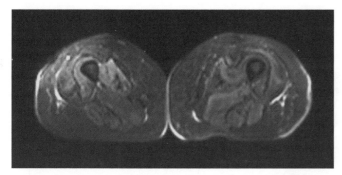

Fig. 36.1 Fat-suppressed magnetic resonance imaging (short TI inversion recovery sequence) in a 73-year-old patient on ciclosporin after kidney transplant who developed rhabdomyolysis after increasing of her dosage of pravastatin,

be useful in certain circumstances (e.g. in a search for vasculitis), but is best left until more than 4 weeks after an episode of rhabdomyolysis. Figure 36.2 shows the 'rhabdomyolysis protocol' used by Cambridge University Hospitals to avoid secondary complications in patients with severe rhabdomyolysis.

Acute/fulminant intrinsic muscle disease

Acute intrinsic muscle disorders may necessitate ICU admission though respiratory compromise or cardiac dysfunction, or may be part of a multisystemic disturbance. The neurologist's role here is to make sure that diagnostic investigations are conducted in a timely and efficient manner. In critically ill patients alternative strategies to secure tissue diagnosis may be necessary (Fig. 36.3).

ICU management of complications in chronic neuromuscular disease

Patients with a chronic neuromuscular disease may require critical care treatment through progression of the primary disease with respiratory or cardiac involvement or through secondary complications due to skeletal deformity or lack of mobility. The neurologist must help other treating teams to understand the specifics of the underlying neuromuscular condition, in particular the expected long-term survival and quality of life specific to the neuromuscular condition, to better estimate the benefits of potential treatments (which in turn depend on the patient's own understanding of quality of life and perception of independence) [11]. Patients' wishes regarding invasive treatments should be known before critical care treatment is begun. Neurologists should become involved early, before significant options have already been missed or decisions on ICU treatment have been made based on inadequate information.

Infrequently, chronic myopathies in adults, such as acid maltase deficiency or myofibrillar myopathy, may come to attention though cardiorespiratory complications before muscle weakness is recognized. Good appreciation of the type and severity of cardiac or respiratory impairment associated with specific muscle conditions is needed in order to advise on the correct management. For example, pacing may be appropriate in some forms of myopathy that cause cardiomyopathy, such as Emery–Dreifus muscular dystrophy Type 1 due to mutations in the emerin gene, whereas in Emery–Dreifuss muscular dystrophy Type 2 due to a lamin A/C mutation a pacemaker will not prevent arrhythmia and a cardioverter–defibrillator is required.

A newly recognized risk is that of liver failure with standard doses of paracetamol in patients with reduced muscle volume [12].

Critical care aspects and emergency management in Duchenne muscular dystrophy (DMD) and other muscular dystrophies

Modern multidisciplinary care using carefully planned protocols including timely interventions such as non-invasive positive pressure ventilation [13] has almost doubled life expectancy for patients with DMD. The margin for patients with DMD to benefit from critical care treatment is therefore much wider than it was in the early 1990s. Patients with borderline respiratory function are more likely to develop respiratory failure through intercurrent infections. Many features that influence the chance of recovery after ICU treatment, such as the baseline respiratory rate or nutritional status, are determined by the quality of care and whether non-invasive ventilation and cough-assist techniques have been instituted in a timely fashion [14]. Although it is still true that patients with advanced neuromuscular disease are difficult to wean from the ventilator, the option of long-term home ventilation means that this is a less central concern before ICU treatment is initiated. Conversely, appropriate discussions with the patient earlier in the course of management have become even more important, and good long-term care includes discussion of issues such as ventilation and tracheotomy with the patient before an emergency situation occurs.

Cardiac involvement in DMD can add to the complexity of ICU treatment, increasing the risk of dysrhythmia and of cardiac failure. Newer techniques such as multigated cardiac radionuclide ventriculography (MUGA) in addition to echocardiography allow better cardiac assessment of DMD patients, but their practical benefit is unclear. Further anaesthetic complications in patients with DMD include intra-operative heart failure, inhaled anaesthetic-related rhabdomyolysis and a malignant hyperthermia-like syndrome, and succinylcholine-induced rhabdomyolysis and hyperkalaemia, on account of which depolarizing muscle relaxants are contraindicated [15]. In general, however, experience of using anaesthetics for these patients has improved with increasing frequency of spinal surgery, and long postoperative ventilation is now rare.

Cardiac disease and transplantation in muscle disease

In some cases cardiac dysfunction or intra-operative cardiac failure may be the presenting symptom of a muscular dystrophy. A number of myopathies (e.g. Becker muscular dystrophy and some myofibrillar myopathies) typically develop cardiomyopathy and may require transplantation, while in others dysrhythmia is more common (e.g. Emery–Dreifuss muscular dystrophy and myotonic dystrophy). Patients with Becker-type dystrophinopathy constitute approximately 50% of the muscular dystrophy patients who undergo cardiac transplantation. Wu et al. [16] reported that outcomes of transplantation in 29 consecutive patients with muscular dystrophy were comparable to controls, with similar rates of infection and rejection, which suggests that transplantation should be considered where the cardiac situation is appropriate and not deferred on account of the muscle disease until late complications such as secondary pulmonary hypertension reduce the chances of success. Similar considerations may apply to patients with myofibrillar myopathy.

Adult Critical Care
Rhabdomyolysis Algorithm

Addenbrooke's Hospital NHS
Cambridge University Hospitals NHS Foundation Trust

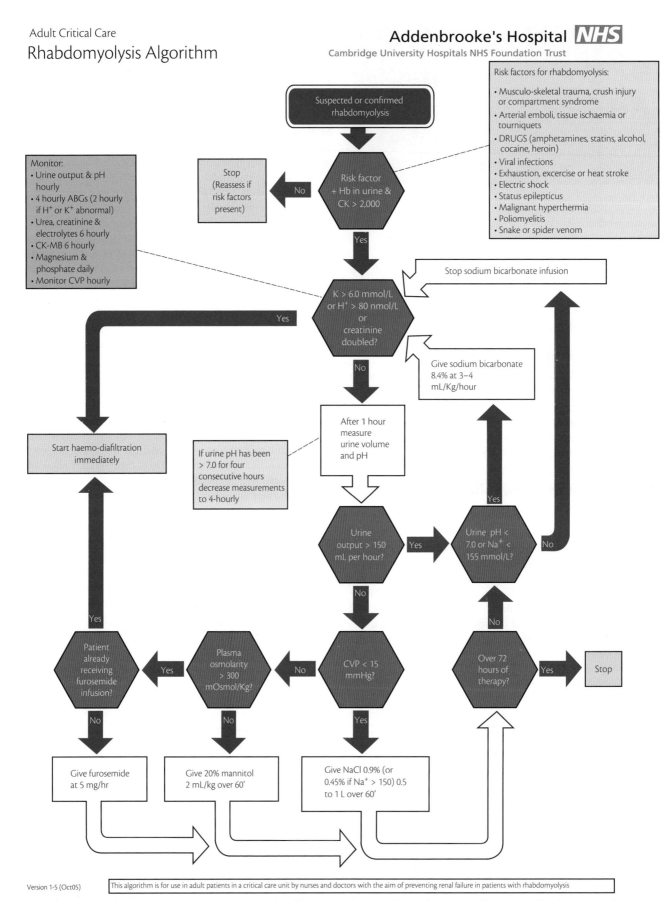

Fig. 36.2 The rhabdomyolysis protocol used in critical care units of Cambridge University Hospitals, UK. The majority of patients needing this treatment have massive rhabdomyolysis after trauma. Abbreviations: ABG, arterial blood gas; CK, creatine kinase; CVP, central venous pressure; Hb, haemoglobin. (Courtesy of Cambridge University Hospitals, Cambridge, UK.)

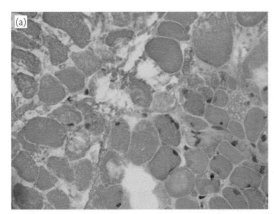
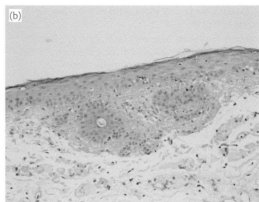

Fig. 36.3 (a) A case of paraneoplastic acute necrotizing myopathy in a patient admitted to ICU with respiratory failure and there found to have a breast tumour; muscle tissue from the pectorals was obtained at mastectomy. (b) A biopsy from a skin rash confirming dermatomyositis in a patient with respiratory failure, coagulopathy, and septic shock unable to undergo muscle biopsy. (Courtesy Dr D. O'Donovan and Dr E. Rytina, Cambridge University Hospitals, Cambridge, UK). (See also figure in colour plate section)

ICU-acquired weakness and critical illness neuromyopathy

Flaccid paralysis of the limbs may develop during treatment in the ICU, and some patients who fail to wean appropriately from mechanical ventilation are found to be awake but with little movement due to neuromuscular weakness. A careful search to exclude acute cerebral and spinal disorders, as well as toxic metabolic myopathy, is always needed, as multiple drugs used on the ICU may cause acute neuropathy or myopathy, or unmask underlying conditions. GBS is often suspected, but GBS rarely arises during treatment of unrelated illness, apart from variants such as inflammatory neuropathy during acute graft-versus-host disease. In the absence of an identifiable cause, patients with symmetric weakness, often sparing the facial muscles, most often have a combination of critical illness polyneuropathy (CIP) and critical illness myopathy (CIM). Neuropathy used to be considered more common, but now myopathic abnormalities are recognized to predominate. Both CIP and CIM appear to be associated with the same risk factors: about a third of patients who are ventilated for over 7 days have some degree of neuromuscular disturbance, rising to 60–70% in those with sepsis/systemic inflammation response syndrome (SIRS) or acute respiratory distress syndrome (ARDS) and up to 100% in those surviving septic shock and multiple organ failure. Abnormal sensory nerve action potentials are typical for CIP, and reduced response to direct muscle stimulation is typical for CIM, but the two entities are often difficult to separate by routine electrophysiological examination and there is considerable overlap, so that the term 'ICU-acquired weakness' (ICU-AW) is now commonly preferred.

A recent series of 33 Spanish patients [17] showed myopathic findings in 79% of electrophysiological studies, evidence of neuropathy in 33%, and a combination in 21%. Muscle biopsies showed significant muscle cell necrosis in 58%, loss of myosin in 36%, and mitochondrial abnormalities in 52%. Muscle biopsy reports indicate three major subtypes of CIM: a diffuse non-necrotizing myopathy affecting Type 2 fibres predominantly; an acute myosin-loss myopathy; and acute necrotizing myopathy [18]. Acute myosin-loss myopathy with selective loss of the thick (myosin) filaments has a more specific association, being most frequently described in patients receiving a combination of steroids and neuromuscular blocking agents, but it can also be seen when steroids are used without

neuromuscular blocking drugs. New data suggest that plasma from patients in the early phase of septic shock may reduce the amount of myosin in experimental animals and suggests a specific role of cytokines in proteolysis [19]. In current clinical practice, muscle biopsy is rarely required: no treatments other than supportive care are available once non-neuromuscular conditions or an intercurrent or coincidental demyelinating neuropathy have been excluded by neuroimaging and neurophysiological investigations, and histological differentiation of subtypes within ICU-AW does not allow a better prediction of outcome.

Ways to prevent ICU-AW remain unclear; there have been reports that strict glycaemic control may reduce its incidence [20], but the overall benefit of intensive insulin therapy on survival is currently controversial. Bedrest and prolonged immobility, sepsis, and corticosteroid exposure are recognized risk factors [21]. There is no known specific treatment. Approximately 50% of patients with ICU-AW recover fully, but half of the rest may retain significant long-term disability. Rigorous long-term follow-up studies are not yet available.

References

1. Damian MS, Ben-Shlomo Y, Howard R, et al. The effect of secular trends and specialist neurocritical care on mortality for patients with intracerebral haemorrhage, myasthenia gravis and Guillain–Barré syndrome admitted to critical care. *Intensive Care Med* 2013; **39**: 1405–12.
2. Plasma Exchange/Sandoglobulin Guillain–Barré Syndrome Trial Group. Randomised trial of plasma exchange, intravenous immunoglobulin, and combined treatments in Guillain–Barré syndrome. *Lancet* 1997; **349**: 225–30.
3. Wijdicks EF, Roy TK. BiPAP in early Guillain–Barré syndrome may fail. *Can J Neurol Sci* 2006; **33**: 105–6.
4. Flachenecker P, Toyka KV, Reiners K. Cardiac arrhythmias in Guillain–Barré syndrome. An overview of the diagnosis of a rare but potentially life-threatening complication [in German]. *Nervenarzt* 2001; **72**: 610–17.
5. Fletcher DD, Lawn ND, Wolter TD, Wijdicks EF. Long-term outcome in patients with Guillain–Barré syndrome requiring mechanical ventilation. *Neurology* 2000; **54**: 2311–15.
6. Burns TM, Conaway M, Sanders DB, MG Composite and MG-QOL15 Study Group. The MG Composite: a valid and reliable outcome measure for myasthenia gravis. *Neurology* 2010; **74**: 1434–40.
7. Seneviratne J, Mandrekar J, Wijdicks EF, Rabinstein AA. Noninvasive ventilation in myasthenic crisis. *Arch Neurol* 2008; **65**: 54–8.

8. Hatheway CL. Botulism: the present status of the disease. *Curr Top Microbiol Immunol* 1995; **195**: 55–75.

9. Bleck TP. *Clostridium botulinum (botulism)*. In: Mandell GL, Bennett JE, Dolin R (ed), *Principles and Practice of Infectious Diseases*, 5th edn, pp. 2543–8. Philadelphia, PA: Churchill Livingstone, 2000.

10. Kongsaengdao S, Samintarapanya K, Rusmeechan S, et al. An outbreak of botulism in Thailand: clinical manifestations and management of severe respiratory failure. *Clin Infect Dis* 2006; **43**: 1247–56.

11. Dreyer PS, Steffensen BF, Pedersen BD. Living with severe physical impairment, Duchenne's muscular dystrophy and home mechanical ventilation. *Int J Qual Stud Health Well-being* 2010; **5**(3): doi: 10.3402/qhw.v5i3.5388.

12. Ceelie I, James LP, Gijsen V, et al. Acute liver failure after recommended doses of acetaminophen in patients with myopathies. *Crit Care Med* 2011; **39**: 678–82.

13. Bushby K, Finkel R, Birnkrant DJ, et al. Diagnosis and management of Duchenne muscular dystrophy, part 2: implementation of multidisciplinary care. *Lancet Neurol* 2010; **9**: 177–89.

14. Hill NS. Neuromuscular disease in respiratory and critical care medicine. *Respir Care* 2006; **51**: 1065–71.

15. Gurnaney H, Brown A, Litman RS. Malignant hyperthermia and muscular dystrophies. *Anesth Analg* 2009; **109**: 1043–8.

16. Wu RS, Gupta S, Brown RN, et al. Clinical outcomes after cardiac transplantation in muscular dystrophy patients. *J Heart Lung Transplant* 2010; **29**: 432–8.

17. Fernández-Lorente J, Esteban A, Salinero E, et al. Critical illness myopathy. Neurophysiological and muscular biopsy assessment in 33 patients. *Rev Neurol* 2010; **50**: 718–26.

18. Hermans G, De Jonghe B, Bruyninckx F, et al. Clinical review: critical illness polyneuropathy and myopathy. *Crit Care* 2008; **12**: 238.

19. van Hees HW, Schellekens WJ, Linkels M, et al. Plasma from septic shock patients induces loss of muscle protein. *Crit Care* 2011; **15**: R233.

20. Hermans G, Wilmer A, Meersseman W, et al. Impact of intensive insulin therapy on neuromuscular complications and ventilator dependency in the medical intensive care unit. *Am J Resp Crit Care Med* 2007; **175**: 480–9.

21. Griffiths RD, Hall JB. Intensive care unit-acquired weakness. *Crit Care Med* 2010; **38**: 779–87.

Index

Note: page numbers in *italics* refer to figures, tables, and boxes.